S0-BQM-100

HANDBOOK OF CARCINOGEN TESTING

HANDBOOK
OF
CARCINOGEN TESTING

Edited by

Harry A. Milman

Office of Toxic Substances
U.S. Environmental Protection Agency
Washington, DC

and

Elizabeth K. Weisburger

Division of Cancer Etiology
National Cancer Institute
National Institutes of Health
Bethesda, Maryland

RC268.65
H35
1985

np **NOYES PUBLICATIONS**
Park Ridge, New Jersey, U.S.A.

Copyright © 1985 by Noyes Publications
No part of this book may be reproduced in any form
without permission in writing from the Publisher.
Library of Congress Catalog Card Number: 85-4930
ISBN: 0-8155-1035-7
Printed in the United States

Published in the United States of America by
Noyes Publications
Mill Road, Park Ridge, New Jersey 07656

10 9 8 7 6 5 4 3 2 1

Library of Congress Cataloging in Publication Data
Main entry under title:

Handbook of carcinogen testing.

Includes bibliographies and index.
1. Carcinogenicity testing--Handbooks, manuals, etc.
I. Milman, Harry A. II. Weisburger, Elizabeth K.
[DNLM: 1. Biological Assay. 2. Carcinogens--toxicity.
3. Carcinogens--United States--legislation.
4. Toxicology--methods. QZ 202 H2355]
RC268.65.H35 1985 616.99'4071 85-4930
ISBN 0-8155-1035-7

Preface

Over 20 years ago the National Cancer Institute (NCI) initiated a program to conduct bioassays of selected compounds to determine their possible carcinogenicity. There are some similarities and many differences between the situation in 1961 and the present. The basic technique remains the same—administer a compound to rats and mice to determine whether it causes cancer in the test animals. However, it soon was realized that there are many confounding factors in the process. Experience over the years has led to the expansion of means to aid in making better decisions of what to test, what to anticipate, how to conduct the test, and how to interpret and apply the results.

For example, structure-activity relationships have been expanded to the stage where better correlations between structure and carcinogenicity are possible. When the NCI Bioassay Program was initiated, there were no systematic short-term tests available to aid in narrowing the selection of compounds. Now, the Ames/*Salmonella* assay, mouse lymphoma and cytogenetics tests, tests for DNA damage plus others have been reasonably well standardized. Background data on spontaneous tumors in rats and mice of various strains have been tabulated; certainly such information is more readily available now than in 1961. More experience on the actual logistics of conducting a study, as well as quality control procedures have aided the progress of bioassay programs. More appropriate statistical methods to evaluate the data have been developed as well as better concepts on how to apply the results in risk analysis.

It seemed that the time was appropriate for a book dedicated to these various points. Furthermore, most other books on testing for carcinogenicity have emphasized short-term or long-term methods alone, without considering all the other facets of the operation. It thus seemed propitious to attempt such a volume, affording a total view of a bioassay, from initial phases to its application.

Harry A. Milman
Elizabeth K. Weisburger

DISCLAIMER

This book was edited by Harry A. Milman and
Elizabeth K. Weisburger in their private capacity.
No official support or endorsement by the U.S.
Environmental Protection Agency or the National Cancer Institute or any other agency of
the U.S. Federal Government is intended or should
be inferred.

Contributors

Richard A. Adams, Ph.D.
Bio-Research Institute, Incorporated
Cambridge, Massachusetts

Joseph C. Arcos, D.Sc.
Assessment Division
Office of Toxic Substances
U.S. Environmental Protection Agency
Washington, D.C.

and

Department of Medicine
Tulane University School of Medicine
New Orleans, Louisiana

Angela Auletta, Ph.D.
Health and Environmental Review Division
Office of Toxic Substances
U.S. Environmental Protection Agency
Washington, D.C.

Charles Aylsworth, Ph.D.
Department of Pediatrics and Human
  Development
Michigan State University
East Lansing, Michigan

Robert P. Beliles, Ph.D.
Office of Risk Assessment
Occupational Safety and Health Administration
Department of Labor
Washington, D.C.

Herbert Blumenthal, Ph.D.
Divison of Toxicology
Center for Food Safety and Applied
  Nutrition
Food and Drug Administration
Washington, D.C.

Gary A. Boorman, D.V.M., Ph.D.
National Toxicology Program
National Institute of Environmental
  Health Sciences
National Institutes of Health
Research Triangle Park, North Carolina

Daniel A. Casciano, Ph.D.
Department of Health and Human Services
National Center for Toxicological Research
Food and Drug Administration
Jefferson, Arkansas

Bruce C. Casto, D.Sc.
Department of Health and Human Services
National Center for Toxicological Research
Food and Drug Administration
Jefferson, Arkansas

Chia-cheng Chang, Ph.D.
Department of Pediatrics and Human Development
Michigan State University
East Lansing, Michigan

David L. Coffin, V.M.D.
Health Effects Research Laboratory
U.S. Environmental Protection Agency
Research Triangle Park, North Carolina

Kenny S. Crump, Ph.D.
K.S. Crump and Company, Incorporated
Ruston, Louisiana

Paul F. Deisler, Jr., Ph.D.
Health, Safety and Environment
Shell Oil Company
Houston, Texas

Harold A. Dunsford, M.D.
Department of Pathology and Laboratory Medicine
University of Texas Medical School
Houston, Texas

Scot L. Eustis, Ph.D.
National Toxicology Program
National Institute of Environmental Health Sciences
National Institutes of Health
Research Triangle Park, North Carolina

William H. Farland, Ph.D.
Health and Environmental Review Division
Office of Toxic Substances
U.S. Environmental Protection Agency
Washington, D.C.

W. Gary Flamm, Ph.D.
Center for Food Safety and Applied Nutrition
Food and Drug Administration
Washington, D.C.

Dawn G. Goodman, V.M.D.
PATHCO Inc.
Potomac, Maryland

Thomas E. Hamm, Jr., D.V.M., Ph.D.
Department of General and Biochemcal Toxicology
Chemical Industry Institute of Toxicology
Research Triangle Park, North Carolina

Jerry F. Hardisty, D.V.M.
Experimental Pathology Laboratories, Incorporated
Research Triangle Park, North Carolina

John Higginson, M.D.
Universities Associated for Research and Education in Pathology, Incorporated
Bethesda, Maryland

Richard N. Hill, M.D., Ph.D.
Office of the Assistant Administrator for Pesticides and Toxic Substances
U.S. Environmental Protection Agency
Washington, D.C.

Freddy Homburger, M.D.
Bio-Research Institute, Incorporated
Cambridge, Massachusetts

Cy Jone, Ph.D.
Department of Pediatrics and Human Development
Michigan State University
East Lansing, Michigan

Richard J. Kociba, D.V.M., Ph.D.
Toxicology Research Laboratory
Dow Chemical U.S.A.
Midland, Michigan

David Y. Lai, Ph.D.
Environmental Toxicology and Ecological Assessment Division
JRB Associates
Science Application, Incorporated
McLean, Virginia

Narendra D. Lalwani, Ph.D.
Department of Pathology
Northwestern University Medical School
Chicago, Illinois

Robert R. Maronpot, D.V.M.
National Toxicology Program
National Institute of Environmental
  Health Sciences
National Institutes of Health
Research Triangle Park, North Carolina

Ernest E. McConnell, D.V.M.
National Toxicology Program
National Institute of Environmental
  Health Sciences
National Institutes of Health
Research Triangle Park, North Carolina

David L. McCormick, Ph.D.
Life Sciences Division
IIT Research Institute
Chicago, Illinois

Charlene A. McQueen, Ph.D.
Naylor Dana Institute for Disease Prevention
American Health Foundation
Valhalla, New York

Harry A. Milman, Ph.D.
Health and Environmental Review Division
Office of Toxic Substances
U.S. Environmental Protection Agency
Washington, D.C.

Charles A. Montgomery, Jr., D.V.M.
National Toxicology Program
National Institute of Environmental
  Health Sciences
National Institutes of Health
Research Triangle Park, North Carolina

Richard C. Moon, Ph.D.
Life Sciences Division
IIT Research Institute
Chicago, Illinois

Suzanne M. Morris, Ph.D.
National Center for Toxicological Research
Food and Drug Administration
Jefferson, Arkansas

C.S. Muir, Ph.D.
Division of Epidemiology and Biostatistics
International Agency for Research on Cancer
Lyon, France

Stephen Nesnow, Ph.D.
Carcinogenesis and Metabolism Branch
Health Effects Research Laboratory
U.S. Environmental Protection Agency
Research Triangle Park, North Carolina

Lalita D. Palekar, Ph.D.
Northrop Services, Incorporated
Research Triangle Park, North Carolina

Colin N. Park, Ph.D.
Health and Environmental Sciences
Dow Chemical U.S.A.
Midland, Michigan

Michael A. Pereira, Ph.D.
Toxicological Assessment Branch
Health Effects Research Laboratory
U.S. Environmental Protection Agency
Cincinnati, Ohio

J. David Prejean, Ph.D.
Chemotherapy Research
Southern Research Institute
Birmingham, Alabama

Peter W. Preuss, Ph.D.
Directorate for Health Services
Consumer Product Safety Commission
Bethesda, Maryland

Janardan K. Reddy, M.D.
Department of Pathology
Northwestern University Medical School
Chicago, Illinois

Joseph V. Rodricks, Ph.D.
ENVIRON Corporation
Washington, D.C.

Diane H. Russell, Ph.D.
Department of Pharmacology
University of Arizona College of Medi-
cine
Tucson, Arizona

Robert J. Scheuplein, Ph.D.
Office of Toxicological Sciences
Center for Food Safety and Applied
Nutrition
Food and Drug Administration
Washington, D.C.

Stewart Sell, M.D.
Department of Pathology and Labora-
tory Medicine
University of Texas Medical School
Houston, Texas

Michael B. Shimkin, M.D.
Department of Community Medicine
University of California at San Diego
LaJolla, California

Abe Silvers, Ph.D.
Electric Power Research Institute
Palo Alto, California

Andrew Sivak, Ph.D.
Biomedical Research and Technology
Section
Arthur D. Little, Incorporated
Cambridge, Massachusetts

Thomas J. Slaga, Ph.D.
The University of Texas System
Cancer Center, Science Park–Research
Division
Smithville, Texas

Donald E. Stevenson, Ph.D.
Toxicology Laboratory
Westhollow Research Center
Shell Development Company
Houston, Texas

Gary D. Stoner, Ph.D.
Department of Pathology
Medical College of Ohio
Toledo, Ohio

John D. Strandberg, D.V.M., Ph.D.
Division of Comparative Medicine
Department of Pathology
School of Medicine
Johns Hopkins University
Baltimore, Maryland

James E. Trosko, Ph.D.
Department of Pediatrics and Human
Development
Michigan State Unjversity
East Lansing, Michigan

Alice S. Tu, Ph.D.
Biomedical Research and Technology
Section
Arthur D. Little, Incorporated
Cambridge, Massachusetts

Duncan Turnbull, D.Phil.
ENVIRON Corporation
Washington, D.C.

Andrew G. Ulsamer, Ph.D.
Directorate for Health Services
Consumer Product Safety Commission
Bethesda, Maryland

Elizabeth K. Weisburger, Ph.D.
Division of Cancer Etiology
National Cancer Institute
National Institutes of Health
Bethesda, Maryland

Paul D. White, B.A.
Directorate for Health Services
Consumer Product Safety Commission
Bethesda, Maryland

Gary M. Williams, M.D.
American Health Foundation
Naylor Dana Institute for Disease Prevention
Valhalla, New York

Marilyn J. Wolfe, Ph.D.
National Toxicology Program
National Institute of Environmental
  Health Sciences
National Institutes of Health
Research Triangle Park, North Carolina

Yin-Tak Woo, Ph.D.
Environmental Toxicology and Ecological Assessment Division
JRB Associates
Science Application, Incorporated
McLean, Virginia

Errol Zeiger, Ph.D.
Cellular and Genetic Toxicology Branch
National Institute of Environmental
  Health Sciences
National Institutes of Health
Research Triangle Park, North Carolina

Abbreviations

AACN	Atypical acinar cell nodules
AAF	N-2-Acetylaminofluorene
A/B	Alveolar/bronchiolar
4-ABP	4-Aminobiphenyl
ACGIH	American Conference of Governmental Industrial Hygienists
ADP	Adenosine-5'-diphosphate
AF_2	2-(Furyl)-3-(5-nitro-2-furyl)acrylamide
2-AF	2-Aminofluorene
AFP	Alphafetoprotein
AHH	Aryl hydrocarbon hydroxylase
AIHC	American Industrial Health Council
AIN	American Institute of Nutrition
AISI	American Iron and Steel Institute
AMP	Adenosine monophosphate
AN	Acrylonitrile
ANSI	American National Standards Institute
API	American Petroleum Institute
ATPase	Adenosine-5'-triphosphatase
AZQ	2,5-Bis(1-aziridinyl)-3,6-bis(2-methoxyethoxy)-p-benzo-quinone
B(a)P	Benzo(a)pyrene
BBN	N-Butyl-N-(4-hydroxybutyl)nitrosamine
BCME	Bis(chloromethyl) ether

BHA	Butylated hydroxyanisole
BHT	Butylated hydroxytoluene
BPL	β-Propiolactone
BUdR	Bromodeoxyuridine
BUF	Buffalo
BZQ	Benzidine
CAG	Carcinogen Assessment Group
CD	Choline-deficient
C/D	Cesarean derived
CHAP	Chronic Hazard Advisory Panel
CHO	Chinese hamster ovary
CIIT	Chemical Industry Institute of Toxicology
ClUdR	Chlorodeoxyuridine
CMA	Chemical Manufacturers Association
CMME	Chloromethyl methyl ether
Con-A	Concanavolin-A
CPSA	Consumer Product Safety Act
CPSC	Consumer Product Safety Commission
CR	Charles River
CS	Choline-supplemented
CTPV	Coal tar pitch volatiles
DAB	4-Dimethylaminobenzene
DBCP	1,2-Dibromo-3-chloropropane
DCB	3,5-Dichloro-(N-1,1-dimethyl-2-propynyl)benzamide
DDPM	Diaminodiphenylmethane
DDT	Dichlorodiphenyltrichloroethane
DEHP	Diethylhexyl phthalate
DEN	Diethylnitrosamine
DES	Diethylstilbestrol
DFMO	α-Difluoromethylornithine
DHHS	Department of Health and Human Services
DMBA	7,12-Dimethylbenz(a)anthracene
DMH	1,2-Dimethylhydrazine dihydrochloride
DMNA	N-Nitrosodimethylamine
DMSO	Dimethylsulfoxide
DNA	Deoxyribonucleic acid

DOC	Deoxycholate
DPPC	Dipalmitoyl phosphatidylcholine
DTNB	5,5'-Dithiobis(2-nitrobenzoate)
EDB	Ethylene dibromide
EDTA	Ethylenediaminetetraacetic acid
EGTA	Ethylene glycol-bis(β-aminoethylether)-N,N'-tetraacetic acid
ELISA	Enzyme linked assays
EMTD	Estimated maximum tolerated dose
ENU	2-Ethyl-N-nitrosourea
EPA	Environmental Protection Agency
ETO	Ethylene oxide
ETS	Emergency temporary standard
FAD	Flavine-adenine dinucleotide
FANFT	N-[4-(5-Nitro-2-furyl)-2-thiazolyl]-formamide
FDA	Food and Drug Administration
FD&C Act	Food, Drug, and Cosmetic Act
FHA	Follicle stimulating hormone
FHSA	Federal Hazard Substances Act
FIFRA	Federal Insecticide, Fungicide, and Rodenticide Act
FSC	Food Safety Council
GGT	Gamma glutamyl transpeptidase
GLP	Good Laboratory Practices
GMP	Guanosine monophosphate
G-6-Pase	Glucose-6-phosphatase
GRAS	Generally recognized as safe
H and E	Hematoxylin and Eosin
HAT	Hypoxanthine-aminopterin-thymidine
HBB	Hexabromobiphenyl
HDZ	Hydralazine
HEP	Hepatectomy
Hepes	2-Hydroxyethylpiperazine-N'-2-ethanesulfonic acid
HG-PRT	Hypoxanthine-guanine-phosphoribosyl transferase
HPC	Hepatocyte primary culture
HSA	Human serum albumin
IARC	International Agency for Research on Cancer
IBT	Industrial Bio-Test Laboratories

ICPEMC	International Commission for Protection Against Environ- mental Mutagens and Carcinogens
IEF	Isoelectric focusing
i.p.	Intraperitoneal
IRLG	Interagency Regulatory Liaison Group
IUdR	Iododeoxyuridine
i.v.	Intravenous
LE	Long Evans
LGL	Large granular lymphocyte
LH	Luteinizing hormone
MBOCA	4,4'-Methylenebis(2-chlorobenzeneamine)
MC	Metabolic cooperation
3-MC	3-Methylcholanthrene
MDA	4,4'-Methylenedianiline
2MDAB	2-Methyl-4-dimethylaminoazobenzene
3'-MDAB	3'-Methyldimethylaminoazobenzene
MGBG	Methylglyoxal-bis(guanylhydrazone)
MLE	Maximum likelihood estimate
MNNG	N-Methyl-N'-nitro-N-nitrosoguanidine
MNU	N-Methyl-N-nitrosourea
MoAb	Monoclonal antibodies
mRNA	Messenger ribonucleic acid
MTD	Maximum tolerated dose
MTV	Mammary tumor virus
1-NA	1-Naphthylamine
2-NA	2-Naphthylamine
NAD	Nicotine adenine dinucleotide
NADH	Nicotine adenine dinucleotide, reduced form
NAS	National Academy of Sciences
NCI	National Cancer Institute
NEPA	National Environmental Policy Act
NGS	Normal goat serum
NIH	National Institutes of Health
NIOSH	National Institute for Occupational Safety and Health
NNK	4-(Methyl-nitrosamido)-1-(3-pyridyl)-1-butanone
NNN	N-nitrosonornicotine

NRC	National Research Council
NTP	National Toxicology Program
O.D.	Optical density
ODC	Ornithine decarboxylase
OECD	Organization for Economic Cooperation and Development
OM	Osborne-Mendel
OMB	Office of Management and Budget
OSHA	Occupational Safety and Health Administration
OSH Act	Occupational Safety and Health Act
OPCS	Office of Population Censuses and Surveys of England and Wales
OPSPA	Bis(1-aziridinyl)morpholino-phosphine sulfide
PAAB	p-Aminoazobenzene
PAH	Polycyclic aromatic hydrocarbons
PBB	Polybrominated biphenyls
PBS	Phosphate buffered saline
PCB	Polychlorinated biphenyls
PE	Perchloroethylene
PEL	Permissible exposure limit
PH	Partial hepatectomy
PHC	Primary hepatocellular carcinoma
PNA	Polynuclear aromatic hydrocarbons
PNS	Peripheral nervous system
p.o.	By mouth
PWG	Pathology Working Group
QA	Quality assurance
RE	Rat embryo
RER	Rough endoplasmic reticulum
RIA	Radioimmunoassay
RLV	Rauscher leukemia virus
RNA	Ribonucleic acid
SA7	Simian adenovirus 7
SAR	Structure activity relationships
SBD	Substituted benzenediamines
SCD	Sister-chromatid differentiation
SCE	Sister-chromatid exchange

SDS	Sodium dodecyl sulfate
SHE	Syrian hamster embryo
SIR	Standardized incidence ratio
SMR	Standardized mortality ratio
SOM	Sensitivity of method
SOPs	Standard Operating Procedures
SPF	Specific pathogen free
STIC	System for Tracking the Inventory of Chemicals
STR	Skin tumor resistant
STS	Skin tumor sensitive
TCDD	2,3,7,8-Tetrachlorodibenzo-p-dioxin
TCE	Trichloroethylene
TEB	Terminal end bud
6TG	6-Thioguanine
THF	Tetrahydrofuran
thio-TEPA	Tris(1-aziridinyl)phosphine sulfide
TK	Thymidine kinase
TLV	Threshold Limit Value
TPA	12-O-Tetradecanoylphorbol-13-acetate
TRIS	Tris(2,3-dibromopropyl)phosphate
TSCA	Toxic Substances Control Act
TWA	Time weighted average
UDS	Unscheduled DNA synthesis
UFFI	Urea-formaldehyde foam insulation
UICC	Union International Contra Cancrum (International Union Against Cancer)
U.S.D.A.	United States Department of Agriculture
UV	Ultraviolet
UVB	Ultraviolet B
VC	Vinyl chloride
VRB	Veterinary Research Branch
VSD	Virtually safe dose
WF	Wistar/Furth
WHO	World Health Organization
WME	Williams' Medium E
WMES	Williams' Medium E containing 10% serum and 50 μg/ml gentamicin

Contents

Preface v
Contributors. vii
Abbreviations. xiii

PART I
PREDICTING CARCINOGENICITY OF
CHEMICALS FROM THEIR STRUCTURE

1. Structural and Functional Criteria for Suspecting Chemical Compounds
   of Carcinogenic Activity: State-of-the-Art of Predictive Formalism 2
   Yin-Tak Woo, Joseph C. Arcos and David Y. Lai
   Introduction. 2
   Criteria for Suspecting a Chemical of Carcinogenic Activity. 3
   General Principles of Chemical Carcinogenesis. 3
   Physicochemical Factors Which May Modify the Carcinogenic
   Potential of a Chemical. 7
   　Molecular Weight. 7
   　Physical State 7
   　Solubility. 7
   　Chemical Reactivity. 7
   Structural Criteria 8
   　Aromatic Amines and Azo Dyes. 8
   　Polynuclear Compounds. 11
   　Alkylating and Acylating Agents 14
   　　Nitrogen Mustards. 15
   　　Haloethers 15
   　　Epoxides 15
   　　Aziridines, Lactones and Sultones. 16
   　　N-Nitroso Compounds 16
   　　Hydrazo-, Aliphatic Azo- and Azoxy-Compounds and
   　　Aryldialkyltriazenes. 16
   　　Carbamates 16
   　Halogenated and Polyhalogenated Hydrocarbons. 16
   　　Haloalkanes 16
   　　Haloalkenes 17
   　　Polyhalogenated Pesticides 17
   　　Polyhalogenated Aromatics and Dibenzodioxins 17
   　Miscellaneous Epigenetic Carcinogens 18
   　Foreign-Body Carcinogens. 18
   　Conclusions to Structural Criteria. .18

Functional Criteria 19
References. 23

PART II
EPIDEMIOLOGICAL INVESTIGATIONS

2. Role of Epidemiology in Identifying Chemical Carcinogens. 28
   C.S. Muir and John Higginson
   Introduction. 28
   Causes of Cancer. 29
     Evidence of Causality. 30
   Discrete Exogenous Chemicals. 31
     Methodological Approaches. 33
     Mapping and Correlation. 36
       Mapping 36
       Group Correlation. 36
       Occupational Mortality. 36
     Cohort 36
     Case-Control. 37
     Studies of Occupational Carcinogenesis 37
       The Significance of a Raised SMR. 38
       Occupation and the Cancer Registry 39
     Group and Individual Comparison 40
     Case-Control Studies 41
     Cohort Studies 42
       Follow-Up: Record Linkage 43
       Industrial Records. 43
       Management. 44
       Labor: Administrative Lists 44
   Other Exposures (Waste Disposal, Accidents, Ambient
    Pollution). 44
   Childhood Cancer 45
   Medication. 46
   Diet and Lifestyle: Endogenous Carcinogenesis 46
     Diet 47
     Lifestyle 48
   Low Levels of Exposure 49
     Extrapolation. 49
     The "Negative" Study 50
   Comment. 50
   References. 51

PART III
IN VITRO TESTS

3. Overview of *In Vitro* Tests for Genotoxic Agents. 58
   Angela Auletta
   Introduction. 58
   Assays for Gene Mutation. 61

Assays for Chromosomal Damage 61
Assays for DNA Damage and Repair 63
Assays for Cellular Transformation 63
Other Limitations of Short-Term Tests 73
   Metabolic Activation Systems 73
   Extrapolation to Humans 74
   Statistical Methodology 75
   Limitations of the Data Base 76
   Assay Selection 76
Systematic Attempts to Evaluate Test Performance 77
   The Gene-Tox Program 77
   The International Collaborative Program for the Evaluation of
   Short-Term Tests for Carcinogenicity 78
Use 79
Future Directions 79
References 80

4. The *Salmonella* Mutagenicity Assay for Identification of Presumptive
   Carcinogens 83
   Errol Zeiger
       Introduction 83
       Description of *Salmonella* Strains 84
       Metabolic Activation 86
           Host-Mediated Systems 86
           Metabolizing Mammalian Cells in Culture 86
           Organ Homogenates 87
       Test Procedure 88
       Variations of the Test 90
           Preincubation Test 90
           Volatile Chemicals 91
           Reductive Metabolism 91
           Conjugated Mutagens 91
           Spot Test 91
           Suspension Assay 92
       Testing Strategy 92
       Statistical Evaluation of *Salmonella* Test Data 92
       Data Reporting 93
       Correlations with Carcinogenicity 94
       Summary 95
       References 96

5. Detection of Carcinogens Based on *In Vitro* Mammalian Cytogenetic
   Tests 100
   Suzanne M. Morris, Daniel A. Casciano and Bruce C. Casto
       Introduction 100
       Background 101
           Chromosomal Aberrations 101
           Sister-Chromatid Exchange 102

Rationale. 103
Testing Methods 103
  Chromosomal Aberrations. 103
    Staining Regimes. 103
    Assay Protocols. 104
  Sister-Chromatid Exchange 104
    SCE Visualization 104
    Assay Protocols. 105
Cell Systems. 105
Classes of Chemicals. 106
Advantages and Disadvantages 107
  Chromosomal Aberrations. 107
    Advantages. 107
    Disadvantages 108
  Sister-Chromatid Exchange 108
    Advantages. 108
    Disadvantages 108
Significance 108
References. 109

6. **Methods and Modifications of the Hepatocyte Primary Culture/DNA
  Repair Test** 116
  Charlene A. McQueen and Gary M. Williams
  Introduction. 116
  Rat Hepatocyte Primary Culture (HPC)/DNA Repair Test. 117
    Preparation of Hepatocyte Primary Cultures. 117
    Hepatocyte Primary Culture/DNA Repair Test 118
    Evaluation of Genotoxicity 118
    Genotoxicity of Xenobiotics in the Rat HPC/DNA Repair Test . 120
  Modifications of the Rat Hepatocyte Primary Culture/DNA
  Repair Test. 120
    Addition of Exogenous Metabolizing Systems. 120
    In Vivo Exposure 121
    Vapor Exposure 121
    Utilization of Mouse, Hamster, and Rabbit Hepatocytes 121
    Genotoxicity of Xenobiotics in the Mouse, Hamster, or Rabbit
    HPC/DNA Repair Test 122
    Effect of Intraspecies Differences on Chemical Genotoxicity . . . 124
  Conclusions 124
  References. 124

7. **Cell Transformation Assays.** 130
  Andrew Sivak and Alice S. Tu
  Introduction. 130
  Methods in Contemporary Use. 131
    Transformation Assays with Early Passage Cells. 131
    Syrian Hamster Embryo Clonal Assay 131
    Syrian Hamster Embryo Focus Assay 133

Human Cell Focus Assay. 133
Epithelial Cell Transformation Assays 134
Transformation Assays with Cell Lines 134
BALB/c-3T3 Focus Assay. 134
C3H-10T½ Focus Assay 135
Other Cell Line Assays 136
Transformation Assays Using Cells Infected with Viruses 138
Rauscher Leukemia Virus—Fischer Rat Embryo (RLV/RE). . 138
Simian Adenovirus SA7—Syrian Hamster Embryo Cells
(SA7/SHE). 139
Comparison of Cell Transformation Systems. 140
Assay Modifications for Problem Chemicals 143
Volatile and Gas Samples 143
Procarcinogens 143
Promoters of Carcinogenicity. 144
Discussion 144
References. 146

PART IV
LIMITED BIOASSAYS

8. Rat Liver Foci Assay 152
Michael A. Pereira
Introduction. 152
Stages of Experimental Hepatocarcinogenesis 153
Initiation. 153
Promotion 156
Protocols of the Rat Liver Foci Assay 156
General Comments About the Protocols 158
Use of Altered-Foci 158
Use of 2-Acetylaminofluorene 160
Quantitation of the Incidence of Foci 160
Species, Strain, Sex and Route of Administration 161
Results 163
Relationship of Altered-Foci to Hepatocellular Carcinoma 168
Conclusion. 171
References. 171

9. Lung Tumors in Strain A Mice as a Bioassay for Carcinogenicity. 179
Gary D. Stoner and Michael B. Shimkin
Introduction. 179
Background 179
Materials and Methods 183
Animals. 183
Chemicals 184
Preliminary Toxicology 184
Bioassays. 184
Data Evaluation 185
Results 186

Pulmonary Tumors in Control Mice 186
Pulmonary Tumors in Chemically-Treated Mice. 186
    Polycyclic Hydrocarbons 198
    Carbamates 198
    Aziridines 198
    N-Nitroso Compounds 198
    Nitrogen Mustards. 199
    Organohalide Compounds. 199
    Metals. 199
    Food Additives. 200
    Chemotherapeutic Drugs. 200
    Silylating Agents. 200
    Nitrotoluenes and Derivatives 201
    Naphthylamines and Derivatives. 201
    Miscellaneous Chemicals 201
Relative Carcinogenicity of Selected Compounds. 202
Comparison of Lung Tumor Data with Results from Two-Year
    Rodent Bioassays. 202
Discussion 206
References. 208

10. **Tumorigenesis of the Rat Mammary Gland**. 215
   David L. McCormick and Richard C. Moon
   Introduction. 215
   Methodology for Screening of Compounds as Mammary
      Carcinogens 216
    Experimental Animals 216
      Strain 216
      Age. 216
      Reproductive Status. 217
    Administration of Test Compounds 218
    Observation of Animals 219
    Necropsy and Histopathology 219
   Characteristics of the Rat Mammary Carcinoma Model System. . . 220
    Attributes and Limitations 220
    Possible Modifications 222
   Chemical and Physical Agents with Carcinogenic Activity in the
      Rat Mammary Gland 224
    Polycyclic Aromatic Hydrocarbons (PAH's) 224
    Aromatic Amides and Derivatives. 225
    Nitrosamides 225
    Ethyl Methanesulfonate 226
    Radiation. 226
   References. 226

11. **SENCAR Mouse Skin Tumorigenesis**. 230
   Thomas J. Slaga and Stephen Nesnow
   Introduction. 230

Complete *vs* Two-Stage Skin Carcinogenesis 232
SENCAR Mouse Skin Tumorigenesis Model 236
    Derivation 236
    Comparison to Other Stocks and Strains of Mice 236
    Carcinogens and/or Initiators Used in SENCAR Mice 239
    Promoters Used in SENCAR Mice. 240
    Experimental Protocol 243
Two-Stage Promotion in SENCAR Mice. 245
Tumor Progression in SENCAR Mice. 245
Anticarcinogens 246
Conclusion. 247
References 247

PART V
LONG-TERM ANIMAL BIOASSAYS

12. Design of a Long-Term Animal Bioassay for Carcinogenicity 252
    Thomas E. Hamm, Jr.
    Introduction. 252
    The Design of the "Standard" Bioassay 253
    Factors to be Considered When Designing a Bioassay 254
        Test Substance 254
        Dosage 254
        Route 255
        Animal Selection. 255
        Duration of Exposure. 256
        Number of Animals 256
        Animal Husbandry. 257
            Genetic Monitoring 257
            Health Quality 257
            Feed. 257
            Water 258
            Temperature and Humidity 259
            Lighting. 259
            Caging. 259
            Sanitation 260
        Randomization 260
        Clinical Observations 261
        Necropsy 261
            Clinical Pathology Tests 261
            Organ Weights. 261
            Histopathology 261
        Quality Assurance 263
        Safety 263
    Conclusion. 263
    References 264

13. Conduct of Long-Term Animal Bioassays. 268
    J. David Prejean
    Introduction. 268
    Preliminary Planning 269
    Initiation. 271
        Protocol/Final Scheduling. 272
        Randomization. 274
        First Dosing 276
    Execution (In-Life Activities) 276
    Completion 277
        Necropsy. 278
        Histologic Processing 279
        Microscopic Evaluation. 280
        Reporting 280
    References. 281

14. Selection and Use of the B6C3F1 Mouse and F344 Rat in Long-Term
    Bioassays for Carcinogenicity. 282
    Dawn G. Goodman, Gary A. Boorman and John D. Strandberg
    Introduction. 282
    Selection of the B6C3F1 Mouse and F344 Rat for Carcino-
    genicity Studies. 283
        Selection of the B6C3F1 Mouse. 286
        Selection of the F344 Rat. 288
    Origin of the B6C3F1 Mouse and F344 Rat 288
        Origin of the B6C3F1 Mouse. 289
        Origin of the F344 Rat. 289
    Characteristics of the B6C3F1 Hybrid Mouse 289
        Common Spontaneous Neoplasms 290
            Hepatocellular Neoplasms. 290
            Lymphoreticular Neoplasms 294
            Alveolar/Bronchiolar Neoplasms. 296
        Common Age-Associated Lesions 298
        Common Induced Tumors. 299
    Characteristics of the F344 Rat 300
        Common Spontaneous Neoplasms 300
            Interstitial Cell Tumors of the Testis. 301
            Anterior Pituitary Neoplasms. 304
            Mammary Gland Neoplasms 305
            Mononuclear Cell Leukemia 305
        Common Age-Associated Lesions 308
        Common Induced Neoplasms. 310
            Hepatocellular Neoplasms. 310
            Urinary Bladder Neoplasms. 311
    Comparison of Carcinogenic Responses Between Strains and
    Species 312
        Comparison of the B6C3F1 Mouse with Other Strains 313
        Comparison of the F344 Rat with Other Rat Strains 314

Comparison of the B6C3F1 Mouse and F344 Rat with
   Other Species 317
Conclusions 318
References 319

15. **Adequacy of Syrian Hamsters for Long-Term Animal Bioassays** 326
   Freddy Homburger and Richard A. Adams
   Reasons for Species Selection 326
      Comparative Studies in Different Species 329
      Long-Term Bioassays in Hamsters of Various Substances
         Without Simultaneous Testing in Other Species 330
      Respiratory Carcinogenesis 331
      Nitrosamines and Other Nitroso Compounds as Carcinogens
         for the Respiratory Tract and Other Organs 332
      Asbestos and Other Particulates as Respiratory Carcinogens. . . 332
      Inhaled Radioactive Substances 333
      The Direct Application of N-Methyl-N-Nitrosourea to a Well
         Defined Segment of the Hamster Trachea 333
      Peculiar Behavior of Hamster Kidney Suggesting Suitability
         for Certain Bioassays for Carcinogenicity 333
      Hamster Pancreas as Target Organ for Certain Nitrosamines. . . 334
      The Gallbladder as a Susceptible Site for Methylcholanthrene
         Carcinogenesis. 334
      Species-Specific Properties of Hamster Skin Possibly Useful
         in Long-Term Bioassays 334
      The Hamster Cheek Pouch as a Bioassay for Carcinogenicity . . 335
   Discussion 335
   References 337

16. **Quality Assurance in Pathology for Rodent Carcinogenicity Studies** ... 345
   *Gary A. Boorman, Charles A. Montgomery, Jr., Scot L. Eustis,
   Marilyn J. Wolfe, Ernest E. McConnell and Jerry F. Hardisty*
   Introduction. 345
   Quality Assurance Through Quality Control and Quality
      Assessment. 346
   Laboratory Quality Control. 346
      Professional Personnel 346
      Necropsy Examination 347
      Histology Procedures 349
      Tissue Trimming 350
      Tissue Embedding and Slide Preparation 351
      Histopathologic Evaluation 353
   Sponsor Quality Assessment 353
   Preliminary Review of Pathology Data. 354
   Review of Pathology Materials. 355
   Pathology Diagnostic Quality Assessment. 356
   Summary. 357
   References. 357

17. Statistical Evaluation of Long-Term Animal Bioassays for
Carcinogenicity..358
   Colin N. Park and Richard J. Kociba
     Introduction..358
     Pairwise Tests......................................361
     Trend Tests...363
     Mortality Adjustments...............................367
     Differential Mortality Tests........................370
     "Time to Tumor" Analyses............................370
     References..371

18. Considerations in the Evaluation and Interpretation of Long-Term
Animal Bioassays for Carcinogenicity 372
   Robert R. Maronpot
     Introduction..372
     Considerations in the Evaluation of Long-Term Rodent Studies
      for Carcinogenicity 372
      Study Audit......................................372
      Peer Review Process..............................373
       Pathology Review Process.......................373
       Peer Review of Findings from Long-Term Studies ...374
      Considerations in the Conduct of Pathology.......374
       Gross Examination 374
       Histologic Evaluation..........................375
     Interpretation of the Study.........................375
      Route of Administration of the Test Substance....375
      Chronic Toxicity and Other Study Results.........375
      Significance 376
      Historic Controls................................377
      False Positives..................................378
      False Negatives 378
      Decreased Tumor Incidences 379
      Evidence of Carcinogenicity 379
      Qualified Conclusions............................380
     References..381

PART VI
BIOASSAYS FOR INSOLUBLE MATERIALS

19. Bioassays for Asbestos and Other Solid Materials.............384
   David L. Coffin and Lalita D. Palekar
     Introduction..384
     Asbestos and Other Mineral Fibers 386
     Influence of Mineralogical Properties on Biological Activities....387
      Tumorigenicity and Fiber Size....................387
      Tumorigenicity and Magnesium (Acid Leaching) ...388
     In Vitro Bioassays................................388
      Influence of Surface Property 388

Genetic Manifestations.............................390
Morphologic Transformation........................391
Bacterial Mutagenic Response 391
Asbestos as a Co-Carcinogen 392
In Vitro Interactions with Human Bronchial Cells 394
Foreign Body Tumorigenicity 394
In Vivo Bioassays 395
Inhalation Exposure..............................395
Intratracheal Instillation........................398
Intrapleural Injection............................400
Intraperitoneal Injection.........................401
Subcutaneous Injection 402
Ingestion Exposure 402
Bioassay for Foreign Body Tumorigenicity............403
Evaluation of Bioassay Methods........................403
Risk Assessment 406
Current Use 406
Asbestos in Place................................407
Natural Environment 407
Asbestos Substitutes 408
References...410

PART VII
ASSAYS WITH POTENTIAL UTILITY

20. *In Vitro* Assay to Detect Inhibitors of Intercellular Communication . . . 422
James E. Trosko, Cy Jone, Charles Aylsworth and Chia-cheng Chang
Intercellular Communication: An Important Biological
Process 422
Metabolic Cooperation: *In Vitro* Means to Measure Inter-
cellular Communication 424
Experimental Protocol to Measure Metabolic Cooperation......425
Rationale.......................................425
Cytotoxicity and Range-Finding Studies 425
Assay for Inhibition of Metabolic Cooperation 427
Interpretation of Results: Potential and Limitations of the
Assay 428
References....................................432

21. Alpha-Fetoprotein: A Marker for Exposure to Chemical Hepato-
carcinogens in Rats 438
Harold A. Dunsford and Stewart Sell
Introduction.....................................438
Chemistry 438
Function.......................................439
Regulation of Production 439
Purification of AFP 440

Preparation of Anti-Rat AFP. 440
Radiolabeling of AFP. 441
Antibody Dilution Curve 441
Radioimmunoassay 441
Application of AFP in Experimental Carcinogenesis. 442
    Hepatocellular Proliferation. .443
    N-2-Acetylaminofluorene (AAF) 443
    Ethionine. 451
    3'-Methyl-4-Dimethylaminoazobenzene (3'MDAB) 451
    Diethylnitrosamine (DEN) 454
    Wy-14,643. 454
    Diaminodiphenylmethane (DDPM). 456
Chemical Carcinogens in Mice 456
Discussion 456
Summary. 459
References. 459

22. Ornithine Decarboxylase as a Marker of Carcinogenesis. 464
    Diane H. Russell
    Introduction. 464
    The Role of Ornithine Decarboxylase in Carcinogenesis 465
    Ornithine Decarboxylase as a Marker of Promotion of
        Carcinogenesis. 467
    Ornithine Decarboxylase Activity as a Marker of the
        Carcinogenic and Promoting Properties of Ultraviolet Light. . . .470
    Effects of Analogs of Vitamin A on Ornithine Decarboxylase
        Activity. 471
    References. 473

23. Assay for Hepatic Peroxisome Proliferation to Select a Novel Class
    of Non-Mutagenic Hepatocarcinogens 482
    Janardan K. Reddy and Narendra D. Lalwani
    Introduction. 482
    Peroxisomes and Peroxisome Proliferation 482
    The Hypothesis. 485
    Experimental Approach 485
        General 485
        Choice of Species and Route of Administration. 485
    Morphological Alterations in Liver Parenchymal Cells. 490
        Light and Electron Microscopy .490
        Cytochemical Localization of Peroxisomal Catalase 490
        Morphometry. 491
    Biochemical Alterations in Liver. .491
        Catalase. 493
            Procedure 493
        Carnitine Acetyltransferase 494
            Procedure 494
        Peroxisomal-β-Oxidation of Fatty Acids. 494

Procedure 494
Other 496
Carcinogenicity Studies 496
Summary. 497
References. 497

PART VIII
RISK ESTIMATION

24. Examination of Risk Estimation Models 502
Abe Silvers and Kenny S. Crump
Introduction. 502
Experimental Design 503
Models 505
Tolerance Distribution Models. 505
Stochastic Models 506
Types of Dose-Response Functions. 506
Threshold 507
Low Dose Linear. 507
Low Dose Sublinear. 508
Low Dose Supralinear 508
Dose-Response Function Tail Behavior at Low Doses 508
Spontaneous Rates 512
Confidence Intervals 513
Limits Based Upon the Asymptotic Distribution of the
Likelihood Ratio. 514
Bootstrap Methods for Confidence Intervals. 516
Goodness-of-Fit 517
Examples of Calculations 517
Toxicokinetics and Risk Assessment 519
References. 524

25. Risk Assessment: Biological Considerations. 526
Joseph V. Rodricks and Duncan Turnbull
Introduction. 526
Elements of Carcinogenesis Risk Assessment. 527
Evaluation of Total Data Base 527
Introduction. 527
Factors in Evaluation. 528
The Evaluative Process 529
Formal Schemes for Ranking Evidence of Carcinogenicity. . . . 531
Selection of Data for Risk Assessment. 533
Introduction. 533
Options for Data Selection 533
Merits and Limitations of Data Selection Options 534
Commonly Used Procedures for Data Selection. 535
Use of Negative Data 535
Uncertainty Introduced into Risk Assessment by Data
Selection 536

Utilization of Selected Data. 536
Considerations in Extrapolation of Risks from Animals to
  Humans. 536
    Introduction: Issues Involved in Dose Adjustment and
      Interspecies Scaling 536
    Measure of Dose 537
    Routes of Absorption. 540
    Metabolism and Pharmacokinetics Data 540
    Approaches to Defining the Uncertainty of Interspecies
      Extrapolation 542
  Biological Thresholds. 543
  Presentation of Risk Assessment. 544
  References. 545

PART IX
REGULATORY IMPLICATIONS

26. Regulatory Implications: Perspective of the U.S. Environmental
  Protection Agency. 548
    Richard N. Hill
    Introduction. 548
    Early Encounters with Carcinogenicity 549
    Assessment Guidelines 549
    Assessment in Practice 550
      Weight-of-the-Evidence. 550
      Dose Extrapolation Models 550
      Genotoxic *versus* Non-Genotoxic 550
      Other Assessments. 551
    The Assessment Future. 551
    Uncertainties 552
    References. 554

27. New Approaches to the Regulation of Carcinogens in Foods: The
  Food and Drug Administration 556
    Robert J. Scheuplein, Herbert Blumenthal and W. Gary Flamm
    Introduction. 556
    Historical Overview of Food Safety Regulation in the United
      States 557
      1906–1957. 557
      1958–Present 559
    The Regulation of Carcinogens. 560
      Regulatory History 560
      Changing Perceptions of the Carcinogenic Hazard 561
      Risk Assessment of Carcinogens. 564
      Risk Assessment—Its Value 566
    References. 567

28. Workplace Carcinogens: Regulatory Implications of Investigations. . . . 569
   Robert P. Beliles
      Introduction. 569
      History of Federal Regulations of Workplace Carcinogens 570
         Asbestos 570
         "Fourteen Carcinogens". 571
         2-Acetylaminofluorene. 572
         4-Aminobiphenyl 573
         4-Nitrobiphenyl 573
         Benzidine. 573
         3,3'-Dichlorobenzidine. 573
         β-Propiolactone. 573
         4-Dimethylaminoazobenzene. 574
         2-Naphthylamine. 574
         1-Naphthylamine. 574
         Bis(chloromethyl) Ether. 574
         Chloromethyl Methyl Ether. 574
         N-Nitrosodimethylamine. 575
         Ethyleneimine 575
         4,4'-Methylenebis(2-chlorobenzenamine). 575
         Vinyl Chloride 575
         Coke Oven Emissions. 576
         1,2-Dibromo-3-Chloropropane. 577
         Arsenic 578
         Acrylonitrile. 578
         Ethylene Oxide. 579
         Ethylene Dibromide. 580
         Beryllium and Trichloroethylene 580
         Benzene. 581
      The Future and Implications of Carcinogenicity Testing 581
      References. 585

29. Evaluation of Carcinogens: Perspective of the Consumer Product
   Safety Commission 587
   Andrew G. Ulsamer, Paul D. White and Peter W. Preuss
      Introduction. 587
      Regulatory Authority. 588
      Carcinogen Policy—Past and Present 589
         Historical Aspects 589
         Interagency Carcinogen Evaluation Efforts. 589
         Chemical Screening Process. 590
         In-Depth Chemical Evaluation 591
      Chemical Carcinogens Evaluated by CPSC 593
         Vinyl Chloride 593
         Tris(2,3-Dibromopropyl) Phosphate 594
         Benzene. 594
         Benzidine Congener Dyes 595
         Asbestos 596

Formaldehyde 596
Diethylhexyl Phthalate and Nitrosamines. 598
Summary and Conclusions 599
References.. 600

30. International Aspects of Testing for Carcinogenicity and
    Regulation: A Selected Bibliography 603
    William H. Farland
    Introduction..................................... 603
    Selected Bibliography.............................. 605

PART X
INDUSTRY PERSPECTIVE

31. An Industrial Perspective on Testing for Carcinogenicity. 608
    Donald E. Stevenson and Paul F. Deisler, Jr.
    Introduction..................................... 608
    The Growth of Industry's Involvement in Carcinogenicity
      Testing 609
    Testing: Needs, Strategies and Approaches 612
    The Use of Test Results in Characterizing and Abating
      Carcinogenic Risks................................ 614
    Areas for Future Consideration 620
    References....................................... 622

Index 625

Part I

Predicting Carcinogenicity of Chemicals from Their Structure

1

Structural and Functional Criteria for Suspecting Chemical Compounds of Carcinogenic Activity: State-of-the-Art of Predictive Formalism*

Yin-Tak Woo

JRB Associates
McLean, Virginia

Joseph C. Arcos

U.S. Environmental Protection Agency
Washington, D.C.

Tulane University School of Medicine
New Orleans, Louisiana

David Y. Lai

JRB Associates
McLean, Virginia

INTRODUCTION

Every year, over 400,000 new organic compounds are synthesized throughout the world, and it is estimated that well over 1,000 of these compounds will

*This project has been funded in part with Federal funds from the U.S. Environmental Protection Agency under Contract No. 68-01-6644. The conclusions reached and scientific views expressed in this review are solely those of the authors. The content of this publication does not necessarily reflect the views or policies of the U.S. Environmental Protection Agency, nor does mention of trade names, commercial products, or organizations imply endorsement by the U.S. Government.

eventually be introduced into economic use, and, thus, into the environment world wide. Although not all of these economically used compounds may be suspected of carcinogenic activity, owing to cost and time limitations actually only a small portion of these new commercial products can be adequately assayed for carcinogenicity. Hence, a significant number of untested or inadequately tested chemicals may find their way into consumer items or industrial uses. Moreover, a considerable number of chemicals that are now in use in industralized countries were introduced before the present relatively stringent criteria for carcinogen testing and risk assessment were established. The safety of at least some of these compounds is questionable in the light of current knowledge about carcinogens. Formalized schemes have been established to detect chemical compounds which may be suspected of carcinogenic activity, to provide the basis for an initial evaluation of the potential carcinogenicity risk, to set the priority list for bioassay testing, and to help the designing of meaningful batteries of screening tests. The aim of this chapter is to present the state-of-the-art of this predictive formalism.

CRITERIA FOR SUSPECTING A CHEMICAL OF CARCINOGENIC ACTIVITY

There are essentially three categories of criteria for suspecting chemical compounds of carcinogenic activity: (1) structural criteria, (2) functional criteria, and (3) "guilt by association" criterion.

(1) *Structural criteria* are based on structure-activity relationship (SAR) analysis, which is the essential component of any scheme for assessing the potential carcinogenicity of a chemical compound. Basically, SAR analysis may use two approaches that are based on: (a) structural *analogies* with established types of chemical carcinogens, and/or (b) consideration of molecular size, shape and symmetry, and of electron distribution and steric factors in or around functional group(s), *independently* from any possible analogy with other compounds.

(2) *Functional criteria* represent the sum of the pharmacological and/or toxicological capabilities which—irrespective of structural type—have been correlated with carcinogenic activity (*e.g.*, mutagenicity, induction of DNA repair, immunosuppression). Functional criteria are used in a complementary manner to structural criteria because structural considerations alone cannot forecast *entirely new* structural types of carcinogens.

(3) The *"guilt by association" criterion* points to the possible carcinogenic potentiality of compounds which—although found inactive under some "standard" conditions of animal bioassay (and/or mutagenicity testing)—belong to chemical classes in which several other compounds were found to be potent and multi-target carcinogens, for example the 5-nitrofuran type urinary antibacterials. These compounds should be reevaluated to determine if retesting *under more stringent conditions* is warranted.

GENERAL PRINCIPLES OF CHEMICAL CARCINOGENESIS

To gain a better insight into the significance of the criteria, a brief outline of the general principles of chemical carcinogenesis is needed. Carcinogenesis is a complex process involving many etiological factors. Figure 1 depicts the principal identified relationships. Chemical compounds may affect one or more of these factors and contribute to the overall effect of the induction of cancer.

From the point of view of mechanism of action, carcinogens may be loosely classified as: (1) genotoxic carcinogens, (2) epigenetic carcinogens, and (3) foreign-body carcinogens. *Genotoxic carcinogens* produce DNA damage through covalent binding (or, in some cases, through strand scission). They act as electrophilic reactants either directly or after metabolic activation. The genotoxic capability of a chemical can, in most cases, be evaluated by determining the extent of covalent binding to DNA or by short-term testing for genetic damage (*e.g.*, unscheduled DNA synthesis, mutagenesis, chromosomal aberrations). Reactivity-wise, genotoxic carcinogens have also been classified as "soft" and "hard" electrophiles (*see* Table 1). *Epigenetic carcinogens* are those that do not damage DNA directly, but may act by a variety of not clearly defined extrachromosomal mechanisms, such as inhibition of intercellular communication, production of endocrine imbalance, chronic tissue injury, immunosuppression, peroxisome proliferation, etc. *Foreign-body carcinogens* are those which, by virtue of their critical size and shape, induce carcinogenesis probably by disrupting intercellular homeostasis or by mechanically interfering with DNA conformational changes. By truly rigorous criteria they cannot be regarded as *chemical* carcinogens because there is no requirement for any specific chemical structure for carcinogenicity. There are two subclasses of foreign-body carcinogens: (a) self-penetrant fibers epitomized by asbestos fibers, and (b) sheets and platelets implanted in tissues.

Table 1: Summary of Concept of "Soft" and "Hard" Electrophiles and Their Respective Points of Attack in Macromolecules*

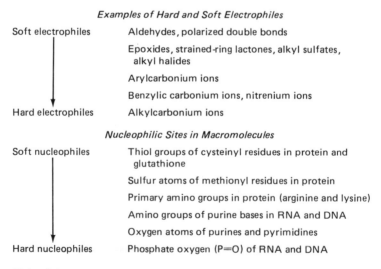

Examples of Hard and Soft Electrophiles

Soft electrophiles — Aldehydes, polarized double bonds; Epoxides, strained-ring lactones, alkyl sulfates, alkyl halides; Arylcarbonium ions; Benzylic carbonium ions, nitrenium ions

Hard electrophiles — Alkylcarbonium ions

Nucleophilic Sites in Macromolecules

Soft nucleophiles — Thiol groups of cysteinyl residues in protein and glutathione; Sulfur atoms of methionyl residues in protein; Primary amino groups in protein (arginine and lysine); Amino groups of purine bases in RNA and DNA; Oxygen atoms of purines and pyrimidines

Hard nucleophiles — Phosphate oxygen (P=O) of RNA and DNA

*Brian Coles, personal communication; for the origination of the concept *see* reference 1.

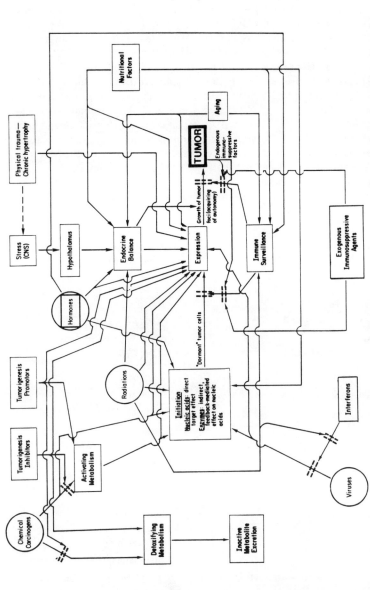

Figure 1: Principal identified relationships in the multifactorial etiology of carcinogenesis. A pathway linking one factor to another symbolizes the relationship that the latter is influenced by the former in a positive or negative sense. A pair of broken lines across a pathway symbolizes inhibition or blockage of the pathway by factor(s) pointing to the broken line-pair. Pathways which link factors to "Initiation" or "Expression" specify those factors that contribute to or bring about the completion of these two major phases of carcinogenesis.

Carcinogens which act as electrophilic reactants may be further classified as: (1) direct-acting carcinogens, (2) carcinogens which require simple acid- or alkali-catalyzed hydrolysis, and (3) carcinogens which require metabolic activation. Direct-acting carcinogens tend to be locally active, whereas those which are activated are carcinogenic mostly toward tissue(s) where activation occurs. The mixed-function oxidases are the chief activating enzyme systems for most carcinogens. Other enzymes which may contribute to metabolic activation are exemplified by aldehyde dehydrogenase, prostaglandin synthetase and for compounds such as dihaloalkanes, glutathione transferase. A compound should be suspected of being carcinogenic if its metabolic split products are known or suspected of being carcinogenic. The types of electrophilic, reactive intermediates which are believed to be potentially carcinogenic include: carbonium, episulfonium, aziridium, oxonium, nitrenium or arylamidonium ions, free radicals, epoxides, lactones, aldehydes, semiquinones/quinoneimines, acylating moieties, and peroxides. Compounds which yield reactive intermediates that can be stabilized by resonance (Fig. 2) often have higher carcinogenic potential because their reactive intermediates have a better chance of remaining reactive during transport from the site of activation to target macromolecules.

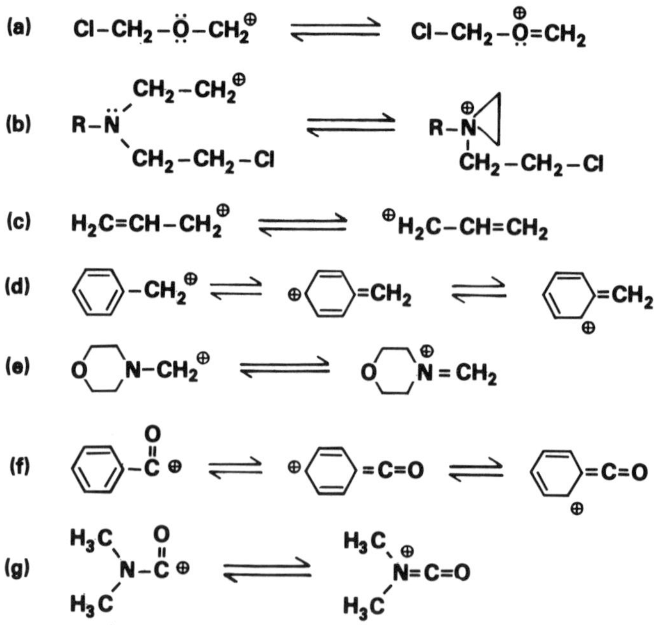

Figure 2: Resonance stabilization of reactive intermediates from (a) bis-(chloromethyl)ether, (b) aliphatic nitrogen mustards, (c) allyl chloride, (d) benzyl chloride, (e) bis-(morpholino)methane, (f) benzoyl chloride, and (g) dimethylcarbamyl chloride.

PHYSICOCHEMICAL FACTORS WHICH MAY MODIFY THE CARCINOGENIC POTENTIAL OF A CHEMICAL

Irrespective of its chemical structure, the carcinogenic potential of a chemical compound is dependent on its physicochemical properties which determine its "bio-availability", that is, its ability to reach target tissues. The most salient factors are discussed below.

Molecular Weight

Compounds with very high molecular weight (over 1,000–1,500) have little chance of being absorbed in significant amounts; in general, they do not pose any appreciable carcinogenic risk. There are at least two important exceptions to this rule: (a) The potential absorption of high molecular weight compounds which can be degraded in the gastrointestinal tract (*e.g.*, by simple hydrolysis or bacterial action) should be assessed considering their probable degradation products. A case in point is the polyazo dyes which may be split into component aromatic amines by bacterial azo reductase *if* the azo bonds are not sterically hindered or involved in coordination to metals. (b) Some moderately high molecular weight water-soluble polymers are known which appear to be carcinogenic toward intestinal tissues by direct contact. For example, several polysaccharide sulfates (dextran sulfate sodium, degraded carrageenan) with molecular weights ranging from 20,000 to 54,000 have been reported to induce tumors of the small intestine in experimental animals.[2-4]

Physical State

The physical state of a chemical compound may, to some extent, determine its capability to reach target tissues. Compounds which are volatile, or which can be inhaled as dust particles, may have "direct access" to nasopharyngeal and/or pulmonary tissues. They should be used with caution particularly if they are chemically reactive (*e.g.*, bis-chloromethyl ether, formaldehyde). Compounds which are nonviscous liquids or are in solution are expected to be absorbed more readily than those which are viscous or solid.

Solubility

In general, compounds which are highly hydrophilic are poorly absorbed and, if absorbed, are readily excreted. Thus, the introduction of hydrophilic groups (*e.g.*, sulfonyl, carboxyl, hydroxyl, glucuronyl) into an otherwise carcinogenic compound usually mitigates and sometimes even abolishes its carcinogenic activity. Compounds which are not soluble in water also have limited bioavailability because compounds which are not in solution are not readily absorbed. The correlation of gastric or skin absorption with the liposolubility (usually expressed as partition coefficient, log P) of chemical compounds has been extensively studied (*see* references 5 and 6) and has been the basis of numerous structure-activity studies.

Chemical Reactivity

Compounds which are "too reactive" are not carcinogenic. By "too reactive" is meant that the compounds polymerize spontaneously, hydrolyze instantaneously, or react with noncritical cellular constituents *before* they can reach target tissues and react with key macromolecules. For example, the introduction of an exocyclic double bond into β-propiolactone (which is reactive and carcinogenic) yields an extremely reactive compound, diketene, which is not carcinogenic (*see* reference 7). It is important to point out that the route of exposure is a key factor in considering whether the compound is "too reactive." For example, bis-chloromethyl ether may be considered "too reactive" if administered orally in aqueous solution ($t_{1/2}$ approximately 40 seconds); however, the compound is a potent nasal/pulmonary carcinogen if inhaled as vapor ($t_{1/2}$ in humid air may be as long as 25 hours) (*see* reference 7).

STRUCTURAL CRITERIA

The structural criteria for suspecting chemical compounds of carcinogenic activity are based on structural analogy with established types of chemical carcinogens along with considerations of molecular size, shape, and symmetry and of electron distribution and steric factors around functional group(s). A general perspective of the established types of chemical carcinogens and some of the noted structure-activity relationships in each class are presented below.

Aromatic Amines and Azo Dyes

The class of compounds in which the structural and molecular basis of carcinogenic activity is the most clearly understood is the aromatic amines. Extensive, analytic reviews of this area have been given by Arcos and Argus,[8] Clayson and Garner,[9] and Sontag.[10] A synoptic summary depicting the types of aromatic amines which are carcinogenic is shown in Figure 3. The typical aryl moieties present in carcinogenic aromatic amines include (from the top, clockwise): phenanthrene, fluorene, anthracene, naphthalene, acenaphthene, fluoranthene, perylene, chrysene, benz(a)anthracene, benzalindene, triphenylmethane, 2,2-bisphenylpropane, toluene, biphenyl, pyrene and stilbene. The unconnected bond(s) on these moieties indicate the positions where attachment of one or more amine or "amine-generating" group(s) yield carcinogenic compounds. Owing to the possible metabolic interconversion of the amine group with hydroxylamine and nitroso groups and the metabolic reduction of the nitro to nitroso (*see* center block in Figure 3), the latter three groups are often termed amine-generating groups. In some but not all instances a dimethylamino group may replace an amino group without significant loss of carcinogenic activity. The dimethylamino group may also be considered amine-generating because metabolic N-demethylation readily occurs *in vivo*. It is important to note in Figure 3 that in the most highly carcinogenic aromatic amines the amine or amine-generating group(s) is linked to the aromatic frame in position(s) corresponding to the terminal end(s) of the longest conjugated system in the molecule.

Aromatic amines require a two-stage metabolic activation for carcinogenicity and the mechanism of activation is now known in considerable detail. The first stage involves N-hydroxylation and N-acetylation to yield an acyl hydroxylamine (hydroxamic acid). The second stage involves O-acylation (the acyl group

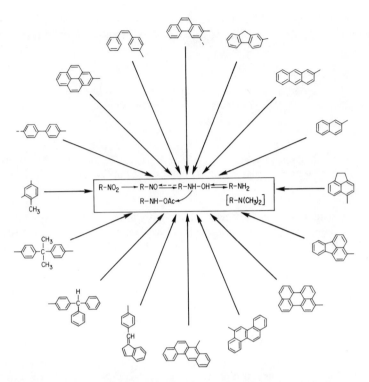

Figure 3: Typical aryl moieties present in carcinogenic aromatic amines. The unconnected bond(s) on these moieties indicate the position(s) where attachment of amine or amine-generating group(s) yield carcinogenic compounds (*see* text for detail).

may be sulfonyl, phosphoryl or acetyl) to yield acyloxy amines which are highly reactive and may readily bind covalently to (arylate) cellular nucleophiles. The arylation of DNA and/or RNA is the critical initiating step in carcinogenesis by aromatic amines. This mechanism of activation provides the rationale for the structural requirement that the amine or amine-generating group(s) be linked to the aromatic frame in position(s) corresponding to the terminal end(s) of the longest conjugated system in the molecule. This is because the molecular mechanism, which is common to seemingly all aromatic amines, is the anionic departure of the N-linked acyloxy grouping leading to an arylamidonium ion and its resonance-stabilized carbonium ion tautomer (*e.g.*, Figure 4), which represent the ultimate carcinogenic form of the aromatic amines. The carcinogenic potency is therefore a function of the leaving potential of the acyloxy anion which, in turn, depends on the bond strength of the O-ester linkage. This facet of the mechanism of action is critically governed by the π-electronic properties of the aryl moiety. That is, the reactivity of the acyloxy compound toward nucleophiles depends on the force of conjugation of (electron donation by) the aryl moiety, labilizing the ester linkage and facilitating the departure of the acyloxy

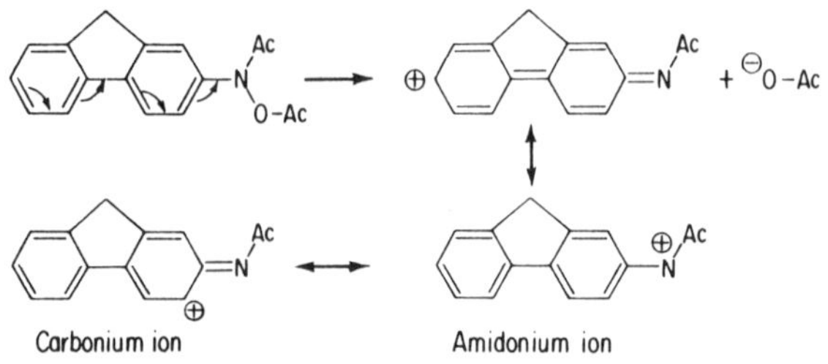

Carbonium ion   Amidonium ion

Figure 4: Molecular mechanism for the generation of resonance-stabilized reactive intermediates from N-acyloxy aromatic amines.

group. Electron donation is much weaker with a phenyl than with the higher aryl groups, and, *within a given molecule*, increases with the length of the conjugated double-bonded system involved. This also explains the apparent lack of carcinogenic activity of phenylhydroxylamine and of the nonaromatic N-hydroxy compounds tested so far. It is consistent with the role of the aryl moiety that substituents which influence the electron density by positive or negative inductive or mesomeric effect, will also, often drastically, affect the carcinogenic potency; moreover, substituents of the aryl moiety often have a modifying effect on the tissue target specificity of carcinogenic action.

It is important to note that since the role of the aromatic moiety is to provide π-electron shift of sufficient strength to facilitate the departure of the leaving group, homocyclic aryl moieties may be replaced by a variety of other aromatic groupings containing heteroatoms (nitrogen, sulfur, oxygen), often without loss of carcinogenic activity *per se*, but often with a significant change of tissue target specificity. A variety of aromatic amines containing heteroatomic moieties (*e.g.*, aminotriazole, auramine, 4-acetylaminodiphenylsulfide, acridine orange, 2-aralkyl-5-nitrofurans, 4-dimethylaminoazobenzene) has been found to be carcinogenic (*see* reference 8).

For solely historical reasons azo dye carcinogens are often treated as a class separate from such aromatic amines as 2-naphthylamine and 2-acetylaminofluorene; however, it is evident that amino azo dyes, at least, behave as true aromatic amines, as indicated by the general identity of the activation mechanism of 4-dimethylaminoazobenzene and its derivatives with that of the other aromatic amines. Nevertheless, it is not known whether all heteroatomic amines require the same type of activation. For example, there is some evidence that acridine orange which, besides being a potent frame-shift mutagen is also a hepatic carcinogen, may not require activation involving N-hydroxylation, but reacts with DNA by intercalation between base-pairs. Unlike polycyclic hydrocarbons, acridine mutagens form highly stable intercalation complexes with DNA. Moreover, several azo compounds which bear no amine substituent display carcinogenic activity; these are methyl-, hydroxy-, methoxy- and sulfonic acid-substituted phenylazonaphthalenes and azonaphthalenes. The metabolic activation of these compounds has not been investigated. A number of non-amine azo compounds, the relative safety of which has been established, are used as food colors and solvent dyes.

Polynuclear Compounds

The next class of carcinogens whose mechanism of action is best known are the polynuclear aromatic hydrocarbons and heteroaromatics. The structure-activity relationships of these compounds have been reviewed by Arcos and Argus,[11] Dipple,[12] and Thakker *et al.*[13] Phenanthrene and pyrene are the recurring ring patterns in most potent carcinogenic hydrocarbons such as benzo[a]pyrene, dibenzo[a,h]pyrene, dibenzo[a,i]pyrene, dibenz[a,h]anthracene, 3-methylcholanthrene and benzo[f]fluoranthene. None of the linearly condensed polynuclear hydrocarbons appear to be carcinogenic. The lowest angular ring structure, phenanthrene, is inactive. A tetracyclic ring system is the lowest level of complexity among the unsubstituted hydrocarbons to confer some carcinogenicity: benz[a]anthracene and benzo[a]phenanthrene are weak to moderately active agents and chrysene is marginally active or inactive. The typical strong hydrocarbon carcinogens are found among the penta- and hexacyclic structures. Hexacyclic ring systems represent the highest molecular complexity compatible with strong carcinogenic activity. However, this does not mean that beyond six condensed cycles there is a sudden, sharp cutoff of carcinogenicity, since a few heptacyclic hydrocarbons (*e.g.*, 1,2,4,5,8,9-tribenzopyrene) have weak-to-moderate activity. Methyl substituent(s) can considerably enhance the activity level of the tri- and tetracyclic structures. However, methyl substitution generally lowers the activity of the penta- and especially of the hexacyclic hydrocarbons because it increases the molecular size beyond the optimal range. Carcinogenic activity is often fully maintained in polynuclears in which a ring –C= is replaced by –N= or a –CH=CH– group is replaced by a –NH–, –S– or –O– bridge.

The angular ring pattern of phenanthrene (present also in pyrene) directed attention in the late 1930's to the potential significance of the *meso*-phenanthrenic double bond for carcinogenic activity. This sterically exposed double bond became known as the "K-region" (*see* Figure 5). Various electronic indexes have been calculated to characterize the reactivity of the K-region, and the indexes have been correlated with the respective carcinogenicities with some degree of success. However, beginning in the 1960's, several lines of investigations prompted a reexamination of the role of the K-region. The discovery of the "NIH" shift led to the recognition of arene oxides (epoxides) as reactive electrophilic intermediates in the metabolism of polycyclic hydrocarbons to phenols and dihydrodiols, as well as in the covalent binding of the hydrocarbons to cellular nucleophiles. Hydrocarbons may be epoxidated in different positions along the periphery of the molecular skeleton and these different epoxides yield polynuclear phenols and dihydrodiols (detected as excreted metabolites) following the NIH shift and the action of epoxide hydrase, respectively. A number of K-region epoxides have been tested and found to be less carcinogenic than the parent hydrocarbons suggesting that the K-region is not involved in the reactions leading to carcinogenesis. Instead, model studies using benzo[a]pyrene established 7,8-dihydrodiol-9,10-epoxide, a "bay region" diol epoxide (*see* Figure 5) as the proximate or ultimate carcinogen of the hydrocarbon. A "bay region" in a polynuclear structure exists when two nonadjacent benzene rings (one of which is a benzo ring) are in close proximity. Thus, the sterically hindered area between the 4- and 5-positions of phenanthrene, 9- and 10- of benzo[a]pyrene, 1- and 12- of benz[a]anthracene, both the 4- and 5-positions and 10- and 11-positions of chrysene, are all "bay regions." The "bay region" diol epoxides of several polycyclic hydrocarbons have been shown to be proximate carcinogens of the parent compounds (*see* reference 13).

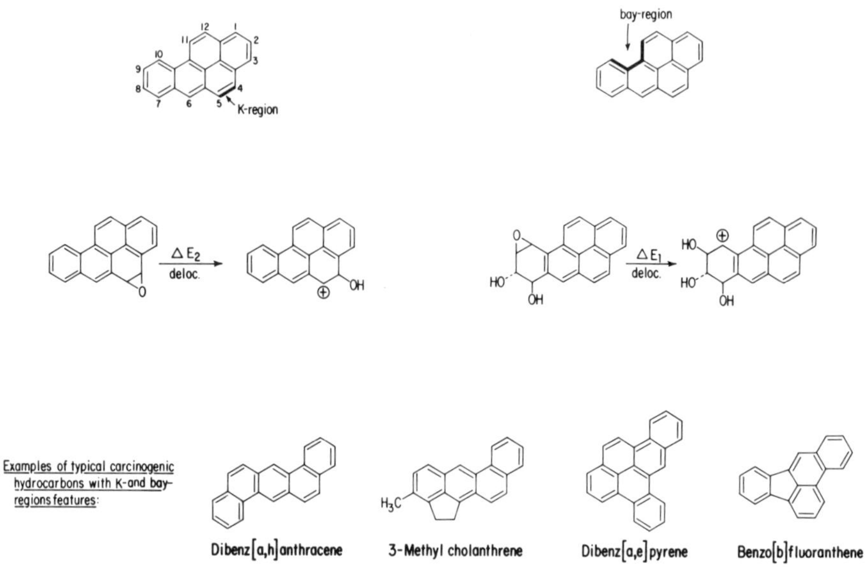

Figure 5: Examples of typical carcinogenic polynuclear hydrocarbons with K-region and bay-region features.

The basis for the much higher chemical reactivity, mutagenicity and carcinogenicity of "bay region" diol epoxides than those of the corresponding K-region epoxides has been established using molecular orbital calculations. Since cleavage of the benzylic oxirane C–O bond and formation of a carbonium ion is involved in the heterolytic reactions of the arene oxides, the more rapidly the carbonium ion is formed from its epoxide precursor, the higher will be the reactivity of the compound. The ease of carbonium ion formation, calculated by Jerina and coworkers in terms of delocalization energy, indicated that ΔE_{deloc} is much higher for a diol epoxide than for a K-region epoxide. The calculations predict that in general "bay region" carbonium ions are more readily formed than "non-bay region" carbonium ions, at benzylic positions of saturated benzo rings, for a given hydrocarbon (*see* reference 13).

Besides the ease of metabolic activation, the overall size of the polynuclear molecule is a determining factor in carcinogenic activity (*see* reference 11). Figure 6 shows the carcinogenicity of a series of hydrocarbons as a function of the molecular size calculated in terms of the "incumbrance area," which represents the minimum rectangular surface area occupied by the molecule in two dimensions. The incumbrance area is a good approximation of the size of the planar

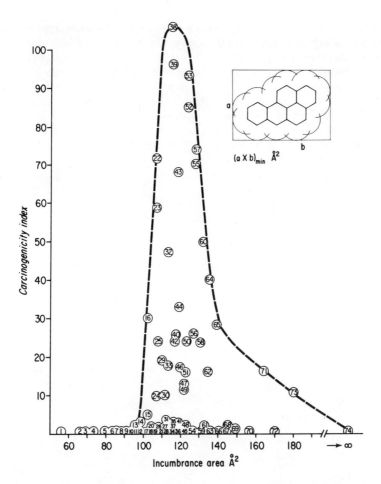

Figure 6: The relationship between the carcinogenic activity and molecular size (as incumbrance area) of a series of polynuclear hydrocarbons. For identification of the hydrocarbons, *see* reference 11.

molecules as long as the structure does not involve overlap between van der Waals radii of nonbonded atoms or groups. As Figure 6 indicates, the optimal size range for highly active compounds is between 100 and 135 Å^2 with no sharp cutoff point toward higher molecular sizes. Not all hydrocarbons in this size range display carcinogenicity, however, since molecular size is a factor which limits membrane transport, steric fit, and molecular interactions, rather than a structural or π-electronic feature which is actually responsible for interaction with macromolecules.

The success in elucidating the metabolic activation mechanism and principal structural requirements of polycyclic hydrocarbons of the phenanthrene and pyrene pattern should not lure us into believing, however, that the basis of carcinogenic activity of *all* polynuclears is now clearly understood. Figure 7 exemplifies the variety of other structural types of polynuclear aromatic carcinogens where a region resembling a "bay region" is barely distinguishable or clearly absent. Moreover, several partially hydrogenated polycyclic hydrocarbons are markedly carcinogenic despite the absence of a bay (or K-) region in the π-electronic sense. The activation mechanism of the variety of polynuclears exemplified in Figure 7 (and of the partially hydrogenated hydrocarbons) may also involve epoxidation. It is possible, however, that the activation of these odd structural types is via a simpler mechanism, by one-electron oxidation at carbon, directly resulting in carbonium ion formation.

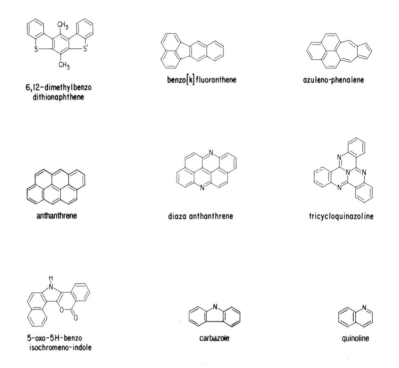

6,12-dimethylbenzo
dithionaphthene

benzo[k]fluoranthene

azuleno-phenalene

anthanthrene

diaza anthanthrene

tricycloquinazoline

5-oxo-5H-benzo
isochromeno-indole

carbazole

quinoline

Figure 7: Examples of carcinogenic polynuclear hydrocarbons without "bay-region" features.

Alkylating and Acylating Agents

The largest and structurally most heterogeneous class of carcinogens are the carcinogenic alkylating agents. This class displays a virtually unlimited structural variety (*see* Figure 8) and there is no **clearly** discernible relationship among them. The only apparent relationship is that they are, or can be, metabolically transformed into electrophilic reactive intermediates which have the capability to alkylate DNA and other cellular nucleophiles. Most of them contain a good leaving group (*e.g.*, sulfate, methanesulfonate, chloride) or strained ring structure (*e.g.*, epoxide, aziridine, lactone). In general, compounds with two or more reactive functional groups are often more carcinogenic than the monofunctional compounds because of their capability to act as cross-linking agents. An extensive, analytic review of this class of compounds has been given by Arcos *et al.*[7] Some of the important subclasses are exemplified in Figure 8.

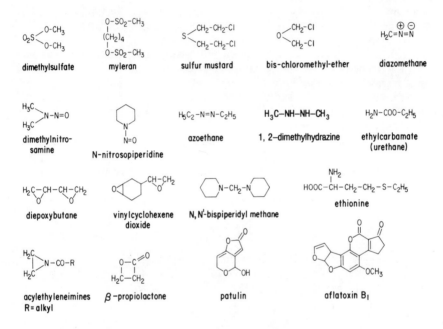

Figure 8: Examples of typical carcinogenic alkylating agents.

Nitrogen mustards. Aliphatic nitrogen mustards are generally more carcinogenic than their aromatic counterparts because the electron-withdrawing capacity of the aromatic ring tends to hinder the formation of the reactive aziridium intermediate. However, aromatic mustards can be potent carcinogens if the mustard group is attached to a molecular moiety representing a normal cellular constituent (*e.g.*, uracil mustard, melphalan, estradiol mustard). Attachment of a mustard group to molecules with favorable size and shape for intercalation also yields potent carcinogens (*e.g.*, acridine mustards).

Haloethers. α-Haloethers (*e.g.*, bis-chloromethyl ether) are substantially more carcinogenic than their β-counterpart probably because of the possibility of the formation of reactive carbonium ions that can be stabilized by resonance involving the oxonium ion form.

Epoxides. Aliphatic epoxides which are carcinogenic are often bifunctional or contain a double bond which may be metabolically activated to become an additional epoxide group. Features such as the position and accessibility (terminal or interdispersed; *cis* or *trans*; sterically hindered or open), the reactivity and stability, the intergroup distance, and the molecular flexibility of the epoxide groups (attached to a rigid ring or freely rotating at the terminal ends of an alkyl chain) all play a role in determining the carcinogenic potency of the compound.

Aziridines, lactones and sultones. Most aziridines, β-lactones and γ-sultones, which all have highly strained ring structures, are carcinogenic (direct-acting) unless the ring has bulky or hydrophilic substituents or substituents that make the compound too reactive. Among the less strained γ-, and δ-lactones, most of the carcinogenic compounds have an α-β double bond which conjugates with the carbonyl group.

N-Nitroso compounds. The majority of the over 200 N-nitroso compounds, which have been tested for carcinogenicity are carcinogenic. The noncarcinogenic nitrosamines either have sterically or electronically hindering substituents at the presumed site of metabolic activation (*e.g.*, α-carbon) or have highly hydrophilic substituents. Moreover, two C-nitroso compounds have been shown to be carcinogenic in experimental animals.

Hydrazo-, aliphatic azo- and azoxy-compounds and aryldialkyltriazenes. The majority of the close to 50 hydrazine derivatives tested are carcinogenic. 1,2-Dialkylhydrazines are metabolically activated through the formation of azoalkanes and azoxyalkanes, which are themselves carcinogenic when tested directly. Thus, these three subclasses of compounds may be considered metabolically equivalent. Virtually all the 1-aryl-3,3-dialkyltriazenes tested are also carcinogenic; substitution or replacement of an alkyl group with a polar substituent greatly diminishes the carcinogenicity of the triazene.

Carbamates. Simple alkyl carbamates appear to have quite specific structural requirements for optimal carcinogenic activity: (a) a two-carbon moiety (ethyl or vinyl) at the carboxyl end, and (b) a relatively free amino end available for N-hydroxylation and N-acyloxylation. 1,1-Diaryl-2-acetylenic carbamates, with the chemical structure:

$$R_1R_2N-CO-O-\underset{\underset{R_4}{|}}{\overset{\overset{R_3}{|}}{C}}-C\equiv C-R_5$$

(where R_3, R_4 = aryl; R_1, R_2, R_5 = hydrogen, alkyl or aryl), are potent carcinogens.

Halogenated and Polyhalogenated Hydrocarbons

Another important and large class of carcinogens of great economic and environmental importance are the halogenated and polyhalogenated hydrocarbons. They include both genotoxic and epigenetic carcinogens and probably act by a variety of mechanisms. An in-depth review of this class of compounds has recently been presented by Woo *et al.*[14] The major subclasses, some aspects of the mechanisms of action, and a general perspective of their structure-activity relationships are summarized below.

Haloalkanes. The carcinogenic potential of simple monohaloalkanes (alkyl halides) appears to correlate with their alkylating capability which is dependent on the leaving potential of the halogen as halide ion and the nature of the alkyl group. Trihalomethanes (*e.g.*, chloroform) and tetrahalomethanes (*e.g.*, carbon tetrachloride) are metabolically activated leading to the formation of a dihalocarbonyl (*e.g.*, phosgene), a highly reactive intermediate; in addition, trichloromethyl free radical is also a reactive intermediate of carbon tetrachloride. However, these intermediates appear to be too reactive to cause direct DNA damage and they possibly exert their carcinogenic effect indirectly, through interaction with membrane lipids or proteins at the immediate vicinity of the site of metabolic activation. Among the carcinogenic haloethanes with two or more halogen substituents (*e.g.*, 1,2-dibromoethane), a common structural requirement is vicinal substitution which allows metabolic activation to highly reactive electrophilic α-haloaldehyde and episulfonium intermediates. 1,2,3-Trihalopropanes (*e.g.*, 1,2-dibromo-3-chloropropane) are carcinogenic probably through metabolic activation to epihalohydrins.

Haloalkenes. The carcinogenic potential and the mechanisms of action of haloalkenes are greatly dependent on the position of the halogen relative to the double bond. Vinylic compounds (*e.g.*, vinyl chloride) require metabolic activation yielding haloalkene epoxide, haloaldehyde and haloacyl halide as electrophilic reactive intermediates. Compounds with allylic structures (as well as benzyl halide) act as alkylating agents in the absence of metabolic activation; their mutagenic potency (and putative carcinogenic potential) correlates reasonably well with their alkylating activity as measured in the 4-NBP (4-nitrobenzylpyridine) test (*see* reference 15).

Polyhalogenated pesticides. These include polyhalogenated cycloalkanes (*e.g.*, lindane, mirex, kepone), cycloalkenes (*e.g.*, aldrin, heptachlor, chlordane), and bridged aromatics (*e.g.*, DDT). Most of these compounds have little or no mutagenic activity, no clear-cut mechanism of action, and are mostly regarded to act epigenetically if carcinogenic. There is some evidence that many of these compounds interfere with the intercellular transfer of growth regulatory factors (*see* Functional Criteria[8]).

Polyhalogenated aromatics and dibenzodioxins. These include polyhalogenated biphenyls (PCBs, PBBs) and dibenzodioxins (*e.g.*, TCDD). Their mechanism of action is poorly understood. There is some evidence that lower chlorinated biphenyl congeners (*e.g.*, 4-chlorobiphenyl) bind covalently to cellular macromolecules and exert a mutagenic effect.[16] However, the more persistent higher chlorinated biphenyls appear to have little or no mutagenic activity. Poland and Knutson[17] have studied the biochemical and toxic effects of a variety of isosteric structural analogs of PCB and TCDD (polyhalogenated dibenzofurans, naphthalenes, azoxybenzenes and biphenylenes). Compounds with a planar, rectangular molecular skeleton, a size of approximately 6 x 11 Å^2* and the presence of at least three halogen substituents in the four lateral ring positions (*e.g.*, 2,3,7,8-positions of dibenzodioxin, 3,4,3',4'- of biphenyl, 2,3,6,7- of naphthalene) all have virtually the same spectrum of toxic effects and are potent inducers of microsomal mixed-function oxidases. Poland and Knutson postulated

---

*These values are at variance with those given by Poland and Knutson. Recalculation of the molecular sizes of biphenyl and dibenzodioxin (involving inclusion of the van der Waals radii) gave the above-quoted molecular size.

that these compounds bind to a common cellular receptor and evoke a sustained gene expression which leads to a pleiotropic response including the promotion of carcinogenesis.

The extraordinary structural variety among carcinogenic alkylating and cross-linking agents, and the fact that arylation by aromatic amines and polynuclear compounds also leads to carcinogenesis, point to the important concept that the chemical nature of the xenobiotic molecular moieties attached to key informational macromolecules is probably immaterial as long as these attachments effectively interfere with the normal functioning of synthetic templates. There is a growing indication that some *acylating agents* are carcinogenic. Indeed, dimethylcarbamyl chloride is a potent carcinogen in animals,[18,19] and there is some epidemiological evidence for an increased cancer incidence among benzoyl chloride manufacturing workers.[20] It is interesting to note that the acylating intermediate of both compounds is resonance-stabilized.

Miscellaneous Epigenetic Carcinogens

Besides the polyhalogenated hydrocarbons described above, there are a variety of other compounds which do not appear to exert their carcinogenic effect through a genotoxic mechanism, that is they do not bind covalently to DNA and do not cause DNA damage directly. Compounds which belong in this category are exemplified by *p*-dioxane, acetamide, thiourea, saccharin, triethanolamine, clofibrate and di-2-ethylhexyl phthalate. Possible epigenetic mechanisms for these compounds are discussed under the section on Functional Criteria.

Foreign-Body Carcinogens

As indicated in the section "General Principles of Chemical Carcinogenesis," for this class of substances there is no requirement for any specific chemical structure for carcinogenicity. The only determining factor is the physical shape and size of the foreign body. For self-penetrant fibers (*e.g.*, asbestos fibers and other mineral fibers) to be carcinogenic, they must have diameters of $<1.5\ \mu$ and lengths $>8\ \mu$. Tumorigenicity increases with the decrease of fiber diameter and the increase of the length (*see* references 21 and 22). All respirable fibrous materials with these fiber dimensions are potentially carcinogenic. For implanted sheets or platelets the chemical composition is immaterial, as they can be plastics, glass, metals, ivory or wood. Carcinogenicity decreases with the decrease of the size of the implant and with the increase of the diameter and number of pores (or holes) if present in the sheets or platelets.

Conclusions to Structural Criteria

The above perspective of the major classes of chemical carcinogens and their structure-activity relationships suggests that compounds which display the following molecular features are prone to show carcinogenic activity:

(1) An amino, dimethylamino, nitroso or nitro group directly linked to an aryl group, that is H_2N–aryl and not H_2N–$(CH_2)_n$–aryl (because a $-CH_2-$ group represents a π-electronically insulating linkage) or possibly linked to an aliphatic conjugated double-bonded

system. Carcinogenic activity is more likely or higher if the directly-linked amine or amine-generating group is at the *terminal* end of the longest conjugated double-bond arrangement in the molecule;

(2) Polycyclic structures with three or more rings, which mimic the angular ring distribution of polynuclear carcinogenic hydrocarbons, if the structure is aromatic, or partially aromatic, or at least contains some double bonds. The likelihood of carcinogenicity of such structures may increase if the molecule bears methyl or ethyl substituent(s) near the double-bonded system;

(3) Aliphatic structures containing conjugated double bonds or isolated double bonds situated at the terminal ends of an aliphatic chain;

(4) N-nitroso, hydrazo-, aliphatic azo- or aliphatic azoxy structures and all 1-aryl-3,3-dialkyltriazenes and 1,1-diaryl-2-acetylenic carbamates. There is also some reason to suspect C-nitroso groupings;

(5) The presence of a sterically strained ring (*e.g.*, epoxide, aziridine, episulfonium, certain lactones and sultones) in any type of structure. The likelihood of carcinogenicity increases if the compound contains two or more of these reactive ring structures;

(6) Any structural type of alkylating, arylating, or acylating agent or larger molecular assemblies incorporating such structures as chemically reactive moieties. The likelihood of carcinogenicity may increase if (a) the reactive intermediate can be stabilized by resonance or by inductive or mesomeric effect, (b) the compound contains two or more of these reactive moieties, and/or (c) the compound has a favorable molecular shape and size for intercalation or is a structural analog of normal cellular constituents;

(7) The presence of a haloalkyl (particularly 1,2-dihalo-), haloalkenyl (both vinylic and allylic), α-haloether, α-haloalkanol, or α-halocarbonyl grouping. All persistent polyhalogenated aromatics, polyhalogenated aliphatics and polyhalogenated aliphatic-aromatic compounds, as well as their structural analogs, are also suspect;

(8) Fibrous materials, irrespective of their chemical nature, with fiber diameters of less than 1.5 μ and lengths of more than 8 μ are potentially carcinogenic.

FUNCTIONAL CRITERIA

Structural criteria alone cannot forecast entirely new structural types of carcinogens. A case in point is the historical example of the nitrosamines. In the mid-1950's, when the carcinogenicity of dimethylnitrosamine was first discovered, there was already a vast body of information available on the carcinogenicity and structure-activity relationships of various polynuclear compounds, aromatic amines, azo dyes and aliphatic alkylating agents. Yet, all this information seemed to be of little help in foreseeing or suspecting the carcinogenicity of nitrosamines which have since emerged as a major class of carcinogens of dietary and environmental significance. Thus, it is critical to complement the structural criteria with functional criteria, that is with the consideration of pharmacological and/or toxicological capabilities which, irrespective of chemical structure, have been correlated with carcinogenic activity or construed as possible component factors in the induction of malignancy. Some of these capabilities have already been put to use in the development of short-term screening tests for carcinogens, while others are less well-known or are in the process of being identified as correlating with carcinogenicity. The types of functional criteria and their rationale are listed below. Compounds which fall in these categories should be suspected of carcinogenic activity.

(1) All compounds which bring about *in vitro cell transformation* either directly or after metabolic activation (*see* Chapter 7 of this monograph for details of cell transformation assay).

(2) All *mutagenic or clastogenic compounds* (*see* Chapters 3, 4 and 5 of this monograph for details on mutagenicity tests and their relevance to carcinogenicity).

(3) All *compounds which trigger DNA repair* as measured by unscheduled DNA synthesis (*see* Chapter 6 of this monograph for details of DNA repair assay and its relevance to carcinogenicity).

(4) Virtually all *teratogenic compounds*, unless their mechanism of teratogenic action is clearly known to be unrelated to the type of chemical reactivity which also leads to carcinogenesis (*e.g.*, prevention of placental nutrient transport).

(5) Compounds which *covalently bind to DNA or RNA* through alkylation, arylation, or acylation. This is particularly pertinent if covalent linkage occurs at sites which can disrupt normal base-pairing (*e.g.*, the O–6 and N–3 positions of guanine, O–4 of thymine, N–7 of adenine, N–3 of cytosine) or disrupt the normal DNA helical structure (*e.g.*, by alkylation of the phosphate backbone) and if the adduct is persistent (*see* reference 23). An attempt to correlate the extent of covalent binding with carcinogenicity of a wide spectrum of compounds has been undertaken by Lutz.[24] Compounds which have a *favorable molecular size and shape for intercalation* (planar, rectangularly-shaped, polynuclear with two to five rings preferably containing hetero-atoms) should also be suspected, particularly if they contain reactive functional groups (*e.g.*, acridine mustards).

(6) *Structural analogs of purine and pyrimidine* which may act as perturbers of nucleic acid replication or transcription, incorporate into nucleic acids, or disturb purine or pyrimidine biosynthesis and metabolism. Also, there is some evidence that the carcinogenic potential of a reactive functional group may be enhanced if attached to purine or pyrimidine bases or to an amino acid. Structural analogs of nucleic acid bases that have been shown to be carcinogenic in animal bioassays or active in cell transformation assays, include a variety of 3-hydroxypurines (tautomeric with purine-N-oxides), thiouracils, 6-mercaptopurine, 1-β-D-arabinofuranosylcytosine, 5-fluorodeoxyuridine, and uracil mustard (*see* references 7, 8, 9 and 14). Structural analogs of some amino acids (*e.g.*, ethionine, azaserine) are also carcinogenic probably through their action on nucleic acid biosynthesis or metabolism.

(7) Potent *inducers of microsomal mixed-function oxidases* (particularly those that induce cytochrome P-448) or, in general, all *stimulators of tissue hyperplasia*. These compounds may promote "dormant" (initiated) tumor cells by triggering gene expression. Certain inducers of microsomal mixed-function oxidases (*e.g.*, benzo[a]pyrene, 3-methylcholanthrene, TCDD, PCBs, phenobarbital) are actually "complete" carcinogens in their own right (*see* references 7, 11 and 14).

(8) *Compounds which affect the structure and functions of the cell membrane and thereby interfere with the intercellular transmission of regulatory factors* are potential "epigenetic" carcinogens or tumorigenesis-promoters (*see* reference 25). Cell-to-cell transfer (through gap junction) of regulatory growth factors is believed to be involved in the control of cell differentiation and proliferation. Inhibition of such intercellular communication is expected to promote tumorigenesis and permit progressive neoplastic growth. A variety of "epigenetically" acting compounds, such as DDT, lindane, dieldrin, kepone, PBBs, saccharin, and phenobarbital[25,28] and classical tumorigenesis-promoters such as phorbol esters[29,30] of diverse chemical structures have been shown, by "metabolic cooperation" or "contact feeding" experiments (*see* Chapter 20 of this monograph), to inhibit intercellular communication. Most of the aforementioned compounds are highly lipophilic (*e.g.*, DDT), some have clathrate-like cage-type structures (*e.g.*, kepone), or may bring about alterations in cell membranes indirectly by triggering gene expression (*e.g.*, phenobarbital).

(9) A variety of *peroxisome proliferators* of diverse chemical structures (*see* Figure 9) (*see* references 7 and 14). Reddy[31] suggested that peroxisome proliferators, as a class, should be considered potentially carcinogenic. The carcinogenic activity of peroxisome proliferators is probably related to the elevation of the intracellular level of hydrogen peroxide and active oxygen species generated by peroxisomal oxidases (*see* reference 7).

(10) Compounds which bring about the *detachment of ribosomes (degranulation) from the rough endoplasmic reticulum (RER)*. Uncontrolled RER degranulation is expected to cause random inhibition of selective protein synthesis which can lead to disturbance of gene expression and a loss of control of nuclear function. A variety of chemical carcinogens (*e.g.*, aflatoxin B_1, 2-acetylaminofluorene, 2-naphthylamine, dimethylnitrosamine, carbon tetrachloride, dieldrin) of diverse chemical structures cause RER degranulation. A reasonably good correlation between RER degranulation and the carcinogenicity of a series of compounds has been demonstrated.[32]

(11) Some suspicion exists regarding *inhibitors of mitochondrial respiration and uncouplers of oxidative phosphorylation*. These compounds decrease the level of ATP available, and this, in turn may lead to faulty DNA repair or faulty transcription and translation. A variety of carcinogenic mycotoxins (*e.g.*, aflatoxin B_1, luteoskyrin, ochratoxin A) inhibit mitochondrial energy metabolism (*see* reference 33). It is unlikely, however, that this property *alone* is sufficient to cause carcinogenesis.

(12) The ambivalence of cancer chemotherapy has been known for decades.[34-36] Virtually all *compounds with antineoplastic activity* are suspected to be carcinogenic. Depending on their mode of action, antineoplastic agents may have different degrees of carcinogenic potency. Alkylators (*e.g.*, cyclophos-

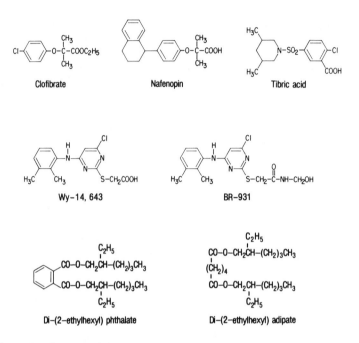

Figure 9: Structural formulas of some carcinogenic peroxisome proliferators.

phamide, mitomycin C, bis-chloroethylnitrosourea) and DNA-binders (*e.g.*, actinomycin D, daunomycin) are relatively potent carcinogens. Antimetabolites (*e.g.*, methotrexate) are marginally active carcinogens. There appears to be no convincing evidence, however, to incriminate mitotic inhibitors (*e.g.*, vinblastine, vincristine) as carcinogens. As noted below, some antineoplastic agents may also be of concern because of their immunosuppressive activity.

(13) Chemical compounds with potent *immunosuppressive activity*. Impairment of host immune competence is often associated with the acceleration of tumor development. A variety of carcinogens, for example, polycyclic hydrocarbons, TCDD (*see* reference 14); urethan (*see* reference 7); and some antineoplastic agents (*see* references 36 and 37) are all immunosuppressive; this effect may be a component factor of the carcinogenic activity of these compounds.

(14) Compounds that cause *hormonal imbalance or overstimulation* are suspected of having carcinogenic activity toward specific target organ(s). A classic example is diethylstilbestrol, a synthetic estrogen which has been linked to the induction of vaginal adenocarcinoma in humans. Estrogen treatment is also suspected to be associated with the induction of endometrial cancer. There is a good correlation between the antithyroid (goitrogenic) activity of thiourea and thioamide compounds (*e.g.*, ethylenethiourea, thiouracil) and their ability to induce thyroid tumors (*see* reference 14). It is noteworthy that a number of "epigenetic" carcinogens (*e.g.*, TCDD, PCBs, DDT) and potent tumorigenesis-

promoters (*e.g.*, phorbol esters, telocidin B) have some hormone-like activity (*see* references 17 and 25).

(15) A number of *inhibitors of spermatogenesis* (*e.g.*, dibromochloropropane, 1,2-dibromoethane, kepone, ethyl methanesulfonate) are well known to be potent carcinogens. Although formal correlative studies are not available, the demonstration of strong antispermatogenic activity of a compound is reason for suspecting it to be a carcinogen. The induction of *sperm abnormalities* (abnormally shaped sperm head) has also been associated with the dosing of animals with carcinogens. The abnormal sperm assay has been developed as an auxiliary predictive screening test for carcinogens with reasonably good success rate.[38]

(16) There is a growing list of compounds (*e.g.*, carbon tetrachloride, chloroform, TCDD, dimethylnitrosamine, thioacetamide) shown to be both *hepatonecrotic* and hepatocarcinogenic. Although a causal relationship between chemically-induced necrosis and carcinogenesis is debatable, there appears to be a consensus that cell proliferation occurring as a result of "chemical trauma" may promote carcinogenesis.

(17) *Strong surface-active agents or hydrogen bond reactors* are known to alter the conformation of macromolecules. These compounds are potentially carcinogenic after prolonged exposure at high doses, particularly if their physicochemical properties allow them to reach target tissues at a sufficiently high level. A number of weak to moderately active carcinogens, such as *p*-dioxane, acetamide, triethanolamine, and benzethonium chloride, may owe their carcinogenic activity to their surface-active, macromolecular conformation-modifying capability (*see* references 7 and 14). Moreover, a variety of surfactants (*e.g.*, Tweens, bile acids, alkylbenzene sulfonates) are active promoters of tumorigenesis (*see* reference 14).

(18) At least a slight suspicion exists regarding *strong chelating agents*. Conceivably, the chelation of critical metal atoms in key enzymes involved in nucleic acid metabolism, cell differentiation, or gene transcription is a possible mechanism of carcinogenesis (*see* reference 39). Chelating agents, such as some dialkyldithiocarbamates (*see* reference 7) are moderately active carcinogens. A recent industry-sponsored study (*see* reference 40) has shown that ethylene diamine tetra(methylenephosphonic acid), a powerful chelating agent, is carcinogenic in rats, inducing osteogenic sarcomas in a relatively short period of time. Further research on the potentiality of chelators as carcinogens is needed.

REFERENCES

1. Pearson, R.G., and Songstad, J., Application of the principle of hard and soft acids and bases to organic chemistry. *J. Am. Chem. Soc.* 89: 1827–1836 (1967)
2. Hirono, I., Kuhara, K., Hosaka, S., Tomizawa, S., and Golberg, L., Induction of intestinal tumors in rats by dextran sulfate sodium. *J. Natl. Cancer Inst.* 66:579–583 (1981)
3. Oohashi, Y., Ishioka, T., Wakabayashi, K., and Kuwabara, N., A study on carcinogenesis by degraded carrageenan arising from squamous metaplasia of the rat colorectum. *Cancer Lett.* 14:267–272 (1981)

4. Wakabayashi, K., A study on carcinogenesis of degraded carrageenan, a polysaccharide-sulfate, derived from seaweeds (Japanese). *Juntendo Med. J.* 27:159-171 (1981)
5. Lien, E., Structure-activity relationships and drug disposition. *Ann. Rev. Pharmacol. Toxicol.* 21:31-61 (1981)
6. Albert, A., *Selective toxicity. The physico-chemical basis of therapy*, 6th edn., London:Chapman and Hall (1981)
7. Arcos, J.C., Woo, Y.T., and Argus, M.F. (with the collaboration of Lai, D.Y.), *Chemical Induction of Cancer*, Vol. IIIA, New York:Academic Press (1982)
8. Arcos, J.C., and Argus, M.F., *Chemical Induction of Cancer*, Vol. IIB, New York:Academic Press (1974)
9. Clayson, D.B., and Garner, R.C., in: *Chemical Carcinogens* (C.E. Searle, ed.), pp. 367-461, American Chemical Society, Washington, DC (1976)
10. Sontag, J.M., Carcinogenicity of substituted-benzene diamines (phenylenediamines) in rats and mice. *J. Natl. Cancer Inst.* 66:591-602 (1981)
11. Arcos, J.C., and Argus, M.F., *Chemical Induction of Cancer*, Vol. IIA, New York:Academic Press (1974)
12. Dipple, A., in: *Chemical Carcinogens* (C.E. Searle, ed.), pp. 245-314, American Chemical Society, Washington, DC (1976)
13. Thakker, D.R., Yagi, H., Nordqvist, M., Lehr, R.E., Levin, W., Wood, A.W., Chang, R.L., Conney, A.H., and Jerina, D.M., in: Appendix I of *Chemical Induction of Cancer* (Arcos, J.C., Woo, Y.T., and Argus, M.F.), Vol. IIIA, pp. 727-747, Academic Press, New York (1982)
14. Woo, Y.T., Lai, D.Y., Arcos, J.C., and Argus, M.F., *Chemical Induction of Cancer*, Vol. IIIB, Academic Press, New York (1985)
15. Eder, E., Henschler, D., and Neudecker, T., Mutagenic properties of allylic and α,β-unsaturated compounds: consideration of alkylating mechanisms. *Xenobiotica* 12:831-848 (1982)
16. Wyndham, C., Devenish, J., and Safe, S., The *in vitro* metabolism, macromolecular binding and bacterial mutagenicity of 4-chlorobiphenyl, a model PCB substrate. *Res. Commun. Chem. Pathol. Pharmacol.* 15:563-570 (1976)
17. Poland, A., and Knutson, J.C., 2,3,7,8-Tetrachlorodibenzo-*p*-dioxin and related halogenated aromatic hydrocarbons: examination of the mechanism of toxicity. *Ann. Rev. Pharmacol. Toxicol.* 22:517-554 (1982)
18. Van Duuren, B.L., Goldschmidt, B.M., Katz, L., Seidman, I., and Paul, J.S., Carcinogenic activity of alkylating agents. *J. Natl. Cancer Inst.* 53:695-700 (1974)
19. Sellakumar, A.K., Laskin, S., Kuschner, M., Rusch, G., Katz, G.V., Snyder, C.A., and Albert, R.E., Inhalation carcinogenesis by dimethylcarbamyl chloride in Syrian golden hamsters. *J. Environ. Pathol. Toxicol.* 4:107-115 (1980)
20. Sakabe, H., Matsushita, H., and Koshi, S., Cancer among benzoyl chloride manufacturing workers. *Ann. N.Y. Acad. Sci.* 271:67-70 (1976)
21. Stanton, M.F., in: *Biological Effects of Asbestos* (P. Bogovski, J.C. Gilson, V. Timbrell, and I.C. Wagner, eds.), pp. 289-294, International Agency for Research on Cancer, Lyon, France (1973)
22. Stanton, M.F., Layard, M., Tegeris, A., Miller, E., May, M., and Kent, E., Carcinogenicity of fibrous glass: pleural response in the rat in relation to fiber dimension. *J. Natl. Cancer Inst.* 58:587-603 (1977)

23. Singer, B., N-Nitroso alkylating agents: formation and persistence of alkyl derivatives in mammalian nucleic acids as contributing factor in carcinogenesis. *J. Natl. Cancer Inst.* 62:1329-1340 (1979)
24. Lutz, W.K., *In vivo* covalent binding of organic chemicals to DNA as a quantitative indicator in the process of chemical carcinogenesis. *Mutat. Res.* 65:289-356 (1979)
25. Williams, G.M., Liver carcinogenesis: the role for some chemicals of an epigenetic mechanism of liver tumor promotion involving modification of the cell membrane. *Food Cosmet. Toxicol.* 19:577-583 (1981)
26. Tsuchimoto, G., Trosko, J.E., Chang, C.C., and Matsumura, F., Inhibition of intercellular communication by chlordecone (kepone) and mirex in Chinese hamster V79 cells *in vitro. Toxicol. Appl. Pharmacol.* 64:550-556 (1982)
27. Tsuchimoto, G., Trosko, J.E., Chang, C.C., and Aust, S.D., Inhibition of metabolic cooperation in Chinese hamster V79 cells in culture by various polybrominated biphenyl (PBB) congeners. *Carcinogenesis* 3:181-185 (1982)
28. Trosko, J.E., Dawson, B., Yotti, L.P., and Chang, C.C., Saccharin may act as a tumor promoter by inhibiting metabolic cooperation between cells. *Nature (London)* 285:109-110 (1980)
29. Fitzgerald, D.J., and Murray, A.W., Inhibition of intercellular communication by tumor-promoting phorbol esters. *Cancer Res.* 40:2935-2938 (1980)
30. Umeda, M., Noda, K., and Ono, T., Inhibition of metabolic cooperation in Chinese hamster cells by various chemicals including tumor promoters. *Gann* 71:614-620 (1980)
31. Reddy, J.K., in: *Drugs Affecting Lipid Metabolism* (R. Fumagalli, D. Kritchevsky, and R. Paoletti, eds.), pp. 301-309, Elsevier/North Holland, Amsterdam (1980)
32. Wright, A.S., Akintonwa, D.A.A., and Wooder, M.F., Studies on the interactions of dieldrin with mammalian liver cells at the subcellular level. *Ecotoxicol. Environ. Safety* 1:7-16 (1977)
33. Hayes, W., *Mutagenicity and Teratogenicity of Mycotoxins*, CRC Press, Boca Raton, Florida (1981)
34. Haddow, A., Mode of action of chemical carcinogens. *Br. Med. Bull.* 4:331-342 (1947)
35. Grundmann, E., and Gross, R. (eds.), *The Ambivalence of Cytostatic Therapy*, Recent Results Cancer Res. Vol. 52, Springer-Verlag, Berlin and New York (1975)
36. International Agency for Research on Cancer, *Some Antineoplastic and Immunosuppressive Agents*, IARC Monog. No. 26, International Agency for Research on Cancer, Lyon, France (1981)
37. Schmähl, D., Experimental investigations with anti-cancer drugs for carcinogenicity with special reference to immune depression. *Recent Results Cancer Res.* 52:18-28 (1975)
38. Heddle, J.A., and Bruce, W.R., in: *Origins of Human Cancer* (H.H. Hiatt, J.D. Watson, and J.A. Winsten, eds.), Book C, pp. 1549-1560, Cold Spring Harbor Laboratory, Cold Spring Harbor, New York (1977)
39. Furst, A., *Chemistry of Chelation in Cancer*, Springfield, Illinois: C.C. Thomas (1963)
40. U.S. Environmental Protection Agency, Status Report 8EHQ-0683-0483S, on ethylenediamine tetra(methylenephosphonic acid). Washington, DC (1983)

Part II

Epidemiological Investigations

2

Role of Epidemiology in Identifying Chemical Carcinogens

C.S. Muir

International Agency for Research on Cancer
Lyon, France

John Higginson

Universities Associated for Research and Education in Pathology, Inc.
Bethesda, Maryland

INTRODUCTION

The historical background of cancer epidemiology has been reviewed by Clemmesen.[1] There had long been evidence that both lifestyle[2] and occupation[3] could influence the risk of cancer. As industrial hazards[4] became better known, experimental animal studies with coal tar began.[5] It was not long before chemically pure carcinogens were isolated.[6] Despite the early discovery of oncogenic viruses[7,8] and of the effects of radiation from x-rays and radium, the thinking concerning carcinogenesis was strongly influenced by the concept that *most* cancer in humans, as well as in experimental animals, was likely to be due to discrete exogenous chemicals found as contaminants of air, water or food, or following exposure at the place of work. The discovery of the carcinogenic effects of tobacco seemed to have little influence on this viewpoint. It is only recently that it has become accepted that "natural" chemical constituents or metabolites of food may influence cancer risk and that there may be endogenous formation of carcinogens from apparently innocuous precursors.

In this chapter we confine ourselves to consideration of exogenous and endogenous chemical exposures in humans. While recognizing that everything that increases cancer risk, even a virus, is chemical, or, if in the form of radiation, exerts its effect through chemical pathways, neither viral nor radiation carcinogenesis will be examined. Although the concepts of initiation and promotion have been extensively studied in the experimental animal, and shown over the years to probably be valid for humans, in view of present uncertainties, no attempt will be made to discuss the classification of chemical carcinogens according to their assumed mechanisms of action.[9]

It is convenient for the epidemiologist to use a general term such as "carcinogenic factor" or "carcinogenic stimulus" to cover all types of agents which increase the risk of cancer. It is preferable to limit the term "carcinogen" to stimuli which can be described as initiators (*e.g.*, vinyl chloride) or promoters (*e.g.*, estrogens) to distinguish them from other less readily defined factors associated with cancer induction. The latter, sometimes referred to as "carcinogenic risk factors", include high intake of saturated fat and calories, dietary fiber deficiency and behavioral patterns such as late age at first pregnancy. Their epidemiological investigation tends to be complex since their role in human carcinogenesis is probably indirect and their effects are frequently still difficult to measure in objective biochemical terms. However, there is essentially no difference in the epidemiological methods used to identify either type of carcinogenic stimulus.

The first portion of this chapter will emphasize the classical epidemiological approach to the investigation of risk, notably in the workplace, and address the problems of endogenous carcinogenesis; the latter part examines some of the unresolved questions relating to identification of effects at very low levels of exposure.

CAUSES OF CANCER

From an etiological and public health viewpoint a carcinogenic factor may be so predominant that for practical purposes it is regarded as the cause. Thus, cigarette smoking may be regarded as the cause of 85% of lung cancers in males, regardless of the relative roles of initiation or promotion or other factors, because in the absence of this habit that proportion of lung cancer would be avoided.

Several authors have recently assessed the relative importance of broad categories of avoidable cause in the above sense.[10-12] The conclusions of all three papers are remarkably consistent (*see* Table 1).

The figures in Table 1, being based on the concept of predominant cause, do not take into account the multifactorial origin of cancer; they result from consideration of temporal, international and regional differences in risk, the evidence from the change in cancer mortality that occurs in migrants, and from case control and cohort studies.

The causes fall into three main groups:

(1) Causes such as tobacco, excess sunlight, excess alcohol, and radiation and several at-work exposures for which avoidance of the exposure can be guaranteed to result in a fall in risk.

(2) Dietary and lifestyle factors such as (a) lack of dietary fiber (colon cancer) or fresh fruit and vegetables (stomach cancer); (b) excess dietary fat (colon and breast cancer); (c) age at first full term preg-

nancy (breast cancer) and coitus (cancer of the cervix). For this group, the consequences of intervention are as yet unknown and may prove to have undesirable side-effects. It is such factors, however, which are believed to be the determinants of the common cancers of the digestive and genital tracts.

(3) Viruses and parasites, *e.g.*, Hepatitis B (liver cancer) and *Schistosoma haematobium* (bladder cancer), which, if controlled by vaccination or interruption of the life cycle, may be followed by a reduction in incidence.

Bearing in mind the induction period, which in adults is typically over 20 years and rarely less than five years, for a risk to be demonstrable by epidemiological means implies that a reasonable number of persons have to be exposed for a considerable time to a carcinogen of some potency. The lack of quantitative precision in the adjectives used in the preceding sentence underscores the problems.

Table 1: Proportion of Avoidable* Cancers

	United States Deyhs . . . (Doll & Peto[12]) . . .		Birmingham, U.K. Incident Cases (Higginson & Muir[11])	
	Both Sexes	Range	M	F
Tobacco	30	25–40	30	7
Alcohol	3	2–40	5	3
Lifestyle				
Diet	35	10–70		
Reproductive habits	7	7–13	30	63
Food additives	<1	0.5–2	–	–
Occupation	4	2–8	6	2
Iatrogenic	1	0.5–3	1	1
Pollution	2	<1–5	–	–
Industrial products[a]	<1	<1–2	–	–
Geophysical (including ultraviolet light and ionizing radiation)	3[b]	2–4	11	11
Infection	10?[c]		–	–
Congenital			2	2
Unknown	?		15	11

See text.
[a]These were included under "unknown" by Higginson and Muir.[11]
[b]Much lower than for incidence as few skin cancers cause death.
[c]Includes hepatitis B virus and parasites which are not an important factor in the United Kingdom.

Evidence of Causality

Several criteria, pertinent to any epidemiological study, are usually applied:

(1) Can positive bias and positive confounding be excluded? (An ex-

ample of positive bias in a case-control study would be better documentation of exposure in cases than in controls. An example of positive confounding would be the association between alcohol and lung cancer which results from their joint association with cigarette smoking. Negative bias and negative confounding would tend to conceal an effect.)

(2) Has, or can, the association be demonstrated in different studies? Does the association occur consistently for different subgroups within the same study?

(3) Does the association link a single, clearly defined exposure to a specified disease?

(4) Is there a dose-response relationship?

(5) Is the association strong?

(6) Is the association unlikely to be due to chance alone?

(7) Does exposure precede disease?

(8) Is the association biologically plausible?

(9) Does removal of the agent result in a reduction in the disease in question?

No single criterion can establish causality—the evidence has to be assessed as a whole. For further discussion *see* Rothman.[13]

DISCRETE EXOGENOUS CHEMICALS

Because occupational groups may be exposed to levels of chemicals which are much higher than those experienced by the general population, carcinogenic risk to humans from discrete chemicals has hitherto been largely studied in the workplace. This is not because chemical exposures do not occur elsewhere but rather because they are much easier to characterize and to estimate in the workplace than in the general population. While the proportion of all cancers due to exposures at work is small (Table 1), these cancers are preventable. In Japan, Hirayama,[14] in a cohort study of 250,000 randomly selected Japanese, considered that at-work exposures accounted for 1.1% of all cancers, a figure which would be increased to 3.3% if the enhancing or synergistic effect of cigarette smoking were taken into consideration.

More recently, risk has been examined in patients given chemotherapeutic agents mainly for tuberculosis and malignant disease, and in those taking medicaments over long periods of time for the control of epilepsy or fertility.

Supplement 4 to the IARC Monographs[15] summarizes the evaluations of the carcinogenic risk of chemicals to humans for the 585 chemicals, groups of chemicals, industrial processes and occupational exposures considered in the first 29 IARC Monographs. For 44 of these (Table 2) the international working groups found that there was "positive evidence of, or a suspicion of, an association with

Table 2: Industrial Processes and Occupational Exposures: Chemicals and Groups of Chemicals Causally Related with Cancer in Humans[9]

Industrial Processes and Occupational Exposures

Auramine manufacture
Boot and shoe manufacture and repair (certain occupations)
Furniture manufacture
Isopropyl alcohol manufacture (strong-acid process)
Nickel refining
Rubber industry (certain occupations)
Underground haematite mining (with exposure to radon)

Chemicals and Groups of Chemicals

4-Aminobiphenyl
Analgesic mixtures containing phenacetin
Arsenic and arsenic compounds
Asbestos
Azathioprine
Benzene
Benzidine
N,N-Bis(2-chloroethyl)-2-naphthylamine (Chlornaphazine)
Bis(chloromethyl)ether and technical-grade chloromethyl methyl ether
1,4-Butanediol dimethanesulfonate (Myleran)
Certain combined chemotherapy for lymphomas (including MOPP)
Chlorambucil
Chromium and certain chromium compounds
Conjugated estrogens
Cyclophosphamide
Diethylstilbestrol
Melphalan
Methoxsalen with ultraviolet A therapy (PUVA)
Mustard gas
2-Naphthylamine
Soots, tars and oils
Treosulfan
Vinyl chloride

*Chemicals, Groups of Chemicals or Industrial Processes
Which Are Probably* Carcinogenic to Humans*

Acrylonitrile
Aflatoxins
Benzo(a)pyrene
Beryllium and beryllium compounds
Combined oral contraceptives
Diethyl sulfate
Dimethyl sulfate
Manufacture of magenta
Nickel and certain nickel compounds
Nitrogen Mustard
Oxymetholone
Phenacetin
Procarbazine
o-Toluidine

*See IARC[15] for definition.

human cancer. For the remaining 541 exposures, epidemiological data were either unavailable or were considered to be inadequate to evaluate carcinogenicity to humans. For 147 of the exposures there was considered to be *sufficient evidence* of carcinogenicity in animals, and for a further 157 exposures there was *limited evidence*. The data were inadequate to evaluate the presence or absence of a carcinogenic effect for the remaining 236 exposures". This publication explains in detail the methods of evaluation and the definitions of sufficient and limited evidence. Most of the exposures in Table 2 are industrial or therapeutic. It is worth emphasizing that for many of the exposures held to be carcinogenic for animals epidemiological data were either not available or inadequate.

Methodological Approaches

In the following discussion, emphasis is given to industrial and occupational risks. The same methods are frequently applicable to other situations (for summary *see* Table 3).

Table 3: Techniques Used in Epidemiological Investigation of
Chemical Carcinogens: Advantages and Disadvantages*

Characteristics or Study Type	Advantage	Disadvantage: Comment
. . . . General Considerations . . . .
Relevance	Deals with human experience directly not with that of another species—animal or bacterial.	Relevance outweighs drawbacks.
Rapidity of answer		Usually slow due to long induction period of cancer. Answers may be "accelerated", if latent period has elapsed, by case-control or retrospective cohort study. Prospective cohort study may take 20 or more years.
Sensitivity		In general, poor unless exposure affects 30% to 70% of population.
Predictive ability		Significance of small increase in relative risk difficult to assess. Cannot predict whether newly introduced agent is likely to be carcinogenic. Extrapolation from dose-response information based on moderate and high level exposure to low dose very inexact and probably of little value.

(continued)

Table 3: (continued)

Characteristics or Study Type	Advantage	Disadvantage: Comment
. . . . Descriptive Epidemiology		
Mapping of cancer incidence mortality levels by small area.	May point to existence of unsuspected "hot-spots".	Reasons for raised level usually or needs to be assessed by other geographical studies. If areas considered are very small many could be significantly higher by chance; if too large effects of localized exposure may be diluted out.
Correlation between cancer levels and various environmental factors or attributes such as occupation.	Frequently based on data already available. May be useful to check on existing hypotheses. May show that an association is unlikely.	Correlations obtained frequently indirect being due to other associated factors, such as smoking. No chemical carcinogen has been identified by this method.
Case reports	May indicate cause if exposure and/or resulting cancer are unusual.	Rarely applicable.
. . . . Analytical Epidemiology		
Case-control	Latent period has elapsed and exposures have had their effects.	Requires a causal hypothesis: Exposures responsible may be unknown, or difficult to recognize or measure *e.g.*, previous dust levels, prior diet, past hormone levels.
	Carcinogenicity of several chemicals established by this method.	For many chemicals, proportion of cancers of a given site due to that substance may be very small and hence effect difficult to detect.
	"Rapid" answer as normally takes two to three years. Economical for common exposures as only 50 to 200 cases with one to four controls per case need be interviewed. May be possible to assess past chemical exposures by detailed enquiry (*see* text).	Control group may be difficult to find. Cases and controls may have differential recollection of past events (memory bias). Same difficulties obtained in studies of childhood cancer (*see* text).
	Other factors can be taken into account. Very important in view of multiple interactions with tobacco.	Does not permit assessment of absolute risk—only relative risk.

(continued)

Table 3: (continued)

Characteristics or Study Type	Advantage	Disadvantage: Comment
. . . . Analytical Epidemiology		
Retrospective cohort	Latent period has elapsed and exposures have had their effects. May be fairly rapid— about two years.	Numbers with over 20 years exposures in a large cohort may be quite small. Exposures may not be measurable in retrospect and may change in nature and intensity over years. Rarely possible to assess effects of other exposures. May not be possible to ensure that all potentially exposed are in cohort and follow-up may be incomplete.
	May be economical if suitable records are available and can be readily and unequivocally linked with outcome in cancer registry or death certificates.	Death certificates frequently inaccurate. Appropriate comparison groups not always easy to identify.
	Study of wide range of cancer sites and other health effects possible.	
Prospective cohort	Cohort usually easier to assemble than for retrospective cohort approach.	Latent period has still to elapse hence long wait for answer. Numbers needed may be very large, in order of 20,000 to 30,000, to yield reasonable number of even common cancers.
	Permits assessment of absolute risk in terms of rates per 100,000 exposed.	
	Economical only if records can be readily and unequivocally linked to outcome. Study of wide range of cancer sites and other health effects possible.	Follow-up may be difficult and expensive. Losses to follow-up may seriously impair value of study.
	Possible to estimate exposures currently and during course of study. Biological and other material can be collected and stored.	Storage and chemical estimation of material collected may be costly.
	Case-control study within the cohort may be feasible, which would permit assessment of effects of factors on which information was not collected at cohort assembly.	Cases may be "lost" or if recognized interview may not be practicable due to migration or death.

*Adapted from Muir.[16] For further details, *see* text.

From time to time industrial and occupational risks have been identified by the alert clinician, *e.g.*, adenocarcinoma of the sinuses and nasal passages of workers in sectors of the furniture and leather industries, angiosarcoma of the liver in vineyard workers spraying arsenic-containing solutions and in vinyl chloride kettle cleaners, and leukemia in artisan shoe repairers using benzene as a solvent. It is very unlikely that this partly intuitive clinical approach, essentially based on the recognition of the coincidence of unusual exposure and rare tumor, could uncover more than a fraction of all risks. This being so, it is necessary to develop systematic methods to look for cancer due to exposure at work.

There are several standard methods for assessing occupational cancer risk, each with its advantages and limitations.[16] These fall into three broad groups, the first of which is suitable for routine exploratory study; the second and third have usually not been used until there was a suggestion of increased risk and are designed to test specific hypotheses. In practice, the methods that are useful for high levels of exposure in small populations may be ineffective when studying ambient environmental risks.

Mapping and Correlation

Mapping. The incidence or mortality of cancer may be mapped by small geographical areas to assess whether unsuspected "hot spots" or clusters exist (after taking account of differences in the age-structure of the populations of the areas considered). Such maps have pointed to areas of high risk, *e.g.*, lung cancer in coastal Georgia. Local inquiry showed that risk coincided with areas where shipbuilding and concomitant asbestos exposure were common and case-control studies confirmed the association.[17]

If the areas mapped are very small, rates may be unstable and a proportion will be significantly higher than expected by chance alone; if too large, a localized increase of risk may be diluted.

Group correlation. While it is possible to correlate cancer incidence or mortality with indicators of exposure, consumption or production, between and within countries, the results are frequently uninterpretable in that any demonstrated correlation may reflect the effect of other linked exposures (for discussion of pitfalls *see* Breslow and Enstrom[18]).

Hypothesis-testing correlation studies contemporaneously measuring aflatoxin intake in African populations and liver cancer incidence in the same areas have been undertaken.[19] These are open to the criticism that there is no assurance that it is the individuals with a high intake of aflatoxin who develop liver cancer and latent period is not considered.

Occupational mortality. This technique involves systematic or ad hoc linkage at the national level of statements of occupation on census records with information on occupation and cause of death given on death certificates. Determination of whether the mortality for a given occupation *taken as a group* is significantly higher or lower than the national average constitutes a form of correlation.

Cohort

In this form of investigation, the numbers of cancers which occur in those

working in a given workplace or occupation over a defined period of time is assessed and compared with the numbers that would have been expected if these
individuals had experienced the national average risk, taking into account age
and calendar time. In such studies, the group of interest may be followed from
some time in the past to the present (retrospective cohort) or from the present
to some time in the future (prospective cohort).

Case-Control

Among the questions asked of individuals with a specific cancer are those
about occupation and possible workplace exposures. Similar questions are posed
to persons, usually of the same age and sex, without this cancer. The results are
compared to see whether there are more cases of cancer among individuals with
a particular occupation or exposure than in controls.[20]

Studies of Occupational Carcinogenesis

It should be emphasized that correlations examine the risk of a group as a
whole. The cohort (exposure oriented) and the case-control (cancer oriented)
approach assess the experience of a series of individuals. Before looking at these
methods more closely it is essential that the reader reminds himself that:

(1) Occupation implies much more than a series of exposures at work.
    Occupation determines income, and income to a major degree in-
    fluences the place of residence, the type and quantity of food con-
    sumed, choice of friends and of leisure activities and, frequently,
    personal habits such as alcohol and tobacco consumption—factors
    which often influence the risk of cancer. Demonstration of an in-
    creased risk in an occupation does not necessarily mean that the
    only cause was in the workplace.

(2) While an occupation is frequently accompanied by a common set
    of exposures, this is not inevitably so. A plumber employed in the
    chemical industry may have a different series of exposures than
    one dealing with the plumbing of buildings. The nature of the ex-
    posure which is associated with a particular occupation may change
    over time and levels of exposure may vary. Many occupations may
    share several exposures.

(3) Although there are exceptions (vinyl chloride monomer, for ex-
    ample), it usually requires 20 or more years of exposure before
    the effect of any carcinogen, occupational or otherwise, can be
    detected. This implies that it is of little value to correlate the ex-
    posures of today and contemporary cancer patterns unless the na-
    ture of the exposures can be assumed to have changed very little.

(4) Not all persons exposed to a carcinogenic stimulus will develop
    cancer in their lifetime. Carcinogenic exposures do not inevitably
    result in cancer; they, however, increase the probability of getting
    cancer.

(5) Cancers caused by workplace exposure are not yet readily dis-

tinguishable from those provoked by other agents. Exposure to the solvent bischloromethyl ether increases the risk of lung cancer as does cigarette smoking. Skin cancer may be caused by cutting oil contaminants and by sunlight. It may require several epidemiological studies to separate the effects of the two exposures.

The Office of Population Censuses and Surveys of England and Wales (OPCS) each ten years examines the risk of dying from cancer, and other causes of death, in persons aged 15 to 64. This age-span is used because these are the ages of employment and a usable statement of occupation is likely to appear on the death certificate: after 65 "retired" may be the only information given. A Standardized Mortality Ratio (SMR), which takes into account the frequency of the disease in a given group and the age at which it occurs is computed for each disease and occupation of interest. The risk for a given disease for the whole population aged 15 to 64 is considered to be 100. Gaffey[21] reviews the properties of the SMR in some detail.

The long latent period for cancer makes it likely that some cancers due to occupational exposures will occur after retirement, and although in England and Wales, and elsewhere, such analyses have been undertaken, they are often held to be less reliable. There are many sources of bias in such analyses which are well described in the most recent publication.[22] These include inaccuracies in stated cause of death, stated occupation, and the effects of early retirement. Further, the classification of occupation used may not reflect changes in industry.

The significance of a raised SMR. Coal miners in England and Wales have a very high SMR for stomach cancer (SMR 171) and indeed for all cancers combined their risk is 19% above the national average (SMR 119). As might be expected from the nature of their occupation SMRs from chest diseases (*e.g.*, pneumoconiosis) and accidents, 252 and 156 respectively, are also raised. The question arises whether the large excess risk of stomach cancer is also due to at-work exposures. There is a marked social class gradient for stomach cancer—a gradient which has persisted since at least 1921.[23] The observation that a large proportion of those belonging to the same social class from which coal miners are drawn also have a raised SMR for this cancer, casts doubts on the occupational specificity of the association. Indeed, when the various occupations within this social class are compared, coal miners are at no more risk from stomach cancer than any other group within the social class, although their overall mortality from all causes (SMR 132) is considerably greater.

Examination of the risk in miners' wives is most instructive in that they too have very high stomach cancer risks, although they do not work in coal mines. This evidence suggests that it is the social class, and all that goes with it in terms of lifestyle (diet, personal habits, etc.) that is important, rather than the exposure at work. Such a conclusion is valid where women do not work or are not exposed to occupational hazards. While it may be true that occupational influences were not present in married women twenty years ago, it is not so today, when a considerable proportion of married women are in active employment. Indirect influences, such as way of life, are assumed to be the same for husband and wife, but there are, nevertheless, large sex differences in, for example, cigarette and alcohol consumption, which cause certain cancers.

The parallel between lung cancer mortality and the smoking pattern of an occupational group is quite remarkable (Table 4).

Fox and Adelstein (1978) summarize this type of evidence thus ". . . surprisingly, only 12% of cancer variation appeared to be associated with work. For other causes, such as circulatory and respiratory diseases, the proportion was nearer 30%".

It will be apparent that as a method for the routine detection of increased risk in an occupation, let alone determining whether the increase was due to exposure at work, this group correlation approach is full of pitfalls and uncertainties. The finer the division of the occupations, the more likely are associations which emerge to be due to statistical chance; the broader the categories, the greater the chance of missing an increased risk in a small group.

Any association found should nonetheless be examined for biological plausibility and if an association seems possible the hypothesis should be tested by a cohort or case-control study. Mistakes will inevitably occur. For example, the OPCS[22] analysis shows an increased risk of cancer of the nose and nasal sinuses in butchers. As an unsupported finding this would probably be dismissed as a chance association. With prior knowledge that furniture workers exposed to wood dust also have a high risk of these cancers, a common exposure—sawdust—seems a plausible explanation.

In summary, this approach is useful to confirm known or suspected associations. By itself it is of comparatively little value for the detection of carcinogens. Indeed, none of those listed by the IARC monographs (Table 2) was detected in this manner.

Table 4: Relationship Between Lung Cancer Mortality and Smoking Habits
for Males Aged 15 to 64 in England and Wales, 1970-1972,
in Selected Occupational Units

Code No.	Occupational Unit	Lung Cancer SMR*	Smoking Index*
002	Farmers, farm managers, market gardeners	57	65
007	Coal-mine workers, underground	114	131
027	Electricians	100	105
039	Machine tool operators	164	116
177	Managers in mining and production	60	67
181	Medical practitioners (qualified)	32	33

*National average is 100.
Table abstracted from OPCS.[22]

Occupation and the cancer registry. Ideally, one would like to know not only about the fatal cancers associated with an occupation but about all those diagnosed. For some sites of cancer, such as those arising in the esophagus, there are very few survivors even after treatment, and death rates give a very good indication of the incidence of the disease. The outlook in lung and stomach cancer is also poor, whereas about half of those with a colon cancer will survive, and, for many kinds of skin cancer, about 98% will do so. For cancers in which treatment results in a considerable proportion of cures, incidence or the number of newly diagnosed cancers is clearly of much greater interest than mortality.

Incidence statistics are collected by cancer registries. Unlike death statistics which are national in coverage, the population covered by a cancer registry may range from a nation such as the German Democratic Republic (17 million), to a region such as Birmingham and the West Midlands in England (5 million), to quite small areas such as Iceland (200,000). About 10% of the population of the United States is currently covered by cancer registries.[25]

Data from reliable registries are published in Monographs of the Cancer Incidence in Five Continents series.[26] Of these, about 75% record information on occupation. However, unlike occupation which appears on all death certificates in many countries and which is one of a series of standard questions asked by the official registering death, the cancer registry has to depend on a series of persons to enter this item of information on the case notes, and eventually the cancer registry notification forms. This may be the hospital admission clerk, a ward nurse or a medical officer and the information may well be missing. It may also be impossible or difficult to obtain information on the numbers and ages of the various occupational groups for the district covered by the cancer registry. For these reasons there has been comparatively little use made of the occupational information stored in cancer registry files. However, Pukkala *et al.*[27] who examined Standardized Incidence Ratios (SIR) for lung cancer in the Finnish population aged 35 to 69 years concluded that the variation in the prevalence of smoking closely corresponded to that of the SIR for lung cancer.

The cancer registry is an invaluable adjunct for economical detection of risk in members of a cohort.

Group and Individual Comparison

Occupational cancer analyses of the type conducted by OPCS are cross sectional and do not take into account the fact that the occupation at the time of death may not have been that followed for most of the deceased's working life. Indeed, the illness leading to death may have resulted in a change of occupation. It must also be stressed that the OPCS approach deals with the average experience of groups of persons, not with individuals, and that no attempt is made to link an individual's death certificate with *his* census returns.

In Norway and Denmark annual statements of occupation are required for all employees and, as these are identified by the unique personal identification number of the employee, they can be readily linked with cancer registry notifications and death certificates. This resource enables estimates to be made of the years-at-risk ensuing from each employment for an individual and in effect makes a cohort study of the entire work force possible. In Sweden it is possible to link, subject to the approval of the Data Inspection Board, census data with death certificate data for individuals and hence assess the level of risk associated with a given employment, taking into account factors such as residence, income, education, etc.[28]

Case-Control Studies

In the case-control approach persons with a given cancer are interviewed and asked about their past exposures including those at work. Their answers are compared with answers to the same questions posed to controls, frequently other hospital patients, who do not suffer from the cancer in question. This is the most widely used epidemiological technique.[29] It is usual to test a series of hypotheses taking into account other factors considered to influence risk, such as tobacco. When many factors have to be considered or the risk factor is either very rare or very common, large numbers of cases are needed and pooling of material from several centers may be required[30]—a procedure which increases the complexity of the study.

The results for occupational exposures are often disappointing in that for a given study the number of persons with a particular cancer who follow a specific occupation is likely to be rather small. Routine case-control studies including questions on occupation and work exposures have been undertaken at the Roswell Park Memorial Institute in Buffalo, New York, with rather meager results.[31] In Los Angeles, California, effort was concentrated on young persons with selected cancers in the belief that at-work exposures were most likely to be detected at ages when other causes were not likely to be so important; the results were again disappointing. However, in a region where there is a relatively high prevalence of the occupation under study the case-control approach may be rewarding. Extending this concept, if cases arising within an industrial cohort study population (which by definition is likely to have considerable numbers in one occupation) and appropriate controls from the same cohort can be interviewed, this constitutes a powerful and effective method of analysis as the effect of confounding factors such as smoking can be taken into account. Obviously cases arising in cohorts followed from some time in the past may have died by the time the study is mounted and under such circumstances information may be limited to that obtainable from surviving relatives.

The analysis of case-control studies permits estimation of the proportion of a given cancer due to a given exposure. Thus, Cole[32] attributed 18% of bladder cancer in males to occupational exposures, 39% to smoking, 24% to coffee drinking and 43% to unidentified causes (such attributable risks may total more than 100%).

Siemiatycki *et al.*[33] have proposed a method "which combines the breadth of studies based on routine reviews of occupation distributions and death certificates with the depth of studies (case-control or cohort) attempting to relate specific exposure to cancer occurrence." Reviewing correlation studies and analysis of cause of death and occupation recorded on death certificates, they proposed case-control studies based on common exposure rather than common job title suggesting that the contrast would be sharper and more *relevant*.

In Montreal, Canada, a patient with one of a series of selected cancers is asked, through a series of questionnaires and personal interviews, to provide detailed descriptions of the activities of the firm(s) with which he worked, the industrial processes in which he was involved, and his specific duties. Although the patient may not be able to identify chemical compounds, experts in engineering and chemistry can frequently establish a list of chemicals to which he may have been exposed in each of his jobs. This is not a simple task, nor can it be done with precision, as it requires not only detailed knowledge of each job but also a knowledge of the evolution of industrial processes.

The selection of controls poses many problems. General population controls can be exceedingly expensive and may not always be suitable. Hospital controls may not be suitable either because of other occupationally-related diseases and the fact that occupational exposures may correlate with socio-economic standing which is known to affect many cancer rates. The authors suggested that each cancer site be controlled by comparison with other cancer sites. There is, however, the disadvantage that chemicals that produce cancer at several sites could be less easily detected.

The authors present tables of the minimum relative risk detectable in a case-control monitoring system of the type they propose, for a region with a population of 500,000 males 35 to 69 years old, for various values of exposure frequency, annual incidence rate and person-years of exposure, assuming equal number of cases and controls. Other useful tables give the statistical sensitivity of different monitoring systems and a checklist of the problems that may reduce sensitivity or increase risk of bias. Whether the pioneering endeavor will be successful in terms of uncovering new risks is not yet clear. Preliminary results[34] show that the system works and that job histories can be translated into chemical exposures. The effect of cigarette smoking was detectable using both population and cancer patients control series. Nonetheless should it fail, the exercise will have been worthwhile by demonstrating most clearly that other methods must be used to decide whether substances are to be admitted to the general environment.

For the statistical analysis of case-control studies *see* Breslow and Day.[35]

Cohort Studies

There are industries which by their very nature are more likely than others to result in the exposure of the work force to possibly hazardous substances (for a general review *see* Simonato and Saracci[36]). Under such circumstances it becomes highly desirable not only to identify each employee but also his work stations and the exposure associated with each work station. As processes and equipment change over time it is essential to keep a record of the exposure levels associated with a particular task. Several large companies have instituted such schemes, notably for petrochemicals. Such environmental measurements need to be linked to possible health effects, including cancer.

Such large scale monitoring of exposure and health effect, in other words a continuing cohort study, is comparatively easy for large companies.[37] However, even within very large companies the number of persons exposed to a particular chemical may be small, and to obtain a valid estimate of the effect of exposure it may be necessary to combine the experience of several companies. A similar problem arises for industries characterized by small production units (thus, Gibson *et al.*[38] describe the foundry industry as almost a cottage industry—80% of American foundries employing less than 100 people). For reasons of commercial secrecy it becomes difficult for any one company to conduct such a study and under these circumstances an outside independent organization, such as a university or research institute, should undertake the work. Independent investigation of a potential hazard is desirable as the results, particularly if negative, are less likely to be impugned by third parties. Thus, the man-made mineral fiber industry in Europe requested the International Agency for Research on Cancer to carry out a multinational, multifactory study on the risk, if any, associated with exposure to these widely used substitutes for the carcinogenic insulating material asbestos.[39]

Nonetheless the results of such enquiries, even though follow-up is excellent, are often disappointing in that even for large cohorts the number with 30 or more years of exposure may be very small. Thus, in the IARC coordinated study of man-made mineral fibers the number of person years in 13 plants in seven countries was 309,353, but only 9,075 (2.9%) of these occurred 30 or more years after first employment, after which 191 deaths (11.5% of the total) took place. Retrospective cohorts that are heterogeneous with respect to the era in which exposure to a hazard began are subject to chronology bias and those assembled sometime after onset of exposure are also subject to selection bias through attrition of the original populations prior to the time of registration.[40]

If numbers permit, it may be possible to demonstrate risk differentials between segments of a plant as in nickel refining.[41] Yet while several studies suggest an association between excess lung cancer and work in iron foundries the exposures responsible are not known. Differences in the mutagenicity of air particulate samples in one foundry paralleled risk.[38]

If an effect is demonstrated, it may not be clear whether this was due to a chemical at work or to some other influence such as smoking (*see* Table 4). In such circumstances, the case-control study within the cohort mentioned above is particularly valuable. An unexpected finding should, if at all possible, be re-examined in a different cohort. Nearly all human carcinogens were first identified by anecdotal data and case control studies, a few by retrospective cohorts. In contrast, despite their cost, no new carcinogens have yet been found in prospective cohort studies although some have elegantly confirmed known causal associations.

Follow-up: record linkage. For a cohort study to be credible it is of the greatest importance that *all* eligible cohort members be identified and followed until death, the diagnosis of cancer, or the end of the study. Thus, Jensen[42] was able to account for 99.3% of cohort members: Less than 95% is hardly acceptable. It must be stressed that the follow-up process includes not only those who remain in the industry for the duration of the study but also those who have left it for any reason, including change of employment or retirement.

The key to a cohort study is the ability to match unequivocally and at low cost the list of persons exposed and the health consequences of such exposures. Traditionally, death certificates have been used but death certificates are frequently inaccurate, even when cancer has been diagnosed in life (*see* Percy et al.[43]), and linkage with cancer registries is to be preferred. Unfortunately in much of the world such linkages are either impossible or becoming increasingly difficult to undertake, due to considerations of confidentiality.

Industrial records. The foregoing discussion of cohort studies, and the long induction period for cancer, implies that records must be kept for at least 60 years for all employees *no matter how short the period of employment.* While employment for less than two years might be regarded as of little import, Newhouse et al.[44] have shown that two years of exposure to asbestos in high concentration increased risk of lung cancer and mesothelioma.

Management. From time to time employee records may be removed from the main files for a particular purpose, *e.g.*, compensation claims, frequent sickness or absenteeism or on retirement. It is such persons who are of the greatest interest from the point of view of health effects and in consequence a system must be devised to ensure that such records are not "lost" when needed. In this connection the old-fashioned bound ledger with serial entries of the name of each new recruit to the company, date of commencement, etc., is invaluable as this is much less likely to be lost or misplaced than an index card or computer file and can serve to check that other files are complete. For cohort studies changes of job station within a factory are of great importance. If such changes entail a change in salary they are usually noted, otherwise regrettably they are not.

Labor: administrative lists. Trade unions can contribute significantly by maintaining and conserving membership records. The recent study of cancer incidence and causes of death in Danish brewery workers was based entirely on union records.[42] This particular study was technically elegant in that union members either worked in a brewery or bottled mineral water, and as only the former had access to a free beer ration the two groups served to control each other.

In many countries the pattern of employment is changing. Fewer gain their livelihood from heavy manufacturing industry, there being a substantial movement into what are termed "service industries", frequently composed of small dispersed units. Although exposures may be substantial and similar in, say, the hairdressing salon, the detection of occupational risk under such circumstances becomes much more difficult and is probably most easily accomplished by the trade union for the occupation in question. When a license is required to exercise a profession or where persons following a particular activity need to be registered, *e.g.*, beauticians, the task is much easier.

The solution of the Swedish building trades is worth careful examination. Under this scheme (Bygghaelsan) management and labor contribute to a joint nationwide environmental health service, which undertakes the measurement of potential hazards in the work place and provides a health service. Such arrangements for industries with a widely dispersed workforce are of capital importance in that users of chemicals and insulating material[45] are frequently much more heavily exposed than those producing them, where the processes may be largely closed.

Employment of a seasonal nature associated with a high turnover of the workforce and a high proportion of migrant labor, frequently illegal, is likely to result in failure to detect risk.

It is likely that in the future, industrial cancer risk will be increasingly detected using records, and unless these are meticulously preserved, carcinogens will perforce remain unrecognized.

OTHER EXPOSURES (WASTE DISPOSAL, ACCIDENTS, AMBIENT POLLUTION)

There are exceptions to the generalization on the concentration of exposure in the workplace in the shape of accidents (*e.g.*, Seveso), human consumption of mercury treated seed grain, the wide-spread use of defoliants, pesticides and herbicides and the careless disposal in dumps, by accident or design, of toxic chemicals which have resulted or are believed to have resulted in human exposure. Many of these events are possibly too recent for any detectable number of cancers to have risen. Nonetheless, it is prudent to lay the groundwork to facilitate a future assessment of the effect of such exposures which are likely to affect women and children as well as men. Landrigan[46] and Heath[47] have listed the steps that should be taken for assessment of dumps but their proposals are applicable to a wider range of circumstances.

(1) The nature and extent of exposure must be documented.

(2) The exposed population must be precisely defined.

(3) Disease and dysfunction in the exposed populations must be diagnosed as unequivocally as possible, and the expected baseline frequency of a given health effect known.

(4) The relationship between exposure and disease must be evaluated with rigorous statistical methodology with particular attention paid to the detection of any dose-response relationship. If the health outcome is relatively rare, such as cancer, the population to be studied will need to be relatively large.

To take account of confounding factors would imply collecting data on past occupational exposures, personal habits such as cigarette smoking and the use of alcohol and possibly drugs as well as characteristics such as gender, race, age and socio-economic status. The more variables a study addresses the more complex its eventual analysis becomes, and the greater the size of the population needed to adequately assess health effects.

In the analysis of dump exposures, special attention is frequently given to reproductive outcomes since latency considerations and limited sample size preclude rapid conclusions regarding the possible oncogenic effects of low doses. For example, for women living close to the Love Canal and for women living elsewhere in the canal area there was no clear increased risk for abortion, birth defects or low birth weight. Pregnancy outcomes, however, are also influenced by birth order, maternal age and maternal history of smoking, hence interpretation of findings is difficult.

Heath[47] comments on the diversity of dump exposures indicating for selected examples the toxic materials involved, the nature of the dump and the principal routes of potential human exposure. In the absence of a biological marker for exposure, the prospective cohort study is the sole method available to detect risk. If untoward effects take a long time to appear those exposed may have dispersed; hence the need for a central national death and, if feasible, cancer incidence index.

CHILDHOOD CANCER

Despite the wide variation in the global environment, levels of childhood cancer, apart from Burkitt's Lymphoma, show little international variation. Although levels are not as uniform as once imagined,[48] this generalization is still broadly true. If most childhood cancers are environmentally induced many of the exposures responsible are likely to have taken place *in utero*, a supposition strengthened by demonstration of the leukemogenic effects of prenatal radiation and of transplacental carcinogens[49] in humans (*i.e.*, adenocarcinoma of the vagina in women aged 14 to 23 years whose mothers had been given diethylstilbestrol (DES) for threatened abortion, a risk estimated to be between 14 and 140 per 100,000 DES-exposed females).

Yet, studies of pregnancy events and exposures of women whose children developed cancer, and comparison with controls, have been disappointing. Smoking by the pregnant mother does not seem to increase risk. The sperm of smokers, however, contains more abnormal forms. A suggestion that the offspring of fathers exposed occupationally to hydrocarbons were at higher risk has not been confirmed.

MEDICATION

Certain chronic diseases are treated over long periods of time by drugs: epilepsy by barbiturates (potent enzyme inducers) and phenytoin; renal transplant patients by immunosuppressives; tuberculosis by isoniazid; malignant disease by chemicals which may themselves have carcinogenic properties. In parts of Sweden and Australia long-term self medication by phenacetin-containing analgesics has been common. Cohort and case-control studies have shown these drugs to be associated with increased risk—hence the importance of trying to follow groups on long-term regimens.

DIET AND LIFESTYLE: ENDOGENOUS CARCINOGENESIS

The foregoing discussion has concentrated on exposures, usually in an industrial setting, to discrete chemical substances. Yet "pure" chemical exposures are probably relatively very rare. While the carcinogenic effect of the cigarette is universally recognized, it is less clear which of the large number of the chemicals in cigarette smoke is responsible for the increased risk. Interaction between carcinogens occurs and may be synergistic (*i.e.*, tobacco and asbestos) and, probably, antagonistic. The effects of some carcinogens may be inhibited in part by dietary components such as Vitamin-A-containing green and yellow vegetables. It may not be possible to analyze the effect of such risk modifiers, many of which probably remain to be discovered.

Much of the burden of cancer today, mainly those tumors arising in the digestive and genital tracts, is, on current evidence, held to be linked to diet and lifestyle (*see* Tables 1 and 5 and the section on Causes of Cancer). For breast, large bowel and endometrial cancer, risk is believed to derive from increases, or alterations, in the levels of substances which are normal cell products or metabolites.

Table 5: Diet and Lifestyle Factors Associated with an Increased Risk of Cancer in Humans

Factor	Cancer Site
Aflatoxin*	Liver
Alcoholic drinks	Mouth, pharynx, larynx, esophagus, liver
Chewing tobacco (with or without betel nut, lime, etc.)	Mouth, pharynx, esophagus
Cholesterol (low serum)	Colon (males)
Dietary fat (? cholesterol)	Breast, endometrium, colon
Dietary fiber (low)	Colon
Vitamin A (low)	Lung
Vitamin C (low) Fresh fruit and vegetables (low)	Stomach
Obesity	Endometrium, gallbladder
Reproductive history Late age at first pregnancy	Breast
Low parity	Breast, ovary
Sexual promiscuity	Cervix uteri
Smoking tobacco	Virtually all sites but skin and large bowel
Snuff	Mouth
Ultraviolet light	Skin

*See Table 2.

Diet

It is unlikely that food additives[12] or even "natural" contaminants such as aflatoxin are now of much importance in occidental countries. Studies in animals strongly suggest that restriction of caloric intake increases lifespan and the frequency of "spontaneous" tumors.[50] It has been claimed that a high fat intake is associated with increases in large bowel, breast and endometrial cancer. The mechanisms are not known; however, a high fat intake results in an increased output of bile acids considered to have promoting activity. Dietary fiber probably reduces risk by increasing fecal bulk and, hence, concentration of bile acid (*see* also Miller[51]).

The smoking and grilling of foods has long been suspected of resulting in increased concentrations of carcinogens in the form of polycyclic aromatic hydrocarbons. Sugimura[52] and his collaborators have more recently shown that the charring of amino acids, proteins and proteinaceous food, especially meat, results in strongly mutagenic heterocyclic amines which are carcinogenic for mice and rats—the latter exhibiting adenomas and carcinomas of the intestine. It remains to be shown that these substances are dangerous for man. It is quite possible that if the relative risk is low, the case-control approach will fail to demonstrate an increased risk. Indeed, Sugimura remarks that the actual amounts in food are very small in comparison with the carcinogenic dose in animals.

It has been shown that chemicals which are not themselves carcinogens may combine to form compounds which have carcinogenic potential, for example, nitrosamines from nitrite and secondary amines in the stomach. This reaction is influenced by pH and the presence of other naturally occurring substances such as Vitamin C, etc. Indicators of nitrosation potential have been developed[53] but these have not yet been modified for use in large population groups.

Investigation of dietary hypotheses is not easy. Diet itself is very difficult to measure objectively and is usually recorded as frequency of use of items rather than in terms of weight. The presence of malignant disease may alter food intake and somatic levels of the chemicals under study and hence the results of the case-control approach may be difficult to interpret. Hoping to avoid such biases, several workers are now concentrating on precancerous lesions such as adenomatous polyps (large bowel cancer) and leukoplakia (oral cavity cancer).

While group correlations have shown an association between dietary items such as fat and colon cancer,[54] the shortcomings of such correlations have been mentioned above. A few investigators have used a modification of this approach by estimating current diet in a small probability, *i.e.*, representative, sample of populations of known and contrasting risks,[55] in other words the diet associated with a given level of risk. Such studies assume that current diet reflects that of the prior ten or more years fairly well. As the numbers are usually small this method cannot yield information on the characteristics of the individuals in these populations who eventually develop a cancer. Nonetheless, the approach is very useful for refining hypotheses.

Prospective studies of "normals" in whom the dietary intake has been measured and biological samples have been taken are probably the best way to advance knowledge in this difficult area. Such investigations require large numbers (*i.e.*, 25,000 in the age-group 50 to 59 to be followed for 10 or more years) and should take into account possible dietary (seasonal) and hormonal (menopause) variation. The crux of such inquiries is the ability to follow cohort members economically until death or diagnosis of cancer. In other words, record linkage must be feasible and there must be a good cancer registry if follow-up costs are to be contained. The use of the case-control within the cohort approach minimizes the expense of chemical estimation but may give rise to large storage costs for the biological and food samples.

It is known that many food components serve as anticarcinogenic factors in both promotion and initiation.[56] Thus, quercitin, a plant flavenoid, can suppress experimental hepatocarcinogenesis in rats although it is mutagenic to microbes and cultured mammalian cells. It is quite possible that a dietary component could be associated with risk in one study, the risk being nullified or attenuated by other components elsewhere. Alteration of intake in one component of food may be associated with changes in others.

To advance in this area, epidemiologists and laboratory scientists must work closely together. The recent epidemiological interest in dietary fiber has resulted in the separation of fiber into a series of non-starch polysaccharides[57] and indeed, reappraisal of the nature of feces.

Lifestyle

One aspect of lifestyle is the age at which women have their first child. In many countries, it has been shown that regardless of overall incidence of breast cancer, the risk is increased in nulliparae and in those having their first full-term pregnancy over the age of 25.[58] There are several explanatory hypotheses relating risk to the balance of several steroid hormones, the length of time in a woman's life during which steroids are unopposed by progesterone, and prolactin levels.

Risk for breast (and endometrial) cancer is similarly affected when these hormones are administered in the form of oral contraceptives and estrogen replacement therapy. The latter and sequential oral contraceptives increase risks of endometrial cancer whereas combination oral contraceptives lower risk. Breast cancer risk may be increased in those using oral contraceptives at an early age or around the menopause. These findings, reviewed by Henderson *et al.*[59] are based on case-control studies. Studies of these important questions have been bedeviled by the fact that oral contraceptives have varied in composition over the years.

Cohort studies of Guernsey women have yielded interesting results. Urinary dehydroepiandrosterone levels were lower in women who subsequently developed ovarian cancer, but the cause for these lower levels is still not known.[60]

LOW LEVELS OF EXPOSURE

When chemicals used industrially spread into the general environment, the levels of exposure are usually likely to be lower and the relative risks smaller. The term "weak association" is usually used for relative risks below two. Nonetheless, it is easy to fall into the relative risk trap. The four-hundred-fold excess risk in vinyl chloride kettle cleaners seems much more clamant than a relative risk of 1.3 affecting half the population, although the latter would result in many more cancers.

Extrapolation

There have been many attempts to extrapolate backwards from dose-response curves based on medium and high levels of exposure to estimate the magnitude of the likely effect at lower doses and/or to conjecture whether a threshold exists. To quote Moolgavkar[61] "In view of the different modes of action of initiators and promoters it is clear that single statistical prescriptions for extrapolation of risk to low doses cannot possibly apply in all situations. Sensible extrapolation can only be made when the mode of action of the specific agent under study is known." In our opinion such exercises are bound to be inconclusive given the complications introduced by the long induction period, the multistage and multifactorial nature of carcinogenesis, the rarity of "pure" exposures and the possible influence of diet and lifestyle factors. The weaker the carcinogenic stimulus the more likely are modulating factors to obscure the effect. Hirayama's data suggest that the protective effect of green and yellow vegetables for lung cancer is greater for low levels of smoking and is overwhelmed in heavy smokers. While linear extrapolation would be regarded by many as a prudent basis on which to decide on control measures, it must be recognized that calculations on effects of low exposures cannot be based on scientific certainty.

Although for some chemicals current exposure levels may be much lower than in the past, this does not prevent the existence and identification of causal associations. However, risk may be over-estimated since the level of earlier and probably higher exposures is unknown.[62]

The "Negative" Study

A proportion of case-control studies reported in recent years could be considered negative in that the relative risk was not significantly different from unity at the 5% significance level. Yet there has been a curious reluctance to accept negative evidence. Two main reasons are given, namely, size of study and insufficient period of follow-up. Any study, if sufficiently large, could result in a significant difference although the relative risk would presumably remain much the same. The longer it takes for an effect to appear, the less likely it is to be significant. Nonetheless, even this generalization is not universally applicable, *e.g.*, asbestos related mesothelioma.

Because bias, confounding, and chance can easily produce a spurious weak association, the need for supporting evidence is great. Under such circumstances we may establish a relationship when none exists or fail to find one when it does. Indeed, the low relative risk presents virtually intractable problems of interpretation and very large numbers of cases and controls would be needed to establish a level of relative risk of 1.5 with confidence. For discussion of this problem *see* Day.[63] The sensitivity of a study can be enhanced by increasing the numbers involved, by picking out the highly exposed and, should the agent act multiplicatively with tobacco, by assessing risk among exposed smokers. For further discussion of bias, confounding, etc., *see* Schlesselman.[20] It is important to indicate in publications, particularly for investigations involving small numbers of persons, the power of the study. Some would not have an 80% chance of detecting a ten-fold relative risk (*see* also reference 62). In general, the confidence interval of the estimate of the relative risk is more informative than the *p* value.

It is of interest to note that epidemiological studies generally show that atmospheric pollution, although undesirable on many other grounds, is not a major source of increased cancer risk in those who do not smoke.[64]

COMMENT

Although the most pertinent discipline dealing directly with humans, it will be obvious from the foregoing that it is precisely in those areas where an answer is most needed, namely, the effect of low doses, that epidemiology is weakest. The epidemiologist cannot predict which chemicals will prove to be carcinogenic.[16] Such predictions must rest on other criteria (*see* Tomatis *et al.*;[65] Dinman and Sussman[66]) but these, for the most part based on animal and other studies, are difficult to extrapolate to man. With rare exceptions, some 20 or more years of exposure are needed to show that a risk exists for humans and perhaps somewhat longer before it can be shown that a particular substance is not likely to increase risk.

Given the diffuse nature of much exposure to chemicals, the epidemiologist must continue to look for effects in populations which he considers likely to be exposed to high levels. There is as yet no universally applicable routine method for the detection of occupational risk or for the assessment of whether a raised risk in an occupation is due to exposure at work.[67] The detection and prevention of occupation-induced cancer will thus continue to need collaboration of both sides of industry, vital statistics offices, cancer registries, the factory physician and the epidemiologist. A key element for such work is the linkage of an individual's exposures at work and elsewhere to their health consequences, which implies the maintenance and preservation of good linkable records and perhaps information on those personal habits of cohort members which may confound results. Despite this, in several countries confidentiality—medical, administrative and industrial—will continue to make the detection of carcinogenic workplace exposures impossible. Under such circumstances one could ask whom does confidentiality benefit—the exposer or the exposed?

The limitations of the conventional question and answer type of epidemiology are increasingly clear and new objective approaches to classify exposed and non-exposed preferably in a quantitative manner, are needed.

Perera and Weinstein[68] review the contribution that molecular epidemiology and carcinogen-DNA adduct detection may bring to studies of human cancer causation. "By combining epidemiological methods with laboratory procedures that assay for cellular and biochemical markers of host susceptibility, for tissue levels of carcinogens and their metabolites, for biologically effective dose, as well as for early human responses to carcinogens, researchers should be able to predict human risks more precisely than hitherto possible. A particularly promising approach is the use of highly sensitive immunological techniques to check the levels of adducts in tissues, white blood cells, urine and other body fluids of individuals exposed to a specific agent. This technique warrants extensive study since it could provide a dosimeter at the cellular level of the biologically effective dose of a carcinogen under the actual conditions of human exposure." Such investigations are most likely to be productive and economical in the case-control study within the cohort situation, but imply financing for periods of time that most funding bodies are not generally prepared to contemplate. Rapidly metabolized genotoxic carcinogens may not leave such "finger prints."

If the epidemiological identification of discrete chemical carcinogens originating in the external environment is difficult, these are nonetheless recognizable as foreign to the human organism. Yet current evidence suggests that perhaps one-quarter and one-half of cancer in Occidental males and females, respectively, is influenced by "normal" constituents of diet and by chemicals which are "normal" cell products or metabolites. The mechanisms and modifying factors are poorly understood and the epidemiological approach frequently difficult, requiring prospective cohort studies. In our opinion, *it is to this area of chemical carcinogenesis that priority for future research should be accorded.* For this the paths of the epidemiologist and laboratory worker must become closer than ever before—the disciplines are complementary, not alternative.

REFERENCES

1. Clemmesen, J., *Statistical Studies in Malignant Neoplasms. I. Review and Results.* pp. 1–543, Munksgaard, Copenhagen (1965)
2. Ramazzini, B., *De Morbis Artificum Diatriba (1700).* Translated by W.C. Wright, Univ. Chicago Press, Chicago, Illinois (1940)

3. Pott, P., *Chirurgical Observations Relative to the Cataract, the Polyps of the Nose, the Cancer of the Scrotum, the Different Kinds of Ruptures and the Mortification of the Toes and Feet.* Hawes, Clarke and Collins, London (1975)
4. Rehn, L., Blasengeschwuelste bei Fuchsin-Arbeitern. *Arch. Klin. Chir.* 50: 588 (1895)
5. Yamagiwa, K., and Ichikawa, K., Ueber die kuenstliche Erzeugung von Papillom. *V. jap. path. Ges.* 5: 142 (1915)
6. Kennaway, E.L., and Hieger, I., Carcinogenic substances and their fluorescence spectra. *Br. Med. J.* i: 1044-1046 (1930)
7. Ellerman, V., and Bang, O., Experimentalle Leukaemie bie Huehnern. *Zentb. f. Bakt.* 46: 595-609 (1908)
8. Rous, P., Transmission of a malignant new growth by means of a cell-free filtrate. *JAMA* 56: 198 (1911)
9. IARC, *Approaches to Classifying Chemical Carcinogens According to Mechanism of Action.* Joint IARC/IPCS/CEC Working Group Report. IARC Internal Technical Report 83/001, pp. 11-69, International Agency for Research on Cancer, Lyon, France (1983)
10. Wynder, E.L., and Gori, G.B., Contribution of the environment to cancer incidence: An epidemiologic exercise. *J. Natl. Cancer Inst.* 58: 825-832 (1977)
11. Higginson, J., and Muir, C.S., Environmental carcinogenesis: Misconceptions and limitations to cancer control. *J. Natl. Cancer Inst.* 63: 1291-1298 (1979)
12. Doll, R., and Peto, R., The causes of cancer: Quantitative estimates of avoidable risks of cancer in the United States today. *J. Natl. Cancer Inst.* 66: 1191-1308 (1981)
13. Rothman, K.J., in: *Cancer Epidemiology and Prevention* (D. Schottenfeld and J.F. Fraumeni, eds.), pp. 15-22, Saunders, Philadelphia (1982)
14. Hirayama, T., in: *Quantification of Occupation and Cancer* (R. Peto and M. Schneiderman, eds.), pp. 631-649, Banbury Rep. No 9., Cold Spring Harbor (1981)
15. IARC, IARC Monographs Supplement 4. *Chemicals, Industrial Processes and Industries Associated with Cancer in Humans.* IARC monographs Volumes 1-29. International Agency for Research on Cancer, Lyon, France (1982)
16. Muir, C.S., Limitations and advantages of epidemiological investigations in environmental carcinogenesis. *Ann. N.Y. Acad. Sci.* 329: 153-164 (1979)
17. Blot, W.J., Harrington, J.M., Toledo, A. *et al.*, Lung cancer after employment in shipyards during World War II. *New Engl. J. Med.* 299: 620-624 (1978)
18. Breslow, N.E., and Enstrom, J.E., Geographic correlations between cancer mortality rates and alcohol-tobacco consumption in the United States. *J. Natl. Cancer Inst.* 53: 631-639 (1974)
19. Peers, F.G., and Linsell, C.A., Dietary aflatoxins and liver cancer in a population-based study in Kenya. *Br. J. Cancer* 27: 473-484 (1973)
20. Schlesselman, J.J., *Case Control Studies—Design, Conduct, Analysis*, pp. 7-354, Oxford University Press, New York (1982)
21. Gaffey, W.R., A critique of the standardized mortality rates. *J. Occup. Med.* 18: 157-160 (1976)
22. Office of Population Censuses and Surveys, *Occupational Mortality. The Registrar General's Decennial Supplement for England-Wales, 1970-72.* Series DS No. 1, pp. 1-224, Her Majesty's Stationary Office, London, England (1978)

23. Logan, W.P.D., *Cancer Mortality by Occupation and Social Class 1851-1971.* IARC Scientific Publications No 36. International Agency for Research on Cancer, pp. 1-252, Lyon, France (1982)
24. Fox, J., and Adelstein, A.M., Occupational mortality 1970-72:Work or way of life. *J. Epid. Comm. Hlth.* 32: 73-78 (1978)
25. Young, J.L., Percy, C.L., and Asire, A.J., *Surveillance, Epidemiology and End Results: Incidence and Mortality Data, 1973-77.* NIH Publications 81-2330, pp. 1-1082, Govt. Print. Office, Washington, DC (1981)
26. Waterhouse, J.A.H., Muir, C.S., Powell, J., and Shanmugaratnam, K. (eds.), *Cancer Incidence in Five Continents.* Vol. IV. Lyon, France: International Agency for Research on Cancer. IARC Scientific Publication No 42, pp. 5-806 (1982)
27. Pukkala, E., Teppo, L., Hakulinen, T., and Rimpela, M., Occupation and smoking as risk determinants of lung cancer. *Int. J. Epidemiol.* 12: 290-296 (1983)
28. Bolander, A.M., (1975): *Linkage of Census and Death Records to Obtain Mortality Registers for Epidemiological Studies in Sweden.* Proc. XIth Int. Cancer Congress, Vol. 3, pp. 36-39: Cancer Epidemiology, Environmental Factors (P. Bucalossi, U. Veronesi, and N. Cascinelli, eds.) Florence (1974)
29. Cole, P., The evolving case-control study. *J. Chron. Dis.* 32: 15-27 (1979)
30. Hoover, R.N., and Strasser, P.H., Artificial sweeteners and human bladder cancer. Preliminary Results. *Lancet* i: 837-840 (1980)
31. Decoufle, P., Stanislawczyk, K., Houten, L., *et al.*, *A Retrospective Survey of Cancer in Relation to Occupation.* DHEW (NIOSH) Publication No 77-178, pp. 1-215, Cincinnati, Ohio (1977)
32. Cole, P., in: *Host Environment Interactions in the Etiology of Cancer in Man* (R. Doll and I. Vadopija, eds.), IARC Scientific Publications No.7, Fogarty International Center Proceedings No 18, pp. 83-87, International Agency for Research on Cancer, Lyon, France (1973)
33. Siemiatycki, J., Day, N.E., Fabry, J., and Cooper, J.A., Discovering carcinogens in the occupational environment: A novel epidemiologic approach. *J. Natl. Cancer Inst.* 66: 217-225 (1981)
34. Siemiatycki, J., Gerin, M., Richardson, L., *et al.*, Preliminary report of an exposure-based, case-control monitoring system for discovering occupational carcinogens. *Teratogenesis Carcinog. Mutagen.* 2: 169-171 (1982)
35. Breslow, N.G., and Day, N.E., *Statistical Methods in Cancer Research. Vol. 1. The Analysis of Case-Control Studies.* IARC Scientific Publications No 32, pp. 84-119, International Agency for Research on Cancer, Lyon, France (1980)
36. Simonato, L., and Saracci, R., in: *Encyclopaedia of Occupational Health and Safety* (L. Parmeggiani, ed.), 3rd Edition, Vol. 1, pp. 369-375, International Labor Organization, Geneva (1983)
37. Pell, S., O'Berg, M.T., and Karrh, B.W., Cancer epidemiologic surveillance in the Du Pont Company. *J. Occup. Med.* 20: 725-740 (1978)
38. Gibson, E.J., McCalla, D.R., Kaiser-Farrell, C., *et al.*, Lung cancer in a steel foundry: A search for causation. *J. Occup. Med.* 25- 573-578 (1983)
39. Saracci, R., *et al.*, Proc. Conference on Biological Effects of Man-Made Mineral Fibers, Copenhagen 20-22 April 1982, WHO, EURO, Reports and Studies No. 81, pp. 80-83, Copenhagen
40. Weiss, W., Heterogeneity in historical cohort studies: A source of bias in assessing lung cancer risk. *J. Occup. Med.* 25: 290-294 (1983)
41. Pedersen, E., Hogtveit, A.C., and Andersen, A., Cancer of respiratory organs among workers at a nickel refinery in Norway. *Int. J. Cancer* 12: 32-41 (1973)

42. Jensen, O.M., Cancer morbidity and causes of death among Danish brewery workers. International Agency for Research on Cancer, pp. 9-143, Lyon, France (1980)

43. Percy, C., Stanek, E., and Gloeckler, L., Accuracy of cancer death certificates and its effect on cancer mortality statistics. *Am. J. Publ. Hlth* 71: 242-250 (1981)

44. Newhouse, M.L., Berry, G., Wagner, J.C., and Turok, M.E., A study of the mortality of female asbestos workers. *Br. J. Industr. Med.* 29: 134-141 (1972)

45. Engholm, G., Englund, A., Hallin, N., and Von Schmalensee, G., Respiratory cancer incidence in Swedish construction workers exposed to man-made mineral fibers (MMMF). Proc. Conference on Biological Effects of Man-Made Mineral Fibers. Copenhagen 20-22 April 1982. WHO EURO, Reports and Studies No. 81, pp. 1-90, Copenhagen

46. Landrigan, P.J., Epidemiologic approaches to persons with exposures to waste chemicals. *Environ. Health Perspect.* 48: 93-97 (1983)

47. Heath, C.W., Field epidemiologic studies of populations exposed to waste dumps. *Environ. Health Perspect.* 48: 3-7 (1983)

48. Breslow, N.E., and Langholz, B., Childhood cancer incidence: Geographical and temporal variations. *Int. J. Cancer* 32: 703-716 (1983)

49. Herbst, A.L., Ulfelder, H., and Poskanzer, D.C., Adenocarcinoma of the vagina—association of maternal stilbestrol therapy with tumor appearance in young women. *New Engl. J. Med.* 284: 878-881 (1971)

50. Bras, G., and Ross, M.H., Tumor incidence patterns and nutrition in the rat. *J. Nutr.* 87: 245-260 (1965)

51. Miller, A.B., in: *Host Factors in Human Carcinogenesis* (H. Bartsch, and B. Armstrong, eds.), IARC Scientific Publications No. 39, pp. 117-192, International Agency for Research on Cancer, Lyon, France (1982)

52. Sugimura, T., in: *Recent Advances in Cancer Control* (S. Yamagata, T. Hirayama, and S. Hisamichi, eds.), pp. 63-72, Int. Congr. Ser. 622. Excerpta Medica, Amsterdam (1983)

53. Oshima, H., and Bartsch, H., Quantitative estimation of endogenous nitrosation in humans by monitoring N-nitrosoproline excreted in the urine. *Cancer Res.* 41: 3658-3662 (1981)

54. Armstrong, B., and Doll, R., Environmental factors and cancer incidence and mortality in different countries, with special reference to dietary practices. *Int. J. Cancer* 15: 617-631 (1975)

55. Jensen, O.M., MacLennan, R., and Wahrendorf, J., Diet, bowel function, fecal characteristics, and large bowel cancer in Denmark and Finland. *Nutr. Cancer* 4: 5-19 (1982)

56. Wattenberg, L.W., Inhibitors of chemical carcinogenesis. *Adv. Cancer Res.* 26: 197-226 (1978)

57. Englyst, H., Wiggins, H.S., and Cummings, J.H., Determination of the non-starch polysaccharides in plant foods by gas-liquid chromatography of constituent sugars as alditol acetates. *Analyst* 107: 307-318 (1982)

58. MacMahon, B., Cole, P., Lin, T., *et al.*, Age at first birth and breast cancer risk. *Bull. Wld Hlth Org.* 43: 209-221 (1970)

59. Henderson, B.E., Ross, R.K., and Pike, M.C., in: *Recent Advances in Cancer Control* (S. Yamagata, T. Hirayama, and S. Hisamichi, eds.), pp. 73-85, International Congress Series 622. Excerpta Medica. Amsterdam, Oxford, Princeton (1983)

60. Cuzick, J., Bulstrode, J.C., Stratton, I., *et al.*, A prospective study of urinary androgen levels and ovarian cancer. *Int. J. Cancer* 32: 723-726 (1983)

61. Moolgavkar, S.H., Model for human carcinogenesis: Action of environmental agents. *Environ. Health Perspect.* 50: 285-291 (1983)
62. Haines, T., and Shannon, H., Sample size in occupational mortality studies. *J. Occup. Med.* 25: 603-608 (1983)
63. Day, N.E., The assessment of negative epidemiological evidence: Some statistical considerations. Proc. of meeting on negative evidence held in Green College, Oxford, July 1983 (in press)
64. Vena, J.E., Air pollution as a risk factor in lung cancer. *Am. J. Epidemiol.* 116: 42-56 (1982)
65. Tomatis, L., Breslow, N.E., and Bartsch, H., in: *Cancer Epidemiology and Prevention* (D. Schottenfeld, and J.F. Fraumeni, eds.), pp. 44-73, Saunders, Philadelphia (1982)
66. Dinman, B.D., and Sussman, N.B., Uncertainty, risk and the role of epidemiology in public policy development. *J. Occup. Med.* 25: 511-516 (1983)
67. Muir, C.S., and Demaret, E., in: *Encyclopaedia of Occupational Health and Safety* (L. Parmeggiani, ed.), 3rd edition, Vol. 1, pp. 377-383, International Labor Organization, Geneva (1983)
68. Perera, F.P., and Weinstein, I.B., Molecular epidemiology and carcinogen-DNA adduct detection: New approaches to studies of human cancer causation. *J. Chron. Dis.* 35: 581-600 (1982)

Part III

In Vitro Tests

3

Overview of *In Vitro* Tests for Genotoxic Agents*

Angela Auletta

U.S. Environmental Protection Agency
Washington, D.C.

INTRODUCTION

This chapter on *in vitro* tests for genotoxic agents will focus only on assays used to detect potential carcinogens. These tests include assays for mutation, chromosomal aberrations, DNA damage and repair, sister chromatid exchange and cellular transformation (Table 1). This chapter will not review methods to determine heritable germ cell mutations nor will it include a discussion of the use of *in vitro* assays to predict mutation *per se* or endpoints other than cancer. For a discussion of the use of both *in vitro* and *in vivo* assays for genotoxic agents to identify potential mutagens (as separate from potential carcinogens) the reader is referred to the recent report from the National Academy of Sciences entitled *Identifying and Estimating the Genetic Impact of Chemical Environmental Mutagens.*[1]

Prior to the late 1960's and early 1970's there seemed to be little or no correlation between mutagenicity and carcinogenicity. Few mutagens had been shown to be carcinogens and, with a few exceptions, carcinogens which had been tested for mutagenicity, primarily in microbial assays which lacked the capacity for metabolic activation, had been designated as nonmutagenic. As basic understanding of the metabolism of carcinogenic chemicals increased, it was discovered that many carcinogens undergo activation by mammalian enzyme systems to an ultimate carcinogenic moiety. This discovery was followed by the development of *in vivo* systems, such as the host-mediated assay for potential mutagen-

*This article was written by Angela Auletta in her private capacity. No official endorsement by the U.S. Environmental Protection Agency or any other agency of the U.S. Federal Government is intended or should be inferred.

Table 1: Currently Available Short-Term Assays for Genotoxicity*

	Gene Mutation	Chromosomal Aberrations	DNA Damage and Repair	Cellular Transformation
Prokaryotes	1. *Salmonella* reverse mutation assay 2. *E. coli* reverse mutation assay 3. Host-mediated assay 4. Body fluid analysis		1. *E. coli* polA$^+$/polA$^-$ assays 2. *B. subtilis* rec$^+$/rec$^-$ assay	
Lower Eukaryotes	1. Forward and reverse mutation assays in *Aspergillus nidulans, crassa, Saccharomyces cerevisiae* and *Schizosaccharomyces pombe*	1. Aneuploidy in *Aspergillus, Saccharomyces,* and *Neurospora*	1. Recombination or crossing over in *Aspergillus nidulans* 2. Gene conversion in *Saccharomyces cerevisiae*	
Plants	1. Assays for gene mutation in several species including *Arabidopsis, Hordeum, Tradescantia* and *Zea mays*	1. Assays for chromosomal aberrations in several species including *Allium, Tradescantia, Hordeum,* and *Vicia faba*		
Insects	1. Sex-linked recessive lethal assay in *Drosophila melanogaster*	1. Assays for sex-chromosome loss or gain, aneuploidy and heritable translocation in *Drosophila melanogaster*		
Higher Eukaryotes	1. Mutation at the TK locus in L5178Y cells 2. Mutation at the HGPRT or Na$^+$/K$^+$ ATPase locus in V79 cells 3. Mutation at the HGPRT locus in CHO cells	1. *In vitro* and *in vivo* assays for chromosomal aberrations 2. *In vitro* and *in vivo* assays for SCE formation 3. Micronucleus assay	1. Assays for UDS performed in *in vitro, in vivo* or *in vivo/in vitro* systems	1. Assays for cellular transformation in SHE cells, BALB/c-3T3 cells or C$_3$H10T½ cells 2. Assays for enhancement of viral transformation

*Does not include *in vivo* assays which are used for detecting mutagenicity *per se*, such as the dominant lethal assay, the heritable translocation assay, the mouse spot test and the mouse specific locus test.

icity;[2] and by *in vitro* testing of reactive forms of carcinogenic chemicals.[3-6] As a result, the mutagenicity of many known carcinogens was demonstrated and an empirical correlation between mutagenicity and carcinogenicity became evident.

With the development of exogenous mammalian metabolic activation systems for use with microbial assays[7,8] the empirical correlation between mutagenicity and carcinogenicity increased still further. For example, McCann *et al.,*[9] using a preselected list of carcinogens and noncarcinogens most of which were tested by the authors, reported a 90% correlation between carcinogenicity and mutagenicity in *Salmonella typhimurium.*

Several hypotheses have been put forward to explain the correlation between mutagenicity and carcinogenicity, for example:

(1) The somatic cell mutation theory proposes that interaction of the carcinogenic moiety with DNA to produce a cellular mutation is crucial to the carcinogenic process. This mutation is believed to occur at the site in the cell which controls differentiation. Release of the altered cell from the differentiated state is accompanied by uncontrolled growth and subsequent formation of a tumor mass.

(2) A closely related theory suggests that the carcinogen enters the cell and causes chromosomal alterations which are responsible for the transition of the cell from a normal to a transformed or cancerous state. Although cells from certain human tumors do show an increased incidence of chromosomal aberrations,[10,11] it is not known if these alterations are the cause or the result of the cancer.

(3) The two-stage theory of carcinogenesis states that during the first stage of tumor formation, interaction of the carcinogen with DNA results in an altered cell. This process has been termed *initiation* and the carcinogen is called an *initiator*. Initiation is followed by exposure to an agent which although not carcinogenic in itself, enhances the body's response to the carcinogen and leads to an increased rate of tumor formation. This type of agent is known as a promoter. Some carcinogens function as both initiators and promoters and are known as complete carcinogens.

Carcinogens such as hormones, some metals, and inert physical agents are believed to act by mechanisms other than interaction with DNA or other cellular macromolecules. These mechanisms may include suppression of the immune system or other host-defense mechanisms or local irritation. Carcinogens which act through such mechanisms are generally negative when tested in *in vitro* assays for genotoxicity.

Whatever the mechanism of carcinogenicity, there appears to be an empirical correlation between mutagenicity and carcinogenicity which is worth exploiting in the identification of potential carcinogens. Assays for mutation or other indicators of genetic damage, such as increased DNA repair, are designed to detect agents which are capable of macromolecular interaction and which hence are considered potential carcinogens. Several short-term *in vitro* assays have been developed for the detection of genotoxic agents. These assays measure different genetic endpoints and employ prokaryotes, lower eukaryotes, insects, cells in culture, and whole animal systems. Assays have also been developed for the detection of promoters of carcinogenicity.[12-14] These assays measure different endpoints than those used to detect genotoxic carcinogens because, for the most part promoting agents are negative in assays which measure genotoxicity.

ASSAYS FOR GENE MUTATION

Assays for gene mutation include tests for mutation in bacteria, lower eukaryotes such as fungi and yeast, mammalian somatic cells in culture, insects, plants, and mammals.

The most widely used gene mutational assay is the *Salmonella typhimurium*/mammalian microsomal assay (Ames assay[15]) which detects reverse mutation in the histidine operon of specially constructed strains of the bacterium *S. typhimurium*. Mammalian metabolic capabilities are provided by the use of an exogenous metabolic activation system prepared from cofactor supplemented post-mitochondrial fractions from rodent liver (S-9 fractions). Currently, five strains of *Salmonella* are recommended for use in the assay. Two strains (*i.e.*, TA 100 and TA 98) carry a plasmid, pkM-101, which confers resistance to ampicillin and at the same time increases sensitivity to mutagenic agents. Four of the five strains (*i.e.*, TA 1535, TA 1537, TA 1538 and TA 98) specifically detect either base-pair or frameshift mutagens, while the fifth strain (*i.e.*, TA 100) detects both types of agents.

A second bacterial assay for gene mutation uses strains of *Escherichia coli* WP2 to detect reverse mutation in the tryptophan synthesis operon.[16] Three strains are commonly used, of which two (WP2 and WP2 uvrA), detect base-pair mutagens. A third strain, WP2 uvrA pkM-101, contains a plasmid which increases sensitivity to mutation in this organism much as it does in *S. typhimurium*. This strain may detect frameshift as well as base-pair mutagens.

Assay systems for mutation in mammalian cells in culture include mutation at the thymidine kinase (TK) locus of L5178Y mouse lymphoma cells,[17] at the hypoxanthine-guanine-phosphoribosyl transferase (HGPRT) locus of Chinese hamster ovary (CHO)[18] and lung (V-79) cells[19,20] and at the Na^+/K^+ ATPase (measured by resistance to ouabain) locus in V-79 cells.[21] These systems are forward mutational assay systems. The TK and HGPRT systems detect base-pair, frameshift, and deletion mutagens and agents which repress these genes; the ouabain system detects base-pair mutagens only. Since cells in culture either do not possess innate metabolic capabilities or have lost them through prolonged culture, exogenous metabolic activation systems, including S-9 fractions and co-cultivation techniques, are used.

Assays which detect gene mutation in lower eukaryotes, insects, plants, and rodents are not routinely used to predict carcinogenic potential.

ASSAYS FOR CHROMOSOMAL DAMAGE

In vitro assays for detecting chromosomal effects include assays for chromosomal aberrations (cytogenetics assays) or sister chromatid exchange (SCE) in mammalian cells in culture. *In vivo* assays for chromosomal aberrations, SCE or micronucleus formation in rodents are also used to detect potential carcinogens but they are more time consuming, and therefore, are not routinely used as *in vitro* assays. In general, assays for chromosomal damage are not as widely accepted as predictors of carcinogenic potential as are assays for gene mutation.

In vitro cytogenetics tests are short-term mutagenicity test systems for the detection of chromosomal aberrations in cultured mammalian cells. Chromosomal aberrations may be either structural or numerical. However, because cytogenetics assays are usually designed to analyze cells at their first post-treatment mitosis and numerical aberrations require at least one cell division to be visualized, this type of aberration is generally not observed in a routine cytogenetics assay. Structural aberrations may be of two types: chromosome or chromatid. Chromosome-type aberrations are induced when a compound acts in the G1 phase of the cell cycle. Chromatid-type aberrations are induced when a chemical acts in the S phase or G2 phase of the cell cycle. The majority of chemicals, including those which act in G1 phase, induce only chromatid-type aberrations because the damage, although induced in the G1 phase, does not become manifest until S phase. Radiation and radiomimetic agents, however, induce damage in all phases of the cell cycle.

The SCE assay detects the ability of a chemical to enhance the exchange of DNA between two sister chromatids of a duplicating chromosome. Sister chromatid exchanges represent reciprocal interchanges of the two chromatid arms within a single chromosome. These exchanges are visualized during the metaphase portion of the cell cycle and presumably require enzymatic incision, translocation and ligation of at least two DNA helices. The precise mechanism of SCE formation is unknown, however.

Both the cytogenetics and SCE assays may be performed *in vitro*, using, for example, rodent or human cells, or *in vivo* using mammals (*i.e.*, rodents such as mice, rats and hamsters).

In vitro cytogenetics and SCE assays may be performed in continuous cell lines or strains or in primary cultures of human or rodent peripheral lymphocytes. Metabolic activation systems are used with these assays and with assays for gene mutation in cells in culture.

In vitro cytogenetics and SCE assays performed with human peripheral lymphocytes may be used to monitor human exposure to environmental contaminants. Although these assays may be used in screening programs, their relationship to human health has not been established. A more complete discussion of the use of cytogenetics and other assays in screening programs is presented in the U.S. Congress Office of Technology report, *The Role of Genetic Testing in the Prevention of Occupational Illness*.[22]

The micronucleus test is a mammalian *in vivo* assay which detects damage of the chromosome or mitotic apparatus by chemicals. Micronuclei are small particles consisting of acentric fragments of chromosomes or entire chromosomes, which lag behind at anaphase of cell division. After telophase, these fragments may not be included in the nuclei of daughter cells and form single or multiple micronuclei in the cytoplasm. Polychromatic erythrocytes in the bone marrow of rodents are used in this assay. When the erythroblast develops into an erythrocyte, the main nucleus is extruded and may leave a micronucleus in the cytoplasm. The visualization of micronuclei is facilitated in these cells because they lack a nucleus. Micronuclei form under normal conditions. The assay is based on an increase in the frequency of micronucleated polychromatic erythrocytes in bone marrow of carcinogen-treated animals.

Cytogenetics assays in lower eukaryotes, insects and plants and some *in vivo* techniques which detect chromosomal damage, such as the dominant lethal and heritable translocation assays, are not routinely used to identify potential carcinogens.

ASSAYS FOR DNA DAMAGE AND REPAIR

The most commonly used DNA damage and repair assays include DNA-repair tests in bacteria and unscheduled DNA synthesis (UDS) assays in mammalian cells in culture.

Bacterial assays for DNA damage measure differential growth inhibition of repair-proficient *versus* repair-deficient isogenic bacteria such as polA⁺/polA⁻ strains of *E. coli*[23] or rec⁺/rec⁻ strains of *Bacillus subtilis*.[24] These assays measure neither mutagenic events *per se* nor DNA repair. They are used as an indication of chemical interaction with DNA. Repair of the resulting lethal events is taken as an indication of potential genotoxicity.

UDS assays measure the repair of DNA damage over the entire genome. Since it is believed that misrepair or incomplete repair of damage may be an initial step leading to a permanent alteration of the genetic material, UDS assays are presumably measuring premutational or precarcinogenic events. However, since UDS assays do not distinguish between error-free and error-prone repair, an increase in UDS following chemical treatment should not be unequivocally equated with potential carcinogenicity.

UDS assays are usually performed in continuous lines of human diploid fibroblasts (*e.g.*, WI-38 cells) or in primary cultures of rat hepatocytes[25] although they need not be limited to these cell types. Assays performed in primary rat hepatocytes do not require an exogenous source of metabolic activation since it is presumed that the cells possess endogenous capabilities to metabolize xenobiotics. Metabolic activation has not been routinely used with human cells.

DNA repair may also be measured *in vivo*.[26,27] *In vivo/in vitro* assays for DNA repair have also been used to identify potential genotoxic agents[28] although these assays are still in the developmental stage.

ASSAYS FOR CELLULAR TRANSFORMATION

Morphologic transformation of cells in culture by chemicals is generally regarded to be a reliable indicator of *in vivo* carcinogenicity because such cells usually produce tumors when inoculated into syngeneic or immunosuppressed hosts. Although the mechanism of action by which cells become morphologically transformed is not known, it is thought to be a multi-phased process analogous to tumor formation, *in vivo*. The endpoint of assays for cellular transformation is the development of foci of transformed cells, recognizable by visible alterations in growth pattern, against a background of normal cells. This morphologic transformation is generally correlated with the ability of the cells to grow in soft agar and to produce tumors *in vivo*. Heidelberger *et al.*[29] concluded that the ability to produce tumors is the ultimate criterion in determining transformation. Assays for cellular transformation may be divided into three categories: (1) transformation in cells with a finite lifespan, such as Syrian hamster embryo (SHE) systems,[30,31] (2) transformation of cells with an indefinite lifespan, predominantly BALB/c-3T3[32] and C3H10T½ systems;[33] and viral-chemical interactive systems.[34,35]

Although assays for cellular transformation show promise as tools for predicting carcinogenicity, they require further development and validation before they can be considered for routine use in screening programs. Of particular importance is the need for development of metabolic activation systems which can be used routinely with these methods.

The advantages and disadvantages of each of the *in vitro* assays described are shown in Table 2. There are other general limitations, however, which apply to the field of short-term testing as a whole and which should be mentioned here.

Table 2: Advantages and Limitations of Short-Term Assays
for Detecting Genotoxic Agents

Assay System	Genetic Endpoint Detected	Advantages	Limitations
Salmonella/ microsomal assay	Gene mutation	1. Rapid, relatively easy to perform, less expensive than lower eukaryotic or mammalian cell systems. 2. Measures gene mutation; detects both base-pair and frame-shift mutagens with a degree of specificity. 3. Known correlation with carcinogenesis for certain classes of chemicals. 4. Has a relatively wide data base of tested chemicals. 5. Test methodology relatively standardized; test is widely used and available. 6. Can test volatiles and gases.	1. Prokaryotic system thereby raising questions of relevance to humans. 2. Tester strains lack repair capacity raising further questions of extrapolation to systems with intact repair capability. 3. Requires use of exogenous metabolic activation. 4. Insensitive to certain classes of chemical carcinogens, *e.g.*, steroids, metals.

(continued)

Table 2: (continued)

Assay System	Genetic Endpoint Detected	Advantages	Limitations
E. coli WP2 and WP2 uvrA reverse mutation assay	Gene mutation	This is a prokaryotic assay with most of the same advantages and limitations as the *Salmonella* assay. Only those advantages or limitations which differ from the *Salmonella* assay are presented. 1. May be particularly suited to testing some classes of chemicals, *e.g.*, hydrazines, nitrofurans, nitrosamines and some metals such as soluble chromates.	1. Smaller data base than the *Salmonella* assay; has not been widely used with metabolic activation systems. 2. Not as widely available for routine use as the *Salmonella* assay.
Assays for mutation and chromosomal effects in lower eukaryotes (includes yeast, *Aspergillus* and *Neurospora* test systems)	Gene mutation (forward and reverse); aneuploidy; gene conversion and crossing over.	1. Eukaryotic systems which makes extrapolation to man easier than with prokaryotic systems. 2. Relatively rapid and inexpensive to perform.	1. Non-mammalian systems which complicate extrapolation to man. 2. Presence of a cell wall may interfere with ability of chemical to enter the cell and interact with target macromolecules. 3. Significance of aneuploidy and endpoints such as gene conversion and crossing over is not known. 4. Assays are not widely used nor readily available. 5. Ability of these assays to detect accurately mutagens/carcinogens from a variety of chemical classes has not been determined.

(continued)

Table 2: (continued)

Assay System	Genetic Endpoint Detected	Advantages	Limitations
Specific locus mutation in mammalian cells in culture 1. L5178Y TK system 2. CHO HGPRT System 3. V-79 HGPRT and Ouabain systems	Gene mutation	1. Mammalian systems thereby negating some concerns about extrapolation to man. 2. Measure forward mutation; TK and HGPRT systems detect base-pair and frameshift mutagens and gene repressors. 3. It may be possible to measure both gene mutation and chromosomal effects in the same assay or to compare them in the same system. 4. Test methodology for L5178Y cells is fairly well standardized; use of metabolic activation with L5178Y is relatively routine. Test methodology for CHO cells is less routine but there is agreement between laboratories. 5. Tests for mutation in L5178Y and CHO cells are readily available. 6. Can test volatiles and gases.	1. Require an exogenous source of metabolic activation. 2. The V-79 ouabain system detects base-pair mutagens only. 3. L5178Y cells are mouse lymphoma cells. This raises some questions about their use in testing for mutagens/carcinogens. 4. Limited data base of validity of tested chemicals for the CHO and L5178Y cells. None have been adequately tested with a variety of chemical classes. 5. Limited availability of assay systems using V-79 cells.
Host-mediated assay and body fluid analysis	Gene mutation	1. Both assays take advantage of whole animal metabolism in detecting mutagens/carcinogens. 2. Host-mediated assay may be useful for detecting mutagens/carcinogens which are difficult to activate *in vitro*, such as azo dye compounds.	1. Test methodologies for the host-mediated assay and body fluid analysis have not been standardized. The effect of variables in protocol on ultimate results in the assay is not known.

(continued)

Table 2: (continued)

Assay System	Genetic Endpoint Detected	Advantages	Limitations
		3. Body fluid analysis may be used to screen at risk populations for exposure to mutagenic agents.	2. Assays for body fluid analysis have not been widely used and have a small data base of chemicals and chemical classes tested. 3. The predictive value of body fluid analysis assays has not been determined. 4. Host-mediated assays are relatively expensive. Neither the host-mediated assay nor the body fluid analysis are widely available. The body fluid analysis is used so seldom no cost estimates could be determined.
Drosophila melanogaster sex-linked recessive lethal assay	Gene mutation	1. Germ cell mutagenesis assay capable of detecting point mutations and small deletions. 2. May be used to determine mutagenic events over different phases of the germ cell cycle. 3. Takes advantage of *in vivo* metabolic capabilities. 4. Molecular dosimetry techniques allow precise quantitation of dose to target tissue and correlation with mutagenic event.	1. Insect system raising questions of extrapolation to mammals. 2. Test has not been widely used to screen for potential carcinogens. 3. Although methodology is fairly well standardized, test is not widely used or easily available and is somewhat expensive.

(continued)

Table 2: (continued)

Assay System	Genetic Endpoint Detected	Advantages	Limitations
		5. May be used to test volatile substances or gases.	
Assays for chromosomal effects in *Drosophila melanogaster*	Sex-chromosome loss or gain; aneuploidy; heritable translocation.	1. Germ cell assays capable of detecting heritable chromosomal events. 2. Translocation assay may be used to determine mutagenic events over different phases of the cell cycle. 3. Takes advantage of *in vivo* metabolic capabilities. 4. May be used to test volatile liquids and gases.	1. Insect system raising questions of extrapolation to mammals. 2. Assays have not been widely used to screen for potential carcinogens. Therefore, their predictive value is not known. 3. Assays are not readily available.
In vitro cytogenetics assays	Structural and numerical chromosomal aberrations.	1. Employ mammalian assay systems thereby reducing problems of extrapolation to man. May also employ cultures of human lymphocytes. 2. Appears to correlate well with *in vivo* carcinogenic potential. 3. Assays with cultured human lymphocytes employ synchronized or partially synchronous cell populations. 4. Since cytogenetics assays may be performed *in vivo* as well as *in vitro* a direct comparison of *in vitro* and *in vivo* results is possible. 5. The assay is readily available.	1. Require exogenous source of metabolic activation. 2. Assays are time-consuming and relatively expensive; multiple harvest times are necessary to determine effects on various stages of the cell cycle. 3. Special training is required to read slides and interpret test results. Some training is needed for slide preparation.

(continued)

Table 2: (continued)

Assay System	Genetic Endpoint Detected	Advantages	Limitations
In vivo cyto-genetics assay	Structural and numerical chromosomal aberrations	1. Take advantage of whole animal metabolism. 2. Chromosomal aberrations may be detected in both somatic and germ cells. 3. Chromosomal aberrations may be detected in circulating white cells of the human population. These assays may be used for population monitoring studies. 4. Assay seems to have good predictive value for detecting potential carcinogens. 5. May be used to test volatile liquids and gases.	1. Assays are labor-intensive and expensive. Multiple sacrifice times are necessary to insure sampling of all stages of the cell cycle. 2. Specialized training is required to read slides, score and interpret test results. Some training is needed for slide preparation. 3. The significance in terms of human health of an increased number of chromosomal aberrations in the circulating white blood cells of an exposed population is not known.
Micronucleus assay	Believed to be damage to the chromosome or mitotic apparatus.	1. *In vivo* assay which takes advantage of whole animal metabolism. 2. Easier to score and evaluate than *in vivo* cytogenetics assays. 3. May be used to test volatile liquids and gases. 4. Test is readily available and less expensive than the *in vivo* cytogenetics assay.	1. Assay is relatively time consuming and expensive. Requires multiple sacrifice times to sample all stages of cell cycle. 2. Relevance of micronucleus formation to human health is unknown. 3. Assay appears to lack a degree of sensitivity and does not appear to be of predictive value.

(continued)

Table 2: (continued)

Assay System	Genetic Endpoint Detected	Advantages	Limitations
Differential growth inhibition of repair deficient bacteria—"Bacterial DNA damage and repair tests."	Unknown; used as an indication of chemical interaction with genetic material.	1. Rapid, easy to perform, inexpensive 2. Has a large data base of tested chemicals. 3. Certain bacterial pairs may be particularly suited for use with certain classes of chemicals.	1. Prokaryotic system which raises questions of relevance to humans. 2. Requires an exogenous source of metabolic activation. 3. Relevance of the endpoint detected to human health is unknown. 4. Positive results are difficult to evaluate in the absence of a positive result in another test system.
Unscheduled DNA synthesis in cells in culture	Enhanced DNA synthesis (as measured by ^{3}H-thymidine uptake into DNA) in cells that are not in S (DNA-synthetic) stage of the cell cycle.	1. Mammalian cell systems which facilitates extrapolation to man. 2. Tests may be performed in human cells in culture or rat hepatocytes. 3. Rat hepatocyte cultures do not need an exogenous source of metabolic activation. 4. Human cells used in the assay are diploid. 5. Techniques for determination of UDS in germ cells are available. 6. Relatively rapid and not overly difficult to perform.	1. Human cell systems require metabolic activation but this has not been used routinely and requires additional development. 2. Relevance of UDS to human health is unknown. 3. Does not distinguish between error-prone and error-free repair. 4. Only amount of repaired damage is measured. 5. Alterations in nucleotide pools could influence results.

(continued)

Table 2: (continued)

Assay System	Genetic Endpoint Detected	Advantages	Limitations
In vitro assays for sister chromotid exchange formation	DNA damage visualized as enhanced exchange of DNA between two sister chromatids of a duplicating chromosome.	1. Employ mammalian assay systems thereby reducing problems of extrapolation to man. May also employ cultures of human lymphocytes. 2. Since SCE assays may be performed *in vivo* as well as *in vitro*, direct comparison of results in the two systems is possible. 3. Shows promise as a predictive tool for detecting carcinogens. 4. Assay is widely available.	1. If established cell lines are used in these assays, they may no longer be diploid and may have undergone other genetic alterations. This may raise questions about their use in a screening program for potential mutagens/carcinogens. 2. Requires an exogenous source of metabolic activation. 3. Requires some specialized training to prepare and read slides and evaluate data. 4. Relevance of SCE formation to human health is unknown. 5. Alterations in nucleoside pools could influence results.
In vivo assays for sister chromatid exchange	DNA damage visualized as enhanced exchange of DNA between two sister chromatids of a duplicating chromosome.	1. Takes advantage of whole animal metabolism. 2. SCE may be detected in circulating white cells of human population. These assays may be used for population monitoring studies. 3. Assay shows promise as a predictive tool for detecting carcinogens. 4. May be used to test volatile liquids and gases. 5. Test is readily available.	1. Assay is relatively expensive and somewhat labor intensive. 2. Requires some specialized training to prepare and read slides and evaluate data. 3. The significance to human health of increased SCE levels in exposed populations is not known. 4. Alterations in nucleoside pools could influence results.

(continued)

Table 2: (continued)

Assay System	Genetic Endpoint Detected	Advantages	Limitations
Cellular transformation assays	Unknown; multiphase process analogous to tumor formation *in vivo*.	1. Detects morphologic transformation which appears to be directly correlated with the ability to produce tumors *in vivo*. 2. Some systems have a considerable data base of tested chemicals. 3. Shows promise as a predictive tool for detecting carcinogens. 4. Can test volatiles and gases. 5. Can use human diploid fibroblasts and epithelial cells.	1. Assays are not widely available and there are problems of reproducibility of results between laboratories. 2. Assays require an exogenous source of metabolic activation. However, the use of metabolic activation systems with cellular transformation assays is still in the developmental stage. 3. Not all cells are transformable. Clones suitable for use must be isolated periodically from cell lines; systems such as the Syrian hamster embryo system must be screened for transformable clones which are then frozen for future use. 4. Spontaneous transformation does occur in untreated cultures and can affect interpretation of results. 5. Different degrees of transformation can occur and it requires some training and skill to differentiate types of transformed foci.

(continued)

Table 2: (continued)

Assay System	Genetic Endpoint Detected	Advantages	Limitations
			6. Ultimate proof of transformation is production of tumors in syngeneic or immunosuppressed hosts. This increases time and cost of assay.
			7. All systems need additional development and validation.

OTHER LIMITATIONS OF SHORT-TERM TESTS

Metabolic Activation Systems

The indicator organisms or cell culture systems used for *in vitro* assays are generally unable to metabolize promutagens/procarcinogens to their ultimate reactive forms. To circumvent this, an exogenous source of metabolic activation must be added.

Such activation systems are often prepared from liver S-9 fractions according to the method of Ames *et al.*[8] who demonstrated their usefulness in activating promutagens and procarcinogens in the Ames assay.

Although these systems are useful and necessary additions to *in vitro* assays, they do not completely mimic the *in vivo* situation. Since enzyme systems are usually fractional sediments of tissue homogenates, they do not represent the actual enzymatic conditions found in the whole animal; co-factor complements are artificially manipulated, and complex interactions such as tissue distribution, organ specificity, repair processes and excretion patterns are missing and are not accounted for in *in vitro* activation systems.

For routine screening programs, S-9 fractions are generally prepared from the livers of male rats which have been treated with nonspecific enzyme inducers such as phenobarbital or Arochlor 1254. Liver is chosen for its ability to metabolize a wide variety of chemical substances; inducers are used to elevate levels of enzymes known to be involved in the metabolic processes. Although some effort has been made to use tissue from organs other than liver (generally selected on the basis of known target organs for chemical carcinogens) for metabolic activation, there doesn't appear to be any good reason for not using liver in general screening programs.

Enzymatic activity of S-9 preparations can be influenced by several factors including species, strain, sex and age of the animal used to prepare the enzyme extract; tissue specificity; choice of inducer; co-factor "cocktail"; media composition; incubation times and temperatures; length and temperature of storage of the S-9 preparation; and test chemical solvent. Mutagenic activity is also affected by the amount of S-9 added to the reaction mixture. To obtain maximum activity several concentrations of test chemical should be used with varying concentrations of S-9. In routine screening, this is not common practice and a single concentration of S-9 is usually all that is used.

Tissue culture systems are very susceptible to toxic effects of S-9 activation systems and technical difficulties may sometimes preclude the use of such systems in these assays. Alternatives to the use of S-9 preparations include the use of primary cultures of rodent hepatocytes, co-cultivation techniques and the selection of clones or lines of cells with metabolic capability for use in assays for mutation and cellular transformation. The primary advantage to the use of cellular systems is that they are enzymatically intact and their metabolism more closely approximates the *in vivo* situation. It is not known, however, if cellular activation systems will detect as broad a spectrum of genotoxic agents as S-9 preparations do. They, therefore, may not be ideally suited for use in a general screening program.

Human tissue, such as human alveolar macrophages and human tissue homogenates obtained from biopsy or autopsy material, has also been used for metabolic activation but restricted availability and variation in metabolic capacities limit its usefulness.

Techniques such as the host-mediated assay, analysis of body fluids for the presence of mutagenic metabolites and transplacental assays for the detection of mutations, cellular transformation or chromosomal aberrations combine whole animal metabolism with *in vitro* detection techniques. These assays are subject to limitations in sensitivity, technical difficulties and, in some instances, need further development and validation before they will be ready for routine use.

Extrapolation to Humans

Phylogenetic differences between humans and prokaryotes, lower eukaryotes, insects and plants raise questions about the use of assays which employ these systems as indicator organisms to identify agents which may prove harmful to humans. Immediately obvious differences include those in structure and function, metabolic capabilities and repair systems. The use of tissue culture systems brings one phylogenetically closer to man but questions of relevance to the human situation exist for these systems also.

In vitro assays, whether they employ prokaryotes, lower eukaryotes or cells in culture, are subject to limitations in metabolic capability which are partially overcome by the metabolic activation systems discussed above.

Tissue culture assays are also influenced by physical factors such as pH, incubation conditions and composition of the media used for cell growth and treatment.

Source of cells used in tissue culture assays can also influence results. Embryonic epithelial tissue responds differently from adult tissue, and there are innate metabolic pathways or repair capabilities specific to the organ or species from which the cells were derived which also influence response to a genotoxic agent. Because of this, certain tissue culture systems may accurately identify some agents as genotoxins and be totally inappropriate for others. Some established cell lines are no longer diploid in nature and may have undergone other biochemical or morphologic changes which make them remote not only from whole animal models or the human situation but even from the tissue from which they were derived. The L5178Y cell culture system is derived from a murine leukemia and, in a sense, has already undergone the transition from a normal to a transformed or genetically altered state. It may be that chemical interaction with genetic material is different in these cells from what it is in untransformed cells.

Most importantly, studies with cells in culture do not reflect the complex pattern of uptake, distribution, organ specificity and excretion seen in the whole animal.

The use of whole animal systems brings one closer to the human situation. Repair systems, metabolic capacity to activate and detoxify xenobiotics, and tissue distribution and excretion factors more closely resemble the human situation. Nevertheless, there are well-known species differences in metabolism which can influence the response of the organism to a test agent. The animal test model is usually a genetically defined individual, maintained in a controlled environment, fed a controlled diet and exposed to one agent at a time under carefully controlled conditions. Humans are genetically diverse and exposed to a complex environment of multiple agents. Their response to a given agent is governed by their physiological status, immune responsiveness, diet and stress in addition to the pattern of exposure to a given agent. There is also evidence that different tissues may have different repair capabilities which may affect response to a given agent. The importance of this evidence in determining response to a genotoxic agent has not been fully investigated and the animal models now in use to identify both genotoxic and carcinogenic agents do not take these complex differences into account.

At this time, direct extrapolation is not made from results in short-term assays to effects in man. Extrapolation is made, however, from results in short-term assays to effects in whole animal systems. Results from *in vitro* assays are used to predict animal carcinogenicity and, by inference, to identify potential human carcinogens.

Statistical Methodology

In analyzing the results from short-term assays for genotoxicity, it must be determined that the magnitude of the response seen in the treated population is significantly different from the response seen in the control population. Whereas in chronic bioassays, the significance of the observed response is determined by statistical analysis, there are no generally accepted statistical techniques for analyzing data from *in vitro* assays. "Rule-of-thumb" criteria have gradually been developed to aid in analyzing such data. These include items such as reproducibility of response; dose-response relationships; and the designation of arbitrary minimum responses (*e.g.*, 2X or 3X background) as being indicative of a positive response. This interjects an element of subjectivity into the analysis which can sometimes result in confusion and disagreement about the reactivity of a chemical in a given assay system. There is a need for generally accepted, uniform statistical methods for analyzing short-term test data which would facilitate not only data interpretation but also would aid in experimental design by influencing sample size for both treatment and analysis.

Limitations of the Data Base

Short-term assays are also limited by the number of chemicals or chemical classes which have been tested in each assay. Often only a few chemicals or chemicals from only a limited number of classes have been tested in a particular assay. This is illustrated by the data base for the cellular mutation assays discussed above. Hsie *et al.*[36] reported that a total of 18 chemicals had been tested in CHO cells. Of these, all but one was a direct-acting alkylating agent. Bradley *et al.*[37] reported that 191 chemicals were tested in V-79 cells of which 119 were polycyclic aromatic hydrocarbons. Clive *et al.*[38] reported that of 48 chemicals tested in L5178Y cells, 25 were anthraquinones. The ability of any one of these assays to detect mutagens/carcinogens from a variety of chemical classes, and the ability of CHO cells to detect chemicals other than direct-acting mutagens has not been adequately demonstrated.

Assay Selection

Selection of assays to be used in screening programs for potential carcinogens is dependent upon factors such as assay reliability and reproducibility, level of development, and correlation with carcinogenicity.

Reliability of the test system may be defined as its ability to predict accurately the *in vivo* activity of the test agent. To determine reliability, it is necessary to demonstrate that the test shows agreement to an identified standard. In this instance, the standard against which test performance is measured is the rodent bioassay. Tests are validated by comparison of test results in the two systems. A test which accurately identifies a high percentage of known carcinogens is assumed to predict the carcinogenicity of chemicals of unknown activity with the same degree of accuracy.

In determining reliability, it is assumed that the standard against which the test is measured accurately predicts carcinogenicity. Since the ultimate concern is with human carcinogenicity, it is further assumed that the ability of a chemical to produce cancer in animals is a reflection of its ability to induce cancer in man. Although there may be inherent errors in both of these assumptions, they are essential if *in vitro* testing is to be used for identification of carcinogens.

Equally important to the process of identification of carcinogens is the ability of *in vitro* tests to identify accurately noncarcinogens. A test which does not discriminate between carcinogens and noncarcinogens but gives positive results with the universe of tested chemicals, is virtually useless.

The ability of a test system to identify carcinogens is called sensitivity; the ability to identify noncarcinogens is called specificity; sensitivity and specificity together are called accuracy. Unfortunately, reliable negative carcinogenicity data are scarce. A review of the test results for reported negative carcinogens sometimes shows technical or data insufficiencies which cast doubt on the validity of negative results.

In a review performed for the U.S. EPA's Gene-Tox Program a panel of experts reviewed the published literature on 510 chemicals, including 277 previously evaluated by the International Agency for Research on Cancer (IARC). Of these, only two were considered to have been adequately tested to be considered as noncarcinogens. An additional seven chemicals were designated as "limited negatives". Limited in this context means that the test chemical did not induce a significant positive response in one or more independent studies using optimal duration of treatment, dose range and numbers of animals. The two chemicals designated as noncarcinogens were found not to cause a significant number of tumors in an adequate number of animals in lifetime studies in at least two species at the maximum tolerated dose. The need for strict standards in designating a chemical as a noncarcinogen is self-evident. However, it is also immediately obvious that such a limited data base of noncarcinogens presents real problems in evaluating test systems for their ability to predict accurately both carcinogens and noncarcinogens.

Reproducibility of test results applies not only to reproducibility within the same laboratory but also to agreement of results in the same assay performed in different laboratories. For screening purposes, qualitative reproducibility is more crucial than quantitative reproducibility. Quantitative differences may be attributed to differences in S-9 preparations and other protocol variations. Qualitative differences are more serious. A carcinogen which is active in a particular test should be active in that assay each time it is tested. Not only should results be consistent from laboratory to laboratory but any given laboratory should also be able to reproduce its own results on a given sample.

The degree of development of a particular assay system should also be taken into consideration when selecting tests for use in a screening program. This includes a consideration of the number of laboratories performing the assay, degree of protocol standardization and a consideration of the number of chemicals and chemical classes which have been tested. A test which is highly suitable for polycyclic aromatic hydrocarbons may not be as well-suited for testing arylamines, for example.

It is generally agreed that the use of several tests in a battery is a better approach to carcinogen screening than the use of a single test for this purpose. The tests used in a battery should not be limited to prokaryotic or lower eukaryotic test systems and should include assays for more than one genetic endpoint. In selecting tests to be used in a battery, consideration should also be given to the physical and chemical nature of the test agent. Although not now routinely performed, tests for promoters of carcinogenicity should also be included in the ideal battery.

Unless results are uniform, analysis of data from a battery of tests can be difficult. Brusick[39] has proposed a system of data analysis which assigns weights to each test on the basis of test performance and endpoint measured. Potency, defined as the lowest positive or highest negative dose tested, is also factored into the analysis. A combined score for the chemical is calculated and agents are classified as having insufficient response to be categorized as genotoxic agents, or they are classified as suspect, confirmed or potent genotoxic agents. Other schemes for assessing multi-test data have been proposed[40,41] each of which is a significant attempt to resolve the problem of data analysis and interpretation.

SYSTEMATIC ATTEMPTS TO EVALUATE TEST PERFORMANCE

The Gene-Tox Program

The Gene-Tox Program sponsored by the U.S. Environmental Protection

Agency is a multi-phased effort to review and evaluate, using the published literature, selected bioassays for mutagenicity and related endpoints. During Phase I, Work Groups of experts in 23 areas of genetic toxicology evaluated literature published in the ten year period from 1969-1979 to assess system performance, chemicals tested and the ability of the assay to discriminate between carcinogens and noncarcinogens. The 23 Work Groups yielded a total of 36 state-of-the-art reviews (published in *Mutation Research Reviews in Genetic Toxicology*) which include lists of chemicals tested, suggested protocols and guidelines for data presentation.

As a result of the Phase I effort, a data base of evaluated test results on over 2,600 chemicals was established and analyzed to determine which tests or combination of tests could be used for: (1) routine screening; (2) testing specific classes of chemicals for their ability to induce genetic damage; (3) discriminating between carcinogens and noncarcinogens; and (4) to predict heritable mutagenic risk. In addition, the data gathered in Phase I were also used to assess the extent of assay development and to distinguish those tests which could be considered to be "routine" from those which should be considered to be developmental. The results of this phase of the Program will also be published in *Mutation Research Reviews in Genetic Toxicology*.

The International Collaborative Program for the Evaluation of Short-Term Tests for Carcinogenicity

The International Collaborative Program was a laboratory study to determine the ability of a series of assays, ranging from bacterial assays to *in vivo* mammalian studies, to correctly identify carcinogens and noncarcinogens. In this study, 42 chemicals—25 carcinogens, 12 noncarcinogens and 5 chemicals classified as neither carcinogens nor noncarcinogens—were tested in 35 assays in 58 to 60 laboratories (not all laboratories performed all assays so the total number varies). All laboratories used coded samples of chemicals supplied from a common source. Each laboratory, however, used the protocol in place at that facility at the time the study was conducted. Because of variations in protocol, the 35 assays yielded 63 sets of test results.

Analysis of the data led to the following conclusions: (1) there was a wide inter-laboratory variation in both qualitative and quantitative response of the same agent when tested in the same system; (2) there appears to be a need for inclusion of mammalian assay systems in any battery approach to testing. For example, the majority of chemicals which gave negative results in the Ames assay, were correctly identified by one or more of the *in vitro* mammalian systems studied; (3) there is probably a maximum number of tests which should be used in a screening battery. Although the detection of carcinogens increased as the number of tests in the battery increased, so too did the number of noncarcinogens which gave a positive response in one or more test systems.

At the end of the Program, 11 carcinogens were identified as being difficult to detect in short-term assays and five noncarcinogens had given a sufficient number of positive responses to be considered presumptive carcinogens which should be retested in a long-term animal bioassay.

A second phase of this program has been initiated. In this phase, multiple laboratories will concentrate on testing ten chemicals which are known to be difficult to detect in short-term bioassays. All chemicals will be from a common source, but chemicals will not be coded. Choice of protocol has been left to the investigator.

For a complete discussion of Phase I, *see* reference 42.

Other systematic approaches to the evaluation of short-term assays have been undertaken, including an analysis of the ability of short-term assays to detect pesticides[43] and a series of reports prepared for the International Commission for Protection Against Environmental Mutagens and Carcinogens (ICPEMC).[44] Each of these studies has a common goal of identifying those short-term assays which most efficiently predict carcinogenicity and of determining the most efficient use of these assays to optimize detection of hazard.

USE

There are several current and future uses for data obtained from assays for genotoxicity. A complete discussion of these is outside the scope of this review but some examples of such uses will be given. Short-term assays may be or are being used: to predict biological reactivity other than carcinogenicity; to set priorities for further testing; to support the qualitative case for presumptive carcinogenicity; to elucidate possible mechanisms of action of chemical carcinogens; to aid in the interpretation of available information on chemical carcinogens; to predict risk from mutation to future generations and to predict health effects other than heritable mutation and cancer.

FUTURE DIRECTIONS

Genetic toxicology as a science is entering into its second decade. In the first years following the demonstration that carcinogens also had mutagenic potential which could be detected in short-term, primarily *in vitro* assays, much emphasis was placed on developing assays which would detect carcinogens with a high degree of accuracy, in a relatively short period of time and at a relatively low cost. *In vitro* assay systems were developed which employed indicator organisms and activation systems which were manipulated to emphasize detection rather than to mimic the *in vivo* situation with its complex detoxification mechanisms. Even with the development and use of *in vivo* systems, the emphasis continued to focus on detection of carcinogens with only limited emphasis on mechanism of action. Recently, the importance of the complex interactions in the whole animal, especially the importance of tissue-specific and organ-specific repair capabilities in the response to genotoxic agents has been recognized. While screening programs for the accurate detection of carcinogens are important, and new and improved methodologies in this area are always necessary, future emphasis should be upon the development of *in vivo* models which can be more easily extrapolated to man. Emphasis should be placed on the influence of repair, immune response and hormonal balance in the final outcome of exposure to genotoxic agents. *In vivo* assays for the direct measurement of DNA damage and somatic cell mutation should also be emphasized. Although it is recognized that only germ cell mutation is of consequence to future generations, somatic cell mutation with its implications for cancer, chronic diseases and the aging process should not be ignored.

REFERENCES

1. National Academy of Sciences, *Identifying and Estimating the Genetic Impact of Chemical Mutagens*. Washington, DC: National Academy Press (1982)
2. Gabridge, M.G., and Legator, M.S., A host-mediated assay for the detection of mutagenic compounds. *Proc. Soc. Exptl. Biol. Med.* 130: 831-834 (1969)
3. Huberman, E., Aspiras, L., Heidelberger, C., Grover, P.L., and Sims, P., Mutagenicity to mammalian cells of epoxides and other derivatives of polycyclic hydrocarbons. *Proc. Natl. Acad. Sci. USA* 68: 3195-3199 (1971)
4. Huberman, E., Donovan, P.J., and DiPaolo, J.A., Mutation and transformation of cultured mammalian cells by N-acetoxy-N-2-fluorenylacetamide. *J. Natl. Cancer Inst.* 48: 837-840 (1972)
5. Ames, B.N., Gurney, F.G., Miller, J.A., and Bartsch, H., Carcinogens as frameshift mutagens: Metabolites and derivatives of acetylaminofluorene and other aromatic amine carcinogens. *Proc. Natl. Acad. Sci. USA* 69: 3128-3132 (1972)
6. Ames, B.N., Sims, P., and Grover, P.L., 1972b. Epoxides of polycyclic hydrocarbons are frameshift mutagens. *Science* 176: 47-49 (1972)
7. Malling, H.V., Dimethylnitrosamine: Formation of mutagenic compounds by interaction with mouse liver microsomes. *Mutation Res.* 13: 425-429 (1971)
8. Ames, B.N., Durston, W.E., Yamasaki, E., and Lee, F.D., Carcinogens are mutagens: A simple test system combining liver homogenates for activation and bacteria for detection. *Proc. Natl. Acad. USA* 70: 2281-2285 (1973)
9. McCann, J., Choi, E., Yamasaki, E., and Ames, B.N., Detection of carcinogens as mutagens in the *Salmonella*/microsome test: Part I: Assay of 300 chemicals. *Proc. Natl. Acad. Sci. USA* 72: 5135-5139 (1975)
10. Berger, R., and Bernheim, A., Cytogenetic studies on Burkitt's lymphoma-leukemia. *Cancer Genet. Cytogenet.* 7: 231-244 (1982)
11. Atkin, N.B., and Baker, M.C., Nonrandom chromosome changes in carcinoma of the cervix uteri. I. Nine near-diploid tumors. *Cancer Genet. Cytogenet.* 7: 209-222 (1982)
12. Berenblum, I., and Shubik, P., A new quantitative approach to the study of the stages of chemical carcinogenesis in the mouse's skin. *Brit. J. Cancer* 1: 383-391 (1947)
13. Mondal, S., Brankow, D.W., and Heidelberger, C., Two-stage chemical oncogenesis in cultures of C3H/10T½ cells. *Cancer Res.* 36: 2254-2260 (1976)
14. Yotti, L.P., Chang, C.C., and Trosko, J.E., Elimination of metabolic cooperation in Chinese hamster cells by a tumor promoter. *Science* 206: 1089-1091 (1979)
15. Ames, B.N., McCann, J., and Yamasaki, E., Methods for detecting carcinogens and mutagens with the *Salmonella*/mammalian-microsome mutagenicity test. *Mutation Res.* 31: 347-364 (1975)

16. Green, M.H.L., and Muriel, W.J., Mutagen testing using trp[+] reversion in *Escherichia coli. Mutation Res.* 38: 3–32 (1976)

17. Clive, D., Flamm, W.G., Machesko, M.R., and Bernheim, N.J., A mutational assay system using the thymidine kinase locus in mouse lymphoma cells. *Mutation Res.* 16: 77–87 (1972)

18. Hsie, A.W., Brimer, P.A., Mitchell, T.J., and Gosslee, D.G., Dose response for mutagen-induced mutations to 6-thioguanine resistance in Chinese hamster ovary cells. *Exp. Cell Res.* 95: 416–424 (1975)

19. Chu, E.H.Y., and Malling, H.V., Mammalian cell genetics II. Chemical induction of specific locus mutations in Chinese hamster cells *in vitro. Proc. Natl. Acad. Sci. USA* 61: 1306-1312 (1968)

20. Bridges, B.A., and Huckle, J., Mutagenesis of cultured mammalian cells by X-rays and ultraviolet light. *Mutation Res.* 10: 141-151 (1970)

21. Baker, R.M., Brunette, D.M., Mankovitz, R., Thompson, L.H., Whitemore, G.F., Siminovich, L., and Till, J.E., Ouabain resistant mutants of mouse and hamster cells in culture. *Cell* 1: 9-21 (1974)

22. Office of Technology, *The Role of Genetic Testing in the Prevention of Occupational Illness.* Washington, DC (1983)

23 Slater, E.E., Anderson, M.D., and Rosenkranz, H.S., Rapid detection of mutagens and carcinogens. *Cancer Res.* 31: 970-973 (1971)

24. Kada, T., Tutikawa, K., and Sadaie, Y., *In vitro* and host-mediated "rec-assay" procedures for screening chemical mutagens; and phloxine, a mutagenic red dye detected. *Mutation Res.* 16: 165-174 (1972)

25. Williams, G.M., Carcinogen induced DNA repair in primary rat liver cell cultures: A possible screen for chemical carcinogens. *Cancer Lett.* 1: 231-236 (1976)

26. Mirsalis, J.C., in: *Banbury Report 13: Indicators of Genotoxic Exposure.* Cold Spring Harbor, New York (1982)

27. Sega, G.A., Unscheduled DNA synthesis in the germ cells of male mice exposed *in vivo* to the chemical mutagen ethyl methanesulfonate. *Proc. Natl. Acad. Sci. USA* 71: 4955-4959 (1974)

28. Mirsalis, J.C., Tyson, C.K., and Butterworth, B.E., Detection of genotoxic carcinogens in the *in vivo-in vitro* hepatocyte DNA repair assay. *Env. Mutagen.* 4: 553-562 (1982)

29. Heidelberger, C., Freeman, A.E., Pienta, R.J., Sivak, A., Bertram, J.S., Castro, B.C., Dunkel, V.C., Francis, M.C., Kakunaga, T., Little, J.B., and Schechtman, L.M., Cell transformation by chemical agents: A review and analysis of the literature: A report of the U.S. EPA's Gene-Tox program. *Mutation Res.* 114: 283-347 (1983)

30. Berwald, Y., and Sachs, L., *In vitro* cell transformation with chemical carcinogens. *Nature* 200: 1182-1184 (1963)

31. Berwald, Y., and Sachs, L., *In vitro* transformation of normal cells to tumor cells by carcinogenic hydrocarbons. *J. Natl. Cancer Inst.* 35: 641-661 (1965)

32. Aaronson, S.A., and Todaro, G.J., Basis for the acquisition of malignant potential by mouse cells cultivated *in vitro. Science* 162: 1024-1026 (1968)

33. Reznikoff, C.A., Brankow, D.W., and Heidelberger, C., Establishment and characterization of a cloned line of C3H mouse embryo cells sensitive to postconfluence inhibition of division. *Cancer Res.* 33: 3231-3238 (1973)

34. Freeman, A.E., Price, P.J., Igel, H.J., Young, J.C., Maryak, J.M., and Huebner, R.J., Morphological transformation of rat embryo cells induced by diethylnitrosamine and murine leukemia virus. *J. Natl. Cancer Inst.* 44: 65-78 (1970)

35. Castro, B.C., and DiPaolo, J.A., Virus, chemicals and cancer (A review). *Prog. Med. Virol.* 16: 1–47 (1973)
36. Hsie, A.W., Casciano, D.A., Couch, D.B., Krahn, D.F., O'Neill, J.P., and Whitfield, B.L., The use of Chinese hamster ovary cells to quantify specific locus mutation and to determine mutagenicity of chemicals. A report of the Gene-Tox Program. *Mutation Res.* 86: 193–214 (1981)
37. Bradley, M.O., Bhuyan, B., Francis, M.C., Langenbach, R., Peterson, A., and Huberman, E., Mutagenesis by chemical agents in V-79 Chinese hamster cells: A review and analysis of the literature. A report of the Gene-Tox Program. *Mutation Res.* 87: 81–142 (1981)
38. Clive, D., McKuen, R., Spector, J.F.S., Piper, C., and Mavourin, K.H., Specific gene mutations in L5178Y cells in culture: A report of the U.S. EPA Gene-Tox Program. *Mutation Res.* 115: 225–251 (1983)
39. Brusick, D., in: Health risk analysis: Proceedings of the third life sciences symposium (C.R. Richmond, P.J. Walsh, and E.D. Copenhaver, eds.), The Franklin Institute Press, Philadelphia (1981)
40. Squire, R.A., Ranking animal carcinogens: A proposed regulatory approach. *Science* 214: 877–880 (1981)
41. Weisburger, J.H., and Williams, G.M., Carcinogen testing: Current problems and new approaches. *Science* 214: 401–407 (1981)
42. de Serres, F.J., and Ashby, J., in: *Progress in Mutation Research*, Vol. 1, Elsevier, North Holland, New York (1981)
43. Waters, M., Sandhu, S., Simmon, V., Mortelmans, K., Mitchell, A., Jorgenson, T., Jones, D., Valencia, R., and Garret, D., in: *Genetic Toxicology and Agricultural Perspectives* (F.A. Fleck, and A. Hollaender, eds.), Basic Life Sciences, Vol. 21, Plenum Press, New York (1982)
44. International Commission for Protection Against Mutagens and Carcinogens, Mutagenesis testing as an approach to carcinogenesis. ICPEMC Committee 2 Final Report, Elsevier, North Holland, New York (1982)

4

The *Salmonella* Mutagenicity Assay for Identification of Presumptive Carcinogens

Errol Zeiger

National Institute of Environmental Health Sciences
National Institutes of Health
Research Triangle Park, North Carolina

INTRODUCTION

As a result of early speculations on the relationship of mutation to cancer,[1] a number of investigators attempted to use mutagenicity in bacteria as a means with which to identify chemical carcinogens and antitumor agents.[2,3] These efforts were, for the most part, unsuccessful because the bacterial strain used was capable of detecting only a highly specific base change in its DNA, and because no attempt was made to approximate the metabolism of the chemicals or to test purified metabolites. These two shortcomings were resolved when it was demonstrated that most carcinogenic chemicals required mammalian metabolic activation to produce the ultimate carcinogens,[4-6] and Ames and his colleagues developed and defined a series of mutants of *Salmonella typhimurium*[7-10] which were capable of being mutated by agents which induced base pair substitution and frameshift mutations.

Malling[11] and Ames[12] brought the *in vitro* mammalian metabolic activation systems and the indicator bacteria together and showed that a bacterial test combined with exogenous mammalian metabolic activation was capable of detecting a number of carcinogens as mutagens.[12,13] A number of subsequent studies[14-18] demonstrated that a high proportion of (activated) carcinogens tested in *Salmonella* were mutagens.

Another impetus for the promotion of the *Salmonella* and other short-term tests for identification of carcinogens is their rapidity, ease of performance, and relatively low cost. A chemical can be adequately tested in *Salmonella* by a single technician in two weeks at a cost of approximately $1,000 to $1,500 (the cost will vary according to the protocol used), whereas a carcinogenicity assay using rodents takes upwards of three to four years to run, requires a large staff and animal and laboratory facilities, and costs approximately $500,000. Other short-term tests using cultured mammalian cells or live rodents take longer to run and are more expensive than the *Salmonella* assay, but still cost less than a tenth of a carcinogenicity assay in rodents. As a result of these correlation studies and the rapidity with which the test can be performed, Ames' *Salmonella* test has been proposed and accepted as an initial procedure for identifying potential carcinogens for regulatory purposes and for further testing in genetic toxicity studies *in vitro* and in animals.

DESCRIPTION OF *SALMONELLA* STRAINS

The core of the *Salmonella* test is a series of *Salmonella typhimurium* tester strains developed by Dr. Bruce Ames and his colleagues[7-10] (Table 1). These strains all contain mutations in the histidine operon rendering the bacteria incapable of synthesizing histidine (histidine auxotrophs). When these cells are placed in growth medium lacking histidine, they are unable to grow and divide. They will grow only if histidine is provided to them in the medium or if they back-mutate (revert) to wild type and regain the ability to synthesize histidine (histidine prototrophs). The histidine-requiring strains that have been selected for the tester series contain different histidine mutations which revert to prototrophy by different molecular mechanisms and by different chemicals. For example, the missense mutation (G46) and the ochre mutation (G428) are both reverted by chemicals that induce base-pair substitution mutations, but because G46 contains a:

$$-C-C-C-$$
$$-G-G-G-$$

sequence and G428 contains a:

$$-T-A-A-$$
$$-A-T-T-$$

sequence at the mutated site, they would be expected to be mutated by different classes of chemicals. Strains TA102 and TA104 carry the *his* G428 mutation on a multicopy plasmid (pAQ1) rather than on the bacterial chromosome. The multiple copies of the mutation in the cell provide multiple targets for the mutagen under test and the cells are more likely to be mutated than cells containing a single copy of the gene, thereby increasing the sensitivity of the strain.[10] There are three different frameshift mutants, C3076, D3057, and D6610, that are reverted by frameshift-inducing chemicals of different specificities. The strains do show overlap in their responses to some chemicals, but chemicals exist which revert only one or two of the three mutants.

Additional mutations have been added to these tester strains to enhance their sensitivity to chemicals: A mutation which removes most of the cell wall (*rfa*) thereby making the cell more permeable to large molecules; a deletion of one of the DNA repair pathways (*uvr*B) interferes with the ability of the cells to

Table 1: *Salmonella* Strains Used for Mutagenicity Testing

Salmonella Strain	His Mutation	DNA Target	Mutational Specificity[1]	Excision Repair[2]	R Factor
TA1535	G46	−CCC− −GGG−	BPS	uvrB	−[3]
TA100	G46	−CCC− −GGG−	BPS + FS	uvrB	pKM101
TA1537	C3076	−CCCC− −GGGG−	FS	uvrB	−
TA97	D6610	−CCCCCC− −GGGGGG−	FS	uvrB	pKM101
TA1538	D3052	−CGCGCGCG− −GCGCGCGC−	FS	uvrB	−
TA98	D3052	−CGCGCGCG− −GCGCGCGC−	FS	uvrB	pKM101
TA102	G428	−TAA− −ATT−	BPS + FS	+	pKM101 + pAQ1
TA104	G428	−TAA− −ATT−	BPS + FS	uvrB	pKM101 + pAQ1

[1]BPS: base pair substitution; FS: frameshift
[2]uvrB: does not contain a functional excision repair pathway; +: normal excision repair pathways
[3]−: R factor not present

correctly repair many types of DNA damage, and, incidentally, confers a biotin requirement; and the addition of a defective bacterial virus (plasmid; pKM101) which appears to promote cellular processing of DNA damage by an error-prone repair system, thereby enhancing the levels of induced mutation. One side effect of the plasmid pKM101 is that strains TA100, TA102, and TA104 are no longer specific for base-pair substitution mutagens but are reverted by frameshift mutagens as well. The uvrB mutation appears to confer a disadvantage in the detection of bifunctional alkylating agents such as mitomycin C and malondialdehyde which require a functional ultraviolet-repair system for their mutagenicity.[19] As a result of these additional mutations, the strains respond not only to DNA-damaging events which would be mutagenic in cells with normal repair capabilities, but also to those DNA-damaging events which would not normally be detected at the specific mutant loci, and events occurring at low frequencies which would normally be repaired.

Although the strains used routinely for detecting mutagens have been made "supersensitive" by means of the various added mutations and modifications, their usefulness in testing for mutagens is not compromised by this enhanced sensitivity. Since the primary reason for using the *Salmonella* test system is the identification of chemicals which have the ability to cause genetic damage (measured here as mutation), the "supersensitive" tester cells simply enhance the level of detection and maximize the number of mutagens identified.

METABOLIC ACTIVATION

Many chemicals that exhibit toxicity in animals are not toxic *per se* but must be metabolized to a toxic form. One disadvantage of testing with bacteria is that they do not contain the drug metabolizing enzymes found in mammals. This limitation has been partially overcome by the development of a number of metabolic activation systems which have been designed to compensate for this lack of metabolic capability in the *Salmonella* tester strains. These activation systems can be grouped into three general categories: (a) Host mediated, where intact animals are used to activate the test chemical. In the host-mediated systems, the active mutagen is detected *in situ* in the animal, or in the urine or other body fluids of the animal treated with the test chemical; (b) metabolically competent mammalian cells in culture. These cells are co-cultivated with the tester bacteria and are used to generate active metabolites for the bacteria; and (c) organ homogenates from mammals (usually rodents) are used to metabolize chemicals in the presence of the bacterial tester strain.

Host-Mediated Systems

These systems have recently been discussed in detail[20] and will not be described here. Even though these systems have the advantage of generating metabolites in the intact animal, they have proven too insensitive for routine testing[21] and are probably best suited for studying specific chemicals known to be metabolized to mutagens. One other advantage of the host-mediated assay, as compared to *in vitro* systems, is that it has the capability of detecting metabolites produced by the intestinal flora of the test animal.[22] *In vitro* systems have been developed, however, which are designed to detect chemicals not metabolized by the liver or other organs, but by the animal's intestinal flora (see below). A number of factors must be taken into account when interpreting negative mutagenicity data from the host-mediated assay. Without additional pharmacological studies, it cannot be determined if the mutagenicity results are negative because the chemical is not metabolized to a mutagen or if other factors preclude detection of the mutagen. These other factors include: The distribution of the active chemicals, tissue-specific activation and detoxification mechanisms, and the half-life of the compound and its metabolites.

An assay procedure for mutagens in urine is available. Although such assays are not readily used as routine screening procedures for unknown chemicals, they have been used successfully to demonstrate mutagens in the urine of laboratory animals treated with chemicals that require metabolic activation for their mutagenic activity[20,23,24] and in humans exposed to known or suspected carcinogens.[20,25]

Metabolizing Mammalian Cells in Culture

Another mammalian activation system is the use of "feeder layers" of mammalian cells in culture which are capable of metabolizing chemicals for the bacterial cells which are not, themselves, capable of this metabolic activation.[26,27] In order for a test substance to respond in this system, it must be taken up by the metabolizing cell, metabolized, and the activated product released into the medium where it can be taken up by the bacteria. Thus, a negative response in this system may be a function of the uptake, release, and stability of the test substance and its metabolites rather than the absence of a mutagenic product. It is also possible that the feeder cells do not contain the necessary metabolic capabilities for activation of the particular test compound, since different cell lines start out with different metabolic capabilities and lose specific enzyme systems at different rates. Another disadvantage of using mammalian cell systems for routine testing is that the procedure is more time consuming than use of organ homogenates and the results are subject to more variability from day to day than organ homogenates.

Organ Homogenates

The most widely used systems at this time are those which employ microsomal enzymes, *in vitro*, from the livers (or other organs) of Aroclor 1254-induced rats, in the presence of the test chemical and the indicator organism. This is the simplest activation system to use and it has provided evidence for the mutagenicity of a large number of substances which had previously appeared to be non-mutagenic in other *in vitro* test systems.[11,12]

This *in vitro* activation system can be performed as a plate test with the test chemical, indicator microorganism, organ homogenate, and enzyme co-factors immobilized in agar on a petri dish, or as a suspension test using the above components in the same manner as a standard *in vitro* drug metabolism study. These procedures have been used successfully with bacterial, yeast, and mammalian cells.

There are several ways by which this approach may fail to detect a mutagen; for instance, (a) the chemical may be metabolized by tissues and structures other than liver-derived microsomal enzymes (*e.g.*, intestinal flora); (b) the active metabolite is too labile, or produced too slowly or at too low levels to achieve concentrations which permit diffusion into the indicator cell; and (c) the *in vitro* metabolism of the substance may not mimic the *in vivo* metabolism.

Because this is the system recommended by Ames and his co-workers for routine testing of chemicals,[13,19] it will be discussed in more detail.

The liver homogenate [usually the 9,000 g supernatant fraction (S-9) of rat liver homogenized in buffer] is able to provide the P450-mixed function oxidase metabolic pathways present in the intact liver. In order to enhance the activity of these enzymes in the liver, the animal is treated prior to sacrifice with an enzyme inducer, usually the polychlorinated biphenyl mixture Aroclor 1254, which produces a high, nonspecific induction,[12,28] although a similar spectrum of induction can be obtained by using 3-methylcholanthrene and β-naphthoflavone.[28] Induction with 3-methylcholanthrene or phenobarbital alone has also been used but it is not recommended for routine use since those treatments do not induce as wide a range of enzymes as does Aroclor 1254.

Following enzyme induction, a 9,000 g supernatant (S-9) is prepared from pooled, homogenized livers of the treated animals.[14,19] The S-9 is stored as frozen (-80°C) aliquots until needed. This S-9 contains the microsomal enzymes plus soluble enzymes, but is free of nuclear enzymes and cell debris. The S-9 fraction or purified microsome preparations from other organs have also been used, but there is no evidence that they will detect chemicals not detected with liver S-9. They are useful, however, in studies on the metabolism of chemicals by specific organs.[29,30]

TEST PROCEDURE

The experimental details and compositions of the various media and reagents can be found in Maron and Ames.[19]

To perform a *Salmonella* mutation plate test, the tester strains are grown overnight in nutrient broth. Bacteria, test chemical, and a metabolic activation preparation (S-9) mix or buffer, are added to molten (45°C) top agar containing biotin and a limited amount of histidine in a test tube, and mixed (Figure 1). This mixture is then poured over the surface of a minimal agar plate and incubated 48 hours to 72 hours at 37°C. Histidine-positive (his$^+$) mutants are scored as bacterial colonies arising above a background lawn of histidine-negative cells (Figure 2). The limited amount of histidine is included in the agar to allow the cells to undergo a few divisions (thereby forming the background lawn), but not enough to allow discrete visible colonies to form. These few divisions enhance the sensitivity of the cells to mutagens since dividing cells are more sensitive to DNA insult. The identity of the tester strains and the integrity of the genetic markers should be checked in each experiment.[19,31,32]

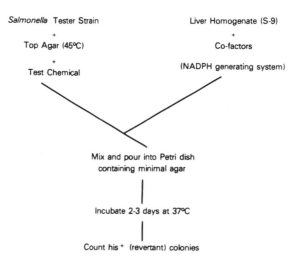

Figure 1: Schematic representation of the various steps in the *Salmonella* plate assay (*see* text for details).

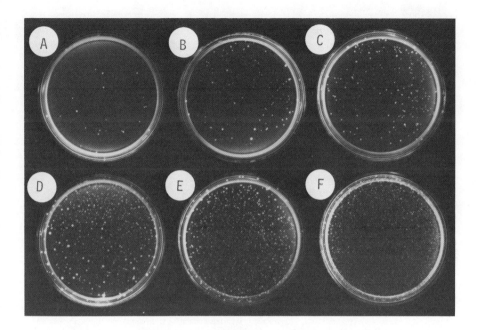

Figure 2: Dose-response in the *Salmonella* test showing his[+] revertant colonies. A: Control, no mutagen; B–F: increasing concentrations of mutagen with increasing numbers of his[+] colonies per plate.

Ideally, one should titrate the S-9 concentrations against chemicals being tested for mutagenicity, since different chemicals require different S-9 concentrations for optimal mutagenicity. This has been demonstrated in studies with benzo(a)pyrene,[33] dimethylnitrosamine,[34] and N,N'-dimethylaminoazobenzene,[35] among others. If chemicals with known structures and/or metabolism are being tested, knowledge of the relevant literature will allow the experimenter to select a low (1% to 5%), high (30% to 50%), or intermediate (5% to 20%) level of S-9 for the initial test. When a large number of chemicals with unknown structures and metabolism routes are being tested, it is impractical to determine the optimal S-9 level for each chemical. In this type of situation, the most effective testing scheme is to use an intermediate level of S-9 and, if a negative or equivocal response is seen, test at a higher, and possibly, a lower S-9 concentration. In the great majority of cases, a higher S-9 concentration (approximately 30%) will be more effective than a lower one.

Testing should be done at multiple doses, the high dose limited by toxicity, solubility, or availability of the test sample. Toxicity is indicated by a thinning or loss of the background lawn of his[-] bacteria, or a reduction in the number of his[+] revertant colonies compared to the solvent control. Two to three plates are run for each dose, and concurrent solvent and positive controls are included. The positive controls are chosen to test the strain and the integrity of the metabolic activation system. The test has usually been run using at least four tester strains

(TA98, TA100, TA1535, and TA1537) both with and without metabolic activation, although Maron and Ames[19] have recommended that TA97 and TA102 replace TA1537 and TA1535, respectively. This will be addressed below. Because the test is so rapid, repeat tests can be run to confirm the original finding or to test at other sample concentrations, depending on the original findings.

VARIATIONS OF THE TEST

A number of variations of the *Salmonella* test have been developed (Table 2) and, in some cases, allow the detection of mutagens which are poorly, or not detected using the standard plate test. Knowledge of the structures and/or properties of the test chemicals can aid in the selection of alternative procedures to the standard plate test.

Table 2: Variations on *Salmonella* Testing Procedures

Test Type	Uses	Reference Number
1. Plate test	General screening	13,19
2. Preincubation	General screening Aliphatic nitrosamines Formaldehyde Pyrrolizidine alkaloids	36-38,41
3. Spot test	Preliminary screening	8
4. Chamber incubation	Volatiles Gases	39,40
5. Reductive metabolism (a) Enzymic (b) Cecal flora/fecal extracts	 Benzidine dyes Benzidine dyes Glycosides	41-44
6. β-Glucuronidase treatment	Urine samples Glycosides	23,24,42,45
7. Suspension assay	Obtaining quantitative mutation frequency data	11,46
8. Host mediated assay	*In vivo* activation of mutagens	20

Preincubation Test

In the preincubation test developed by Yahagi *et al.*,[36] the bacteria, test chemical, and S-9 mix are added to the tube and incubated for 20 minutes to 1 hour at either 25°C or 37°C prior to the addition of the top agar. This procedure has a number of advantages over the standard plate test. Because the test chemical, cells, and S-9 mix are allowed to react prior to the addition of the top agar, both the chemical and the enzymes in the S-9 mix are at higher concentrations than they would be after addition of the agar and pouring onto the plate. This concentration effect has produced positive results with a number of chemicals that were negative in the standard plate test, such as dimethylnitrosamine,[34] pyrrolizidine alkaloids,[37] and formaldehyde.[38] Also, volatile chemicals are less likely to escape at the 25°C preincubation temperature than at the 45°C temperature of the top agar.

Volatile Chemicals

Volatile chemicals and gases have been successfully tested by exposing the bacteria in the petri plate to the vapor phase of the test chemical in a desiccator or other enclosed chamber. This system has worked well for volatile halogenated aliphatic chemicals.[39,40]

Reductive Metabolism

Although the procedures described above are designed for chemicals that require aerobic (oxidative) metabolism for their activation, many substances, such as benzidine dyes, require an initial reduction step. These reductive pathways occur in the mammalian liver *in situ* and in the mammalian gut through the action of the normal gut flora. Therefore, chemicals which may be metabolized to mutagens *in vivo* may appear to be non-mutagenic when tested using the standard (aerobic) metabolic activation protocols.

Procedures have been developed which use an altered S-9 mix in a preincubation protocol,[41] or cultures or extracts of rodent or human fecal bacteria.[42-44] These systems have worked well for benzidine dyes, which require an initial reductive metabolism.[41,44]

Conjugated Mutagens

A number of plant-derived substances are in the form of glycosides, which are not mutagenic directly and cannot be metabolized by liver, or other organ enzymes to a mutagen. Cecal flora, however, contain the glycosidases capable of hydrolyzing these glycosides. Fecal extracts or plant glucosidases used in place of S-9 mix in the plate and preincubation tests have produced active mutagens from these glycosides.[42,43,45]. In intact organisms, many mutagens are conjugated and excreted in their conjugated forms. When testing the urine of individuals or test animals for the presence of mutagens, it is necessary to add glucuronidases to release the active mutagen since *Salmonella* do not contain these enzymes.[20]

Spot Test

A rapid test for initial screening of a large number of chemicals is the spot test, originally developed by Iyer and Szybalski,[3] and adapted to *Salmonella* by Ames.[8] The procedure for this test is described in detail elsewhere.[19] It must be kept in mind that this is strictly a qualitative test and is designed to simply give a yes, no, or no-test answer. Since there are a number of chemicals which are mutagenic in the standard plate incorporation or preincubation tests, but are negative in the spot test, a negative response in the spot test cannot be taken as definitive. The spot test is designed to provide a rapid indication of which chemicals or test samples are likely to be mutagenic. All spot test results, therefore, must be confirmed in either the plate incorporation or preincubation test.

Suspension Assay

Variations of the *Salmonella* test protocol also exist in which cells are treated in suspension and both mutants and the surviving population are measured.[11,46] This procedure is more time consuming, but it does allow the calculation of mutation frequencies.

TESTING STRATEGY

If no information is available on the metabolism or potential mutagenicity of a series of chemicals, or if a series of coded chemicals is to be tested, it is prudent to use at least four tester strains (TA98, TA100, TA1535, and TA1537) with and without metabolic activation in a plate or preincubation procedure. The tester series should include strains that detect base-pair substitutions as well as frameshift mutations. Although Maron and Ames[19] recommend replacing TA1535 and TA1537 with TA102 and TA97, respectively, these strains are relatively new and testing laboratories do not have much experience with them at the present time. Also, there is some question as to whether or not TA97 is more effective than TA1537 in detecting mutagens not detected by the other strains (E. Zeiger, unpublished results). In addition to the strains listed in Table 1, a number of other strains with different characteristics and sensitivities exist and are also available.[19] The preincubation test may be better than the plate test for routine screening of unknown chemicals because it has been shown to be more sensitive than the plate test and better for volatile chemicals as well.[38,47]

If a single chemical, or series of chemicals, related to a known class of mutagens is being tested, then the initial test need be only with the strain and metabolic activation procedure known to be best for those chemicals. Then, if negatives are obtained in this initial scheme, they can be tested further using other strains, activation procedures, protocols, etc. Likewise, a protocol employing reductive metabolism should be used if there is reason to believe that the chemical may require this type of metabolism for its activation, and a desiccator assay should be used for highly volatile substances. In any case, a chemical should not be declared "not mutagenic" unless it has been tested in at least four different tester strains, both with and without metabolic activation under appropriate test conditions.

STATISTICAL EVALUATION OF *SALMONELLA* TEST DATA

The majority of *Salmonella* test data in the literature has not been evaluated statistically. In general, decisions of "positive" and "negative" are made on an *ad hoc* basis. A number of reports in the literature rely on the so-called "two-fold" rule, which states that if a doubling of his[+] revertants over background is seen, the chemical is considered mutagenic, regardless of the number of doses or plates used. This "two-fold" rule can lead to false conclusions because it does not require a dose-related response, and therefore, a chemical can be called a mutagen if it causes a doubling of his[+] revertants, at one dose only. The rule does not require that the effect be reproducible and also ignores the magnitude of the response, giving as much weight to an increase from ten colonies to 20 colonies per plate, regardless of the variation around these counts, as an increase from 100 colonies to 200 colonies per plate.

The most appropriate determinant of a positive, mutagenic response is a reproducible, dose-related increase over background. Likewise, a chemical should not be declared negative in the *Salmonella* test unless it has been tested in a series of strains measuring different endpoints, with and without metabolic activation, and at doses up to toxic levels.

Recently, a number of statistical procedures have been proposed for the *Salmonella* assay,[48-50] but there is no consensus as to which particular procedure(s) should be used for data evaluation. It is clear, however, that regardless of the statistical evaluation procedure used, the data evaluated must meet a number of criteria, such as: The data must be derived from a defined protocol covering a range of doses both with and without metabolic activation; the results must be reproducible; and the anticipated carcinogenicity or non-carcinogenicity of the chemical must not be a consideration in the evaluation. The statistical system selected must be relevant to, and appropriate for, the data to be evaluated. For example, the possibility that the test data may not exhibit a Poisson distribution, or that the dose-response curve may turn down at the high doses, must be factored into the analysis.[48]

DATA REPORTING

Although a number of guidelines have been presented,[19,31] there is no generally agreed-upon format for presentation of *Salmonella* test data. This problem is not limited to the *Salmonella* test, but exists with other short-term tests and for carcinogenicity tests as well. In general, the data should be presented with a description of the test protocol(s) used, rather than simply referencing Ames *et al.*[13] or Maron and Ames,[19] since these protocols offer a number of alternatives, such as S-9 concentration, type and source of S-9, preincubation time, number of replicate plates, etc. Additionally, many laboratories use varying levels of S-9 co-factors, different agar compositions, cell growth conditions, etc., all of which can influence the ultimate response.

Results are best reported as mean plate counts plus or minus the standard error of the mean or standard deviation. Concurrent positive and solvent control data must be reported with the test results. As a rule, the solvent control counts should not be subtracted from the test plate counts; where mean plate counts minus mean control counts are presented, the relevant control values must also be given. Transformed data—*i.e.*, his$^+$ revertants per μg or μmol test chemical, or per ml, g, or unit sample—are not acceptable by themselves. The original plate count values must also be available since transformation of data can tend to exaggerate differences and lead to an incorrect conclusion. Also, fold-increases, by themselves, are misleading, because, for example, while a doubling from 100 his$^+$ colonies per plate to 200 colonies per plate would probably be significant, a doubling from one colony to two colonies would not.

CORRELATIONS WITH CARCINOGENICITY

The primary reason for screening chemicals using *Salmonella* is to obtain information as to the presumptive carcinogenicity of the chemicals. This justification is predicated on the assumption that carcinogens are mutagens, and, conversely, that mutagenic chemicals will be carcinogenic. Implicit in this reasoning is the conclusion that non-mutagens will not be carcinogenic. The fallacy of this latter assumption will be discussed below.

The conclusion, originally put forth by McCann *et al.*[14] and supported by others,[15-18] that carcinogens are mutagens and the majority of non-carcinogens are not mutagens, is based on biased data. The data used to justify this statement come from studies where the identity of the chemicals and their carcinogenicity were known to the investigators before they were tested. Because the investigators knew the identities of the chemicals and their "expected" mutagenicity, the test protocols could be modified or the tests repeated until the desired results were obtained. While these practices lead to a true picture of a chemical's mutagenicity and tend to maximize the carcinogenicity-mutagenicity correlations, they do not reflect the results that would be obtained from testing chemicals whose expected responses are not known.[51] Also, in the past, supporting evidence for a strong positive correlation was obtained from data published in the open literature. This source also maximizes the correlation and does not reflect the proportion of carcinogens that are not mutagenic, since negative data are often not submitted for publication.

An important factor that influences the reported correlations is the inadequate identification of non-carcinogens. Many chemicals have been identified as non-carcinogenic on the basis of their chemical structure or perfunctory tests for carcinogenicity;[52] relatively few chemicals have been tested in lifetime studies using adequate chemical exposures. This uncertainty in identifying non-carcinogens leads to an inaccurate estimate of the proportion of non-carcinogens that are positive in short-term tests, because many chemicals initially identified as non-carcinogens strictly on the basis of chemical structure may be carcinogenic if tested in a sufficient number of animals in lifetime studies. As a result, there are insufficient data available on adequately-tested non-carcinogens to support any statement regarding correlations between non-mutagens and non-carcinogens.

Another problem exists (in the literature) with respect to developing correlations between carcinogenicity and mutagenicity. Often, the chemicals that are tested come from a limited class of chemicals known or expected to be positive, such as direct-acting alkylating agents or polycyclic aromatic hydrocarbons. In such a situation, a strong positive correlation is obtained which is often used to justify the use of the system but, in actuality, reflects the activity of the chemicals rather than the responsiveness or relevance of the test system. This can be an advantage. Where correlations have been performed based on the structures of the chemicals, it was seen that some classes of carcinogens, such as nitro compounds, alkylating agents, and polycyclic aromatic hydrocarbons, exhibit high correlations, whereas chlorinated hydrocarbons and hormones show no correlation.[14,17,51] This lack of correlation may be the result of an inappropriate metabolic activation system, the insensitivity of the *Salmonella* tester strains to the type of DNA lesion produced, or the chemical may not be a mutagen, but exerts its carcinogenic effect through a different mechanism.

The ideal data base to use for establishing correlations between *Salmonella* (or other short-term test) results and rodent (or human) carcinogenicity is one where the carcinogenicity or structure of the chemicals is not known to the investigator beforehand, and the test results are all judged by the same criteria. Therefore, one does not know whether the short-term test results are "right" or "wrong." This approach will minimize the proportion of carcinogens detected, but will also eliminate bias from the correlations. In actual practice, however, additional testing using modified protocols would be done on chemicals whose structure would lead one to believe that the original test conditions were not appropriate. An example would be the need of some benzidine-based dyes for reducing conditions followed by an oxidative system, rather than a strictly oxidative system for their metabolism,[41] or the use of a closed system for alkyl halides which may be volatile under normal test conditions.[39,40]

SUMMARY

The *Salmonella* mutagenicity test has gained wide acceptance as an initial test for the identification of potential carcinogens. This is because the test is rapid and inexpensive to run, and it has demonstrated a positive correlation between mutagenicity and carcinogenicity in rodents. The use of data from the *Salmonella* test for making decisions on the carcinogenicity or non-carcinogenicity of a chemical must be tempered with the knowledge that all correlations with carcinogenicity or non-carcinogenicity developed to date are not perfect. However, based upon chemical class-related correlations, it can be safely assumed that a positive mutagenic response in some chemical classes is sufficient to indict a chemical as a carcinogen, although carcinogenicity still remains to be demonstrated. Alternatively, negative results for other classes of chemicals are not sufficient to support a presumption of non-carcinogenicity; a number of chemical classes also exist for which there are insufficient data to estimate the predictivity of the *Salmonella* test. Finally, it should be noted that there are no data available to show that a negative response with any other short-term test system negates the implications of the original *Salmonella* positive.

It would be desirable to have short-term microbial tests that will tell us not only if a chemical will be carcinogenic in animals but also the extent of carcinogenicity. However, there are problems in making these potency determinations. It is difficult to get agreement on a definition of mutagenic potency and even more difficult to get agreement on what potency in *Salmonella* (or other short-term tests) means in terms of carcinogenicity. A definition of carcinogenic potency is also problematical. Attempts to define carcinogenic and mutagenic potency are underway in many laboratories and the results of these exercises will determine whether it will be possible to extrapolate the potency of a carcinogenic chemical from its activity in a mutagenicity test. It must be kept firmly in mind that the *Salmonella* tests described here measure mutagenicity—not carcinogenicity. Our knowledge of the biology of mutagenicity and carcinogenicity is increasing, but is still sparse; for that reason we can discuss "correlations" but not causal relationships or mechanisms. Therefore, any qualitative or quantitative extension of results from these mutagenicity tests to carcinogenicity is an inference based on parallels in molecular mechanisms and on correlations between the two effects.

Because of the efficiency of the *Salmonella* tests and the ubiquity of potentially hazardous chemicals, far more chemicals will be identified as potential carcinogens than will be confirmed by long-term animal tests. Also, we will be in the position of considering a chemical as a potential human carcinogen years before definitive proof, as determined by long-term animal tests or epidemiological studies, is available. Until a chemical is confirmed as an animal (or human) carcinogen, it is important to minimize, if not eliminate, exposure. In the interim between the short-term mutagenicity test and the confirmatory animal or epidemiologic studies, the potential hazards of the chemical should be considered and attempts made to limit or eliminate exposure where possible.

REFERENCES

1. Burdette, W.J., The significance of mutation in relation to the origin of tumors: A review. *Cancer Res.* 15: 201-226 (1955)
2. Hemmerly, J., and Demerec, M., Tests of chemicals for mutagenicity. *Cancer Res.* Suppl. 3: 69-75 (1955)
3. Iyer, V.N., and Szybalski, W., Two simple methods for the detection of chemical mutagens. *Appl. Microbiol.* 6: 23-29 (1958)
4. Miller, J.A., and Miller, E.C., Chemical carcinogenesis: Mechanisms and approaches to its control. Guest Editorial. *J. Natl. Cancer Inst.* 47: v-xiv (1971)
5. Miller, E.C. and Miller, J.A., in: *Chemical Mutagens: Principles and Methods for Their Detection* (Hollaender, A., ed.), Vol. 1, pp 83-119, Plenum Publishing Corp., New York (1971)
6. Wright, A.S., The role of metabolism in chemical mutagenesis and chemical carcinogenesis. *Mutation Res.* 75: 215-241 (1980)
7. Whitfield, H.J., Jr., Martin, R.G., and Ames, B.N., Classification of aminotransferase (C gene) mutants in the histidine operon. *J. Mol. Biol.* 21: 335-355 (1966)
8. Ames, B.N., in: *Chemical Mutagens: Principles and Methods for Their Detection*, (Hollaender, A., ed.), Vol. 1, pp 267-282, Plenum Publishing Corp., New York (1971)
9. Levin, D.E., Yamasaki, E., and Ames, B.N., A new *Salmonella* tester strain, TA97, for the detection of frameshift mutagens: A run of cytosines as a mutational hot-spot. *Mutation Res.* 94: 315-330 (1982)
10. Levin, D.E., Hollstein, M.C., Christman, M.F., Schwiers, E.A., and Ames, B.N., A new *Salmonella* tester strain (TA102) with A:T base pairs at the site of mutation detects oxidative mutagens. *Proc. Natl. Acad. Sci. USA* 79: 7445-7449 (1982)
11. Malling, H.V., Dimethylnitrosamine: Formation of mutagenic compounds by interaction with mouse liver microsomes. *Mutation Res.* 13: 425-429 (1971)
12. Ames, B.N., Durston, W.E., Yamasaki, E., and Lee, F.D., Carcinogens are mutagens: A simple test system combining liver homogenates for activation and bacteria for detection. *Proc. Natl. Acad. Sci. USA* 70: 2281-2285 (1973)

13. Ames, B.N., McCann, J., and Yamasaki, E., Methods for detecting carcinogens and mutagens with the *Salmonella*/mammalian-microsome mutagenicity test. *Mutation Res.* 31: 347-364 (1975)
14. McCann, J., Choi, E., Yamasaki, E., and Ames, B.N., Detection of carcinogens as mutagens in the *Salmonella*/microsome test: Assay of 300 chemicals. *Proc. Natl. Acad. Sci. USA* 72: 5135-5139 (1975)
15. Sugimura, T., Sato, S., Nagao, M., Yahagi, T., Matsushima, T., Seino, Y., Takeuchi, M., and Kawachi, T., in: *Fundamentals in Cancer Prevention* (P.N. Magee *et al.*, eds.), pp 191-215, University of Tokyo Press, Tokyo (1976)
16. Purchase, I.F.H., Longstaff, E., Ashby, J., Styles, J.A., Anderson, D., Lefevre, P.A., and Westwood, F.R., An evaluation of six short-term tests for detecting organic chemical carcinogens. *Brit. J. Cancer* 37 (Appendix II): 924-930 (1978)
17. Rinkus, S.J., and Legator, M.S., Chemical characterization of 465 known or suspected carcinogens and their correlation with mutagenic activity in the *Salmonella typhimurium* system. *Cancer Res.* 39: 3289-3318 (1979)
18. Bartsch, H., Malaveille, C., Camus, A.-M., Martel-Planche, G., Brun, G., Hautefeuille, A., Sabadie, N., Barbin, A., Kuroki, T., Drevon, C., Piccoli, C., and Montesano, R., Validation and comparative studies on 180 chemicals with *S. typhimurium* strains and V79 Chinese hamster cells in the presence of various metabolizing systems. *Mutation Res.* 76: 1-50 (1980)
19. Maron, D.M., and Ames, B.N., Revised methods for the *Salmonella* mutagenicity test. *Mutation Res.* 113: 173-215 (1983)
20. Legator, M.S., Bueding, E., Batzinger, R., Conner, T.H., Eisenstadt, E., Farrow, M.G., Ficsor, G., Hsie, A., Seed, J., and Stafford, R.S., An evaluation of the host-mediated assay and body fluid analysis. A report of the U.S. Environmental Protection Agency Gene-Tox Program. *Mutation Res.* 98: 319-374 (1982)
21. Simmon, V.F., Rosenkranz, H.S., Zeiger, E., and Poirier, L.A., Mutagenic activity of chemical carcinogens and related compounds in the intraperitoneal host-mediated assay. *J. Natl. Cancer Inst.* 62: 911-918 (1979)
22. Gabridge, M.G., Denunzio, A., and Legator, M.S., Cycasin: Detection of associated mutagenic activity *in vivo. Science* 163: 689-691 (1969)
23. Durston, W.E., and Ames, B.N., A simple method for the detection of mutagens in urine: Studies with the carcinogen 2-acetylaminofluorene. *Proc. Natl. Acad. Sci. USA* 71: 737-741 (1974)
24. Commoner, B., Vithayathil, A.J., and Henry, J.I., Detection of metabolic carcinogen intermediates in urine of carcinogen-fed rats by means of bacterial mutagenesis. *Nature* 249: 850-852 (1974)
25. Yamasaki, E., and Ames, B.N., Concentration of mutagens from urine by adsorption with the nonpolar resin XAD-2: Cigarette smokers have mutagenic urine. *Proc. Natl. Acad. Sci. USA* 74: 3555-3559 (1977)
26. Bos, R.P., Neis, J.M., van Gemert, P.J.L., and Henderson, P.T., Mutagenicity testing with the *Salmonella*/hepatocyte and the *Salmonella*/microsome assays. A comparative study with some known genotoxic compounds. *Mutation Res.* 124: 103-112 (1983)
27. Langenbach, R., and Oglesby, L., in: *Chemical Mutagens: Principles and Methods for Their Detection* (de Serres, F.J., ed.), Vol. 8, pp 55-93, Plenum Publishing Corp., New York (1983)
28. Ong, T.-M., Mukhtar, H., Wolf, C.R., and Zeiger, E., Differential effects of cytochrome P450-inducers on promutagen activation capabilities and enzymatic activities of S-9 from rat liver. *J. Environ. Pathol. Toxicol.* 4: 55-65 (1980)

29. Robertson, I.G.C., Philpot, R.M., Zeiger, E., and Wolf, C.R., Specificity of rabbit pulmonary cytochrome P-450 isozymes in the activation of several aromatic amines and aflatoxin B_1. *Mol. Pharmacol.* 20: 662-668 (1981)
30. Robertson, I.G.C., Sivarajah, K., Eling, T., and Zeiger, E., Activation of some aromatic amines to mutagenic products by prostaglandin endoperoxide synthetase. *Cancer Res.* 43: 476-480 (1983)
31. de Serres, F.J., and Shelby, M.D., Recommendations on data production and analysis using the *Salmonella*/microsome mutagenicity assay. *Mutation Res.* 64: 159-165 (1979)
32. Zeiger, E., Pagano, D.A., and Robertson, I.G.C., A rapid and simple scheme for confirmation of *Salmonella* tester strain phenotype. *Environ. Mutagen.* 3: 205-209 (1981)
33. Zeiger, E., Chhabra, R.S., and Margolin, B.H., Effects of the hepatic S9 fraction from Aroclor 1254-treated rats on the mutagenicity of benzo[a]-pyrene and 2-aminoanthracene in the *Salmonella*/microsome assay. *Mutation Res.* 64: 379-389 (1979)
34. Prival, M.J., King, V.D., and Sheldon, A.T., Jr., The mutagenicity of dialkyl nitrosamines in the *Salmonella* plate assay. *Environ. Mutagen.* 1: 95-104 (1979)
35. Zeiger, E., and Pagano, D.A., Comparative mutagenicity of dimethylamino-azobenzene and analogues in *Salmonella*. *Carcinogenesis* 3: 559-561 (1982)
36. Yahagi, T., Degawa, M., Seino, Y., Matsushima, T., Nagao, M., Sugimura, T., and Hashimoto, Y., Mutagenicity of carcinogenic azo dyes and their derivatives. *Cancer Lett.* 1: 91-96 (1975)
37. Yamanaka, H., Nagao, M., Sugimura, T., Furuya, T., Shirai, A., and Matsushima, T., Mutagenicity of pyrrolizidine alkaloids in the *Salmonella*/mammalian-microsome test. *Mutation Res.* 68: 211-216 (1979)
38. Haworth, S., Lawlor, T., Mortelmans, K., Speck, W., and Zeiger, E., *Salmonella* mutagenicity test results for 250 chemicals. *Environ. Mutagen.* 5 (Suppl. 1): 3-142 (1983)
39. Rannung, U., Johansson, A., Ramel, C., and Wachmeister, C.A., The mutagenicity of vinyl chloride after metabolic activation. *Ambio* 3: 194-197 (1974)
40. Simmon, V.F., Kauhanen, K., and Tardiff, R.G., in: *Progress in Genetic Toxicology* (Scott, D., Bridges, B.A., and Sobels, F.H., eds.), pp 249-258, Elsevier/North Holland, Amsterdam (1977)
41. Prival, M.J., and Mitchell, V.D., Analysis of a method for testing azo dyes for mutagenic activity in *Salmonella typhimurium* in the presence of flavin mononucleotide and hamster liver S9. *Mutation Res.* 97: 103-116 (1982)
42. Brown, J.P., and Dietrich, P.S., Mutagenicity of plant flavinols in the *Salmonella*/mammalian microsome test: Activation of flavinol glycosides by mixed glycosidases from rat cecal bacteria and other sources. *Mutation Res.* 66: 223-240 (1979)
43. Tamura, G., Gold, C., Ferro-Luzzi, A., and Ames, B.N., Fecalase: A model for activation of dietary glycosides to mutagens by intestinal flora. *Proc. Natl. Acad. Sci. USA* 77: 4961-4965 (1980)
44. Reid, T.M., Morton, K.C., Wang, C.Y., and King, C.M., Conversion of Congo red and 2-azoxyfluorene to mutagens following *in vitro* reduction by whole-cell rat cecal bacteria. *Mutation Res.* 117: 105-112 (1983)
45. Matsushima, T., Matsumoto, H., Shirai, A., Sawamura, M., and Sugimura, T., Mutagenicity of the naturally occurring carcinogen cycasin and synthetic methylazoxymethanol conjugates in *Salmonella typhimurium*. *Cancer Res.* 39: 3780-3782 (1979)

46. Zeiger, E., and Sheldon, A.T., Jr., The mutagenicity of heterocyclic N-nitros-amines for *Salmonella typhimurium. Mutation Res.* 57: 1-10 (1978)

47. Rosenkranz, H.S., Karpinsky, G., and McCoy, E.C., in: *Short-Term Test Systems for Determining Carcinogens* (Norpoth, K. and Garner, R.C., eds.), pp 19-57, Springer, Berlin (1980)

48. Margolin, B.H., Kaplan, N., and Zeiger, E., Statistical analysis of the Ames *Salmonella*/microsome test. *Proc. Natl. Acad. Sci. USA* 78: 3779-3783 (1981)

49. Stead, A.G., Hasselblad, V., Creason, J.P., and Claxton, L., Modeling the Ames test. *Mutation Res.* 85: 13-27 (1981)

50. Bernstein, L., Kaldor, J., McCann, J., and Pike, M.C., An empirical approach to the statistical analysis of mutagenesis data from the *Salmonella* test. *Mutation Res.* 97: 267-281 (1982)

51. Zeiger, E., in: *Environmental Mutagens and Carcinogens* (Sugimura, T., Kondo, S., and Takebe, H., eds.), pp 337-344, University of Tokyo Press, Tokyo/Alan R. Liss, Inc., New York (1982)

52. Purchase, I.F.H., Clayson, D.B., Preussmann, R., and Tomatis, L., in: *Evaluation of Short-Term Tests for Carcinogenesis* (de Serres, F.J. and Ashby, J., eds.), pp 21-32, Elsevier/North Holland (1981)

5

Detection of Carcinogens Based on *In Vitro* Mammalian Cytogenetic Tests

Suzanne M. Morris
Daniel A. Casciano
Bruce C. Casto

National Center for Toxicological Research
Jefferson, Arkansas

INTRODUCTION

The induction of the cancerous state by chemical and physical agents is a complex process. According to the somatic cell mutational theory of carcinogenesis, there are at least two phases in the development of a neoplasia. The initiating phase is brought about by direct interaction with DNA, resulting in a mutation, while the promoting phase, operating through an independent mechanism, allows clonal expansion of the initiated cell.[1] Chemical carcinogens, therefore, can be considered to be complete carcinogens, initiating agents or promoters. Complete carcinogens are those agents which are themselves capable of inducing the neoplastic state, in contrast to initiating agents and promoters which must work in concert to induce cancer.

Support for the mutational theory, in part, derives from the demonstration that reactive metabolites of carcinogens damage critical cellular macromolecules, especially DNA[2] and from evidence indicating that many carcinogens are also mutagens.[3,4] Because of these properties of chemical carcinogens, a number of assay systems were developed over the last ten years specifically directed toward detecting the interaction of a chemical with cellular DNA. The interaction of chemical and physical carcinogens with chromatin, either directly or indirectly, can also result in chromosomal rearrangements such as sister-chromatid exchanges and structural chromosomal aberrations. Thus, measurement of the induction of these cellular responses to chemical trauma may also be indicative of damage capable of inducing the neoplastic state.[5]

BACKGROUND

Chromosomal Aberrations

Subsequent to the recognition of chromosomes as carriers of genetic information, Boveri[6] developed the concept that the initiation and the progression of a normal cell to a cancer cell is caused by a change in its genetic material. Evans[7] suggested that the first clear demonstration that exposure of cells to a mutagen results in chromosomal aberrations was made more than seventy years ago when pollen cells from lilies were exposed to radium. Other reports followed demonstrating radiation-induced chromosomal aberrations in roundworms, fish, amphibians, insects and plants[8,9] and, fifty years after the initial observation, radiation-induced aberrations were observed in man.[10] The induction of mutations by chemical substances was first demonstrated by Auerbach[11,12] who found that mustard gas induced the entire array of mutagenic effects known to occur after X-irradiation: dominant lethal and viable mutations, recessive sex-linked and autosomal lethals and viables, large and small deletions, inversions, and translocations. Since then, many mutagenic carcinogens or their reactive metabolic derivatives, have been shown to react with DNA and to produce chromosomal aberrations.[13]

Studies of the human chromosomal breakage syndromes provide additional support for a relationship between chromosomal aberrations and cancer. These diseases, which include Bloom syndrome, ataxia telangiectasia, Fanconi anemia, and Werner syndrome, are associated with chromosomal instability and a predisposition to neoplasia (for a review, *see* Ray and German[14]). Each of these syndromes has specific neoplasias associated with the disease state and specific types of chromosomal alterations produced during the clinical course of the disease. Cells isolated from individuals with these disorders also display hypersensitivity to DNA-damaging agents. This hypersensitivity is manifested in several ways including increased chromosomal instability.[14,15] Heddle *et al.*[16] have further described these disease entities as mutagen-hypersensitive syndromes. In addition to chromosomal instability syndromes, individuals with certain syndromes which are characterized by specific stable anomalies such as Down, have a higher risk of developing cancers than individuals with normal karyotypes. Thus, although the exact nature of the relationship is as yet undefined, there appears to be more than a casual association between chromosomal aberrations and neoplasia.

Sandberg,[17] while recognizing that a relationship might exist between chromosomal abnormalities and human cancer, could observe defects in only about 50% of the cases studied. However, the development of high-resolution (1200 band stage) techniques[18,19] and the systematic study of malignant progression have led to the observations of non-random karyotypic changes associated with specific cancers. Yunis[20] reviewed cytogenetic findings of patients with acute leukemias and found cytogenetically abnormal clones in over 90% of the patients. Specific chromosomal defects have also been associated with certain tumors such as retinoblastoma[21,22] or Wilm's tumor.[23,24] Most commonly, these defects involve deletions of specific band segments but additions or marker chromosomes in certain tumors have also been found. Current studies are localizing the specific band involved in the aberrations associated with the formation of tumors.

High-resolution chromosome banding has also provided evidence for the importance of the specific breakpoints in the induction and progression of the disease state. In certain leukemias and lymphomas associated with specific rearrangements, the breakpoints on the chromosomes consistently map in specific regions or bands. Comparison of the breakpoints to the human gene map has led to observations that the rearrangement of specific genes (*e.g.*, immunoglobulin, oncogenes) may be of great importance in the induction of cancer.[20,25-27]

Sister-Chromatid Exchange

Sister-chromatid exchanges (SCE) were originally described by Taylor *et al.*[28] Cells from plant root tips were allowed to replicate once in the presence of tritiated thymidine followed by a subsequent replication cycle without the isotope. This resulted in mitotic chromosomes with three unlabelled DNA strands and one strand substituted with the radioactively labelled thymidine. SCE were visualized as exchanges of radioactive label from one sister chromatid to the other. The technical difficulties associated with this autoradiographic procedure restricted its experimental application. However, the description by Latt,[29] Wolff and Perry,[30] and Perry and Wolff[31] of procedures using bromodeoxyuridine (BUdR) to differentially label the chromatids gave great impetus to studies of SCE. These procedures were much easier to apply in the laboratory and produced fewer artefacts than those which utilized autoradiography.[32]

The use of analysis of SCE as a screen for genotoxic compounds was first suggested by the work of Latt[33] and Perry and Evans[34] in which cells exposed to known mutagens, carcinogens and clastogens had increased frequencies of SCE when compared to control cells. An increase in frequency of SCE was detected at doses of chemical which had little or no effect on the frequency of chromosomal aberrations.[33] However, as the concentration of chemicals increased, both the frequency of SCE and the frequency of chromosomal aberration also increased. This observation led to the suggestion that SCE might be related to formation of chromosomal aberrations. That is, chromosomal aberrations were the result of incomplete SCE, formed as the system responsible for SCE became saturated. However, subsequent experimental studies have shown no consistent relationship between the induction of SCE and chromosomal aberrations.[35-40] Studies also demonstrated the lack of a strong relationship between the formation of SCE and unscheduled DNA synthesis[41-43] or post-replication repair.[41] These findings suggested that formation of SCE might be related to the presence of damage on the genome at a critical time.[44]

In keeping with the hypothesis that unrepaired DNA damage might be important in the formation of SCE and the elegant demonstration by Perry and Evans[34] that known mutagens induced SCE, Goth-Goldstein[45] and Wolff[46-48] speculated that alkylation-induced SCE might be related to the levels of O^6-alkylguanine in the DNA. This DNA adduct, which is not repaired in either SV40-transformed *Xeroderma pigmentosum* (XP) or Chinese hamster ovary (CHO) cells[45,49] appears important in induction of mutations in mammalian cells, both on a theoretical[50,51] and experimental basis.[52,53] Further, Carrano *et al.*[54] suggested that although the relationship between SCE and frequency of mutation might vary from chemical to chemical, SCE might be useful as an indicator of mutagenesis since many agents induced both endpoints. Subsequent studies, however, have found that while mutagenic DNA damage may induce SCE, there does not appear to be a quantitative, predictive relationship between induction of SCE and mutagenesis or the levels of O^6-alkylguanine.[52,55-57] In fact, depending upon the cell type employed and the class of compounds under study, stronger relationships have been found between induction of SCE and loss of cloning efficiency,[55,56,58] cell transformation,[59,60] or carcinogenic potency.[61]

RATIONALE

Rearrangement of the chromatin as a response to cellular trauma is an observation compatible with elements in current models of carcinogenesis. The formation of structural chromosomal aberrations and the induction of SCE are particularly relevant as cytological markers for these chromosomal alterations. These endpoints are induced by both DNA-damaging agents and those which damage chromatin through more indirect means. Thus, their inclusion in the test battery of carcinogen screening systems appears warranted.

TESTING METHODS

Chromosomal Aberrations

Staining regimes. The most commonly used staining methods for assaying chromosomal aberrations are regular Giemsa or Aceto-orcein staining protocols. With these stains, the chromosomes are uniformly stained and structural aberrations such as breaks and gaps can be observed. Descriptions of chromosomal aberrations and the classification standards for these aberrations have been published (*see e.g.*, references 7, 62 and 63). These staining procedures lend themselves to observation of certain types of aberrations, *i.e.*, chromatid breaks and gaps, di- and multicentric chromosomes, acentric fragments, obvious translocations, etc., which can be ascertained by gross morphological characteristics.

The resolution of these staining procedures, however, may not be sufficient to accurately identify more subtle rearrangements. Reciprocal translocations which involve approximately equal segments of chromosomal material would not be obvious when the chromosomes are uniformly stained. Also, terminal deletions, involving only a small segment of the chromosome, interstitial deletions which minimally shorten the length of the chromosome arm, or inversions which did not involve the centromere could easily be missed using this methodology. Thus, for accurate identification of all chromosomal rearrangements, the application of chromosome banding techniques to the analysis must be considered. Banding analysis is easily applied to cells from many sources including human (for technical protocols for human cell lines, *see* reference 64) and standard karyotypes from most species are available. To obtain accurate karyotypes, both fluorescent and nonfluorescent dyes can be used. In analyses using human cell lines, resolution of the karyotype can be obtained from the classical metaphase chromosome (250 and 320 band stage) to the 1200 band level using cell synchronization techniques. (*See* reference 20 for review of technical procedures and newly recognized chromosomal defects consistently associated with specific neoplasias.)

   Assay protocols. Accurate identification of all chromosomal aberrations may rely upon selection of the appropriate exposure and culture conditions. Two classes of clastogenic agents have been identified: Those that are direct acting, *i.e.*, can induce an aberration in the first mitosis after exposure in the G_2 phase, and those in which the cells must pass through an S-phase after exposure before an aberration is seen (for reviews, *see* references 7, 63, 65 and 66). X-Rays and radiomimetic chemicals are generally of the first class, producing both chromosomal and chromatid aberrations. Those chemicals which produce damage that is repaired by either nucleotide or nucleoside excision repair are generally of the second class and produce chromatid, rather than chromosomal aberrations.[7] Exposure times for chemicals should consider not only the length of the cell cycle and cycle stage during exposure, but also the binding characteristics and decomposition rate of the chemical. For those chemicals which react quickly or have short half-lives, a short exposure, such as two hours, may be adequate to induce aberrations. However, for chemicals which either bind or interact with DNA more slowly (*e.g.*, intercalating agents), exposure times may be increased up to 24 hours to determine the presence of clastogenic damage. It should be recognized, however, that aberration frequencies in cells exposed to chemicals for a longer period may be confounded by several factors. For example, cells are traversing through the cell cycle during exposure and aberration frequencies may be skewed by damage affecting some cells in the G_1 phase and some in the G_2 phase. This same factor also applies in asynchronously growing cultures. And, for those chemicals which induce aberrations only after a cell has passed through an S-phase, the possibility exists that clastogenic damage may be repaired in an error-free manner before the time for aberration induction. Thus, the initial damage may be underestimated.

   These same factors make selection of an appropriate fixation time more difficult. Since the mechanism of action and DNA binding characteristics of a test chemical are usually unknown, there may be no *a priori* reason for selection of a six-hour, 12-hour, or 24-hour harvest time. Thus, multiple timepoints at a particular dose may be necessary to fully assess the actual clastogenic potency of an unknown chemical.

Sister-Chromatid Exchange

   SCE visualization. To produce sister-chromatid differentiation (SCD), cells replicate twice in the presence of a halogenated pyrimidine, the most commonly used of which is the brominated derivative, bromodeoxyuridine (BUdR). SCD can also be accomplished by substituting DNA with iododeoxyuridine (IUdR) and chlorodeoxyuridine (ClUdR), although on an equimolar basis, these derivatives result in a higher background frequency of SCE compared to cells cultured in BUdR.[67-70] The basis for obtaining SCD is the unequal substitution (3:1) of the strands of the DNA which is then reflected in the light-dark staining pattern of the chromosomes. SCD can be visualized by direct staining with fluorescent dyes such as Hoechst 33258[29,33] or acridine orange.[71] Other procedures have been developed which use the more permanent stain, Giemsa to visualize SCD.

These include protocols involving a pretreatment with a fluorescent dye[30-32,72] or a hot alkaline buffer[73-75] before Giemsa staining.

Assay protocols. Many of the components of the culture systems used in analysis of SCE have been shown to affect the final frequency of SCE and should be considered in the experimental design. BUdR, which is necessary for the demonstration of SCD, is itself capable of inducing SCE[30,76] in a dose-dependent manner. This effect appears to be due both to the incorporation of the analog into the DNA[69,70,77] and to an effect on the relative concentrations of cellular nucleotide pools.[78] Also, interactions between the BUdR in the culture system and the test chemical have been reported to result in higher than expected frequencies of SCE.[79,80] Other factors which have been shown to affect the frequency of SCE include composition of the media,[81,82] pH,[83] serum,[84] and temperature,[83,85-87] as well as the individual donor[88] or the species of the cells used in the culture system.[81]

Additional factors which must be considered in the experimental design are the length of exposure to the test chemical and the selection of the fixation time of the culture. The results of liquid holding studies[55,89] have demonstrated that cells given an increased time interval between exposure to the chemical and the first S-phase have reduced frequencies of SCE compared to control cells. This suggests that the damage which induces an SCE can be modulated to a degree and implies that during longer exposure times, the effects of SCE-inducing damage may be lessened. Thus, exposure times should be selected to give an optimum time for action of the chemical, but to minimize other effects. In addition, sequential fixation times should be considered in evaluating the SCE-inducing effects of chemical exposure to cells in various stages of the cell cycle.[90,91]

CELL SYSTEMS

This section will address only those cell systems utilized for *in vitro* analyses of chromosomal damage. However, the reader should be aware that several different cell types are used in *in vivo* analyses of chromosomal damage including germ cells and an array of somatic cells.[13,92] A wide variety of cell types derived from different laboratory animals and man, and originating initially from normal or neoplastic tissue, are available for use as systems to detect chromosomal damage resulting from exposure to chemicals.[93] There are several commonly used established cell lines including Chinese hamster ovary (CHO), Chinese hamster lung (V79), and mouse lymphoid (L5178Y) cells. In addition, normal diploid cell strains, such as human fibroblasts (WI-38) or human lymphocytes, have been used to detect chromosomal damage.

Important criteria for determining the usefulness of a cell type in assaying chromosomal alterations include chromosome number and morphology. For example, Chinese hamster cells have a low number of chromosomes, 18 to 22, depending upon the strain, which are diverse in appearance. Both of these factors make identification of chromosomal aberrations, as well as SCE, less tedious. In addition, CHO and V79 have a stable modal chromosome number, a well-defined gene map, an established banded karyotype, and a short generation time with a well characterized cell-cycle. The development of mutagenicity and cloning ability assays for these lines makes them very useful in studies of multiple endpoints. The disadvantages associated with these cell lines include the necessity for exogenous metabolic activation systems to detect the majority of premutagens and precarcinogens and their non-human origin.

The ultimate endpoint of any carcinogen testing program is the estimation of hazard to man. Thus, the use of cell systems from man should be considered in the test battery. Of the human cell types available for cytogenetic testing, the most widely used is the human peripheral blood lymphocyte. Studies using cells from exposed individuals or cells exposed in culture, have shown that the human peripheral lymphocyte is an extremely sensitive indicator of both *in vivo* and *in vitro* induced chromosomal structural change.[13,92] Evans and O'Riordan[94] suggest that even though there are problems in extrapolating from *in vitro* results to the *in vivo* situation, the lymphocyte offers several advantages as an *in vitro* test system for detecting human genotoxicants. These include the availability of a large number of human cells; the distribution of the cells throughout the body; their circulation in all tissues and the long lifespan of a proportion of the cells; the synchrony of virtually all the peripheral blood lymphocytes in the same G_0 or G_1 stage of the mitotic interphase; the ability of a proportion of the lymphocytes to be stimulated by mitogens to undergo mitosis in culture; the excellent techniques available for making chromosomal preparations; and, the low spontaneous frequency of chromosomal aberrations of these cells. These cells, however, are unable to metabolically activate many precarcinogens and premutagens and are hypersensitive to the toxicity of exogenous metabolic activation systems.[13] Thus, the risk of induced chromosomal abnormalities by certain chemicals may be underestimated.

CLASSES OF CHEMICALS

The classes of chemicals which have been found to induce chromosomal effects include alkylating agents, aromatic amines and amides, chlorinated hydrocarbons, metals, mycotoxins, nitrosamines, nucleic acid antimetabolites, polynuclear aromatic hydrocarbons, and a variety of miscellaneous chemicals.[13,92,95-101] In a recent study[99] a variety of chemicals representative of several classes were tested using a standard protocol in the same cell line and in the presence and absence of an activation system. The following results were obtained: 4-nitroquinoline-N-oxide, 3-methyl-4-nitroquinoline-N-oxide, benzidine, benzo(a)pyrene, dimethylcarbamoyl chloride, 2-naphthylamine, and epichlorohydrin induced both SCE and chromosomal aberrations; hydrazine sulfate and diethylstilbestrol (DES) were positive in the chromosomal aberration test only; while 1-naphthylamine and 4-dimethylaminoazobenzene were weakly positive only in the SCE test; 3,3',5,5'-tetramethylbenzidine, pyrene, dimethylformamide, methionine, ethionine, hexamethylphosphoramide, ethylenethiourea, and safrole were found negative in both tests. The results of this study indicate that both SCE and chromosomal aberration tests should be performed when cytogenetic tests are used in screening carcinogens. It was emphasized, that based on these analyses, the SCE test cannot replace the chromosomal aberration test.

Two major problems in evaluating the *in vitro* cytogenetic effects of chemical mutagens are the different methods of reporting the data and the use of a variety of experimental protocols.[100] As mentioned earlier relative to experimental design, the quality and quantity of the response depends upon the time and duration of exposure and the sampling of the mitotic cells. To optimize the biological response, these parameters must be adjusted to reflect the reactivity of the chemical under study, the proliferation kinetics of the target cell, and the metabolic activity of the homogenate used to activate precarcinogens and premutagens. Another variable to consider when assessing a chemical's potential to induce chromosomal abnormalities is the specie of the target cell used. DES did not induce SCE in the CHO cell line, either in the presence or absence of metabolic activation.[99] However, Rudiger *et al.*[102] and Hill and Wolff[103] demonstrated that DES induced SCE in human fibroblasts and lymphocytes. A possible explanation for this discrepancy may be the differences in inherent metabolic potential of the human cell relative to the rodent cell, or as Hill and Wolff[104] suggest, that the induction of SCE by DES, at least in human lymphocytes, is related to the hormonal state of the individual from which the cell was derived.

Many of the chemicals evaluated in these assay systems are representative of various chemical classes. A majority are direct acting mutagenic carcinogens, but others require metabolic activation to demonstrate their carcinogenic nature. The most commonly used activation system is that described by Ames and his coworkers[3,4,105] which utilizes a 9,000 g supernatant fraction of a liver homogenate (S9). One technical difficulty with S9 is its toxicity to the target cell. This toxicity may be minimized by altering the length of exposure of the target cell to the homogenate. A more serious difficulty may be the inherent problems associated with cell-free preparations in which interlocking pathways of activation and detoxification have been disrupted. This disruption may destroy the specific catalytic activities of enzyme complexes present *in vivo*.[106] This problem may be overcome by using specific intact cells for metabolic activation.[106-109] These intact cells may be isolated from animals which are pre-induced and therefore have greater metabolic capacity[110] or may be isolated from uninduced animals. These systems have the potential of providing important information about target organ specificity.[107,108]

ADVANTAGES AND DISADVANTAGES

Chromosomal Aberrations

Advantages

(a) Direct observation of chromosomal rearrangements can be made.

(b) By using banding analysis, specific chromosomes or specific segments of chromosomes involved in rearrangements can be identified.

(c) Multiple types of aberrations can be identified from one sample, and the same samples can be used to score other cytogenetic phenomena.

(d) The same types of aberrations are found *in vivo* as *in vitro*.

(e) Metabolic activation systems can be used during exposure to chemicals to assess the effects of indirect-acting agents.

Disadvantages

(a) Scoring requires considerable technical expertise and can be somewhat subjective with variation between observers and laboratories.

(b) At concentrations of agents necessary to induce aberrations, few cells may be available for analysis.

(c) Scoring is tedious and time-consuming and a relatively large number of cells must be scored for valid statistical analysis.

Sister-Chromatid Exchange

Advantages

(a) In comparison to classical analysis of cytogenetic aberrations, analysis of SCE is easier to perform. Cell cultures and staining techniques are relatively simple and the mechanics of scoring are much less subjective than those for aberrations.

(b) The technique lends itself more easily to the establishment of dose-response relationships than aberration scoring. That is, the induction of SCE can be monitored at doses of chemical much lower than those which induce chromosomal aberrations. Also, analysis of SCE requires relatively few cells for valid statistical analysis.

(c) The technique is applicable to different cell lines, to a variety of tissues from single species, and to the same tissue from different species, *e.g.*, lymphocytes. Thus, inter-species comparisons, as well as those between target and non-target organs can be made.

(d) By coupling analysis of SCE with metabolic activation regimes, both direct-acting chemicals and those requiring activation can be studied.

Disadvantages

(a) The nature of the cellular damage inducing an SCE and the significance of an increase in frequency of SCE is unknown.

(b) Certain classes of chemicals, *e.g.*, those that are radiomimetic, are poor inducers of SCE.

(c) The nucleoside analogs necessary to produce sister-chromatid differentiation (*e.g.*, BUdR), induce SCE. The metabolism of these compounds and their effects on the frequency of SCE may not be the same in treated cells and control cells.

SIGNIFICANCE

The relationship between alterations in chromosome structure and the induction of neoplasia is an area of wide interest. Structural chromosomal rearrangements obviously involve rearrangement of the cellular genome, and possibly, duplications and deficiencies of specific segments of the chromosomes. The relationship of these alterations to the induction of cancer is being characterized by studies which relate specific chromosomal rearrangements to the induction and course of specific cancers. The significance of induction of SCE is less clear. Several studies indicate a potential relationship with cellular survival, but it is doubtful that an SCE is, of itself, a lethal event. Whether the rearrangement of chromatin between the sister-chromatids which occurs during formation of SCE is itself a significant genotoxic event or whether an SCE is an innocuous event which increases in response to cellular trauma has not been clarified. However, the utility of these tests lies in the observations that known carcinogens can induce these endpoints, and thus, their importance in the test battery is recognized.

Acknowledgements

The authors wish to thank Carolyn Phifer for her assistance in the preparation of this manuscript. We also gratefully acknowledge the comments and suggestions of Drs. Joel Pounds, Robert Morrisey, and Robert Heflich.

REFERENCES

1. Berenblum, I., and Armuth, V., Two independent aspects of tumor promotion. *Biochim. Biophys. Acta* 651:51-63 (1981)
2. Miller, J.A., and Miller, E.C., in: *Origins of Human Cancer* (H.H. Hiatt, J.D. Watson and J.A. Winsten, eds.), Book B, pp 605-627, Cold Spring Harbor Laboratory, Cold Spring Harbor, New York (1977)
3. McCann, J., Choi, E., Yamasaki, E., and Ames, B.N., Detection of carcinogens as mutagens in the *Salmonella*/microsome test: Assay of 300 chemicals. *Proc. Natl. Acad. Sci. USA* 72:5135-5139 (1975)
4. McCann, J., and Ames, B.N., Detection of carcinogens as mutagens in the *Salmonella*/microsome test: Discussion. *Proc. Natl. Acad. Sci. USA* 73:950-954 (1976)
5. Casciano, D.A., Mutagenesis assay methods. *Food Technol.* March: 48-52 (1982)
6. Boveri, T., *The Origin of Malignant Tumors*, Baltimore: Williams and Wilkins (1929)
7. Evans, H.J., in: *Progress in Genetic Toxicology* (D. Scott, B.A. Bridges and F.H. Sobels, eds.), pp 57-74, Elsevier/North-Holland Biomedical Press, New York (1977)
8. Sax, K., An analysis of x-ray induced chromosomal aberrations in *Tradescantia*. *Genetics* 25:41-68 (1940)
9. Muller, H.J., Types of visible variations induced by x-rays in *Drosophila*. *Genetics* 22:494-516 (1930)
10. Bender, M.A., and Gooch, P.C., Types and rates of x-ray-induced chromosome aberrations in human blood irradiated *in vitro*. *Proc. Natl. Acad. Sci. USA* 48:522-532 (1962)
11. Auerbach, C., and Robson, J.M., The production of mutations by chemical substances. *Proc. Roy. Soc. Edinburgh B.* 62:271-283 (1947)

12. Auerbach, C., *Mutation Research: Problems, Results and Perspectives*, London: John Wiley & Sons (1976)
13. Preston, R.J., Au, W., Bender, M.A., Brewen, J.G., Carrano, A.V., Heddle, J.A., McFee, A.F., Wolff, S., and Wassom, J.S., Mammalian *in vivo* and *in vitro* cytogenetic assays: A report of the U.S. EPA's Gene-Tox Program. *Mutat. Res.* 87:143-188 (1981)
14. Ray, J.H., and German, J., in: *Chromosome Mutation and Neoplasia* (J., German, ed.), pp 135-167, Alan R. Liss, New York (1983)
15. Cleaver, J.E., in: *Chromosome Mutation and Neoplasia* (J. German, ed.), pp 235-249, Alan R. Liss, New York (1983)
16. Heddle, J.A., Krepinsky, A.B., and Marshall, R.R., in: *Chromosome Mutation and Neoplasia* (J. German, ed.), pp 203-234, Alan R. Liss, New York (1983)
17. Sandberg, A.A. (ed.), *The Chromosomes in Human Cancer and Leukemia*, Amsterdam: Elsevier/North Holland (1980)
18. Yunis, J.J., Sawyer, J.R., and Ball, D.W., The characterization of high-resolution G-banded chromosomes in man. *Chromosoma* 67:293-307 (1978)
19. Francke, U., and Oliver, N., Quantitative analysis of high-resolution trypsin-giemsa bands on human chromosomes. *Human Genet.* 45: 137-165 (1978)
20. Yunis, J.J., The chromosomal basis of human neoplasia. *Science* 221:227-236 (1983)
21. Francke, U., Retinoblastoma and chromosome 13. *Cytogenet. Cell Genet.* 16:131-134 (1976)
22. Balaban-Malenbaum, G., Gilbert, F., Nichols, W.W., Hill, R., Shields, J., and Meadows, A.T., A deleted chromosome No. 13 in human retinoblastoma cells: relevance to tumorigenesis. *Cancer Genet. Cytogenet.* 3:243-250 (1981)
23. Riccardi, V.M., Sujansky, E., Smith, A.C., and Francke, U., Chromosomal imbalance in the Aniridia-Wilm's tumor association: 11p interstitial deletion. *Pediatrics* 61:604-610 (1978)
24. Francke, U., Holmes, L.B., Athin, L., and Riccardi, V.M., Aniridia-Wilm's tumor association: Evidence for a specific lesion of 11p 13. *Cytogenet. Cell Genet.* 24:185-192 (1979)
25. Cooper, G.M., Cellular transforming genes. *Science* 218:801-806 (1982)
26. Bishop, J.M., in: *Annual Review of Biochemistry* (E.E. Snell, ed.), Vol. 52, pp 301-354, Annual Rev. Inc., Palo Alto (1983)
27. Rowley, J.D., Human oncogene locations and chromosome aberrations. *Nature* 301:290-291 (1983)
28. Taylor, J.H., Woods, P.S., and Hughes, W.L., The organization and duplication of chromosomes as revealed by autoradiographic studies using tritium-labeled thymidine. *Proc. Natl. Acad. Sci. USA* 43: 122-128 (1957)
29. Latt, S.A., Microfluorometric detection of deoxyribonucleotide replication in human metaphase chromosomes. *Proc. Natl. Acad. Sci. USA* 70: 3395-3399 (1973)
30. Wolff, S., and Perry, P., Differential Giemsa staining of sister chromatids and the study of sister chromatid exchange without autoradiography. *Chromosoma* (Berlin) 48: 341-353 (1974)
31. Perry, P., and Wolff, S., New Giemsa method for the differential staining of sister chromatids. *Nature* (London) 251: 156-158 (1974)
32. Wolff, S., and Perry, P., Insights on chromosome structure from sister chromatid exchanges and the lack of both isolabelling and heterolabelling as determined by the FPG technique. *Exp. Cell Res.* 93: 23-30 (1975)

33. Latt, S.A., Sister chromatid exchanges, indices of human chromosome damage and repair: Detection by fluorescence and induction by mitomycin-C. *Proc. Natl. Acad. Sci. USA* 71: 3162-3172 (1974)
34. Perry, P. and Evans, H.J., Cytological detection of mutagen-carcinogen exposure by sister chromatid exchange. *Nature* (London) 258: 121-125 (1975)
35. Ueda, N., Uenaka, H., Akematsu, T., and Sugiyama, T., Parallel distribution of sister chromatid exchanges and chromosome aberrations. *Nature* (London) 262: 581-583 (1976)
36. Ikushima, T., Role of SCE in chromatid aberration formation. *Nature* (London) 268: 235-236 (1977)
37. Galloway, S.M. and Wolff, S., The relation between chemically induced sister chromatid exchanges and chromatid breakage. *Mutation Res.* 61: 297-307 (1979)
38. Raj, A.S. and Heddle, J.A., Simultaneous detection of chromosome aberrations and sister chromatid exchanges. Experience with DNA intercalating agents. *Mutation Res.* 78: 253-260 (1980)
39. van Kesteren-van Leeuwen, A.C., and Natarajan, A.T., Localization of 7,12-Dimethylbenz(a)anthracene induced chromatid breaks and sister chromatid exchanges in chromosomes 1 and 2 of bone marrow cells of rat *in vivo*. *Chromosoma* (Berlin) 81: 473-481 (1980)
40. Gebhart, E., Sister chromatid exchange (SCE) and structural chromosome aberration in mutagenicity testing. *Human Genet.* 58: 235-254 (1981)
41. Wolff, S., Bodycote, J., Thomas, G.H., and Cleaver, J.E., Sister chromatid exchange in xeroderma pigmentosum cells that are defective in DNA excision-repair or post-replication repair. *Genetics* 81: 349-355 (1975)
42. Wolff, S., Rodin, B., and Cleaver, J.E., Sister chromatid exchanges induced by mutagenic carcinogens in normal and xeroderma pigmentosum cells. *Nature* (London) 265: 347-349 (1977)
43. Cleaver, J.E., in: *Molecular Human Cytogenetics*, ICN-UCLA Symposium on Molecular and Cellular Biology, (R.S. Sparkes, ed.), Vol. 7, pp 341-354 (1977)
44. Cleaver, J.E., Repair replication and sister chromatid exchange as indicators of excisable and nonexcisable damage in human (Xeroderma pigmentosum) cells. *J. Toxicol. Environ. Health* 2: 1387-1394 (1977)
45. Goth-Goldstein, R., Repair of DNA damaged by alkylating carcinogens is defective in xeroderma pigmentosum fibroblasts. *Nature* (London) 267: 81-82 (1977)
46. Wolff, S., Sister chromatid exchange. *Ann. Rev. Genetics* 11: 183-201 (1977)
47. Wolff, S., in: *DNA Repair Mechanisms*, ICN-UCLA Symposium on Molecular and Cellular Biology, Vol. 9, pp 751-760, Academic Press, New York (1978)
48. Wolff, S., in: *Sister Chromatid Exchange* (S. Wolff, ed.), pp 41-57, Wiley, New York (1982)
49. Goth-Goldstein, R., Inability of CHO cells to excise O^6-alkylguanine. *Cancer Res.* 40:2623-2624 (1980)
50. Loveless, A., Possible relevance of O^6-alkylation of deoxyguanine to the mutagenicity and carcinogenicity of nitrosamines and nitrosamides. *Nature* (London) 223: 206-207 (1969)
51. Gerchman, L.L., and Ludlum, D.B., The properties of O^6-methylguanine in templates for RNA polymerase. *Biochim. Biophys. Acta* 308: 310-316 (1973)

52. Heflich, R.H., Beranek, D.T., Kodell, R.L., and Morris, S.M., Induction of mutations and sister-chromatid exchanges in Chinese hamster ovary cells by ethylating agents: Relationship to specific DNA adducts. *Mutation Res.* 106: 147-161 (1982)

53. Beranek, D.T., Heflich, R.H., Kodell, R.L., Morris, S.M., and Casciano, D.A., Correlation between specific DNA-methylation products and mutation induction at the HGPRT locus in Chinese hamster ovary cells. *Mutation Res.* 110: 171-180 (1983)

54. Carrano, A.V., Thompson, L.H., Lindl, P.A., and Minkler, J.L., Sister chromatid exchange as an indicator of mutagenesis. *Nature* (London) 271: 551-553 (1978)

55. Connell, J.R., and Medcalf, A.S.C., The induction of SCE and chromosomal aberrations with relation to specific base methylation of DNA in Chinese hamster cells by N-methyl-N-nitrosourea and dimethyl sulfate. *Carcinogenesis* 3: 385-390 (1982)

56. Morris, S.M., Heflich, R.H., Beranek, D.T., and Kodell, R.L., Alkylation-induced sister-chromatid exchanges correlate with reduced cell survival, not mutations. *Mutation Res.* 105: 163-168 (1982)

57. Morris, S.M., Beranek, D.T., and Heflich, R.H., The relationship between sister-chromatid exchange induction and the formation of specific methylated DNA adducts in Chinese hamster ovary cells. *Mutation Res.* 121: 261-266 (1983)

58. Tofilon, P.J., Williams, M.E., and Deen, D.F., Nitrosourea-induced sister chromatid exchanges and correlation to cell survival in 9L rat brain tumor cells. *Cancer Res.* 43: 473-475 (1983)

59. Popescu, N.C., Amsbaugh, S.C., and DiPaolo, J.A., Relationship of carcinogen-induced sister chromatid exchange and neoplastic cell transformation. *Int. J. Cancer.* 28: 71-77 (1981)

60. Turnbull, P., Popescu, N.C., DiPaolo, J.A., and Myhr, B.C., Cis-platinum(II) diamine dichloride causes mutation, transformation and sister chromatid exchanges in cultured mammalian cells. *Mutation Res.* 66: 267-275 (1979)

61. Parodi, S., Zonino, A., Ottaggio, L., DeFerrari, M., and Santi, L., Quantitative correlation between carcinogenicity and sister-chromatid exchange induction *in vivo* for a group of 11 N-nitroso derivatives. *J. Toxicol. Env. Health* 11: 337-346 (1983)

62. Hsu, T.C., in: *Mammalian Chromosomes Newsletters*, 20 Vol. 3, pp 60-69 (1979)

63. Bender, M.A., in: *DNA Repair and Mutagenesis in Eucaryotes*, (Generoso *et al.*, eds.), Basic Life Sciences, Vol. 15, pp 245-265, Plenum Press, New York (1980)

64. Priest, J.H., in: *Medical Cytogenetics and Cell Culture*, Lea and Febiger, Philadelphia (1977)

65. Wolff, S., in: *Research in Photobiology* (A. Castellani, ed.), pp 721-732, Plenum Press, New York (1977)

66. Wolff, S., in: *Chromosomes Today* (Bennett, Bobrow and Hewitt, eds.), Vol. 7, pp 226-241, George Allen and Univin, London (1981)

67. Ikushima, T., and Wolff, S., Sister chromatid exchanges induced by light flashes to 5-bromodeoxyuridine and 5-iododeoxyuridine substituted Chinese hamster chromosomes. *Exp. Cell Res.* 87: 15-19 (1974)

68. DuFrain, R.J., and Garrand, T.J., The influence of incorporated halogenated analogues of thymidine on the sister-chromatid exchange frequency in human lymphocytes. *Mutation Res.* 91: 233-238 (1981)

69. Heartlein, M.W., O'Neill, J.P., and Preston, R.J., SCE induction is proportional to substitution in DNA for thymidine by CIdU and BrdU. *Mutation Res.* 107: 103-109 (1983)

70. O'Neill, J.P., Heartlein, M.W., and Preston, R.J., Sister-chromatid exchanges and gene mutations are induced by the replication of 5-bromo- and 5-chlorodeoxyuridine substituted DNA. *Mutation Res.* 109: 259-270 (1983)

71. Tice, R., Chaillet, J., and Schneider, E.L., Evidence derived from sister chromatid exchanges of restricted rejoining of chromatid subunits. *Nature* (London) 256: 642-644 (1975)

72. Goto, K., Akematsu, T., Shimazu, H., and Sugiyami, T., Simple differential Giemsa staining of sister chromatids after treatment with photosensitive dyes and exposure to light and the mechanism of staining. *Chromosoma* (Berlin) 53: 223-230 (1975)

73. Takayama, S., and Sakanishi, S., Sister chromatid differential staining by direct staining in Na_2HPO_4-Giemsa solution and the mechanism involved. *Chromosoma* (Berlin) 75: 37-44 (1979)

74. Takayama, S., Utsumi, K.R., and Sasaki, Y., Topographic examination of sister chromatid differential staining by Nomarski interference microscopy and scanning electron microscopy. *Chromosoma* (Berlin) 82: 113-119 (1981)

75. Korenberg, J.R., and Freedlender, E.F., Giemsa technique for the detection of sister chromatid exchanges. *Chromosoma* (Berlin) 48: 355-360 (1977)

76. Kato, H., Spontaneous sister chromatid exchanges detected by a BrdU-labelling method. *Nature* (London) 251: 70-72 (1974)

77. Mazrimas, J.A., and Stetka, D.G., Direct evidence for the role of incorporated BUdR in the induction of sister chromatid exchanges. *Exp. Cell Res.* 117: 23-30 (1978)

78. Davidson, R.L., Kaufman, E.R., Dougherty, C.P., Ouellette, A.M., DiFalco, C.M., and Latt, S.A., Induction of sister chromatid exchanges by BudR is largely independent of the BUdR content of DNA. *Nature* (London) 284: 74-76 (1980)

79. Stetka, D.G. and Carrano, A.V., The interaction of Hoechst 33258 and BrdU substituted DNA in the formation of sister chromatid exchanges. *Chromosoma* (Berlin) 63: 21-31 (1977)

80. Speit, G., Wolf, M., and Vogel, W., Synergistic action of cysteamine and BrdU-substituted DNA in the induction of sister chromatid exchanges. *Chromosoma* (Berlin) 81: 461-471 (1980)

81. Sharma, T., and Das, B.C., Culture media and species-related variations in the requirement of 5-bromodeoxyuridine for differential sister-chromatid staining. *Mutation Res.* 81: 357-364 (1981)

82. Morgan, W.F., and Crossen, P.E., Factors influencing sister-chromatid exchange rate in cultured human lymphocytes. *Mutation Res.* 81: 395-402 (1981)

83. Littlefield, L.G., Colyer, S.P., and DuFrain, R.J., Physical, chemical and biological factors affecting sister-chromatid exchange in human lymphocytes exposed to mitomycin C prior to culture. *Mutation Res.* 81: 377-386 (1981)

84. Kato, H., and Sandberg, A.A., The effect of sera on sister chromatid exchanges *in vitro. Exp. Cell Res.* 109: 445-448 (1977)

85. Speit, G., Effects of temperature on sister chromatid exchanges. *Human Genet.* 55: 333-336 (1980)

86. Pandita, T.K., Effect of temperature variation on sister chromatid exchange frequency in cultured human lymphocytes. *Human Genet.* 63: 189-190 (1983)

87. Gutierrez, C., Schvartzman, J.B., and Lopez-Saez, J.F., Effect of growth temperature on the formation of sister-chromatid exchanges in BrdUrd-substituted chromosomes. *Exp. Cell Res.* 134: 73-79 (1981)

88. Carrano, A.V., Minkler, J.L., Stetka, D.G., and Moore, D.H., Variation in the baseline sister chromatid exchange frequency in human lymphocytes. *Environ. Mutagen.* 2: 325-337 (1980)

89. Jostes, R.F., Sister chromatid exchanges but not mutations decrease with time in arrested Chinese hamster ovary cells after treatment with ethyl nitrosourea. *Mutation Res.* 91: 371-375 (1981)

90. Carrano, A.V., Thompson, L.H., Stetka, D.G., Minkler, J.L., Mazrimas, J.A., and Fong, S., DNA crosslinking, sister-chromatid exchange and specific-locus mutations. *Mutation Res.* 63: 175-188 (1979)

91. Ockey, C.H., Differences between "spontaneous" and induced sister-chromatid exchanges with fixation time and their chromosome localization. *Cytogen. Cell Genet.* 26: 223-235 (1980)

92. Latt, S.A., Allen, J., Blood, S.E., Carrano, A., Falke, E., Kram, D., Schneider, E., Schreck, R., Tice, R., Whitfield, B., and Wolff, S., Sister-chromatid exchanges: A report of the Gene-Tox Program. *Mutation Res.* 87: 17-62 (1981)

93. Evans, H.J., in: *Chemical Mutagens: Principles and Methods for Their Detection* (A. Hollaender, ed.), Vol. 4, pp 1-29, Plenum Press, New York (1976)

94. Evans, H.J., and O'Riordan, M.L., in: *Handbook of Mutagenicity Test Procedures* (B.J. Kolbey, M. Legator, W. Nichols and C. Ramel, eds.), pp 261-274, Elsevier, North Holland, New York (1977)

95. Gebhart, E., in: *Chemical Mutagenesis in Mammals and Man* (F. Vogel and G. Rohrborn, eds.), pp 367-382, Springer-Verlag, New York (1970)

96. Fishbein, L., in: *Mutagenic Effects of Environmental Contaminants* (H.E. Sutton and M.I. Harris, eds.), pp 129-170, Academic Press, New York (1972)

97. Fishbein, L., in: *Chemical Mutagens: Principles and Methods for Their Detection* (A. Hollaender, ed.), Vol. 4, pp 219-319, Plenum Press, New York (1976)

98. Wolff, S., in: *Genetic Damage in Man Caused by Environmental Agents* (K. Berg, ed.), pp 229-246, Academic Press, New York (1979)

99. Natarajan, A.T., and van Kestteren-van Leevween, A.C., in: *Evaluation of Short-Term Tests for Carcinogens, Progress in Mutation Research* (F.J. deSerres and J. Ashby, eds.), Vol. 1, pp 551-559, Elsevier/North Holland, New York (1981)

100. Brewen, J.G., Natarajan, A., and Obe, G., in: *Comparative Chemical Mutagenesis* (F.J. deSerres and M.D. Shelby, eds.), pp 433-486, Plenum Press, New York (1981)

101. Wolff, S., Perry, P., and Natarajan, A.T., in: *Comparative Chemical Mutagenesis* (F.J. deSerres and M.D. Shelby, eds.), pp 539-548, Plenum Press, New York (1979)

102. Rudiger, H.W., Haenisch, F., Metzler, M., Oesch, F., and Glatt, H.R., Metabolites of diethylstilbestrol induce sister chromatid exchange in human cultured fibroblasts. *Nature* (London) 281: 392-394 (1979)

103. Hill, A., and Wolff, S., Sister chromatid exchange and cell division delays induced by diethylstilbestrol, estradiol, and estriol in human lymphocytes. *Cancer Res.* 43: 4114-4118 (1983)

104. Hill, A., and Wolff, S., Increased induction of sister chromatid exchange by diethylstilbestrol in lymphocytes from pregnant and premenopausal women. *Cancer Res.* 42: 893-896 (1982)

105. Ames, B.N., McCann, J. and Yamasaki, E., Methods for detecting carcinogens and mutagens with the *Salmonella*/mammalian-microsome mutagenicity test. *Mutation Res.* 31: 347-364 (1975)

106. Casciano, D.A., in: *Banbury Report* (A.W. Hsie, J.P. O'Neill, and V.R. McElheny, eds.), Vol. 2, pp 125-130, Cold Spring Harbor Laboratory, Cold Spring Harbor (1979)

107. Langenbach, R., Freed, J.H., and Huberman, E., Liver cell-mediated mutagenesis of mammalian cells with liver carcinogens. *Proc. Natl. Acad. Sci. USA* 75: 2864-2867 (1978)

108. Langenbach, R., and Nesnow, S., in: *Basic Life Sciences: Organ and Species Specificity in Chemical Carcinogens* (R. Langenbach, S. Nesnow, and J.M. Rice, eds.), Vol. 24, pp 377-390, Plenum Press, New York (1983)

109. Casciano, D.A., and Shaddock, J.G., Carcinogenic non-hepatocarcinogens can be detected as mutagens in the liver cell-mediated CHO/HGPRT assay. *Environ. Mutagen.* 4: 354-355 (1982)

110. Casciano, D.A., Farr, J.A., Oldham, J.W., and Cave, M.D., 2-Acetylaminofluorene-induced unscheduled DNA synthesis in hepatocytes isolated from 3-methylcholanthrene treated rats. *Cancer Lett.* 5: 173-178 (1978)

6

Methods and Modifications of the Hepatocyte Primary Culture/DNA Repair Test

Charlene A. McQueen
Gary M. Williams

American Health Foundation
Naylor Dana Institute for Disease Prevention
Valhalla, New York

INTRODUCTION

A principal function of the liver is the biotransformation of xenobiotics. The development of techniques for the isolation and maintenance of intact liver cells has provided cell culture systems that can be utilized for toxicologic and pharmacologic investigations of chemicals.[1-4] Uptake of xenobiotics as well as a variety of reactions including aromatic and aliphatic hydroxylation, N-demethylation, glucuronide and sulfate conjugation, and N-acetylation are performed by hepatocytes.[5-12] Comparison of isolated hepatocytes and tissue homogenates demonstrates that metabolism in hepatocytes closely resembles *in vivo* metabolism.[8,13-17]

One use of isolated hepatocytes has been to identify genotoxic chemicals.[18-20] Genotoxicity, defined as damage to DNA, can be measured either as alteration of DNA or DNA excision repair.[21] DNA repair, when determined by reliable techniques, has an advantage in that it is not produced by non-specific cytotoxicity; in fact, it is inhibited under such conditions. Numerous conditions for hepatocytes in culture and methods of measuring DNA repair have been proposed. Hepatocytes can be cultured as suspensions[22-25] or monolayers on plastic or collagen.[18-20,23,26-28] Methods that are used for measuring DNA repair in hepatocytes include incorporation of ^{3}H-thymidine as determined by autoradiography,[18-20] acid precipitation of macromolecules[23,27,29,30] or isolation of DNA on a gradient.[23,27]

The hepatocyte primary culture (HPC)/DNA repair test developed in this laboratory combines monolayer cultures of hepatocytes with autoradiographic determination of unscheduled DNA synthesis (UDS).[18,19] There are several advantages to this approach:

(1) Unlike suspension cultures which consist of both viable and non-viable cells, monolayer cultures initially comprise virtually only viable cells;[31]

(2) There is no requirement for inhibitors of DNA synthesis, since less than 0.1% of these cells are in S-phase;[32]

(3) When autoradiography is used, the few S-phase cells present are readily identified; and

(4) With autoradiography, the percentage of cells undergoing repair synthesis can be quantified.

The HPC/DNA repair test was developed and validated using rat hepatocytes,[18,33] but has been extended to use hepatocytes from other species.[34-39] This broadens the spectrum of genotoxins that are detected, and a positive result in several species increases the likelihood of hazard to humans. A particularly important development is the use of human cells.[40,41]

RAT HEPATOCYTE PRIMARY CULTURE (HPC)/DNA REPAIR TEST

Preparation of Hepatocyte Primary Cultures

Hepatocytes are isolated from adult animals by a two-step perfusion of the liver.[18,42] Males are preferred because of their greater metabolic capability.

Animals are anesthetized with Nembutal Sodium solution given intraperitoneally at 50 mg/kg body weight. A ventral midline incision is made from the pubic bone to the xiphisternum and the portal vein is cannulated with a 21 gauge butterfly needle. A 37°C sterile solution of 0.5 mM ethylene glycol-bis(β-aminoethyl ether)-N,N'-tetraacetic acid (EGTA) in calcium and magnesium-free Hanks' balanced salt solution containing 10 mM 2-hydroxyethylpiperazine-N'-2-ethanesulfonic acid (Hepes) adjusted to pH 7.35 with 1N NaOH is perfused for approximately one minute at a rate of 8 ml/min. The subhepatic inferior vena cava is immediately severed to prevent excessive swelling of the liver. Uniform blanching of the liver should be observed. The incision is then extended through the diaphragm and the thoracic vena cava is cut, allowing the perfusate to run to waste. The system is then closed by clamping the proximal segment of the subhepatic inferior vena cava and the pump speed is increased to 40 ml/min. Perfusion of the liver with EGTA should be done for a total of four minutes.

The EGTA solution is followed by Solution II consisting of 100 units collagenase/ml Williams' Medium E (WME) (Gibco, Grand Island, NY)[31] (buffered with 10 mM Hepes and adjusted to pH 7.35 with 1N NaOH). This solution is perfused for ten minutes at a rate of 20 ml/min. The liver is covered to keep it moist, and a 40 watt bulb is positioned above the liver.

Following perfusion, the liver is removed to a sterile dish containing WME and extraneous tissue is trimmed. The liver is next placed in a dish containing

Solution II, and the capsule is stripped away. Cells are detached by gently brushing the liver with a hog bristle paint brush or a wide-tooth stainless steel dog comb. The fibrous connective tissue which remains is discarded. A wide bore pipet is used to transfer the cell suspension to a 50 ml centrifuge tube and the volume brought to 50 ml with WME containing 10% calf serum and 50 μg/ml gentamicin (WMES). The cells are sedimented for 2.5 minutes at $50g$ and resuspended in WMES. Cell viability is determined on a diluted aliquot of the cell suspension by trypan blue exclusion. Only cell preparations having a viability greater than 80% are used.

An aliquot containing 5 x 10^5 viable cells/ml WMES is seeded onto a 25 mm round Thermanox coverslip in a 6 well dish containing 2 ml of WMES and placed in a 5% CO_2 incubator at 37°C. Glass coverslips and Petri dishes can also be used.

Hepatocyte Primary Culture/DNA Repair Test

After an attachment interval of two hours (three hours if glass coverslips are used), the monolayer cultures are washed with one ml of WME. Two ml of WME containing 10 μCi methyl-^{3}H-thymidine (60 to 80 Ci/mM) are added to each culture followed by the test compound. At least five concentrations, each separated by a factor of ten, are tested. A known genotoxic chemical, a structurally related nongenotoxic analogue, and the solvent as well as an untreated cell control are run simultaneously with the test chemical. Triplicate coverslips are done for each concentration of the test chemical and the controls.

The cultures are incubated for 18 to 20 hours at 37°C in a 5% CO_2 incubator. Following exposure, the coverslips are washed by dipping in three successive beakers each containing 100 ml of phosphate buffered saline, pH 7.4. The cells are first swollen to allow for better quantification of the grains by immersing the coverslips in 1% sodium citrate, then fixed in three changes of ethanol: acetic acid (4:1). The air dried coverslips are mounted, cell side up, on glass slides and dipped in NTB (Kodak, Rochester, NY) emulsion. The slides are dried overnight before placing in a light-tight box for ten days at 4°C.

The slides are developed in D19 for four minutes then placed in a stop bath of acidified tap water for 30 seconds, followed by immersion in fixer for ten minutes and washing in tap water for ten minutes. The developed slides are stained with hematoxylin and eosin.

Evaluation of Genotoxicity

Grains in the emulsion are counted using an Artek electronic counter. Grains occur both over the nucleus and the cytoplasm. Several sources contribute to the grains that are observed over the cytoplasm, including nonspecific binding of ^{3}H-thymidine or its metabolites[43] as well as incorporation into mitochondrial DNA.[44] In HPC, in which a positive result is observed, the count in a nuclear area is due both to incorporation of ^{3}H-thymidine into nuclear DNA during repair and binding of radioactive products to cellular macromolecules in the nucleus and cytoplasm covering the nucleus. In order to correct for the cytoplasmic contribution to the counts obtained in the nuclear area, grain counts are determined in three cytoplasmic areas adjacent to that nucleus. The highest of these three cytoplasmic counts is subtracted from the nuclear count to calculate the net nuclear grain count for an individual nucleus. The number of nuclei to be counted is a function of the ratio of net nuclear grains to cytoplasmic grains.[45] As the ratio decreases, the number of nuclei that must be counted to meet statistical significance increases. Generally, at least 20 nuclei are counted for each slide. The mean and standard deviation of the average net nuclear count of triplicate samples are determined.

With unexposed or solvent-exposed HPC and those exposed to nongenotoxic chemicals, the major source of the grain count obtained in the nuclear area is due to binding of ^{3}H-thymidine in the cytoplasm overlying the nucleus. This results in the net nuclear count being a negative number. Originally, negative grain counts have been represented as zero in calculating the average net nuclear grain count.[18,42] Using this method, a test chemical is considered positive if a net nuclear count of greater than five is observed, since, historically, the upper limit for solvent-exposed cultures was five.[18] However, other investigators use the negative number in the calculation,[20,46,47] while continuing to use a value of greater than five as a positive response.[46,47] Another suggestion has been that an increase of at least two standard deviations above the control value in two successive concentrations constitutes a positive result.[20] Additionally, it has been recommended that the percent of positive cells (>5 grains) also be determined.[18,46,47]

Recently, statistical criteria for a positive result in the HPC/DNA repair test have been proposed.[48] With this approach an increase of three grains above the control is statistically significant. The quantification of the number of cells in repair is recommended along with the statistical analysis to fully evaluate a chemical in the HPC/DNA repair test.[48] This method seems promising and data from additional laboratories will be useful in assessing the approach.

The method for assessing positive results in the HPC/DNA repair test should be standardized to facilitate identification of genotoxic chemicals, especially those which are weakly positive. A value of greater than five is currently considered a positive result. Although established genotoxic chemicals are readily identified using this value, it may be too conservative for weak agents. Improvements in the HPC/DNA repair test have now resulted in control values in our laboratory of less than one. Additionally, this positive value of five was determined using negative numbers as zero.

Our recommendations are that: 1) both net nuclear grain counts and the percent of positive cells be considered in evaluating results in the HPC/DNA repair test; 2) negative numbers be used in calculating average grain counts; 3) the value constituting a positive response be re-evaluated; 4) statistical criteria for this test be validated and adopted; and 5) at least two and preferably three positive concentrations be demonstrated before a test chemical is concluded to be genotoxic.

The HPC/DNA repair test depends on the ability of hepatocytes to metabolize xenobiotics and to repair damage to DNA. Since both of these functions are affected by cell viability, it is important to know whether the test chemical is cytotoxic. This can be readily determined by assessing the general morphology of cells; pyknotic or misshapen nuclei indicate toxicity. These observations have been confirmed by other parameters such as the release of intracellular enzymes or trypan blue exclusion. Generally, the concentration that induces maximum DNA repair results in little or no cytotoxicity.[49]

The UDS that is measured by autoradiography has been verified to be DNA repair, *i.e.*, synthesis occurring in nonreplicated DNA.[43,50,51] The quantification of DNA repair in hepatocytes can potentially be complicated by the presence of grains in the cytoplasm as well as in the nucleus. Modifications such as isolation of DNA on gradients, isolation of nuclei or limiting ^{3}H-thymidine[23,27,30,52] have been tried to reduce cytoplasmic counts. However, cytoplasmic grain counts do not hinder the determination of DNA repair.

Genotoxicity of Xenobiotics in the Rat HPC/DNA Repair Test

The rat HPC/DNA repair test has been shown to be sensitive to a wide variety of structural classes of carcinogens.[18-20] In our laboratory, alkylating agents, aminoazo dyes, aza-aromatics, monocyclic and polycyclic aromatic amines and amides, mycotoxins, polycyclic aromatic hydrocarbons, nitrosamines and pyrrolizidine alkaloids have been tested. Approximately 90% of the known carcinogens in these groups were positive and all the noncarcinogens were negative.[53]

The reliability of the rat HPC/DNA repair test has also been assessed by testing a series of coded compounds.[42] All of the compounds that were positive were carcinogens. Half of the chemicals that were negative were noncarcinogens. The remaining nine chemicals that were negative included four whose carcinogenicity probably does not involve DNA damage. An additional series of coded samples included complex environmental mixtures.[54] Diesel emission, roof tar pot emission and cigarette smoke condensate all induced DNA repair in hepatocytes.

Hepatocarcinogens as well as carcinogens that induce tumors in extrahepatic tissue can be identified as genotoxic in the HPC/DNA repair test. Nonhepatocarcinogens administered *in vivo* can induce repairable damage to liver DNA.[55] However, it is possible that tumors do not develop in this tissue because DNA damage in the liver by hepatocarcinogens is more readily repaired than damage in other tissues.

There are several possible reasons to explain the failure of a carcinogen to elicit a positive response in the HPC/DNA repair test. One reason is that the isolated hepatocytes fail to metabolize the carcinogen to its active metabolite. For some chemicals, the rat HPC/DNA repair test can be modified to provide the necessary metabolic steps. This will be discussed in detail below.

A second reason is that some carcinogens do not interact with DNA. These nongenotoxic carcinogens would not be identified in any test that relies on interaction of the chemical with DNA as its endpoint. These negative results are not a false negative, but rather indicate that these carcinogens act by another mechanism.

A third reason is that the carcinogen inhibits DNA repair. Since a positive response requires that DNA repair occur, inhibition of any step in the repair process would cause a negative result. A variety of chemicals including drugs, hormones, vitamins and pesticides can interfere with excision repair.[56]

MODIFICATIONS OF THE RAT HEPATOCYTE PRIMARY CULTURE/DNA REPAIR TEST

Addition of Exogenous Metabolizing Systems

The metabolism of some chemicals to active metabolites can require extrahepatic enzymes. Glycosides, nitroaromatics and benzidine congener-derived azo dyes often require bacterial metabolism. Cycasin is a glucoside which has been shown to induce tumors when fed to conventional[57] but not germ-free animals.[58] When cycasin is tested in the rat HPC/DNA repair test, no DNA repair is induced.[59] However, if the test is supplemented by the addition of bacterial β-glucosidase, cycasin is positive.[59] The response is dependent on both the concentration of cycasin and the amount of bacterial enzyme.

Nitroaromatics such as dinitrotoluene fail to elicit DNA repair in isolated hepatocytes.[46] Dinitrotoluene is primarily metabolized by intestinal bacteria[60] and it will induce DNA repair in hepatocytes following *in vivo* exposure.[47] However, since other nitroaromatics such as 4-nitrobiphenyl are positive in the HPC/DNA repair test, hepatocytes can activate some chemicals of this type.[53]

In Vivo Exposure

As described in the above section, the HPC/DNA repair test can be supplemented with bacterial enzymes.[59] However, an alternative approach is *in vivo* exposure to the test chemical followed by isolation of hepatocytes and detection of DNA repair.[47,55] Most of the chemicals that are positive following *in vivo* exposure are also positive in the HPC/DNA repair test, although 2,4-dinitrotoluene, which requires metabolism by intestinal bacteria, is only positive following *in vivo* exposure. Some nonhepatocarcinogens such as benzo(a)pyrene and 7,12-dimethylbenz(a)anthracene yield negative results in this test[61] while others such as 3,2'-dimethyl-4-aminobiphenyl are positive.[55] All three of these chemicals induce DNA repair in hepatocytes in primary culture. Therefore, given the much greater effort required for this modification,[55,61] the conventional test is recommended as the primary screen.

Vapor Exposure

The HPC/DNA repair test has been performed on chemicals such as chlorinated ethanes and ethylenes that are vaporized at 37°C.[62] The cultures, prepared as described previously, are placed in a chamber that can be sealed. The test chemical is added either in its liquid or vapor phase to the chamber and the cultures are incubated as previously described. Since the exposures are done in an atmosphere that lacks carbon dioxide, it is necessary to substitute L-15 medium, which is phosphate buffered, for WME, which is buffered with bicarbonate. L-15 Medium (Gibco, Grand Island, NY) is only used during the exposure to the chemical and not for cell attachment.

Utilization of Mouse, Hamster, and Rabbit Hepatocytes

Species differences in xenobiotic metabolism and susceptibility to chemical carcinogens have been described.[63-65] Although the rat has been the most widely used species for preparation of hepatocytes, isolation techniques for several species including mouse,[34,36-38,66-70] hamster,[34,36-38,71-73] rabbit,[35,38,74-76] guinea pig[77] and man[40,41,74,78] have been developed. The development of the HPC/DNA repair test in multiple species now permits evaluation of species-specific responses.[34,36,53]

Preparation of hepatocyte primary cultures. The procedures described previously for the rat are modified for mouse,[34,37,38] hamster,[34,37,38] and rabbit.[35,38] The changes in procedures for isolation of hepatocytes are necessary to accommodate differences in the animal size. Cannulation of the portal vein requires a 21 gauge needle for hamster, 25 gauge for mouse and a 2.5 mm Teflon tube for rabbit.[38] The EGTA solution is perfused for three minutes in mouse and hamster at a rate of ten ml/min and 25 ml/min, respectively and for six minutes at 70 ml/min in rabbit.[38] Collagenase perfusion is for 8 minutes to 10 minutes at 5 to 8 ml/min in mouse, 15 ml/min in hamster and 50 ml/min in rabbit.[38] Additionally, the amount of calf serum required for the initiation of cultures is altered to 1% for mouse and hamster cells.[38]

Genotoxicity of Xenobiotics in the Mouse, Hamster, or Rabbit HPC/DNA Repair Test

A concentration dependent induction of DNA repair is seen in rat, mouse, hamster, or rabbit hepatocytes exposed to the aromatic amine 4,4'-methylene-bis-2-chloroaniline (MBOCA) (Table 1). There are differences both in the concentration inducing maximum DNA repair and in the degree of maximum response. Rabbit hepatocytes exhibit maximum repair for MBOCA at 10^{-4} M to 10^{-3} M, concentrations that are toxic to the other three species.[34,39]

Table 1: Species Differences in the Genotoxicity
of Methylenebis-2-Chloroaniline*

Species	Concentration Inducing Maximum Repair (M)	Net Grains/Nucleus
Rat	10^{-5}	64.0 ± 1.9
Mouse	5×10^{-5}	58.5 ± 20.2
Hamster	10^{-5}	21.8 ± 0.7
Rabbit	10^{-4} to 10^{-3}	13.7 ± 1.7

*Data from References 34 and 39.

The value of testing in multispecies is seen when a comparison is made of the results in the rat, mouse, and hamster HPC/DNA repair test. When safrole and procarbazine were initially tested in the rat HPC/DNA repair test, no DNA repair was observed.[20] Subsequently, these two chemicals were retested in the rat as well as two additional species. Positive results were obtained for mouse and hamster (Table 2).[79]

Chemicals from at least six structural classes have now been tested in the mouse and hamster HPC/DNA repair test[36] as well as in the rat HPC/DNA repair test.[19,21] All of the known or presumed carcinogens are positive in at least one species. The known or presumed noncarcinogens are negative in mouse and rat; however, positive results are seen in hamster hepatocytes with aflatoxin G_2 and pyrene. These chemicals have not been tested for carcinogenicity in the hamster and the results suggest that aflatoxin G_2 and pyrene may be potentially carcinogenic in this species.[36]

Table 2: Species Differences in the Genotoxicity of Safrole and Procarbazine

Chemical	Concentration	Rat[1]	Mouse[2]	Hamster[2]
Safrole	$10^{-2}\%$	T[3]	T	T
	$10^{-3}\%$	$-$[4]	T	+++
	$10^{-4}\%$	-	+++	++
	$10^{-5}\%$	-	++	+
Procarbazine	10^{-2}M	T	++	T
	10^{-3}M	-	-	+++
	10^{-4}M	-	-	++
	10^{-5}M	-	-	++

[1]McQueen, C.A., and Williams, G.M.: unpublished observations.
[2]Reference 79
[3]Toxic
[4]– Negative; + positive

To date, a number of chemicals have demonstrated species-specificity in the HPC/DNA repair test (Table 3). Dimethylhydrazine, hydrazine, safrole, and pro-carbazine do not induce DNA repair in rat hepatocytes, but repair is seen in mouse or hamster cells.

Table 3: Species Differences in the Hepatocyte Primary Culture
(HPC)/DNA Repair Test[1]

Chemical	. . . .Rat		. . .Mouse . . .		. .Hamster . .	
	Carc.[2]	DNA Repair	Carc.	DNA Repair	Carc.	DNA Repair
Aflatoxin G_2[3]		$-$[4]		-		+
1,2-Dimethylhydrazine	+	-	+	+	+	+
Hydrazine	+	-	+	+	-	+
Methylhydrazine		-		+		+
Procarbazine	+	-	+	+		+
Pyrene	-	-	-	-		+
Safrole	+	-	+	+		+

[1]References 36, 79 and unpublished observations.
[2]Results from IARC Monographs on the evaluation of the carcinogenic risk of chemicals to humans.
[3]Negative in trout.
[4]– Negative; + positive

In vivo differences in susceptibility can also be reflected in the *in vitro* assay. The mouse is relatively resistant to the tumorigenic effect of aflatoxin B_1.[80] This chemical induces maximum DNA repair in mouse hepatocytes at a concentration ten to 100 times that necessary to elicit the same response in hamster hepatocytes.[36] Preparations from mouse liver are capable of forming aflatoxin B_1 epoxide[81] but are more efficient in inactivating aflatoxin B_1 than rat preparations.[13,81]

Effect of Intraspecies Differences on Chemical Genotoxicity

The effect of a difference in a single metabolic step on genotoxicity can be investigated in the HPC/DNA repair test. N-Acetylation of aromatic amines and hydrazines is under polymorphic genetic control in humans and rabbits and individuals are classified as rapid or slow acetylators.[82-86] Sensitivity to the toxicity, including damage to DNA, of drugs that are metabolized by N-acetyltransferase, has been linked to acetylator phenotype.[87] Rabbit hepatocytes in primary culture allow measurement of N-acetyl transferase activity and DNA damage in the same system.[35,39] Hepatocytes isolated from both acetylator phenotypes maintain their *in vivo* differences in culture.[35] Phenotype-dependent differences in genotoxicity are observed with 2-aminofluorene (2-AF),[35] benzidine (BZD),[35] and hydralazine (HDZ).[35] Hepatocytes from rabbits which are rapid acetylators are more susceptible to the genotoxic effects of 2-AF or BZD. A 10^{-4}M concentration of 2-AF induced maximum repair in hepatocytes from rapid acetylator rabbits while 10^{-3}M of 2-AF was necessary to elicit a maximum response in hepatocytes from slow acetylators. A positive response to hydralazine is only observed in hepatocytes from slow acetylator rabbits. These results provide evidence for the role of the acetylator polymorphism as a factor in determining susceptibility to these genotoxic chemicals.

CONCLUSIONS

The HPC/DNA repair test utilizes the metabolic capacity of intact liver cells and the specificity of DNA repair as an indicator of DNA damage. Extensive validation of the rat HPC/DNA repair test shows that it is a reliable method for evaluating the genotoxic potential of a chemical.[18-21,53] Hepatocytes from a variety of species can be used in the HPC/DNA repair test. Such testing permits establishment of multispecies genotoxicity as well as identification of species specific responses.

REFERENCES

1. Fry, J.R., and Bridges, J.W., in: *Reviews in Biochemical Toxicology* (E. Hudgson, J.R. Bend, and R.M. Philpot, eds.), Vol. 1, p 201, Elsevier: North Holland, New York (1979)
2. Sirica, A.E., and Pitot, H.C., Drug metabolism and effects of carcinogens in cultured hepatic cells. *Pharmacol. Rev.* 31: 205-228 (1980)
3. Thurman, R.G., and Kaufman, F.C., Factors regulating drug metabolism in intact hepatocytes. *Pharmacol. Rev.* 31: 229-251 (1980)
4. Williams, G.M., in: *Proceedings of Symposium on Chemical Indices and Mechanisms of Organ Directed Toxicity* (S.S. Brown, and D. Davies, eds.), p 131, New York: Pergamon Press (1981)
5. Eaton, D.L., and Klaassen, C.D., Carrier-mediated transport of ouabain in isolated hepatocytes. *J. Pharmacol. Exp. Ther.* 205: 408-488 (1978)
6. Galivan, J.H., Transport and metabolism of methotrexate in normal and resistant cultured rat hepatoma cells. *Cancer Res.* 39: 725-733 (1979)

7. Morland, J., and Olsen, H., Metabolism of sulfadimidine, sulfanilamide, *p*-aminobenzoic acid and isoniazid in suspensions of parenchymal and non-parenchymal rat liver cells. *Drug Metab. Disp.* 5: 511-517 (1977)
8. Billings, R.E., McMahon, R.E., Ashmore, J., and Wagle, S.R., The metabolism of drugs in isolated rat hepatocytes. A comparison with *in vivo* metabolism and drug metabolism in subcellular liver fractions. *Drug Metabol. Disp.* 5: 518-526 (1977)
9. Jones, C.A., Moore, B.P., Cohen, G.M., Fry, J.R., and Bridges, J.W., Studies on the metabolism and excretion of benzo(a)pyrene in isolated adult rat hepatocytes. *Biochem. Pharmacol.* 27: 693-702 (1978)
10. Suolinna, E., The metabolism of sulfanilamide and related drugs in isolated rat and rabbit liver cells. *Drug Metab. Disp.* 8: 205-207 (1980)
11. Shirkey, R.J., Kao, J., Fry, J.R., and Bridges, J.W., A comparison of xenobiotic metabolism in cells isolated from rat liver and small intestinal mucosa. *Biochem. Pharmacol.* 28: 1461-1466 (1979)
12. McQueen, C.A., Maslansky, C.J., Glowinski, I.B., Crescenszi, S.B., Weber, W.W., and Williams, G.M., Relationship between the genetically determined acetylator phenotype and DNA damage induced by hydralazine and 2-aminofluorene in cultured rabbit hepatocytes. *Proc. Natl. Acad. Sci. USA* 79: 1269-1272 (1982)
13. Decad, G.M., Hsieh, D.P.H., and Byard, J.L., Maintenance of cytochrome P_{450} and metabolism of aflatoxin B_1 in primary hepatocyte cultures. *Biochem. Biophys. Res. Commun.* 78:279-287 (1977)
14. Dybing, E., Soderlund, E., Timm-Haug, L., and Thorgeirsson, S.S., Metabolism and activation of 2-acetylaminofluorene in isolated rat hepatocytes. *Cancer Res.* 39: 3268-3275 (1979)
15. Vadi, H., Moldeus, P., Capdevila, J. and Orrenius, S., The metabolism of benzo(a)pyrene in isolated rat cells. *Cancer Res.* 35: 2083-2091 (1975)
16. Schmeltz, I., Tosk, J., and Williams, G.M., Comparison of the metabolic profiles of benzo(a)pyrene obtained from primary cell cultures and subcellular fractions derived from normal and methyl-cholanthrene-induced rat liver. *Cancer Lett.* 5: 81-89 (1978).
17. Bates, D.J., Foster, A.B., and Jarman, M., The metabolism of cyclophosphamide by isolated rat hepatocytes. *Biochem. Pharmacol.* 30: 3055-3063 (1981)
18. Williams, G.M., The detection of chemical carcinogens by unscheduled DNA synthesis in rat liver primary cell cultures. *Cancer Res.* 37: 1845-1851 (1977)
19. Williams, G.M., in: *Chemical Mutagens* (F.J. de Serres, and A. Hollaender, eds.), Vol. 6, pp 61-79, Plenum Press, New York (1980)
20. Probst, G.S., McMahon, R.E., Hill, L.E., Thompson, C.Z., Epp, J.K., and Neal, S.B., Chemically-induced unscheduled DNA synthesis in primary rat hepatocyte cultures. *Environ. Mutagen.* 3: 11-32 (1981)
21. Williams, G.M., Classification of genotoxic and epigenetic hepatocarcinogens using liver culture assays. *Ann. N.Y. Acad. Sci.* 349: 273-282 (1980)
22. Nordenskjold, M., Moldeus, P., and Lambert, B., Effects of ultraviolet light and cyclophosphamide on replication and repair synthesis of DNA in isolated rat liver cells and human leukocytes coincubated with microsomes. *Hereditas* 89: 1-6 (1978)
23. Michalopoulos, G., Sattler, G.L., O'Connor, L., and Pitot, H.C., Unscheduled DNA synthesis induced by procarcinogens in suspensions and primary cultures of hepatocytes on collagen membranes. *Cancer Res.* 38: 1866-1871 (1978)

24. Brouns, R.E., Poot, M., deVrind, R., v.Hoek-Kon, Th., and Henderson, P.Th., Measurement of DNA-excision repair in suspensions of freshly isolated rat hepatocytes after exposure to some carcinogenic compounds. *Mutation Res.* 64: 425-432 (1979)

25. Hsia, M.T.S., and Kreamer, B.L., Induction of unscheduled DNA synthesis in suspensions of rat hepatocytes by an environmental toxicant, 3,3', 4,4'-tetrachloroazobenzene. *Cancer Lett.* 6: 207-212 (1979)

26. Seglen, P.O., and Fossa, J., Attachment of rat hepatocytes *in vitro* to substrate of serum protein, collagen, or concanavalin A. *Exp. Cell Res.* 116: 199-206 (1978)

27. Oldham, J.W., Casciano, D.A., and Cave, M.D., Comparative induction of unscheduled DNA synthesis by physical and chemical agents in non-proliferating primary cultures of rat hepatocytes. *Chem. Biol. Interact.* 29: 303-314 (1980)

28. Sirica, A.E., Hwang, C.G., Sattler, G.L., and Pitot, H.C., Use of primary cultures of adult rat hepatocytes on collagen gel-nylon mesh to evaluate carcinogen-induced unscheduled DNA synthesis. *Cancer Res.* 40: 3259-3267 (1980)

29. Williams, G.M., Further improvements in the hepatocyte primary culture DNA repair test for carcinogens: Detection of carcinogenic biphenyl derivatives. *Cancer Lett.* 4: 69-75 (1978)

30. Althaus, F.R., Lawrence, S.D., Sattler, G.L., Longfellow, D.G., and Pitot, H.C., Chemical quantification of unscheduled DNA synthesis in cultured hepatocytes as an assay for the rapid screening of potential chemical carcinogens. *Cancer Res.* 42: 3010-3015 (1982)

31. Williams, G.M., Bermudez, E., and Scaramuzzino, D., Rat hepatocyte primary cultures. III. Improved dissociation and attachment techniques and the enhancement of survival by culture medium. *In Vitro* 13: 809-817 (1977)

32. Laishes, B.A., and Williams, G.M., Conditions affecting primary cell cultures of functional adult rat hepatocytes: II. Dexamethasone-enhanced longevity and maintenance of morphology. *In Vitro* 12: 821-832 (1976)

33. Williams, G.M., Carcinogen-induced DNA repair in primary rat liver cell cultures: A possible screen for chemical carcinogens. *Cancer Lett.* 1: 231-236 (1976)

34. McQueen, C.A., Maslansky, C.J., Crescenzi, S.B., and Williams, G.M., The genotoxicity of 4,4'-methylene-bis-2-chloroaniline in rat, mouse, and hamster hepatocytes. *Toxicol. Appl. Pharmacol.* 58: 231-235 (1981)

35. McQueen, C.A., Maslansky, C.J., Glowinski, I.B., Crescenzi, S.B., Weber, W.W., and Williams, G.M., Relationship between the genetically determined acetylator phenotype and DNA damage induced by hydralazine and 2-aminofluorene in cultured rabbit hepatocytes. *Proc. Nat. Acad. Sci. USA* 79: 1269-1272 (1982)

36. McQueen, C.A., Kreiser, D.M., and Williams, G.M., The hepatocyte primary culture/DNA repair assay using mouse or hamster hepatocytes. *Environ. Mutagen.* 5: 1-8 (1983)

37. Maslansky, C.J., and Williams, G.M., Evidence for an epigenetic mode of action of organochlorine pesticide hepatocarcinogenicity: A lack of genotoxicity in rat, mouse, and hamster hepatocytes. *J. Toxicol. Environ. Health.* 8: 121-130 (1981)

38. Maslansky, C.J., and Williams, G.M., Primary cultures and levels of cytochrome P_{450} in hepatocytes from mouse, rat, hamster, and rabbit liver. *In Vitro* 18: 683-693 (1982)

39. McQueen, C.A., Maslansky, C.J., and Williams, G.M., The role of the acetylation polymorphism in determining susceptibility of cultured rabbit hepatocytes to DNA damage by aromatic amines. *Cancer Res.* 43: 3120-3123 (1983)
40. Strom, S.C., Novicki, D.L., Novotny, A., Jirtle, R.L., and Michalopoulos, G., Human hepatocyte-mediated mutagenesis and DNA repair activity. *Carcinogenesis* 4: 683-686 (1983)
41. Begue, J.M., LeBigot, J.F., Guguen-Guillouzo, C., Kiechel, J.R., and Guillouzo, A., Cultured human adult hepatocytes: A new model for drug metabolism studies. *Biochem. Pharmacol.* 32: 1643-1646 (1983)
42. Williams, G.M., Laspia, M.F., and Dunkel, V.C., Reliability of the hepatocyte primary culture/DNA repair test. *Cancer Lett.* 6: 199-306 (1982)
43. Yager, J.D., and Miller, J.A., DNA repair in primary cultures of rat hepatocytes. *Cancer Res.* 38: 4385-4395 (1978)
44. Lonati-Galligani, M., Lohman, P.H.M., and Berends, F., The validity of the autoradiographic method for detecting DNA repair synthesis in rat hepatocytes in primary culture. *Mutation Res.* 113: 145-160 (1983)
45. Rodgers, A.W., *Techniques in Autoradiography*. New York: Elsevier Scientific Publishing Co. (1973)
46. Bermudez, E., Tillery, D., and Butterworth, B., The effect of 2,4-dinitrotoluene and isomers of dinitrotoluene on unscheduled DNA synthesis in primary rat hepatocytes. *Environ. Mutagen.* 1: 391-398 (1979)
47. Mirsalis, J.C., and Butterworth, B.E., Detection of unscheduled DNA synthesis in hepatocytes isolated from rats treated with genotoxic agents: An *in vivo/in vitro* assay for potential carcinogens and mutagens. *Carcinogenesis* 1: 621-625 (1980)
48. Casciano, D.A., and Gaylor, D.W., Statistical criteria for evaluating chemicals as positive or negative in the hepatocyte/DNA repair assay. *Mutat. Res.* 122: 81-86 (1984)
49. McQueen, C.A., and Williams, G.M., Cytotoxicity of xenobiotics in adult rat hepatocytes in primary culture. *Fundam. Appl. Toxicol.* 2: 139-142 (1982)
50. McQueen, C.A., and Williams, G.M., Characterization of DNA repair elicited by carcinogens and drugs in the hepatocyte primary culture/DNA repair test. *J. Toxicol. Environ. Health* 8: 463-477 (1981)
51. Andrae, U., and Schwarz, L.R., Induction of DNA repair synthesis in isolated rat hepatocytes by 5-diazouracil and other DNA damaging compounds. *Cancer Lett.* 13: 187-193 (1981)
52. Williams, G.M., and Laspia, M.F., The detection of various nitrosamines in the hepatocyte primary culture/DNA repair test. *Cancer Lett.* 6: 199-206 (1979)
53. McQueen, C.A., and Williams, G.M., The use of cells from rat, mouse, hamster, and rabbit in the hepatocyte primary culture/DNA repair test. *Ann. N.Y. Acad. Sci.* 407: 119-130 (1983)
54. Ved Brat, S., Tong, C., and Williams, G.M., in: *Genotoxic Effects of Airborne Agents* (R.R. Tice, D.L. Costa, and K.M. Schaich, eds.), pp 619-631, Plenum Press, New York (1982)
55. Hellemann, A., Maslansky, C.J., Bosland, M., and Williams, G.M., Rat liver DNA damage by the nonhepatocarcinogen 3,2'-dimethyl-4-aminobiphenyl. *Cancer Lett.* 22: 211-218 (1984)
56. Bernheim, N.J., and Falk, H., Chemical, physical and genetic factors interfering with DNA repair—A review. *J. Amer. Coll. Toxicol.* 2: 23-54 (1983)

57. Laqueur, G.L., The induction of intestinal neoplasms in rats with the glycoside cycasin and its aglycone. *Virchows Arch.* 340: 151-163 (1965)
58. Laqueur, G.L., Carcinogenic effects of cycad meal and cycasin, methylazoxymethanol glycoside in rats and effects of cycasin in germ-free rats. *Fed. Proc.* 23: 1386-1388 (1964)
59. Williams, G.M., Laspia, M.F., Mori, H., and Hirona, I., Genotoxicity of cycasin in the hepatocyte primary culture/DNA repair test supplemented with β-glucosidase. *Cancer Lett.* 12: 329-333 (1981)
60. Guest, D., Schnell, S.R., Rickert, D.E., and Dent, J.G., Metabolism of 2,4-dinitrotoluene by intestinal microorganisms from rat, mouse, and man. *Toxicol. Appl. Pharmacol.* 64: 160-168 (1982)
61. Mirsalis, J.C., Tyson, C.K., and Butterworth, B.E., Detection of genotoxic carcinogens in the *in vivo-in vitro* hepatocyte DNA repair assay. *Environ. Mutagen.* 4: 553-562 (1982)
62. Shimada, T., Swanson, A.F., Leber, P., and Williams, G.M., The evaluation for genotoxicity of several halogenated solvents. *Environ. Mutagen.* 5: 447 (1983)
63. Miller, E.C., Miller, J.A., and Enomoto, M., The comparative carcinogenicity of 2-acetylaminofluorene and its N-hydroxy metabolite in mice, hamsters, and guinea pigs. *Cancer Res.* 24: 2018-2031 (1964)
64. Irving, C.C., in: *Carcinogens: Identification and Mechanisms* (A.C. Griffin, and C.R. Shaw, eds.), pp 211-277, Raven Press, New York (1979)
65. Selkirk, J.K., in: *Carcinogenesis* (T.J. Slaga, ed.), Vol. 5, pp 1-31, Raven Press, New York (1980)
66. Crisp, D.M., and Pogson, C.I., Glycolytic and gluconeogenic enzyme activities in parenchymal and nonparenchymal cells from mouse liver. *Biochem. J.* 126: 1009-1023 (1972)
67. Renton, K.W., DeLoria, L.B., and Mannering, G.J., Effects of polyriboinosinic acid, polyribocytidylic acid and a mouse interferon preparation on cytochrome P_{450}-dependent monooxygenase systems in cultures of primary mouse hepatocytes. *Mol. Pharmacol.* 14: 672-681 (1978)
68. Decad, G.M., Doughtery, K.K., Hsieh, D.P.H., and Byard, J.L., Metabolism of aflatoxin B_1 in cultured mouse hepatocytes: Comparison with rat and effects of cyclohexene oxide and diethyl maleate. *Toxicol. Appl. Pharmacol.* 50: 429-436 (1979)
69. Klaunig, J.E., Goldblatt, P.J., Hinton, D.E., Lipsky, M.M., Chasko, J., and Trump, B.F., Mouse liver cell culture I. Hepatocyte isolation. *In Vitro* 17: 913-925 (1981)
70. Klaunig, J.E., Goldblatt, P.J., Hinton, D.E., Lipsky, M.M., and Trump, B.F., Mouse liver cell culture II. Primary culture. *In Vitro* 17: 926-934 (1981)
71. Poiley, J.A., Raineri, R., and Pienta, R.J., Use of hamster hepatocytes to metabolize carcinogens in an *in vitro* bioassay. *J. Natl. Cancer Inst.* 63: 519-523 (1979)
72. Raineri, R., Poiley, J.A., Andrews, A.W., Pienta, R.J., and Lijinsky, W., Greater effectiveness of hepatocyte and liver S9 preparations from hamster than rat preparations in activating N-nitroso compounds to metabolites mutagenic to *Salmonella. J. Natl. Cancer. Inst.* 67: 1117-1122 (1981)
73. Kornbrust, D.J., and Barfknecht, T.R., Comparison of rat and hamster primary culture/DNA repair assays. *Environ. Mutagen.* 6: 1-11 (1984)
74. Reese, J.A., and Byard, J.L., Isolation and culture of adult hepatocytes from liver biopsies. *In Vitro* 17: 935-940 (1981)

75. Corona, G.L., Santagostino, G., Facino, R.M., and Pirillo, D., Cell membrane modifications in rabbit isolated hepatocytes following a chronic amitryptiline treatment. *Biochem. Pharmacol.* 22: 849-856 (1973)

76. Zaleski, J., and Bryla, J., The effects of oleate, palmitate and octanoate on gluconeogenesis in isolated rabbit liver cells. *Arch. Biochem. Biophys.* 183: 553-562 (1977)

77. Arinze, I.J., and Rowley, D.L., Gluconeogenesis by isolated guinea pig liver parenchymal cells. *Biochem. J.* 152: 393-399 (1975)

78. Strom, S.C., Jirtle, R.L., Jones, R.S., Novicki, D.L., Rosenberg, M.R., Novotny, A., Irons, G.P., McLain, J.R., and Michalopoulos, G., Isolation, culture and transplantation of human hepatocytes. *J. Natl. Cancer Inst.* 68: 771-778 (1972)

79. McQueen, C.A., Kreiser, D.M., Hurley, P.M., and Williams, G.M., The hepatocyte primary culture/DNA repair test using mouse and hamster cells. *Environ. Mutagen.* 5: 483 (1983)

80. Wogan, G.N., Aflatoxin carcinogenesis. *Methods Cancer Res.* 7: 309-344 (1973)

81. Degen, G.H., and Neuman, H.G., Differences in aflatoxin B_1-susceptibility of rat and mouse are correlated with the capability *in vitro* to inactivate aflatoxin B_1-epoxide. *Carcinogenesis* 2: 299-306 (1981)

82. Knight, R.A., Selin, M.J., and Harris, H.W., Genetic factors influencing isoniazid blood levels in humans. *Trans. Conf. Chemother. Tuberc.* 18: 52-60 (1959)

83. Evans, D.A.P., Manley, K.A., and McKusick, V.A., Genetic control of isoniazid metabolism in man. *Brit. Med. J.* 2: 485-491 (1960)

84. Frymoyer, J.W., and Jacox, R.F., Investigation of the genetic control of sulfadiazine and isoniazid metabolism in the rabbit. *J. Lab. Clin. Med.* 62: 891-904 (1963)

85. Frymoyer, J.W., and Jacox, R.F., Studies of genetically controlled sulfadiazine acetylation in rabbit livers. Possible identification of the heterozygous trait. *J. Lab. Clin. Med.* 62: 905-909 (1963)

86. Gordon, G.R., Shafizadeh, A.G., and Peters, J.H., Polymorphic acetylation of drugs in rabbits. *Xenobiotica* 3: 133-150 (1973)

87. Drayer, D.E., and Reidenberg, M.M., Clinical consequences of polymorphic acetylation of basic drugs. *Clin. Pharmacol. Therap.* 22: 251-258 (1977)

7

Cell Transformation Assays

Andrew Sivak
Alice S. Tu

Arthur D. Little, Inc.
Cambridge, Massachusetts

INTRODUCTION

Over the last decade, the development and maturation of assays for cellular neoplastic transformation have provided the means to pose specific questions related to the mechanism of carcinogenesis. These methods have also offered a tool to identify potentially carcinogenic chemicals. A number of recent reviews[1-3] have described and evaluated the general methodology for measuring cellular transformation, *in vitro*.[4-7] This chapter will therefore only focus on specific issues dealing with technical problems and modifications in performing several of the assays. The applications of these assays to examine other components related to the carcinogenic process and an assessment of desirable directions for future research will be considered.

The cell transformation assays have their roots in observations made from the earliest availability of cell culture technologies. These early studies reported morphological differences in cultures of cells treated with chemical carcinogens as well as behavioral changes of tumor cells in culture as compared to non-tumor cells.[8-11] Although a wide variety of systems have been described over the years, including studies with human cells, the assay procedures that are in contemporary use are relatively few in number and our primary discussion will be limited to them.

Overall, cell transformation systems can be categorized among three generic types. One variety utilizes primary or early passage cells in culture and is exemplified by the Syrian hamster embryo cell clonal transformation assay originally described by Berwald and Sachs[12] and practiced by a number of investigators in the intervening two decades without substantial change from the originally described protocol. A focus assay with Syrian hamster embryo cells has also been described,[13] and appears to result in a measurable transformation response with known carcinogens. Other focus transformation assays have utilized early passage cells of human origin. The procedures described are more varied and differ in approach from assays using rodent cells which have tended to adhere to fairly rigorous standard methodologies among different laboratories.

The remaining studies demonstrating neoplastic transformation in early passage cells have been carried out with epithelial cells. The largest body of data has been developed for mouse epidermal cells and rat tracheal epithelial cells. The argument is often made that, since the large majority of neoplastic lesions occur in epithelial tissue, the cells from these tissues are the most appropriate for assessment of the carcinogenic potential of chemicals.

A second category of neoplastic transformation assays is that carried out with established cell lines. Of the systems described, three utilize heteroploid mouse lines that exhibit a strong tendency for monolayer growth as a result of density dependent inhibition of cell proliferation with multilayered foci being induced by carcinogenic stimuli. The cells employed in these assays are specific clones of BALB/c-3T3, C3H-10T½ and a mouse prostate line originally developed in the laboratory of Heidelberger. In addition, an assay procedure involving BHK-21 hamster cells has been described which measures the ability of carcinogens to enhance the growth of these cells in soft agar or other suspending matrices.

The third class of neoplastic transformation assays is that which utilizes cells that have been infected by a transforming virus. In one case, Fischer rat embryo cells have been infected with Rauscher leukemia virus and the resultant cells do not exhibit transformed behavior until after many passages in culture, nor do they shed oncornavirus. Treatment of these cells with carcinogens yields morphologically altered foci after several passages. A second cell-virus assay is one that measures the capacity of carcinogens to enhance the transformation of Syrian hamster embryo cells with the simian adenovirus SA7. This assay is markedly different from other transformation assays in that it detects the effect of carcinogens on events induced by a DNA virus interacting with the cell genome rather than the behavior of cells responding directly to carcinogens. To be sure, proponents of oncogene models for neoplastic transformation point out close similarities to oncogene activation in this class of transformation assays.

METHODS IN CONTEMPORARY USE

Transformation Assays with Early Passage Cells

Syrian hamster embryo clonal assay. The prototype assay in this category is the Syrian hamster embryo (SHE) clonal transformation procedure. Either fresh or cryopreserved mixed populations of secondary or tertiary embryo cells, mostly of fibroblast morphology, are employed. The procedure shown below is typical of the methodology usually employed.

Cell Cultures

Primary Syrian hamster embryo cells are prepared by trypsinization of decapitated and eviscerated 12 to 14 day old embryos. Cells are cryo-preserved at 2×10^6 cells/ampule to 5×10^6 cells/ampule.

Medium

Dulbecco's modified Eagle's medium with 10% (or 20%) pretested fetal calf serum and 2mM L-glutamine.

Transformation Assay

(1) Thaw feeder cells from frozen stock, grow and subculture cells for two to five days prior to use.

(2) Irradiate (5000R) feeder cells and plate at 6×10^4 cells/60 mm dish. Thaw and grow target cells one day prior to use.

(3) Seed target cells onto feeder cells at 200 cells or 300 cells per dish.

(4) Add chemicals one day later and incubate for seven days at $37°C$ in 10% CO_2 incubator without feeding.

(5) Fix and stain dishes at end of incubation.

Scoring and Quantitation

Colonies in each dish are counted manually. Cytotoxicity of the test chemical is determined by comparing the mean number of colonies in treated dishes with the untreated control. Colonies of scoreable size are evaluated under the stereomicroscope. Transformation frequency is expressed as number of transformed colonies compared to the total colonies scored.

This assay has several advantages. The target cells are diploid and retain more diverse metabolic capabilities than most established cell lines. The assay can be completed in two weeks. In addition, the clonal nature of this assay also allows the direct measurement of surviving cell fraction at risk and transformation frequency in the same population.

However, procedurally this assay appears to be the most sensitive to operational conditions among the commonly used assays. Beyond the usual needs of good housekeeping and quality control of the constituents used in the assay, the requirement for a lot of fetal calf serum that will be efficacious for demonstration of neoplastic transformation is a major factor in the successful performance of this assay.[14] The reasons for the different behaviors of different serum lots with respect to transformation response are not known, nor has any concerted research effort been reported to address this important problem. Characteristics of cell viability such as growth rate or cloning efficiency in varied serum lots are not diagnostic for determining the transformation efficiency. At the present time, the only viable procedure is to select serum lots that work empirically on a trial and error basis.

The observation by Pienta *et al.*[7] and DiPaolo[15] that frozen pools of cells could be used effectively in the transformation assay was an important finding since it provided the means to obtain pools of cells that could be used over extended time intervals allowing for some consistency from assay to assay over procedures that used fresh cell pools for each assay. However, it was observed that not all cell pools from the embryos of single dams were transformable. Moreover, when cells from individual embryos in the same litter were tested for their capacity to be transformed by carcinogens, a marked heterogeneity was seen.[16] Thus, each cell pool requires verification of its ability to respond to carcinogens prior to storing for later use. As with the problem with fetal calf serum, there are no substantial experimental findings that provide an explanation for this response, and there has been little, if any, effort to explore the reasons for this wide variation in cellular behavior. This facet of the assay deserves further investigation in order to obtain a higher degree of uniformity in transformation response and to understand better, from a mechanistic point of view, what is happening in the cell culture during the transformation process.

The actual performance of the assay as shown presents no major technical problems for those skilled in standard cell culture procedures. In contrast, the evaluation of the stained plates for diagnosis of transformed clones is associated with difficulties in the definitive identification of such clones. Being of mixed origin, the clones, both normal and transformed, display a wide range of morphological characteristics with respect to density and configuration. The effect of this morphological variation is a high degree of uncertainty in the identification of clones outside the range of those that clearly demonstrate altered morphology in terms of multilayering of cells in the clone and the random orientation of cells at the periphery of the clone. Although several diagnostic measures other than morphology have been examined to establish whether clones are normal or transformed,[17] there are no presently available reliable markers to obtain an independent measure of transformation. For example, the occurrence of plasminogen activator resulting in fibrinolytic activity was shown to have no correlation with transformation response.[18,19]

Syrian hamster embryo focus assay. Casto *et al.*[13] have described a focus assay for use with Syrian hamster embryo cells. The report suggested that the cells responded to a similar range of carcinogens in the focus assay as in the clonal assay. Since the quantitation of cytotoxicity and the number of cells at risk is a problem in all focus assays and the morphological diagnosis of transformation is more difficult than in other focus assays due to the mixed cell types of this system, there appears to be no advantage to using this procedure. In fact, beyond the original few descriptions of the assay procedure and the original list of chemicals tested, there are no further reports of its use and no evidence that the assay is being used presently with any frequency as a tool to identify carcinogens.

Human cell focus assay. There is a certain fascination with the use of human cells for neoplastic transformation assays, the argument being that assays with cells from the species of prime interest for the prevention of carcinogenesis would yield the most reliable data for making judgments on human risk. However, the facts as they have evolved suggest that there is no special advantage for identification of potential carcinogens by the use of human cells as compared to rodent cells of a variety of sources.

The studies that have been reported with human cells have employed mostly fibroblasts,[20-23] and the range of chemicals tested is limited in comparison to other assay systems. The assay generally is a multistep procedure that involves intervals of several months before the occurrence of morphologically altered foci. Tests on such foci have shown that they give rise to growths in nude mice[24] or invasive lesions in chicken egg allantoic membranes.[25]

Epithelial cell transformation assays. The development of methods to cultivate epithelial cells from a variety of organs has led to the study of neoplastic transformation in several systems. The studies of Yuspa and his colleagues[26-28] have demonstrated that an alteration of cellular behavior can be induced in mouse epidermal cells exposed to a chemical carcinogen. Modifications of the concentration of calcium have allowed the clonal visualization of morphologic variants that exhibit abnormal behavior characteristic of transformed cells.[29,30] While these procedures provide a strong tool to examine questions relating to the mechanism of the carcinogenic process at the cellular level, their application as a general screening bioassay method for carcinogens does not appear to be feasible at the present time.

An interesting series of investigations by Nettesheim *et al.*[31-34] has been carried out using rat trachea as a source for cellular material. Following a variety of carcinogen exposures to trachea *in situ*, trachea heterotopically transplanted and tracheal cells in culture, there have been clear demonstrations of transformation. In general, the occurrence of transformed cells in culture has required long cultivation times of several months. However, squamous cell carcinomas have resulted from transformed cells implanted into suitable hosts suggesting that the events observed in culture have a direct relationship to the carcinogenic process *in vivo*. Nonetheless, these procedures, like the epidermal system described above, appear to provide a means to study questions of mechanism rather than to have utility as a general bioassay vehicle.

Transformation Assays with Cell Lines

BALB/c-3T3 focus assay. This assay was originally described by Kakunaga in 1973.[35] Its performance remains essentially unchanged, and the general methodology is shown below.

Cell Cultures

Working stock cultures of BALB/c-3T3 clone 1–13 cells are stored in liquid nitrogen at $\sim 1 \times 10^6$ cells/ampule.

Medium

Eagle's minimum essential medium with 10% pretested fetal calf serum. Penicillin and streptomycin are present in 50 units/ml and 50 μg/ml, respectively.

Transformation Assay

(1) Thaw target cells from frozen stock, grow and subculture for two days to five days prior to use.

(2) Plate 10^4 cells/60 mm dish. Add chemicals one day later for a period of three days.

(3) At the end of the treatment period, trypsinize cells from two replicate dishes of each experimental set, pool and count cells to determine cytotoxicity of the test compound. Plate an aliquot of the

counted cells at 100–200 cells/dish to determine cloning efficiency.

(4) Feed the remainder of the dishes with medium containing no test chemicals and incubate for approximately four weeks. Change the medium twice in the first two weeks and then weekly during the last two weeks of the assay.

(5) Fix and stain dishes at end of incubation.

Scoring and Quantitation

Each stained dish is examined under the stereomicroscope. Type III foci (aggregation of multilayered densely stained cells that exhibit criss-cross array at the edge of the focus) over the background monolayer are scored. Transformation frequency is expressed as the number of Type III foci per dish as well as the number of dishes with Type III foci over the total dishes.

Among the neoplastic transformation assays carried out with cell lines, this assay has the largest data base. One of the primary reasons for its relatively wide use is the general availability of the cells, most of which are subclones isolated by Kakunaga from Clone A31 of the BALB/c-3T3 cells. In contrast to the heterogenous population of cells obtained for the clonal Syrian hamster embryo assay, BALB/c-3T3 cells that have been cloned represent a relatively uniform cell pool. However, not all subclones from A31 cells are responsive to induced transformation.[36,37] The reason for this phenomenon is not clear. Metabolic capability is apparently not a factor since variant clones with different induced transformation frequencies exhibited similarities in the formation and removal of benzo(a)pyrene DNA adducts.[38]

An important factor associated with BALB/c-3T3 neoplastic transformation assay is the stability of response of sister pools of cells over an interval of several years in terms of spontaneous and induced transformants. Figure 1 shows the transformation response of seven target cell pools prepared in our laboratory over a period of three years. The similarity in response over this interval allows the historical comparison of data.

Although the transformation assay exhibits some serum dependence (Figure 2), this factor is substantially less limiting than for the Syrian hamster embryo clonal assay. The impact of passage number, plating density, exposure time, and total assay interval have been described previously,[4] and the protocol outline takes into account the optimization of these variables.

C3H-10T½ focus assay. This cell line was developed by Reznikoff *et al.*[39,40] at about the same time the transformation of the BALB/c-3T3 line by carcinogenic chemicals was reported. The transformation assay with the C3H-10T½ cell line is similar in a general manner to the BALB/c-3T3 protocol. The differences applicable to the C3H-10T½ assay as it is usually performed are time of exposure (one day), assay duration (six weeks) and the original cell plating density (10^3 cells per 60 mm dish). Subsequent studies carried out for additional validation data have shown that a plating density of 10^4 cells results in a higher degree of detection sensitivity than the original suggested cell density.

In contrast to the BALB/c-3T3 assay, the sensitivity to the lot of fetal calf

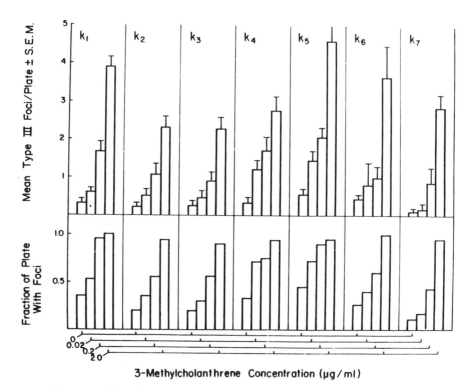

Figure 1: Transformation response of different target cell pools to 3-methylcholanthrene. Each target cell pool (k series) consisting of approximately 60 ampules of cells was expanded from a cryopreserved stock of BALB/c-3T3 clone 1-13 cells originally obtained from T. Kakunaga. The transformation response of each cell pool to 3-methylcholanthrene was validated by conducting a standard transformation assay as described in the text. The data represent a mean of 15 to 20 plates per test condition.

serum for demonstration of transformation is considerably more acute resulting in the need to screen multiple lots to obtain an efficacious serum.[41] In this regard, the C3H-10T½ more resembles the Syrian hamster embryo cell clonal assay in its serum requirement profile.

With an effective lot of fetal calf serum, C3H-10T½ cells exhibit a high degree of stability in behavior with respect to transformation over a larger number of passages than BALB/c-3T3 cells. In addition, the very low spontaneous transformation frequency and uniformity of the monolayer upon which the transformed foci occur makes detection of foci easier than in the BALB/c-3T3 assay.

Other cell line assays. The earliest transformation assay described using established cells was reported by Chen and Heidelberger in 1969,[42] who employed a line of fibroblasts that evolved from a mouse prostate culture. This line shares many of the characteristics of the BALB/c-3T3 and C3H-10T½ lines and was

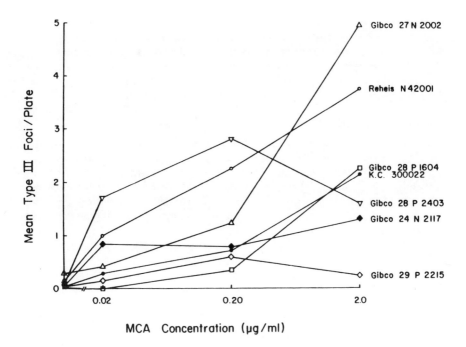

Figure 2: Transformation of BALB/c-3T3 cells by 3-methylcholanthrene in various fetal calf serum lots. The BALB/c target cells were thawed from cryopreserved working stock and adapted to growth in the serum lot under test. The ability of the various serum lots to support transformation was screened by conducting a standard transformation assay as described in the text with 3-methylcholanthrene (MCA). The mean Type III foci/plate represents data from 15 to 20 plates per test condition.

used by Mondal and Heidelberger[43] and later by Marquardt *et al.*[44,45] to explore structure-activity relationships among a wide range of polycyclic aromatic hydrocarbons and their metabolites. However, the assay with mouse prostate fibroblasts has not been widely pursued by different laboratories, and since it offers no unique advantages over the other cell line transformation assays already available and for which large data bases exist, it is unlikely that it will be used as a general tool for detection of carcinogens.

Another assay that had a flurry of activity over the last several years was a procedure using the BHK-21 Syrian baby hamster kidney cell line. The procedure involved the measurement of an increase in cloning efficiency in a suspension culture induced by a chemical in the presence or absence of a metabolic activation system. Although the originators of the assay developed a substantial data base that has been published,[46-48] there has been only limited application of the procedure in other laboratories. One key factor in the successful performance of the assay is the selection of a clone with suitable cloning behavior in soft agar. The observation that BHK-21 cells can give rise to tumors without further alteration suggests that the assay may not be assessing a neoplastic trans-formation, but rather measuring a specific modulation of anchorage-independent growth.[49] Information generated by Bouck and diMayorca supports this view.[50] Given the high likelihood that the assay in reality may be the consequence of a mutation-like procedure, although the frequencies are rather high, this assay does not appear to be a useful adjunct to other available ones.

Transformation Assays Using Cells Infected with Viruses

Rauscher leukemia virus–Fischer rat embryo (RLV/RE). This assay detects transformed foci in a population of Fischer rat embryo cells that were previously infected with Rauscher leukemia virus. Although the mechanism by which the virus infection influences the occurrence of neoplastic transformation by chemi-cal carcinogens is not understood, the range of chemicals tested indicates a broad applicability for the assay. The procedure for conduct of the assay as described by Traul et al.[5] is as follows:

Cell Cultures

Primary cultures of Fischer 344 rat embryo (15-day gestation) cells are prepared by repeated trypsinization of decapitated and eviscerated em-bryo carcasses. At the fourth passage, the cells are infected with Rauscher leukemia virus (RLV) originally derived from JLS-V9 cells. The RLV-infected cells, designated $2FR_450$ are frozen at passages seven to eleven.

Medium

Eagle's minimum essential medium containing Hanks' salts with 10% heat inactivated fetal calf serum, 2 mM L-glutamine, 0.1 mM non-es-sential amino acids and 2 mM pyruvate.

Transformation Assay

(1) Treat flasks of the $2FR_450$ cells, plated at 2.6 x 10^4 cells/cm^2 48 hours earlier, with test chemicals.

(2) After seven days, replace the medium with fresh medium contain-ing no test chemicals.

(3) Refeed one of the duplicate flasks with fresh medium seven to eleven days later and fix and stain after another two weeks of incu-bation. Subculture cells from the other duplicate flask into three flasks at 7 x 10^5 cells/flask.

(4) Stain one of the divided triplicate flasks 14 days later; refeed an-other with medium and stain after an additional two weeks; sub-culture cells from the third again into triplicate flasks.

Scoring and Quantitation

Each stained flask is examined for presence of foci, piled up polar cells against a background of homogenous cobblestone-like monolayer cells. Data are recorded as positive or negative at each concentration tested.

The protocol differs substantially from the previously described assays with

Syrian hamster embryo cells and mouse cell lines in that transformation is generally not observed until after sixteen weeks and several cell passages. Although the number of compounds tested in this system is substantial, the nature of the assay allows for only a positive or negative result which does not permit description of the response on a cells-at-risk basis or allow calculation of chemical potencies with any degree of certainty. In addition, the long duration of the assay sometimes results in transformation of untreated cells so that judicious selection of the assay interval is paramount in obtaining useable assay results.

Ultimately, the primary disadvantage of this assay system is its extensive requirement for time and space to conduct a single assay in comparison to other procedures. Moreover, this expenditure of extensive resources to obtain only a qualitative description of the response does not appear to be desirable with the availability of other assays that yield more definitive responses.

Simian adenovirus SA7–Syrian hamster embryo cells (SA7/SHE). This assay is qualitatively different from the other assays available to assess neoplastic transformation in that it measures the ability of a chemical to enhance the expression of a viral-induced transformation event. This event appears to result from an increased integration of viral DNA into cellular DNA as a result of lesions in cellular DNA produced by chemical and physical agents. The assay is a reasonably facile one in terms of performance and it takes about four weeks to carry out the procedure.

Cell Cultures

Primary Syrian hamster embryo cells are prepared by trypsinization of decapitated and eviscerated embryos between 13 to 15 days old. Continuous lines of monkey kidney cells, VERO, are maintained by weekly subculturing in 100 mm dishes.

Virus

VERO cells in 100 mm dishes are inoculated with Simian adenovirus SA7 at an input multiplicity of two to three plaque-forming units per cell. After a two-hour adsorption period, five ml of medium is added to each dish and about 72 hours later the infected cells are harvested and freeze-thawed four times. The virus is separated from cell debris by low speed centrifugation. Virus stocks are stored in one to two ml aliquots at -65°C.

Medium

Dulbecco's modified Eagle's medium with 10% heat-inactivated fetal calf serum and $NaHCO_3$ (2.2 g/ℓ).

Transformation Assay

(1) Treat duplicate dishes of primary SHE cells (three to four days in culture, 4×10^6 to 6×10^6 cells/60 mm dish) with test chemical for two or 18 hours. Alternately, treat cells with chemicals two to three hours after viral adsorption for 48 hours.

(2) Following chemical treatment, rinse the cells and inoculate with

3×10^7 to 4×10^7 plaque-forming units of SA7 in 0.2 ml medium containing 5% fetal calf serum.

(3) After three hours of adsorption, trypsinize cells and replate at 10^3 cells/dish for survival assay and at 2×10^5 cells/dish for transformation in medium containing 0.1 mM $CaCl_2$ and 1.1 g/ℓ of $NaHCO_3$.

(4) After three days change the medium to one containing 0.1 mM $CaCl_2$ and 2.2 g/ℓ of $NaHCO_3$.

(5) After five to six days, feed the cultures with 3 ml of low calcium medium containing 0.6 g/100 ml of Bacto agar. Add additional 3 ml of agar medium to the dishes at four to five day intervals.

(6) Fix the dishes overnight with 10% buffered formalin 25 to 30 days after the initiation of the experiment. Remove the agar overlay and stain the cells with Giemsa.

Scoring and Quantitation

Adenovirus-transformed foci appear as darkly stained areas of piled-up cells against a background monolayer. The transformation frequency is expressed as number of SA7 foci per 10^6 surviving cells. Enhancement of viral transformation by test chemical is expressed as ratio between the transformation frequency of the treated and control cells.

Unlike other assays, there is little difficulty in identifying transformed foci because of morphological variability since these foci have a uniform and distinct appearance that allows for facile scoring. Also unique for this assay is the reporting mode which expresses activity as an enhancement factor induced by a chemical over that seen in its absence. Since the transformation values are each corrected for survival and the result is expressed as a ratio, certain anomalies can occur as a result of unusual toxicity responses. An additional factor that can cloud the interpretation of the assay as a direct measure of a neoplastic transformation response is the fact that any DNA-perturbing agent would be expected to be active and thus this assay may be more akin to a mutagenesis or DNA damage assay than a transformation assay.

COMPARISON OF CELL TRANSFORMATION SYSTEMS

It is clear that each assay has its attributes as well as deficiencies. Conceptually, the clonal SHE cell strain assay is the most advantageous in its short duration assay period. The subjectivity in scoring however poses a major problem and uncertainty for this assay. Although the cell line assays offer a compromise in less ambiguity in scoring transformants, the target cells may have a narrower spectrum of metabolic capability. On the other hand, the viral transformation assays are technically more time-consuming, labor intensive to perform and may have a different mechanism of action than the presumably more direct measurement of chemically-induced morphological transformation. Ultimately, however, the value of the assays depends on their ability to accurately identify carcinogens and noncarcinogens.

Of the assays described in the previous section, the four transformation assays with the detailed methodologies also have the widest data base. No less than 500 chemicals have been screened in the various assays. However, the number of chemicals which have been assayed in all these systems to allow for a direct comparison is still sparse. Furthermore, in many cases, the chemicals studied have not been adequately tested in *in vivo* carcinogenicity tests. Of the data that are available, the most complete comparison is detailed in an extensive review by Heidelberger *et al.*[1] that was prepared as an activity of the Gene-Tox project of the U.S. Environmental Protection Agency.

As a class, the polycyclic aromatic hydrocarbons and direct-acting agents yield the most consistent responses in the several assays reviewed (Table 1). In most mutation assays, polycyclic aromatic hydrocarbons are not active without the supplement of an exogenous metabolic activation system. Another class that yields consistently positive results in a large proportion of the assays is the carcinogenic metallic salts. This finding is of special significance since many of the metals are not detected in most mutagenicity assays. This difference emphasizes the uniqueness of the transformation assay, *i.e.*, its ability to detect some carcinogens that may not act as direct electrophilic compounds.

Table 1: Examples of Concordant Results Among Transformation Assays

Chemical	. . . . .Transformation Assay			
	SHE	BALB/c-3T3	RLV/RE	SA7/SHE
Polycyclic aromatic hydrocarbons				
7,12-Dimethylbenz(a)anthracene	+	+	+	+
Dibenz(a,h)anthracene	+	+	+	+
Benzo(a)pyrene	+	+	+	+
Benzo(e)pyrene	–	–	–	NT
3-Methylcholanthrene	+	+	+	+
Pyrene	–	–	–	NT
Direct-acting agents				
N-Methyl-N'-nitro-N-nitroso- guanidine	+	+	+	+
4-Nitroquinoline-1-oxide	+	+	+	+
N-Acetoxy-2-acetylaminofluorene	+	+	+	+
Methylazoxymethanol acetate	?	+	+	+
Metals				
Beryllium sulfate	+	+	+	+
Calcium chromate	+	+	+	+
Lead acetate	?	+	+	+
Titanocene dichloride	+	+	+	NT

+ = Positive response
– = Negative response
? = Questionable response
NT = Not tested

With respect to endogenous metabolic activation capability, the virus-infected target cells appear to have a broader range than the other rodent cell assay systems. For example, positive results in the RLV/RE system with a number of aromatic amines and steroids (Table 2) suggest that the cells have a broader range of metabolic capacity than most other cell systems. This particular property is a clear advantage over most other assay systems that require an exogenous metabolic activation system which in many cases has substantial perturbing effects on the assay.

Table 2: Varied Response to Aromatic Amines and Steroids in
Three Transformation Assays

Chemical	Transformation Assay		
	SHE	BALB/c-3T3	RLV/RE
Aromatic amines			
Aniline	–	+	+
p-Rosaniline	?	+	+
2-Methyl-4-(dimethylamino)azobenzene	–	–	+
4-(Dimethylamino)azobenzene	?	–	+
N-Hydroxy-2-acetylaminofluorene	+	+	+
Steroids and related hormones			
Diethylstilbestrol	?	–	+
Ethinylestriol	–	–	+
Lithocholic acid	?	–	+
Progesterone	–	–	+

+ = Positive response
– = Negative response
? = Questionable response

Among the cell line focus assays which measure a morphological endpoint, divergent responses were observed with some of the chemicals tested. Table 3 shows examples of variant responses in the BALB/c-3T3 and C3H-10T½ cells.

Table 3: Examples of Discordant Results in the BALB/c-3T3 and
C3H-10T½ Assays

Chemical	Transformation Assay	
	BALB/c-3T3	C3H-10T½
Aniline	+	–
p-Rosaniline	+	–
Titanocene dichloride	+	–
Beryllium sulfate	+	–
Lead acetate	+	–
p-Phenylenediamine dihydrochloride	+	–
Methylazoxymethanol acetate	+	–
Cinnamyl anthranilate	+	–
5-Nitro-o-toluidine	–	+
p-Quinone dioxime	–	+
Trianthranol	–	+

+ = Positive response
– = Negative response

In some cases, carcinogens that have been detected with BALB/c-3T3 cells have not yielded a positive response with C3H-10T½ cells. In order to overcome this problem, several variations of the assay protocol have been devised to increase the sensitivity of detection in the C3H-10T½ cell system. Nesnow *et al.*[51] have reported that delaying exposure of the target cells for several days until the population has increased is effective in addressing the sensitivity and synchrony issues. An alternative procedure originally described by Schechtman *et al.*[52] is a replating procedure which has been termed a "Level II" assay. In this procedure, treated and control cells are allowed to achieve a monolayer and then split to expand the culture, which is carried for an additional four weeks to determine the transformation response. This protocol appears to increase the sensitivity of the assay and allows the detection of some carcinogens that produce a negative response in the standard assay.

ASSAY MODIFICATIONS FOR PROBLEM CHEMICALS

In the development and validation of a short-term assay as a screening method the initial phases generally involve the optimization of the assay procedure using a set of model compounds. Once standardized, investigations are often directed toward adapting the procedure for improving the assay to detect a wider spectrum of chemicals.

Volatile and Gas Samples

Data on the testing of samples which are not in liquid phase under the normal cell growth conditions are relatively sparse. More recent works have presented an adaption of the assay procedure utilizing chambers which permit the assay of volatile compounds and gases. Hatch *et al.*[53] recently described a method for testing a series of chlorinated hydrocarbons in the SA7/SHE assay. Their results suggest that some highly volatile compounds such as 1,2-dichloroethane and trichloroethylene which are immiscible in cell culture medium, produced a positive response in the modified assay procedure but not in the standard assay.

Our laboratory has also adapted a chamber system originally described by Krahn of E.I. duPont de Nemours and Company (personal communications) for use in the Ames assay for the testing of volatile and gas samples in BALB/c-3T3 cells. The chamber accommodates the simultaneous exposure of a large size sample of twenty culture dishes per test group.

Procarcinogens

The major drawback for many of the assay systems, especially those that measure direct morphological changes induced by carcinogens, is their limited endogenous metabolic capabilities. For the assays that are prime candidates to include in test batteries at the present time (Syrian hamster embryo clonal assay, BALB/c-3T3 and C3H-10T½), there remains a need for the development and validation of one or more efficacious metabolic activation procedures that can aid in the detection of a wide range of chemical classes of carcinogens. Since this need has been identified for many years, and effective procedures are not yet forthcoming, in spite of substantial efforts over that interval, it clearly indicates the technical difficulties involved.

Reports on the successful use of metabolic activation systems have been restricted only to a few chemicals. Pienta and coworkers had reported the use of a hamster microsomal fraction[54] and of hamster hepatocytes[55] in the activation of some procarcinogens in the clonal SHE assay. Metabolic activation of cyclophosphamide was reported by Benedict *et al.*[56] in the C3H-10T½ system. We have also compared the relative efficacy of hepatocytes and microsomal fraction to supplement the cell line assay system.[64] However, data are still only available for reference compounds such as cyclophosphamide, aliphatic nitrosamines and 2-aminoanthracene. The effectiveness of the metabolic activation systems still needs to be examined by screening a large number of chemicals under code with a standard metabolic activation protocol.

Promoters of Carcinogenicity

The multistep nature of carcinogenesis is a generally accepted hypothesis of chemical carcinogenesis. With this recognition, a category of chemicals known as tumor promoters has gained increasing attention because of their potential role in the carcinogenic process. Since the *in vitro* transformation assays utilize an endpoint which mimics the *in vivo* neoplastic process in the conversion of normal cells to transformed phenotype, they occupy a unique position among the available short-term bioassays in having further utility for the screening of promoters.

Procedures for the detection of promoters have been described for the clonal SHE assay,[57,58] for the BALB/c-3T3[59] and C3H-10T½[60,61] cell line assays and for the viral RLV/RE[62] and SA7/SHE assays.[63] The assay procedure used is generally a slight modification of the standard assay. The target cells are initiated with a nontransforming dose of a carcinogen such as 3-methylcholanthrene or N-methyl-N'-nitro-N-nitrosoguanidine. At various times after treatment with the carcinogen, depending on the particular assay, the test promoter is introduced to the cells in the culture medium and is present for the remainder of the assay period. The endpoint measured is an enhancement of transformation that is higher than either induced by treatment with the initiator or promoter alone.

DISCUSSION

The neoplastic transformation assays have several potential uses that should be considered in order to understand their limitations and benefits. Accumulated data over the last few decades have indicated that morphological transformation of cells in culture is one of the characteristics in a generally recognized multistep process of carcinogenesis. This underlies the rationale for the use of transformation as an endpoint for screening carcinogens. No explicit assumption of a genetic event is necessary compared to the other short-term assays utilizing cytogenetic or mutational endpoints. Furthermore, the good correlation of transformation response in several of the assays with *in vivo* carcinogenic activity in rodent bioassays points to the value of the transformation assay as a complement to a battery of short-term *in vitro* tests for screening potential mutagens/carcinogens.

At the present time no single transformation assay system has gained universal acceptance. The three systems with the largest number of chemicals tested are the SHE clonal assay and the two viral transformation assays (RLV/RE and SA7/SHE). Data from all three assays were generated essentially by single laboratories. The interlaboratory reproducibility of results is largely unknown. Currently, these three assays are being evaluated with respect to this key factor under the auspices of the National Toxicology Program.

The absence of an effective metabolic activation system for the cell line assays (BALB/c-3T3 and C3H-10T½) has limited the more general application of these methods. However, based on other factors of the assays, such as resistance to perturbing variables, available data base, simplicity of performance and the similar responses obtained among laboratories, additional research efforts in metabolic activation systems for cell line assays may be worthwhile.

In addition to the identification of potential carcinogens, the assays have been used less frequently to identify limited numbers of cocarcinogens and promoters of carcinogenicity. With the increasing awareness that modifying factors that are not carcinogenic in their own right may play a major role in carcinogenesis, the availability of procedures to identify these modifying factors provides a means to generate data that could be used as a basis for actions to prevent or reduce exposure to such factors. While none of the assays for promotion or cocarcinogenesis have been validated to any significant degree, their availability allows such validation programs to be carried out and makes it possible to explore the potential usefulness of the transformation assays in this arena.

More problematic is the use of cell culture assays to study mechanisms of carcinogenesis. Regardless of the target cell type used, a common characteristic is the high degree of selection that has occurred by the time a transformation assay is performed. For the cell lines, this selection is evident from an examination of the history of each of the lines. However, even in the Syrian hamster embryo clonal assay, the target cells represent a small fraction of robust survivors in comparison to the primary cell pools from which they originated. Thus, imposing mechanistic interpretations from a highly selected cell population *in vitro* to the unselected and complex *in vivo* cell populations that are the precursors of tumors should be done with great caution.

Another factor that has been raised with respect to the use of an aneuploid cell line in studying mechanisms of carcinogenesis is its non-normal character. In fact, such cells bear most of the characteristics of neoplastic cells with the exception of their morphological regularity which gives them their utility in transformation assays.

In summary, several cellular systems are available for identifying potentially carcinogenic substances. If one examines the lists of transformation responses among the assays that have been reported, and adjusts for anomalies caused by the absence of metabolic capacity, the correlation of response with *in vivo* carcinogenic activity in the rodent bioassays correspond to values (80% to 90% accuracy) obtained for mutagenesis assays. Ideally, a reproducible assay employing epithelial cells from the organs most often affected by cancer would be desirable. Although individual descriptions of several epithelial systems have been reported, there appear to be none that are applicable as screening tools, and this area deserves considerable research attention.

REFERENCES

1. Heidelberger, C., Freeman, A.E., Pienta, R.J., Sivak, A., Bertram, J.S., Casto, B.C., Dunkel, V.C., Francis, M.W., Kakunaga, T., Little, J.B., and Schechtman, L.M., Cell transformation by chemical agents—a review and analysis of the literature. *Mutation Res.* 114: 283-385 (1983)
2. Meyer, A.L., *In vitro* transformation assays for chemical carcinogens. *Mutation Res.* 115: 323-338 (1983)
3. Sivak, A., and Tu, A.S., in: *Mutagenicity: New Horizons in Genetic Toxicology* (J.A. Heddle, ed.), pp 143-169, Academic Press, New York (1982)
4. Sivak, A., Charest, M.C., Rudenko, L., Silveira, D.M., Simons, I., and Wood, A.M., in: *Advances in Modern Environmental Toxicology* (N. Mishra, V. Dunkel and M. Mehlman, eds.), Vol. I, pp 133-180, Senate Press, Inc., Princeton Junction, New Jersey (1980)
5. Traul, K.A., Takayama, K., Kachevsky, V., Hink, R.J., and Wolff, J.S., A rapid *in vitro* assay for carcinogenicity of chemical substances in mammalian cells utilizing an attachment-independence endpoint. *J. Appl. Toxicol.* 1: 190-195 (1981)
6. Dunkel, V.C., Pienta, R.J., Sivak, A., and Traul, K.A., Comparative neoplastic transformation responses of BALB/c-3T3 cells, Syrian hamster embryo cells, and Rauscher murine leukemia virus-infected Fischer 344 rat embryo cells to chemical carcinogens. *J. Natl. Cancer Inst.* 67: 1301-1315 (1981)
7. Pienta, R.J., Poiley, J.A., and Lebherz III, W.B., Morphological transformation of early passage golden Syrian hamster embryo cells derived from cryopreserved primary cultures as a reliable *in vitro* bioassay for identifying diverse carcinogens. *Int. J. Cancer* 19: 642-655 (1977)
8. Earle, W.R., and Voegtlin, C., The mode of action of methylcholanthrene on cultures of normal tissues. *Am. J. Cancer* 34: 373-390 (1938)
9. Shelton, E., and Earle, W.R., Production of malignancy *in vitro*. XIII. Behavior of recovery cultures. *J. Natl. Cancer Inst.* 11: 817-837 (1951)
10. Earle, W.R., and Nettleship, A., Production of malignancy *in vitro*. V. Results of injections of cultures into mice. *J. Natl. Cancer Inst.* 4: 229-248 (1943)
11. Earle, W.R., Shelton, E., and Schilling, E.L., Production of malignancy *in vitro*. XI. Further results from reinjection of *in vitro* cell strains into strain C3H mice. *J. Natl. Cancer Inst.* 10: 1105-1113 (1950)
12. Berwald, Y., and Sachs, L., *In vitro* transformation with chemical carcinogens. *Nature* (London) 200: 1182-1184 (1963)
13. Casto, B.C., Janosko, N., and DiPaolo, J.A., Development of a focus-assay model for transformation of hamster cells *in vitro* by chemical carcinogens. *Cancer Res.* 37: 3508-3515 (1977)
14. Schuman, R.F., Pienta, R.J., Poiley, J.A., and Lebherz III, W.B., The effect of fetal bovine serum on 3-methylcholanthrene transformation of hamster embryo cells *in vitro*. *In Vitro* 15: 730-735 (1979)
15. DiPaolo, J.A., Quantitative *in vitro* transformation of Syrian golden hamster embryo cells with the use of frozen stored cells. *J. Natl. Cancer Inst.* 64: 1485-1489 (1980)
16. Poiley, J.A., Raineri, R., Cavanaugh, D.M., Ernst, M.K., and Pienta, R.J., Correlation between transformation potential and inducible enzyme levels of hamster embryo cells. *Carcinogenesis* 1: 323-328 (1980)
17. Barrett, J.C., Crawford, B.D., Mixter, L.O., Schechtman, L.M., Ts'o, P.O.P., and Pollack, R., Correlation of *in vitro* growth properties and tumorigenicity of Syrian hamster cell lines. *Cancer Res.* 39: 1504-1510 (1979)

18. Barrett, J.C., Sheela, S., Ohki, K., and Kakunaga, T., Reexamination of the role of plasminogen activator production for growth in semisolid agar of neoplastic hamster cells. *Cancer Res.* 40: 1438-1442 (1980)

19. Davies, C., Rivedal, E., and Sanner, T., Fibrinolytic activity and morphological transformation of hamster embryo cells. *Carcinogenesis* 3: 21-624 (1982)

20. Kakunaga, T., Neoplastic transformation of human diploid fibroblast cells by chemical carcinogens. *Proc. Nat. Acad. Sci. U.S.A.* 75: 1334-1338 (1978)

21. Milo, G., and DiPaolo, J.A., Neoplastic transformation of human diploid cells *in vitro* after chemical carcinogen treatment. *Nature* (London) 275: 130-132 (1978)

22. Oldham, J.W., Allred, L.E., Milo, G.E., Kinding, O., and Capen, C.C., The toxicological evaluation of the mycotoxins T-2 and T-2 tetraol using normal human fibroblasts *in vitro*. *Toxicol. Appl. Pharmacol.* 52: 159-168 (1980)

23. Zimmerman, R.J., and Little, J.B., Characterization of a quantitative assay for the *in vitro* transformation of normal human diploid fibroblasts to anchorage independence by chemical carcinogens. *Cancer Res.* 43: 2176-2182 (1983)

24. Zimmerman, R.J., and Little, J.B., Characteristics of human diploid fibroblasts transformed *in vitro* by chemical carcinogens. *Cancer Res.* 43: 2183-2189 (1983)

25. Milo, G., Oldham, J., Zimmerman, R., Hatch, G., and Weisbrode, S., Characterization of human cells transformed by chemical and physical carcinogens *in vitro*. *In Vitro* 17: 719-729 (1981)

26. Elias, P.M., Yuspa, S.H., Gullino, M., Morgan, D.L., Bates, R.R., and Lutzner, M.A., *In vitro* neoplastic transformation of mouse skin cells: Morphology and ultrastructure of cells and tumors. *J. Invest. Dermatol.* 62: 569-581 (1974)

27. Yuspa, S.H., Hawley-Nelson, P., Koehler, B., and Stanley, J.R., A survey of transformation markers in differentiating epidermal cell lines in culture. *Cancer Res.* 40: 4694-4703 (1980)

28. Kulesz-Martin, M.F., Koehler, B., Hennings, H., and Yuspa, S.H., Quantitative assay for carcinogen altered differentiation in mouse epidermal cells. *Carcinogenesis* 1: 995-1006 (1980)

29. Hennings, H., Michael, D., Cheng, C., Steinert, P., Holbrook, K., and Yuspa, S.H., Calcium regulation of growth and differentiation of mouse epidermal cells in culture. *Cell* 19: 245-254 (1980)

30. Yuspa, S.H., Koehler, B., Kulesz-Martin, M., and Hennings, H., Clonal growth of mouse epidermal cells in medium with reduced calcium concentration. *J. Invest. Dermatol.* 76: 245-257 (1981)

31. Marchok, A.C., Rhoton, J.C., Griesemer, R.A., and Nettesheim, P., Increased *in vitro* growth capacity of tracheal epithelium exposed *in vivo* to 7,12-dimethylbenz(a)anthracene. *Cancer Res.* 37: 1811-1821 (1977)

32. Terzaghi, M., and Nettesheim, P., The dynamics of neoplastic development in carcinogen-exposed tracheal mucosa. *Cancer Res.* 39: 4003-4010 (1979)

33. Steele, V.E., Marchok, A.C., and Nettesheim, P., Oncogenic transformation in epithelial cell lines derived from tracheal explants exposed *in vitro* to N-methyl-N'-nitro-N-nitrosoguanidine. *Cancer Res.* 39: 3805-3811 (1979)

34. Terzaghi, M., Nettesheim, P., Yarita, T., and Williams, M.L., Epithelial focus assay for early detection of carcinogen-altered cells in various organs of rats exposed *in situ* to N-nitrosoheptamethyleneimine. *J. Natl. Cancer Inst.* 67: 1057-1062 (1981)

35. Kakunaga, T., A quantitative system for assay of malignant transformation by chemical carcinogens using a clone derived from BALB/3T3. *Int. J. Cancer* 12: 463-473 (1973)

36. Sivak, A., and Tu, A.S., in: *The Predictive Value of Short-Term Screening Tests in Carcinogenicity Evaluation* (G.M. Williams, R. Kroes, H.W. Waaijers and K.W. van de Poll, eds.), pp 171-197, Elsevier/North-Holland Biomedical Press, Amsterdam (1980)

37. Kakunaga, T., and Crow, J.D., Cell variants showing differential susceptibility to ultraviolet light-induced transformation. *Science* 209: 505-507 (1980)

38. Lo, K.Y., and Kakunaga, T., Similarities in the formation and removal of covalent DNA adducts in benzo(a)pyrene-treated BALB/3T3 variant cells with different induced transformation frequencies. *Cancer Res.* 42: 2644-2650 (1982)

39. Reznikoff, C.A., Bertram, J.S., Brankow, D.W., and Heidelberger, C., Quantitative and qualitative studies of chemical transformation of cloned C3H mouse embryo cells sensitive to postconfluence inhibition of cell division. *Cancer Res.* 33: 3239-3249 (1973)

40. Reznikoff, C.A., Brankow, D.W., and Heidelberger, C., Establishment and characterization of a cloned line of C3H mouse embryo cells sensitive to postconfluence inhibition of division. *Cancer Res.* 33: 3231-3238 (1973)

41. Oshiro, Y., Balwierz, P.S., and Piper, C.E., Selection of fetal calf serum for use in the C3H-10T½ C18 cell transformation assay system. *Environ. Mutagenesis* 4: 469-574 (1982)

42. Chen, T.T., and Heidelberger, C., Quantitative studies on the malignant transformation *in vitro* of cells derived from adult C3H mouse ventral prostate. *Int. J. Cancer* 4: 166-178 (1969)

43. Mondal, S., and Heidelberger, C., *In vitro* malignant transformation by methylcholanthrene of the progeny of single cells derived from C3H mouse prostate. *Proc. Natl. Acad. Sci. USA* 65: 219-225 (1970)

44. Marquardt, H., Kuroki, T., Huberman, E., Selkirk, J.K., Heidelberger, C., Grover, P.L., and Sims, P., Malignant transformation of cells derived from mouse prostate by epoxides and other derivatives of polycyclic hydrocarbons. *Cancer Res.* 32: 716-720 (1972)

45. Marquardt, H., Sodergren, T.E., Sims, P., and Grover, P.L., Malignant transformation *in vitro* of mouse fibroblasts by 7,12-dimethylbenz(a)anthracene and by their K-region derivatives. *Int. J. Cancer* 13: 304-310 (1974)

46. Ishii, Y., Elliot, J.A., Mishra, N.K., and Lieberman, M.W., Quantitative studies of transformation by chemical carcinogens and ultraviolet radiation using a subclone of BHK 21 clone 13 Syrian hamster cells. *Cancer Res.* 37: 2023-2029 (1977)

47. Styles, J.A., A method for detecting carcinogenic organic chemicals using mammalian cells in culture. *Br. J. Cancer* 36: 558-564 (1977)

48. Purchase, I.F.H., Longstaff, E., Styles, J.A., Anderson, D., Lefevre, P.A., and Westwood, F.R., An evaluation of six short-term tests for detecting organic chemical carcinogens. *Br. J. Cancer* 37: 873-959 (1978)

49. DiMayorca, G., Greenblatt, M., Trauthen, T., Soller, A., and Giordano, R., Malignant transformation of BHK 21 clone 13 cells *in vitro* by nitrosamines; a conditional state. *Proc. Natl. Acad. Sci. USA* 70: 46-49 (1973)

50. Bouck, N., and DiMayorca, G., Chemical carcinogens transform BHK cells by inducing a recessive mutation. *Mol. Cell Biol.* 2: 97-105 (1982)
51. Nesnow, S., Garland, H., and Curtis, G., Improved transformation of C3H-10T½ CL8 cells by direct- and indirect-acting carcinogens. *Carcinogenesis* 3: 377-380 (1982)
52. Schechtman, L.M., Kiss, E., McCarvill, J., Gallagher, M., Kouri, R.E., and Lubet, R.A., A method for amplification of sensitivity of the C3H-10T½ cell transformation assay. *Proc. Am. Assoc. Canc. Res.* 23: 74 (1982)
53. Hatch, G.G., Mamay, P.D., Ayer, M.L., Casto, B.C., and Nesnow, S., Chemical enhancement of viral transformation of Syrian hamster embryo cells by gaseous and volatile chlorinated methanes and ethanes. *Cancer Res.* 43: 1945-1950 (1983)
54. Pienta, R.J., in: *Carcinogens: Identification and Mechanisms of Action* (A.C. Griffin and C.R. Shaw, eds.), pp 131-141, Raven Press, New York (1979)
55. Poiley, J.A., Raineri, R., and Pienta, R.J., The use of hamster hepatocytes to metabolize carcinogens in an *in vitro* bioassay. *J. Natl. Cancer Inst.* 63: 519-524 (1979)
56. Benedict, W.F., Banerjee, A., and Venkatesan, N., Cyclophosphamide-induced oncogenic transformation, chromosomal breakage, and sister chromatid exchange following microsomal activation. *Cancer Res.* 38: 2922-2924 (1978)
57. Poiley, J.A., Raineri, R., and Pienta, R.J., Two-stage malignant transformation in hamster embryo cells. *Br. J. Cancer* 39: 8-14 (1979)
58. Rivedal, E., and Sanner, T., Metal salts as promoters of *in vitro* morphological transformation of hamster embryo cells initiated by benzo(a)pyrene. *Cancer Res.* 41: 2950-2953 (1981)
59. Sivak, A., and Tu, A.S., Cell culture tumor promotion experiments with saccharin, phorbol myristate acetate and several common food materials. *Cancer Lett.* 10: 27-32 (1980)
60. Mondal, S., Brankow, D.W., and Heidelberger, C., Two-stage chemical oncogenesis in cultures of C3H/10T½ cells. *Cancer Res.* 36: 2254-2260 (1976)
61. Frazelle, J.H., Abernethy, D.J., and Boreiko, C.J., Factors influencing the promotion of transformation in chemically-initiated C3H/10T½ C18 mouse embryo fibroblasts. *Carcinogenesis* 4: 709-715 (1983)
62. Traul, K.A., Hink, R.J., Jr., Kachevsky, V., and Wolff, J.S. III, Two-stage carcinogenesis *in vitro*: Transformation of 3-methylcholanthrene-initiated Rauscher murine leukemia virus-infected rat embryo cells by diverse tumor promoters. *J. Natl. Cancer Inst.* 66(1): 171-176 (1981)
63. Fisher, P.B., Mufson, R.A., Weinstein, I.B., and Little, J.B., Epidermal growth factor, like tumor promoters, enhances viral and radiation-induced cell transformation. *Carcinogenesis* 2: 183-187 (1981)
64. Tu, A., Breen, P., and Sivak, A., Comparison of primary hepatocytes and S9 metabolic activation systems for the C3H-10T½ cell transformation assay. *Carcinogenesis* in press (1984)

Part IV

Limited Bioassays

8

Rat Liver Foci Assay*

Michael A. Pereira

Health Effects Research Laboratory
U.S. Environmental Protection Agency
Cincinnati, Ohio

INTRODUCTION

The evaluation of the potential carcinogenic activity of the large numbers of chemicals and complex mixtures present in the workplace, home and environment is a very costly and time consuming task. Many of these chemicals and complex mixtures have demonstrated mutagenic activity in short-term *in vitro* assays such as the Ames test. The correlation between mutagenicity and carcinogenicity is at best very weak. There are many carcinogens that are not mutagens and there are a number of mutagens that possess either weak or no carcinogenic activity. Therefore, assays are needed that can detect the carcinogenicity of a substance whether or not it is a mutagen. Such assays must conclusively demonstrate carcinogenic activity by the appearance, for example, of tumors or preneoplastic lesions that are predictive of malignancy.

Two distinct mechanisms of action, genotoxic and nongenotoxic (epigenetic), have been suggested for chemical carcinogens.[1-4] It is generally assumed that genotoxic carcinogens are mutagens that can initiate carcinogenesis while non-genotoxic carcinogens are not mutagenic and include carcinogens that enhance (promote) the progression of initiated (transformed) cells to cancer. Some carcinogens possess both properties and the estimation of their potential human health hazard requires the determination of the relative contribution of both activities to the carcinogenic hazard. The two proposed mechanisms of carcinogenesis can be operationally distinguished in initiation-promotion assays.

Long-term feeding or exposure bioassays such as those of the National Toxi-

*This article was written by Michael A. Pereira in his private capacity. No official endorsement by the U.S. Environmental Protection Agency or any other agency of the U.S. Federal Government is intended or should be inferred.

cology Program/National Cancer Institute are not suitable for the evaluation of the carcinogenic activity of the large numbers of chemicals and complex mixtures to which humans are potentially exposed even if they are limited only to the testing of mutagenic substances.[5] The long-term bioassay is also not suited for the determination of the mechanism of action of chemical carcinogens. Much shorter and cost effective assays are required. Short-term assays have been proposed[4,5] that include: (a) rat liver foci assay; (b) mouse skin initiation-promotion assay; (c) cell transformation (including an initiation-promotion protocol); (d) initiation-promotion assays in other organs including bladder, kidney, colon, mammary gland, etc.; and (e) strain A mouse lung adenoma assay (of limited usefulness in determining mechanism of action). In this review, I shall evaluate the use of the rat liver foci assay to identify carcinogens and determine mechanism of action. Previous reviews of the rat liver foci assay have been published.[3,6-8]

STAGES OF EXPERIMENTAL HEPATOCARCINOGENESIS

The first demonstration of two-stage hepatocarcinogenesis was reported by Peraino *et al.*[9] in which a limited exposure of 2-acetylaminofluorene (2-AAF) fed to weanling rats for 18 days was followed by phenobarbital in the diet for up to 180 days. While only 20% of the rats that received 2-AAF followed by control diet lacking 2-AAF or phenobarbital developed nodules, 70% of the rats that received 2-AAF followed by phenobarbital in the diet developed these lesions. Rats that did not receive the initial exposure of 2-AAF but received phenobarbital in the diet, did not develop hyperplastic nodules. An increased incidence of nodules compared to rats that received 2-AAF in the diet alone, was seen in rats even when there was a delay of 30 days between the termination of the 2-AAF feeding and the start of the feeding of phenobarbital. In an earlier study, Peraino *et al.*[10] reported that the concurrent feeding of phenobarbital with 2-AAF decreased the incidence of neoplasms induced by 2-AAF, thus demonstrating the importance of the sequence in which phenobarbital is administered relative to 2-AAF. These and other studies[9-12] conclusively demonstrated two-stage hepatocarcinogenesis in which the initial stage, initiation, was accomplished by a limited exposure to 2-AAF and the second stage, promotion, by prolonged exposure to phenobarbital.

Initiation

Initiation of chemical carcinogenesis is believed to be accomplished by the interaction of a carcinogen or a metabolite with DNA followed by fixation during transcription of the alteration into the daughter genome (Figure 1). For initiation to occur, DNA damage must be fixed prior to DNA repair. After a few cycles of cellular replication by the daughter cell, focal changes in phenotype can be observed. These altered-foci have been proposed as the earliest observable evidence of initiation and will be discussed later with respect to their use in the rat liver foci assay to demonstrate carcinogenic activity. Therefore, the extent of initiation is a function of both the extent of DNA damage and the rate of DNA replication and repair.

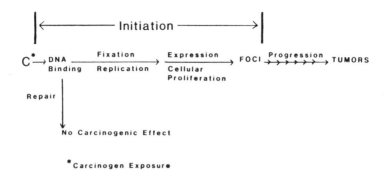

Figure 1: Model for initiation of chemical hepatocarcinogenesis. The time for initiation has been exaggerated. In reality, initiation comprises only a small part of the neoplastic progression from the initial effect of the carcinogen to the occurrence of cancer.

The adult rat liver possesses a very low level of cellular proliferation and turnover. Thus, there is a very limited capacity to fix the DNA damage. The administration of a necrogenic dose of a carcinogen results in regenerative cellular proliferation that fixes the DNA damage and completes the process of initiation. There are numerous genotoxic carcinogens that are not liver carcinogens including polycyclic aromatic hydrocarbons [benzo(a)pyrene and 7,12-dimethylbenz(a)-anthracene][13-15] and methylating agents [N-methyl-N'-nitro-N-nitrosoguanidine and N-methyl-N-nitrosourea],[16-19] that extensively bind and damage DNA in adult rat liver. These carcinogens cause liver cancer when they are administered so that their binding to DNA occurs during regenerative cellular proliferation induced by either $2/3$ partial hepatectomy or by intoxication with carbon tetrachloride.[19-22] The extent of initiation, as measured by the occurrence of altered-foci induced by a carcinogen, is greatly increased when the test substance is administered in association with stimulated cellular proliferation.[23-27] This is the rationale for the use of either a partial hepatectomy or a necrogenic dose of carbon tetrachloride prior to the administration of a test chemical.

The temporal relationship of the stimulus for cell proliferation and the administration of the test substance is critical. For dimethylhydrazine, N-methyl-N-nitrosourea, and diethylnitrosamine which rapidly bind to DNA within two to four hours,[16-18] maximum initiation occurred when the partial hepatectomy was performed 12 to 24 hours prior to the administration of the carcinogens.[25] For benzo(a)pyrene, maximum binding to DNA occurred at approximately 18 hours[13,14] and the optimal time for the partial hepatectomy was six hours prior to the administration of the carcinogen.[25] The first and maximum cycle of DNA replication after a partial hepatectomy occurs at 22 hours, which would be synchronous with the maximum DNA binding. Therefore, the use of a partial hepatectomy in the initiation of hepatocarcinogenesis is optimized when the maximum rate of DNA transcription is synchronized to the time of the appearance of the maximum level of the DNA adduct or damage responsible for initiation. Since the rate of DNA binding and repair is not known for most test substances, it is recommended that substances being tested for initiating activity be administered to one group of rats at six hours after a partial hepatectomy and to a second group of rats at 18 hours after the operation.

Ghoshal and Farber[28] have recently shown that feeding a choline-deficient/methionine-low diet for two to three weeks can substitute for partial hepatectomy during the initiation phase of the assay. This type of diet has been demonstrated previously to promote the hepatocarcinogenicity of 2-AAF,[29,30] diethylnitrosamine,[31] azaserine, and DL-ethionine.[32] Rats treated with benzo(a)pyrene or 1,2-dimethylhydrazine during the three weeks feeding of the deficient diet had the same number of gamma-glutamyltranspeptidase (GGT)-positive foci, a putative preneoplastic lesion, as partially hepatectomized rats fed these carcinogens. It is noteworthy that the deficient diet worked equally well with benzo(a)pyrene and 1,2-dimethylhydrazine which have different optimal relationships between timing of their administration and the conduct of partial hepatectomy (six and 12 to 18 hours, respectively). Administration of the carcinogen as four equal doses to animals fed the deficient diet resulted in the same incidence of foci induction as when the same total dose was administered as a single application. Therefore, a choline-deficient/methionine-low diet can potentially replace partial hepatectomy during the initiation phase of the rat liver foci assay. Its use would also eliminate the necessity for the determination of the optimal time between partial hepatectomy and the administration of the test substance and would allow for the use of multiple doses in order to increase the total administered dose.

Takahashi et al.[33] have shown that 3-aminobenzamide, a specific inhibitor of poly(ADP-ribose)polymerase, when administered to non-hepatectomized rats four hours after diethylnitrosamine, increased the initiation of hepatocarcinogenesis as measured by an enhanced incidence of GGT-positive foci. The extent of enhancement by 3-aminobenzamide was similar to the enhancement by partial hepatectomy performed four hours after the administered diethylnitrosamine, an initiating agent. These results indicate that 3-aminobenzamide might be used instead of partial hepatectomy in some cases. Poly(ADP-ribose)polymerase is involved in excision repair,[34] so that the enhancement by 3-aminobenzamide might be due to a delay in the repair of the diethylnitrosamine-induced damage to DNA. This delay could result in the fixation of the damaged DNA during the limited DNA transcription in the liver. Even though 3-aminobenzamide did not produce any histologically detectable liver cell necrosis at 48 hours after administration of the compound, it is still possible that the enhancement of GGT-positive foci was due to a stimulation of cell proliferation.

The administration of substances with initiating activity, either prenatally, to neonates, or to weanling rats, has been shown to increase the sensitivity of the liver to carcinogens as demonstrated by either an enhancement of the GGT-positive foci or the tumor response.[22,35,36] The greater sensitivity of fetal and weanling liver to initiation by chemical carcinogens probably resides in the rapid rate of cell proliferation. The inconvenience attendant upon using these young animals, especially the need for a colony that can supply timed pregnant animals, is a major limitation in their usefulness for evaluation of a large number of substances. However, the use of fetal and neonatal rats can supply needed information about prenatal and adolescent exposure to chemical carcinogens.

Promotion

Two types of promotion schemes have been employed in experimental hepatocarcinogenesis. One type employs a liver mitogen, such as phenobarbital, in order to stimulate cell proliferation. Phenobarbital and other liver mitogens stimulate cellular proliferation in the liver resulting in an enlarged liver.[11,37,38] However, the stimulation of DNA synthesis by mitogens in non-initiated liver is transitory, lasting only a few days. It has been proposed that mitogenic promoters act by both stimulating DNA replication and preventing the death of initiated cells.[37,38]

The other type of promotion is the result of the apparent resistance of initiated hepatocytes to cytotoxic chemicals. Initiated hepatocytes are stimulated to grow selectively by treating the rats with a low dose (0.02%) of 2-AAF in the diet for two to three weeks.[6,25,39-42] Apparently, the initiated hepatocytes are resistant to the cytotoxicity of 2-AAF so that they have a selective advantage. Since partial hepatectomy is usually performed during initiation, a second type of stimulus for cell proliferation is administered during the feeding of the 2-AAF. Farber and coworkers have used carbon tetrachloride.[25,42] Ito and coworkers[43] have shown that numerous other hepatotoxic carcinogens can substitute for 2-AAF and selectively allow diethylnitrosamine-initiated hepatocytes to grow into nodules. Another modification of the use of selection of resistant hepatocytes is the use of choline-deficient/methionine-low diet for promotion.[29-32] "Normal" hepatocytes are apparently more sensitive to choline deficiency and become very swollen with lipids in contrast to the hepatocytes of altered foci and nodules.

PROTOCOLS OF THE RAT LIVER FOCI ASSAY

Four protocols for the rat liver foci assay are presented in Figure 2. A substance being tested for initiating activity is usually administered to partially hepatectomized young adult rats. In most cases, diethylnitrosamine is used as the positive control for initiation. Commencement of the promotion regimen is delayed for one to two weeks in order to allow recovery of the liver from the partial hepatectomy and any toxicity due to the test substance.

Protocols No. 1[3,44,45] and No. 2[7,8,46] employ phenobarbital as the promoter and are terminated after six to 12 weeks of treatment with phenobarbital. The initiating activity of the test substance is determined by an increased incidence of altered-foci, usually measured as GGT-positive foci (Figure 3). Otherwise, the assay can be continued for 12 to 18 months and initiating activity assessed by the incidence of hyperplastic nodules and hepatocellular carcinoma. Protocols No. 3[25,39-42] and No. 4[29-32] (Figure 2) are examples of promotion accomplished by selective growth of resistant hepatocytes. In Protocol No. 3 (Figure 2), initiating activity is measured by the appearance of GGT-positive foci and nodules (Figure 4). When the assay was allowed to continue for more than five weeks (one week after cessation of the feeding of the 2-AAF-containing diet), the nodules started to undergo remodeling and the majority ultimately reverted to normal-appearing liver.[47-49] Protocol No. 4 (Figure 2) employs a choline-deficient/methionine-low diet for promotion and, after eight weeks of the diet,

Protocol

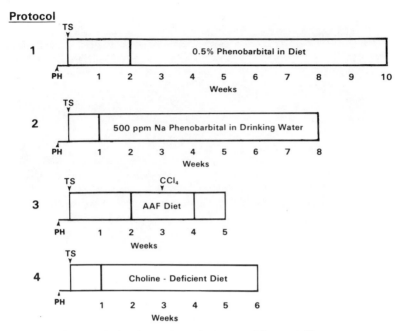

Figure 2: Protocols for the rat liver foci assay. PH, partial hepatectomy; TS, test substance; AAF diet, 0.02% 2-acetylaminofluorene in the diet; and choline-deficient diet, choline-deficient/methionine-low diet.

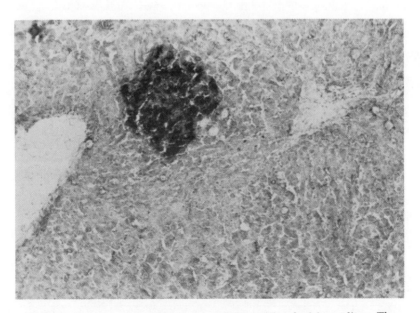

Figure 3: Gamma-glutamyl-transpeptidase-positive foci in rat liver. The animal was initiated with diethylnitrosamine followed by promotion with phenobarbital (Protocol No. 2 of Figure 2).

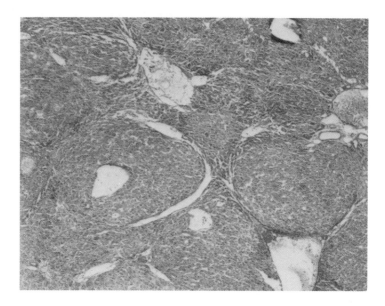

Figure 4: Lobulation of the liver by basophilic hepatocytes in rat liver. The animals were initiated with diethylnitrosamine followed by promotion with 0.02% 2-acetylaminofluorene in the diet (Protocol No. 3 of Figure 2).

determines initiating activity by the appearance of GGT-positive foci or after 12 months by the appearance of hepatocellular carcinoma.[29-32]

A substance can be tested for promoting activity by substituting it for the promotion regimen in Protocols Nos. 1 to 4 (Figure 2) and assessing its ability to enhance the incidence of altered foci, hyperplastic nodules, or hepatocellular carcinoma. Most assays for promoting activity have employed for initiation, diethylnitrosamine administered either 18 hours after a partial hepatectomy or as a necrotic dose.

General Comments About the Protocols

Use of altered-foci. The numerous markers for altered-foci are presented in Table 1. GGT-positive foci have been the most widely used markers. Their maroon color is readily detected against the hematoxylin counterstained liver (Figure 3). In adult liver only the bile ductules contain GGT activity. Other markers that have been used include ATPase and glucose-6-phosphatase (G-6-Pase)-deficient foci and foci of hepatocytes that have lost the ability to concentrate iron. These are negative markers so that they are less readily detected. GGT-positive foci are the most dependable markers in rat liver, detecting about 90% of the foci and nodules in the liver while ATPase, G-6-Pase, or iron-deficient foci detect a smaller number.[50]

A major technical problem in the use of GGT-positive foci in rat liver is that numerous chemicals including phenobarbital,[8,65,66] ethanol,[67] hexachlorobenzene,[8,68] mestranol,[8] and saccharin[8] can induce GGT activity in the periportal region of the liver lobule (Figure 5). Cells in the periportal region that possess induced GGT activity include bile ductules, oval cells, and a few hepatocytes. In some cases, the extent of induced GGT activity is great enough to include zones 2 and 3. Induced GGT activity occurs to the same extent in all periportal regions of the liver and follows a line between the triads, which is distinctive from GGT-positive foci which are round to oval in shape and randomly dispersed throughout all the regions of the lobule. Removal of phenobarbital in Protocol No. 2 (Figure 2) for up to two weeks prior to sacrifice reduced but did not eliminate the periportal-induced GGT activity. Caution must be exercised in the interpretation of GGT activity in the periportal region in order to distinguish between induction of GGT-positive foci and GGT activity.

Table 1: Histochemical Markers for Altered-Foci

A. Increase
1. Gamma-glutamyl transpeptidase[3,7,50]
2. Basophilia[51-53]
3. DT-Diaphorase[54]
4. Epoxide hydratase, preneoplastic antigen[55-58]
5. Glycogen storage[59,60]
6. Glucose-6-phosphate dehydrogenase[59,60]

B. Decrease
1. Adenosine triphosphatase[3,45,50,61]
2. Glucose-6-phosphatase[3,45,50]
3. Serine dehydratase[62]
4. Ability to concentrate iron[51,63]
5. Ribonuclease and deoxyribonuclease[64]

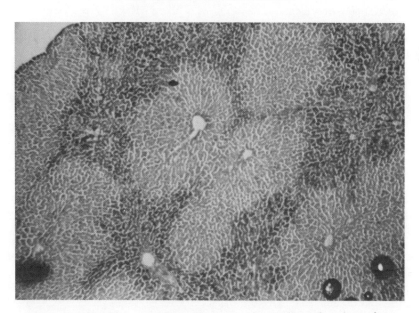

Figure 5: Induction of GGT activity in the periportal region of rat liver. GGT activity was induced by 500 ppm sodium phenobarbital in the drinking water.

Another limitation of the use of GGT-positive foci is that not all initiators and promoters produce GGT-positive foci and tumors that contain GGT activity. Wy-14,643, a peroxisome proliferator, induced altered-foci, hyperplastic nodules, and hepatocellular carcinoma in Fischer-344 rats that were negative for GGT activity.[69] Several other peroxisome proliferators are hepatocarcinogens.[70,71] For peroxisomal proliferators at least, the use of GGT-positive foci appears to be inappropriate when assessing activity as a carcinogen. GGT-positive foci might be appropriate in an assay that employs phenobarbital promotion when assessing the initiating activity of a substance that does not produce GGT positive tumors. Under this circumstance, the phenobarbital could induce GGT activity in otherwise hidden foci so that they are scored.

Phenobarbital has been demonstrated to induce preferentially GGT activity in altered-foci and tumors in the liver of mice[72-74] and rats.[75] Other chemicals might also induce GGT activity in foci and tumors without increasing the tumor incidence. Therefore, when testing a substance for promoting activity, caution is required in the interpretation of an increased incidence of GGT-positive foci without simultaneous increase in tumor incidence.

A carcinogen can induce thousands of altered-foci in the liver while only inducing a few hepatocellular carcinomas.[3,6,7] This large number of foci results in the great sensitivity of the assay. However, it also precludes the use of the incidence of foci to predict the incidence of hepatocellular carcinoma. Before the rat liver foci assay can be used to predict the carcinoma incidence, the quantitative relationship between the incidence of foci and the incidence of cancer has to be determined for a given protocol and for different classes of carcinogens.

Use of 2-acetylaminofluorene. 2-Acetylaminofluorene is a recognized animal carcinogen to which the exposure of workers is strictly regulated in the United States. This limits the use of the 2-AAF diet in Protocol No. 3 (Figure 2). Another limitation of Protocol No. 3 is the concurrent use of two carcinogens, 2-AAF and carbon tetrachloride, in the protocol which can hinder the interpretation of results.

Quantitation of the incidence of foci. Results of the rat liver foci assay have been reported as either foci/unit area or foci/unit volume. The use of foci/cm^2 has been criticized because the ability to detect foci in a cross section is dependent on both the number of foci in the liver and the size of the foci. The larger foci are more likely to be detected. Therefore, the better estimation of the quantity of foci in the liver should be the incidence of foci/cm^3, the calculation of which depends on the incidence of foci intersections in the cross section and their individual size. It should be remembered that the calculated value is only an estimate, and the actual number of foci in the liver has to be determined from serial sections of the liver. Mathematical formulas have been developed using quantitative stereology and assuming a spherical shape for the foci.[76-78] Although most foci in a cross section are either round or oval in shape, this is not always the case especially if degenerative changes and remodeling have occurred. Goldfarb et al.[53] have determined that in mice given a single intraperitoneal injection of 5 μg diethylnitrosamine/gm body weight at 15 days of age, the foci (basophilic) have almost spherical shapes. The correlation between the maximal cross sectional areas of foci and the volumes of the foci was $V = 0.99$. In rats, GGT-positive foci and ATPase- or G-6-Pase-deficient foci appear to contain quite irregular shapes in transection for which the correlation between the maximal cross sectional areas of foci and the volume of the foci has yet to be determined. Thus, in rats, the mathematical derivation of foci/cm^3 is only a best estimate of the quantity of foci.

Despite the uncertainties in the calculation of foci/cm^3, it is a better measure of incidence of foci for evaluating the kinetic and quantitative relationship of foci to hepatocellular carcinoma. Previously, results have been reported as foci/cm^2. The ability now to calculate foci/cm^3 should not invalidate studies that used foci/cm^2 in order to determine whether a test substance possessed initiating activity. Foci/cm^2 is an acceptable determinant to demonstrate activity in the assay where the control level of foci/cm^2 is usually below one and the test substance initiates a statistically significant greater incidence of foci/cm^2. It is also acceptable in ranking substances for initiating activity in the same protocol, especially when the mean and median size of the foci initiated by the different test substances are similar. The sizes of the foci are less dependent on the test substance than on whether partial hepatectomy or a promoter of carcinogenicity was employed. Therefore, in most cases, results of the rat liver foci assay can be reported as foci/cm^2 although calculation as foci/cm^3 would be preferred.

Species, strain, sex and route of administration. In mouse liver, hepatocellular tumors in non-treated control animals were negative for GGT activity.[72-74,79,80] GGT activity was present in all safrole-induced tumors, although the activity was variable between different nodules and between cells within the same nodules.[80] The percentage of nodules induced by 3,5-dichloro(N-1,1-dimethyl-2-propynyl)benzamide (DCB) that contained GGT activity was 5% in the low dose and 64% in the high dose group.[81] Jalanko and Ruoslahti[79] found that there was no GGT activity in nodules from untreated control mice while o-aminoazotoluene-induced nodules did contain the enzyme. Benzo(a)pyrene-induced tumors did not contain GGT activity unless the mice received phenobarbital after the benzo(a)pyrene.[74] Phenobarbital also induced GGT activity in spontaneous tumors.[72-74] Therefore, the presence of GGT activity in hepatic tumors of mice was more related to the type of treatment than to the neoplastic process.

In mouse liver, basophilic[53] and iron-resistant foci[63] are suitable markers for carcinogen-induced preneoplastic lesions. In non-treated control animals and in DCB-,[81] diethylnitrosamine-,[82] and dieldrin-[82] treated mice, benign tumors and carcinomas were found with either increase, decrease or no change in ATPase or G-6-Pase activity with respect to the surrounding tissue (Figure 6 and Figure 7). There was a trend for elevated enzyme activity in the carcinomas compared to benign tumors.[82] Laib et al.[83] did not find an increase in ATPase-deficient foci in diethylnitrosamine-treated mice, guinea pigs and tupaias. It would appear that ATPase- and G-6-Pase-deficient foci are suitable markers for carcinogen-induced preneoplastic lesions in rats but not in mice, guinea pigs and tupaias.

Using Protocol No. 2 (Figure 2) with diethylnitrosamine as the initiator and phenobarbital as the promoter, the incidence of GGT-positive foci between three different strains of rats—Sprague-Dawley, Fischer-344, and Wistar-Lewis—was not significantly different.[84] In rats that did not receive the diethylnitrosamine, a significant background level of GGT-positive foci was found only in the Fischer-344 rats. After repeated administration of diethylnitrosamine, Deml et al.[85] ob-

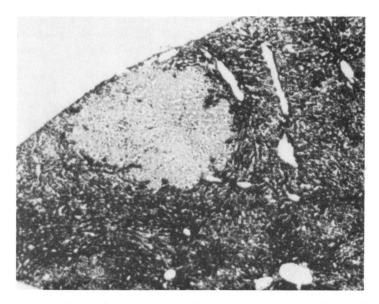

Figure 6: Glucose-6-phosphatase-deficient foci in mouse liver. The animal was initiated with 45 ppm diethylnitrosamine for four weeks in the drinking water followed by promotion with 500 ppm sodium phenobarbital in the drinking water.

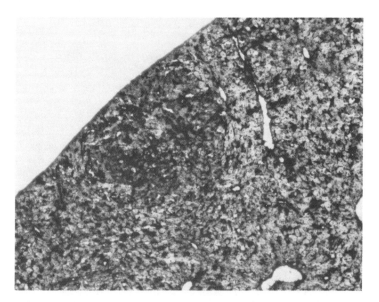

Figure 7: ATPase-increased foci in mouse liver. The animal was initiated with 45 ppm diethylnitrosamine for four weeks in the drinking water followed by promotion with 500 ppm sodium phenobarbital in the drinking water.

tained the same incidence of GGT-positive foci and ATPase-deficient foci in Sprague-Dawley and Wistar rats. Laib *et al.*[83] found Sprague-Dawley rats more sensitive than Wistar rats to a single dose of diethylnitrosamine as measured by ATPase-deficient foci.

The lack of or minimal effect of gender was demonstrated for the initiation by diethylnitrosamine, 7,12-dimethylbenzanthracene and 1,2-dimethylhydrazine of GGT-positive foci in Protocol No. 2 (Figure 2).[84] Deml *et al.*[85] found adult female Sprague-Dawley rats more sensitive than their male counterparts to diethylnitrosamine-induced GGT-positive foci. There no gender-related differences for ATPase-deficient foci in Sprague-Dawley or in Wistar rats for either GGT-positive or ATPase-deficient foci. In weanling rats, female Sprague-Dawley and Wistar rats were more sensitive than the corresponding males. Laib *et al.*[83] found female Sprague-Dawley and Wistar rats more sensitive than the males to diethyl-nitrosamines as shown by induced ATPase-deficient foci. The consensus of the studies on the effect of gender in the rat liver foci assay would be that female rats are of either equal or greater sensitivity than male rats.

The extent of initiation of GGT-positive foci in Protocol No. 2 (Figure 2) by diethylnitrosamine, 7,12-dimethylbenzanthracene, or 1,2-dimethylhydrazine was not affected by the route of administration, *i.e.*, gavage or intraperitoneal injection.[84] 7,12-Dimethylbenzanthracene was more toxic when administered intraperitoneally compared to gavage. The three chemicals were chosen because they represent different chemical classes and possess different water solubility. Hasegawa *et al.*,[86] in a modified Protocol No. 3 (Figure 2), did not observe any differences in the ability of diethylnitrosamine to initiate hyperplastic nodules when it was administered by either gavage, intraperitoneal injection, intravenous injection, or subcutaneous injection. These investigators found, however, that gavage was a more efficient route of administration for N-methyl-N'-nitro-N-nitrosoguanidine and benzo(a)pyrene than intraperitoneal or subcutaneous injection. Pereira *et al.*[84] did not find such differences for another polycyclic hydrocarbon, 7,12-dimethylbenzanthracene. This might be due to the greater toxicity of 7,12-dimethylbenzanthracene administered by intraperitoneal injection than by gavage. In any case, gavage would appear to be a suitable route of administering a test substance in the rat liver foci assay.

RESULTS

The results for the various substances tested in the rat liver foci assay are presented in Table 2. The assay was responsive to both hepatocarcinogens and non-hepatocarcinogens such as benzo(a)pyrene, 7,12-dimethylbenzanthracene, N-methylnitrosourea, and urethan. The sensitivity to non-hepatocarcinogens was especially evident when the carcinogen was administered to (a) rats that had received a partial hepatectomy; (b) neonates; or (c) weanling rats. The assay was insensitive to some hepatocarcinogens including chloroform, p-dioxane, and safrole, and to some non-hepatocarcinogens including benzene, lead acetate, and β-propiolactone. The reason why the assay did not detect all carcinogens could be due to the following: (a) Some of the carcinogens such as chloroform, p-dioxane, benzene and lead acetate might be promoters of carcinogenicity and do not possess initiating activity; (b) the time of the partial hepatectomy did not result in the regenerative DNA replication occurring in the presence of sufficient amounts of DNA adducts; or (c) the carcinogen exhibits tissue specificity for binding to DNA resulting in either insufficient binding to liver DNA or in the formation of non-genotoxic adducts to liver DNA. The mechanism(s) for the insensitivity of the rat liver foci assay to certain carcinogens needs to be investigated further especially to determine whether the timing of the partial hepatectomy was inappropriate.

Table 2: Chemicals Tested in the Rat Liver Foci Assay

| Chemical | Protocol[a] | . . . . Result. . . . . . . | | Reference |
		Rat Liver Foci Assay	Carcinogenicity	
2-Acetyl-aminofluorene	2	+	+	87
	3	+	+	25,88
	A	+	+	23
Aflatoxin B$_1$	2	+	+	87
	3	+	+	88
	A	+	+	23
Aflatoxin B$_2$	2	–	–	87
4-Aminobiphenyl	3	+	+	25
3-Amino-1,4-dimethyl-5H-pyrido(4,3-b)indole	3	+	?	89
2-Aminodipyrido-(1,2-a:3',2'-d)-imidazole	3	+	?	89
2-Amino-6-methyldi-pyrido-(1,2-a:3',2'-d)-imidazole	3	+	?	89
3-Amino-1-methyl-5H-pyrido-(4,3-b)indole	3	–	?	89
2-Amino-3-methyl-9H-pyrido(2,3-b)indole	3	+	?	89
2-Amino-9H-pyrido-(2,3-b)indole	3	+	?	89
Anthracene	3	–	–	25
Auramine	3	+	+	25
Azaserine	4	+	+	30
Benzene	2	–	+	87
Benzo(a)anthracene	3	+	+	25
Benzo(a)pyrene	2	+	+	87
	3	+	+	25,86
	B	+	+	35
Benzo(e)pyrene	2	–	+/–	87
Bromoform	2	–	?	90
N-Butyl-(4-hydroxy-butyl)nitrosamine	3	+	+	91
N-butyl-N-nitrosourea	3	+	+	25
Chlorazepate	1	–	–	92
Chloroform	2	–	+	90
Citrinin	3	+	+	93
Cycasin	1	+	+	94

(continued)

Table 2: (Continued)

Chemical	Protocol[a]	Rat Liver Foci Assay	Carcinogenicity	Reference
3,4-Cyclopenteno-pyrido-(3,2-a)carbazole	3	+	?	89
Cyproterone acetate	3	–	–	95
Diazald	2	–	?	19
Diazepam	1	–	–	92
Dibenzo(a,h)anthracene	3	+	+	25
1,2-Dibromoethane	2	–	+	96
Dieldrin	3	+	+	25
Diethylnitrosamine	2	+	+	87
	3	+	+	86,88
	A	+	+	23
	C	+	+	36
7,12-Dimethylbenz(a)-anthracene	2	+	+	87
	3	+	+	25
	C	+	+	36
1,2-Dimethylhydrazine	2	+	+	87
	3	+	+	25
Dimethylnitrosamine	2	+	+	87
	3	+	+	88
	A	+	+	23
Dimethyl sulfate	2	–	+	19
p-Dioxane	2	–	+	8
Estradiol-17B	3	–	+	95
DL-Ethionine	A	+	+	23
N-Ethylnitrosourea	3	+	+	91
Ethinylestradiol	3	–	+	95
Fluorene	3	–	–	25
Hycanthone methane-sulfonate	3	+	+	25
Lead acetate	2	–	+	8
Lorazepam	1	–	–	92
3-Methylcholanthrene	3	+	+	25
2-Methyl-N,N-dimethyl-4-aminoazobenzene	1	+	–	97
3'-Methyl-4-dimethyl-aminoazobenzene	1	+	+	98
	A	+	+	3,23
3'-Methyl-4-dimethyl-aminobenzene	3	+	+	86,88,99
	2	–	+	19
N-Methyl-N'-nitro-N-nitrosoguanidine	2	+	+	87
	3	+	+	25,86
N-Methyl-N-nitrosourea	2	+	+	19
	3	+	+	24
Morpholine	3	–	–	25
Naphthalene	3	–	–	25
α-Naphthylamine	3	+	+	25
β-Naphthylamine	3	+	+	25

(continued)

Table 2: (Continued)

Chemical	Protocol[a]	Result		Reference
		Rat Liver Foci Assay	Carcinogenicity	
N-[4-(5-Nitro-2-furyl)-2-thiazolyl] formamide	3	+	+	25
N-Nitrosomorpholine	2	+	+	100
	3	+	+	25,101
N-Nitrosopiperidine	3	+	+	25
Norethindrone acetate	3	−	?	95
Norethynodrel	3	−	?	95
Ochratoxin A	3	+	+	93
Oxazepam	1	−	−	92
Patulin	3	+	?	93
Phenanthrene	3	−	−	25
Piperidine	3	−	−	25
Progesterone	3	−	?	95
β-Propiolactone	2	−	+	8
Pyrene	3	−	−	25
Quinoline	3	+	+	91
(+) Rugulosin	3	+	+	93
Saccharin	3	−	+	91
Safrole	2	−	+	8
	3	+	+	25
Sterigmatocystin	3	+	+	93
12-O-Tetradecanoylphorbol-13-acetate	3	−	−	91
Thioacetamide	C	−	+	36
Trichloroethylene	D	−	+	102
2,4,6-Trichlorophenol	2	−	+	8
Urethane	2	+	+	87
	3	+	+	25
	C	−	+	36
Vinyl bromide	D	+	+	103
Vinyl carbamate	3	+	+	25
Vinyl chloride	D	+	+	102,103
Vinyl fluoride	D	+	?	104
Vinylidene fluoride	D	+	?	105
Wy-14,643[[4-chloro-6-(2-3-xylidino)-2-pyr-imidinylthio] acetic acid]	E	−	+	69
Vehicles				
Corn Oil	2	−	−	87
	3	−	−	25,86,88
Dimethyl sulfoxide	3	−	−	25,86,88
Saline	3	−	−	25,86
Tricaprylin	2	−	−	87
Water	2	−	−	87

[a]Protocol Nos. 1–4 (*see* Figure 2); A, the chemical was administered to partial hepatectomized rats without promotion; B, the chemical was administered one day after birth followed by 0.05% phenobarbital in the diet after weaning; C, the chemical was administered prenatally followed at weaning with selection by 2-acetylaminofluorene in the diet and partial hepatectomy; D, the chemical was administered to newborn rats without promotion; E, the chemical was administered in a long-term feeding study.

Some of the proposed uses of the rat liver foci assay include: (a) Identification of chemical carcinogens; (b) confirmation of carcinogenicity of genotoxic chemicals (*i.e.*, mutagens identified by the Ames Test); (c) prioritization of chemicals for long-term animal bioassays; (d) demonstration of the mechanism of action (*i.e.*, initiating activity *versus* promoting activity); and (e) determination of dose-response relationship for initiating activity and possible carcinogenicity. The rat liver foci assay has been used to identify the putative carcinogenic activity of pyrolysis products of amino acids and proteins that are highly mutagenic in the Ames Test.[89] The carcinogenic activity of the products confirmed using Protocol No. 3 (Figure 2) include 3,4-cyclopentenopyrido(3,2-a)-carbazole; 2-amino-9H-pyrido(1,2-b)indole; 2-amino-3-methyl-9H-pyrido(2,3-b)-indole; 3-amino-1,4-dimethyl-5H-pyrido(4,3-b)indole; 3-amino-1-methyl-5H-pyrido(4,3-b)indole; 2-amino-6-methyldipyrido(1,2-a:3',2'-d)imidazole; and 2-amino-dipyrido (1,2-a:3',2'-d)imidazole.[89] This demonstrates the usefulness of the rat liver foci assay in the identification and isolation of the carcinogens present in complex environmental mixtures.

The ability of fluorinated ethylenes to induce ATPase-deficient foci in newborn rats was compared to that of vinyl bromide and vinyl chloride in order to demonstrate and rank their carcinogenic hazard.[102-105] Vinyl fluoride and vinylidene fluoride were weaker inducers of foci suggesting that they are weaker carcinogens than vinyl bromide and vinyl chloride. Their relative ability to induce ATPase-deficient foci compared to vinyl chloride might be used as an estimate of their carcinogenic hazard in the absence of results from a long-term animal bioassay.

The rat liver foci assay has been used to determine the adducts of carcinogenic methylating agents. Only agents that methylate guanine at the O^6-position initiated foci in Protocol No. 2 (Figure 2) while agents that produced N-7 methylguanine did not.[19] O^6-Methylguanine but not N-7 methylguanine, has been shown to result in misreading of the genetic code[16,17] that could result in a mutagenic event. Therefore, the initiation of GGT-positive foci would appear to require a mutagenic event.

Hepatocarcinogens that are not genotoxic do not appear to initiate foci indicating that they might be promoters. Carcinogens such as chloroform,[90] p-dioxane[8] and sex steroids[94] that are not genotoxic and apparently do not significantly bind to DNA, did not initiate foci. Though this supports a non-genotoxic mechanism for these carcinogens, confirmation is still required.

The rat liver foci assay is usually performed at two or more doses of the test substance in order to obtain an indication of the dose-response relationship. The dose-response relationship of diethylnitrosamine in partial hepatectomized rats has been determined over a one thousand-fold range of dose.[23,46] The initiation of ATPase-deficient foci indicated a direct proportionality between the incidence of foci and dose in the range of 0.3 mg to 30 mg of diethylnitrosamine/kg.[23] Using Protocol No. 2 of Figure 2, a direct proportionality was also found between the incidence of GGT-positive foci and dose in the range of 0.01 mg to 10 mg of diethylnitrosamine/kg.[46] At doses of diethylnitrosamine greater than 50 mg/kg, there was a much slower rate of increase in incidence of foci with dose in both studies. Thus, the initiation of carcinogenesis in partially hepatectomized rats exhibited one-hit kinetics and did not appear to possess a thresh-

old. This would indicate that the formation of the responsible structural alteration in the DNA also possesses one-hit kinetics that is proportional to dose without a threshold. The use of partial hepatectomy in the foci assays of diethylnitrosamine eliminated any requirement of initiation for carcinogen-induced
DNA replication. In intact animals at the low, non-necrotic doses of diethylnitrosamine used, only the low endogenous rate of DNA replication would occur. Therefore, although the initiation of foci in partially hepatectomized rats
was linearly related to dose and did not exhibit a threshold, the dose-response
relationship in intact rats could be quite different because of the requirement for
carcinogen-induced DNA replication.

RELATIONSHIP OF ALTERED-FOCI TO HEPATOCELLULAR CARCINOMA

The determination of the relationship of altered-foci to the development of
hepatocellular carcinoma is critical to the use of the rat liver foci assay to predict carcinogenicity. Figure 8 depicts two possible models for the relationship of
carcinogen-initiated foci to the development of hepatocellular carcinoma. In the
precursor model, the carcinogen initiates the altered-foci which can either (a) revert back to the normal hepatocyte phenotype, (b) remain as a stable lesion in
the liver, (c) progress to hepatocellular carcinoma, or (d) progress to hyperplastic
nodules that can then progress to carcinoma. The main characteristic of this
model is that the altered-foci are precursors of hepatocellular carcinoma. The
foci can be a preneoplastic or even a neoplastic precursor depending upon where
in the progression from initiated hepatocyte to hepatocellular carcinoma the
neoplastic transformation occurs. A second model, in which the altered-foci are
ancillary lesions induced by the carcinogen, proposes other initiated hepatocytes
as the precursors for hepatocellular carcinoma. The initiated hepatocyte in some
cases might occur in an altered-focus, however, the focus in this model is only
an associated lesion.

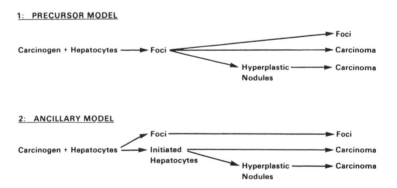

Figure 8: Proposed models for the relationship of carcinogen-initiated
altered foci to the development of hepatocellular carcinoma.

Proof that the altered-foci are direct precursors and not ancillary lesions requires the demonstration that hepatocytes in altered foci have a greater probability of progressing to hepatocellular carcinoma than non-involved hepatocytes. Laishes and collaborators[106,107] have demonstrated that hepatocytes of GGT-positive nodules induced by the 2-AAF selection model of Protocol No. 3 (Figure 2) were transplantable into syngeneic rats treated with 2-AAF. These transplantation or similar cell culture studies need to be repeated with purified populations of GGT-positive hepatocytes obtained from foci, not nodules, induced by either Protocol No. 1 or No. 2 (Figure 2).

There has been a large amount of circumstantial evidence to indicate that altered-foci are precursor and preneoplastic lesions (Table 3). Altered-foci are detected as phenotypic changes in hepatocytes that are also present in hyperplastic nodules and hepatocellular carcinoma. However, no single phenotypic change is presented in all hepatocellular carcinoma and different protocols induce different spectra of phenotypes in foci and hepatocellular carcinoma. For example, Wy-14,643 does not induce GGT-positive foci while inducing hepatocellular carcinoma.[69] Therefore, the phenotypes used to identify altered-foci are associated and not obligatory alterations.

Table 3: Evidence that Altered-Foci Are Preneoplastic/Neoplastic Lesions

1. Foci possess phenotypic changes similar to those found in hyperplastic nodules and hepatocellular carcinoma
2. Reappearance of fetal enzymes (*e.g.*, GGT)
3. Clonal origin of foci
4. Stability of foci
5. Initiated by genotoxic carcinogens and not by noncarcinogens
6. Dose-time-response relationship of induction of foci is consistent with a precursor relationship to hepatocellular carcinoma
7. Initiation of foci requires DNA replication similar to the initiation of hepatocarcinogenesis
8. Promoters of carcinogenicity affect altered-foci consistent with their acceleration of the appearance of tumors

GGT-positive foci represent the reappearance of a fetal enzyme which is absent in matured hepatocytes of adult rats. Although not all altered-foci and tumors contain GGT, phenobarbital has been demonstrated to induce GGT activity in foci and tumors in mice[72-74] and rats.[45,75] It is not known whether phenobarbital will also induce GGT in hidden foci and tumors induced by Wy-14,643. Phenobarbital and other promoters of carcinogenicity can also induce GGT activity in the periportal region of the liver.[8,65,66,68] GGT-positive foci occur in all three zones of the liver which indicates that the normal control of this fetal enzyme in matured hepatocytes has been altered. The reappearance of GGT activity is supportive of the oncodevelopmental theory of cancer and of the preneoplastic nature of GGT-positive foci.

Cancer is believed to be the result of a clonal event and altered-foci also appear to be clonal in origin. Scherer and Hoffman[108] have suggested a monoclonal origin for diethylnitrosamine-induced ATPase-deficient foci. Foci induced by diethylnitrosamine and simultaneous administration of ³H-thymidine, were less labelled at five weeks after induction than the surrounding tissue. The cells of the foci lost the label by the diluting effect of repeated cell division, thus suggesting a monoclonal origin. Multi-hit kinetic analysis of the genesis of diethylnitrosamine-induced ATPase-deficient foci also supports a clonal origin.[61,109] In mice, ATPase-deficient foci were of clonal origin with respect to isozymes of 3-phosphoglycerate kinase.[110]

Diethylnitrosamine initiated- and phenobarbital promoted-GGT-positive foci using Protocols No. 1 and No. 2 (Figure 2) were stable lesions even after the removal of the phenobarbital.[109,111] Schulte-Hermann *et al.*[38] found that approximately 70% of the N-nitrosomorpholine initiated- and phenobarbital promoted-GGT-positive foci regressed after the removal of the phenobarbital. Most, but not all, of the hyperplastic nodules induced by Protocol No. 3 in Figure 2 also regressed.[47-49] Therefore, although some investigators have found GGT-positive foci induced by certain protocols to be stable, a more general finding to include all protocols is that two types of altered-foci and hyperplastic nodules exist. One type of lesion is independent and the other type is dependent on continuous exposure to the promoter to prevent phenotypic reversion.

Numerous genotoxic hepatocarcinogens are positive in the rat liver foci assay (Table 2). Nongenotoxic hepatocarcinogens including p-dioxane, and 2,4,6-trichlorophenol were negative.[8] Only methylating agents that produced O^6-methylguanine, a mutagenic adduct in DNA, initiated GGT-positive foci in Protocol No. 2 (Figure 2) while methylating agents that only produced N-7 methylguanine did not.[19] Therefore, the initiation of altered-foci appears to be dependent on a genotoxic event.

The extent of initiation by diethylnitrosamine[61,109] or N-nitrosomorpholine[112] of ATPase-deficient foci was related to the dose of the carcinogen. The dose-time-response relationship for induction of foci had characteristics identical to that observed for the induction of tumors. The results are consistent with a minimum requirement of two hits in which foci incidence was related to dose by a power of one and time of exposure by a power of two. Therefore, only the first hit is carcinogen-dependent (DNA alteration?) whereas the second-hit for phenotypic alteration is caused by a time-dependent and carcinogen-independent event. Kunz *et al.*[112] have proposed that the second hit could be a promoter sensitive alteration in ploidy status that leads to abnormal chromosomal redistribution so that heterozygous recessive mutations become homozygous. These characteristics of the dose-time-response relationships for induction of altered-foci are consistent with a precursor relationship of foci to hepatocellular carcinoma.

A partial hepatectomy during initiation has been shown to enhance the incidence of altered-foci and tumors by both hepatocarcinogens and non-hepatocarcinogens.[20-27] The relationship of the time of operation to the administration of the carcinogen is very critical and appears to require coincidental occurrence of the increased DNA replication and maximum extent of binding of the carcinogen to DNA.[25] The increased replication of DNA is believed to be required for fixation of the carcinogen-induced damage in the DNA prior to its repair. The requirement of DNA replication for the induction of altered-foci and tumors supports the requirement of a genotoxic event for both foci and tumor induction and thus the precursor role of altered-foci.

ATPase-deficient foci[113] and GGT-positive foci[37,38] have an increased rate of DNA synthesis compared to surrounding hepatocytes. Schulte-Hermann *et al.*[37,38] have demonstrated that promoters such as phenobarbital, cyproteron acetate, and progesterone enhance proliferation and growth of GGT-positive foci. The promoters also increased the lifespan and/or prevented phenotypic reversion of foci. The effects of promoters on altered-foci are similar and consistent to their acceleration of the appearance of tumors.

CONCLUSION

The rat liver foci assay is capable of distinguishing both hepatocarcinogens and non-hepatocarcinogens from non-carcinogens so that it is suitable for inclusion in a battery of tests to identify chemical carcinogens. The rat liver foci assay can identify both pure carcinogens and carcinogens present in complex mixtures of environmental samples. Although the altered-foci used as determinants in the assay have not conclusively been demonstrated to be precursor and preneoplastic lesions, substantial circumstantial evidence exists to support the precursor relationship. Therefore, the assay can confirm and predict carcinogenic activity. Due to the large numbers of altered-foci produced in the assay compared to the incidence of tumor, it is at present impossible to use the assay for a quantitative prediction of hepatocellular carcinoma. Before this is feasible, the quantitative relationship of the incidence of foci to the incidence of tumors would have to be determined for a given protocol and for different chemical classes of initiators. It appears that the assay can be used to rank chemicals within a class when assayed under a single protocol.

Caution is necessary before modifying the rat liver foci assay to assess promoting activity. The assay can not distinguish between an effect that enhances the incidence and growth of altered-foci resulting in promotion from an effect that increases the visualization of foci by the induction of GGT activity in hidden foci which does not result in an increased incidence of tumor.

REFERENCES

1. Boutwell, R.K., The function and mechanism of promoters of carcinogenesis. *CRC Crit. Rev. Toxicol.* 2: 419-447 (1974)
2. Slaga, T.J., Overview of tumor promotion in animals. *Environ. Health Perspect.* 50: 3-14 (1983)
3. Pitot, H.C., and Sirica, A.E., The stages of initiation and promotion in hepatocarcinogenesis. *Biochim. Biophys. Acta* 605: 191-215 (1980)
4. Weisburger, J.H., and Williams, G.M., The distinct health risk analyses required for genotoxic carcinogens and promoting agents. *Environ. Health Perspect.* 50: 233-245 (1983)
5. Bull, R.J., and Pereira, M.A., Development of a short-term testing matrix for estimating relative carcinogenic risk. *J. Amer. Coll. Toxicol.* 1: 1-15 (1982)

6. Farber, E., The sequential analysis of liver cancer induction. *Biochim. Biophys. Acta* 605: 149-166 (1980)

7. Pereira, M.A., Rat liver foci bioassay. *J. Amer. Coll. Toxicol.* 1: 101-117 (1982)

8. Pereira, M.A., Herren, S.L., Britt, A.L., and Khoury, M.M., Initiation/promotion bioassay in liver: Use of gamma glutamyltranspeptidase-positive foci to indicate carcinogenic activity. *Toxicol. Pathol.* 10: 11-18 (1982)

9. Peraino, C., Fry, R.J.M., Staffeldt, E., and Kisieleski, W.E., Effects of varying the exposure to phenobarbital on its enhancement of 2-acetylamino-fluorene-induced hepatic tumorigenesis in the rat. *Cancer Res.* 33: 2701-2705 (1973)

10. Peraino. R.J., Fry, M., and Staffeldt, E., Reduction and enhancement by phenobarbital of hepatocarcinogenesis induced in the rat by 2-acetyl-aminofluorene. *Cancer Res.* 31: 1506-1512 (1971)

11. Peraino, R.J., Fry, M., Staffeldt, E., and Christopher, J.P., Comparative enhancing effects of phenobarbital, amobarbital, diphenylhydantoin, and dichlorodiphenyltrichloroethane on 2-acetylaminofluorene-induced hepatic tumorigenesis in the rat. *Cancer Res.* 35: 2884-2890 (1975)

12. Peraino, R.J., Fry, M., and Staffeldt, E., Effects of varying the onset and duration of exposure to phenobarbital on its enhancement of 2-acetyl-aminofluorene-induced hepatic tumorigenesis. *Cancer Res.* 37: 3623-3627 (1977)

13. Lutz, W.K., Viviani, A., and Schlatter, C., Nonlinear dose-response relationship for the binding of the carcinogen benzo(a)pyrene to rat liver DNA *in vivo. Cancer Res.* 38: 575-578 (1978)

14. Eastman, A., Sweetenham, J., and Bresnick, E., Comparison of *in vivo* and *in vitro* binding of polycyclic hydrocarbons to DNA. *Chem. Biol. Interact.* 23: 345-353 (1978)

15. Daniel, F.B., and Joyce, N.J., DNA adduct formation by 7,12-dimethyl-benz(a)anthracene and its noncarcinogenic 2-fluoro analogue in female Sprague-Dawley rats. *J. Natl. Cancer Inst.* 70: 111-118 (1983)

16. Lawley, P.D., in: *Chemical Carcinogens* (C.E. Searle, ed.), pp 83-151, American Chemical Society, Washington, DC (1976)

17. Lawley, P.D., in: *Chemical Carcinogens and DNA*, (P.L. Grover, ed.), Vol. 1, pp 1-19, CRC Press, Boca Raton (1979)

18. Singer, B., Sites in nucleic acids reacting with alkylating agents of differing carcinogenicity or mutagenicity. *J. Toxicol. Environ. Health* 2: 1279-1288 (1977)

19. Pereira, M.A., Lin, L.-H.C., and Herren, S.L., Role of O^6-methylation in the initiation of GGTase-positive foci. *Chem. Biol. Interact.* 43: 313-332 (1983)

20. Craddock, V.M., Liver carcinomas induced in rats by single administration of dimethylnitrosamine after partial hepatectomy. *J. Natl. Cancer Inst.* 47: 889-896 (1971)

21. Craddock, V.M., Effect of a single treatment with the alkylating carcinogens dimethyl-nitrosamine, diethylnitrosamine and methyl methanesulphonate, on liver regeneration after partial hepatectomy. I. Test for induction of carcinomas. *Chem. Biol. Interact.* 10: 313-332 (1975)

22. Craddock, V.M., in: *Liver Cell Cancer* (M.M. Cameron, D.A. Linsell, and G.P. Warwick, eds.), pp 153-201, Elsevier, North Holland, Amsterdam (1976)

23. Scherer, E., and Emmelot, P., Kinetics of induction and growth of enzyme-deficient islands involved in hepatocarcinogenesis. *Cancer Res.* 36: 2544-2554 (1976)

24. Cayama, E., Tsuda, H., Sarma, D.S.R., and Farber, E., Initiation of chemical carcinogenesis requires cell proliferation. *Nature* 275: 60-62 (1978)

25. Tsuda, H., Lee, G.L., and Farber, E., Induction of resistant hepatocytes as a new principle for a possible short-term *in vivo* test for carcinogens. *Cancer Res.* 40: 1157-1164 (1980)

26. Ishikawa, T., Takayama, S., and Kitagawa, T., Correlation between time of partial hepatectomy after a single treatment with diethylnitrosamine and induction of adenosinetriphosphatase-deficient islands in rat liver. *Cancer Res.* 40: 4261-4264 (1980)

27. Columbano, A., Rajalakshmi, S., and Sarma, D.S.R., Requirement of cell proliferation for the initiation of liver carcinogenesis as assayed by three different procedures. *Cancer Res.* 41: 2079-2083 (1981)

28. Ghoshal, A., and Farber, E., The induction of resistant hepatocytes during initiation of liver carcinogenesis with chemicals in rats fed a choline deficient methionine low diet. *Carcinogenesis* 4: 801-804 (1983)

29. Lombardi, B., and Shinozuka, H., Enhancement of 2-acetylaminofluorene liver carcinogenesis in rats fed a choline-devoid diet. *Int. J. Cancer* 23: 565-570 (1979)

30. Takahashi, S., Katyal, S.L., Lombardi, B., and Shinozuka, H., Induction of foci of altered hepatocytes by a single injection of azaserine to rats. *Cancer Lett.* 7: 265-272 (1979)

31. Shinozuka, H., Sells, M.A., Katyal, S.L., Sell, S., and Lombardi, B., Effects of a choline-devoid diet on the emergence of γ-glutamyl-transpeptidase-positive foci in the liver of carcinogen-treated rats. *Cancer Res.* 39: 2515-2521 (1979)

32. Shinozuka, H., Lombardi, B., Sell, S., and Iammarino, R.M., Early histological and functional alterations of ethionine liver carcinogenesis in rats fed a choline-deficient diet. *Cancer Res.* 38: 1092-1098 (1978)

33. Takahashi, S., Ohnishi, T., Denda, A., and Konishi, Y., Enhancing effect of 3-aminobenzamide on induction of γ-glutamyl transpeptidase positive foci in rat liver. *Chem. Biol. Interact.* 39: 363-368 (1982)

34. Park, S.D., Kim, C.G., and Kim, M.G., Inhibitors of poly(ADP-ribose) polymerase enhance DNA strand breaks, excision repair, and sister chromatid exchanges induced by alkylating agents. *Environ. Mutagen.* 5: 515-525 (1983)

35. Peraino, C., Staffeldt, E., and Ludeman, V.A., Early appearance of histochemically altered hepatocyte foci and liver tumors in female rats treated with carcinogens one day after birth. *Carcinogenesis* 2: 463-465 (1981)

36. Ogawa, K., Uokokawa, K., Tomoyori, T., and Onoe, T., Induction of glutamyltranspeptidase-positive altered hepatocytic lesions by combination of transplacental-initiation and postnatal-selection. *Int. J. Cancer* 29: 333-336 (1982)

37. Schulte-Herman, R., and Parzefall, W. Failure to discriminate initiation from promotion of liver tumors in a long-term study with the phenobarbital-type-inducer α-hexachlorocyclohexane and the role of sustained stimulation of hepatic growth and monooxygenases. *Cancer Res.* 41: 4140-4146 (1981)

38. Schulte-Hermann, R., Schuppler, J., Timmermann-Trosiener, I., Ohde, G., Bursch, W., and Berger, H., The role of growth of normal and preneoplastic cell populations for tumor promotion in rat liver. *Environ. Health Perspect.* 50: 185-194 (1983)

39. Solt, D., and Farber, E., New principle for the analysis of chemical carcinogenesis. *Nature* 263: 701-703 (1976)

40. Solt, D.B., Medine, A., and Farber, E., Rapid emergence of carcinogen-induced hyperplastic lesions in a new model for the sequential analysis of liver carcinogenesis. *Am. J. Pathol.* 88: 595-618 (1977)

41. Farber, E., and Cameron, R., The sequential analysis of cancer development. *Adv. Cancer Res.* 31: 125-226 (1980)

42. Solt, D.B., Cayama, E., Tsuda, H., Enomoto, K., Lee, G., and Farber, E., Promotion of liver cancer development by brief exposure to dietary 2-acetylaminofluorene plus partial hepatectomy or carbon tetrachloride. *Cancer Res.* 43: 188-191 (1983)

43. Ito, N., Tsuda, H., Hasegawa, R., and Imaida, K., Comparison of the promoting effects of various agents in induction of preneoplastic lesions in rat liver. *Environ. Health Perspect.* 50: 131-138 (1983)

44. Pitot, H.C., Barness, L., Goldsworthy, T., and Kitagawa, T., Biochemical characterization of stages of hepatocarcinogenesis after a single dose of diethylnitrosamine, *Nature* 271: 456-458 (1978)

45. Sirica, A.E., Barsness, L., Goldsworthy, T., and Pitot, H.C., Definition of stages during hepatocarcinogenesis in the rat: Potential application to the evaluation of initiating and promoting agents in the environment. *J. Environ. Pathol. Toxicol.* 2: 21-28 (1978)

46. Ford, J.O., and Pereira, M.A., Short-term *in vivo* initiation/promotion bioassay for hepatocarcinogens. *J. Environ. Pathol. Toxicol.* 4: 39-46 (1980)

47. Ogawa, K., Solt, D.B., and Farber, E., Phenotypic diversity as an early property of putative preneoplastic hepatocyte populations in liver carcinogenesis. *Cancer Res.* 40: 725-733 (1980)

48. Enomoto, K., Ying, T.S., Griffin, M.J., and Farber, E., Immunohistochemical study of epoxide hydrolase during experimental liver carcinogenesis. *Cancer Res.* 41: 3281-3287 (1981)

49. Enomoto, K., and Farber, E., Kinetics of phenotypic maturation of remodeling of hyperplastic nodules during liver carcinogenesis. *Cancer Res.* 42: 2330-2335 (1982)

50. Pugh, T.O., and Goldfarb, S., Quantitative histochemical and autoradiographic studies of hepatocarcinogenesis in rats fed 2-acetylaminofluorene followed by phenobarbital. *Cancer Res.* 38: 4450-4457 (1978)

51. Daoust, R., and Calamai, R., Hyperbasophilic foci as sites of neoplastic transformation in hepatic parenchyma. *Cancer Res.* 31: 1290-1296 (1971)

52. Hirota, N., and Williams, G.M., Persistence and growth of rat liver neoplastic nodules following cessation of carcinogen exposure. *J. Natl. Cancer Inst.* 63: 1257-1266 (1979)

53. Goldfarb, S., Pugh, T.D., Koen, H., and He, Y.-A., Preneoplastic and neoplastic progression during hepatocarcinogenesis in mice injected with diethylnitrosamine in infancy. *Environ. Health Perspect.* 50: 149-161 (1983)

54. Schor, N.A., Ogawa, K., Lee, G., and Farber, E., The use of the D-T diaphorase for the detection of foci of early neoplastic transformation in rat liver. *Cancer Lett.* 5: 167-171 (1978)

55. Okita, K., and Farber, E., An antigen common to preneoplastic hepatocyte population and to liver cancer induced by N-2-fluorenylactamide, ethionine or other carcinogens. *Gann. Monogr.* 17: 283-299 (1975)

56. Okita, K., Kligman, L.H., and Farber, E., A new common marker for premalignant and malignant hepatocytes induced in the rat by chemical carcinogens. *J. Natl. Cancer Inst.* 54: 199-202 (1975)

57. Levin, W., Lu, A.Y.H., Thomas, P.E., Ryan, D., Kizer, D.E., and Griffin, M., Identification of EH as the preneoplastic antigen in rat liver hyperplastic nodules. *Proc. Natl. Acad. Sci. U.S.A.* 75: 3240-3243 (1978)

58. Oesch, F., Vogel-Bindel, U., Guenthner, T.M., Cameron, R., and Farber, E., Characterization of microsomal epoxide hydrolase in hyperplastic liver nodules of rats. *Cancer Res.* 43: 313-319 (1983)

59. Bannasch, P., Mayer, D., and Hacker, H.-J., Hepatocellular glycogenesis and hepatocarcinogenesis. *Biochim. Biophys. Acta* 605: 217-245 (1980)

60. Bannasch, P., Moore, M.A., Klimek, F., and Zerban, H., Biological markers of preneoplastic foci and neoplastic nodules in rodent liver. *Toxicol. Pathol.* 10: 19-34 (1982)

61. Emmelot, P., and Scherer, E., The first relevant cell stage in rat liver carcinogenesis: a quantitative approach. *Biochim. Biophys. Acta* 605: 247-304 (1980)

62. Kitagawa, T., and Pitot, H.C., The regulation of serine dehydratase and glucose-6-phosphatase in hyperplastic nodules of rat liver during diethylnitrosamine and N-2-fluorenylacetamide feeding. *Cancer Res.* 35: 1075-1084 (1975)

63. Williams, G.M., The pathogenesis of rat liver cancer caused by chemical carcinogens. *Biochim. Biophys. Acta.* 605: 167-189 (1980)

64. Fontaniere, B., and Daoust, R., Histochemical studies on nuclease activity and neoplastic transformation in rat liver during diethylnitrosamine carcinogenesis. *Cancer Res.* 33: 3108-3111 (1973)

65. Roomi, M.W., and Goldbert, D.M., Comparison of γ-glutamyl-transferase induction by phenobarbital in the rat, guinea pig and rabbit. *Biochem. Pharmacol.* 30: 1563-1571 (1981)

66. Ratanasavanh, A.T., Galteau, M.M., and Siest, G., Localization of gamma-glutamyl-transferase in subcellular fractions of rat and rabbit liver: effect of phenobarbital. *Biochem. Pharmacol.* 28: 1363-1365 (1979)

67. Nishimura, N., Stein, H., Berges, W., and Teschke, R., Gamma-glutamyl-transferase activity of liver plasma membrane: Induction following chronic alcohol consumption. *Biochem. Biophys. Res. Commun.* 99: 142-148 (1981)

68. Adjarov, D., Ivanov, E., and Keremidchiev, D., Gamma-glutamyl-transferase: A sensitive marker in experimental hexachlorobenzene intoxication. *Toxicol.* 23: 73-77 (1982)

69. Rao, M.S., Lalwani, N.D., Scarpelli, D.G., and Reddy, J.K., The absence of γ-glutamyl-transpeptidase activity in putative preneoplastic lesions and in hepatocellular carcinomas induced in rats by hypolipidemic peroxisome proliferator Wy-14,643. *Carcinogenesis* 3: 1231-1233 (1982)

70. Cohen, A.J., and Grasso, P., Review of the hepatic response to hypolipidaemic drugs in rodents and assessment of its toxicological significance to man. *Fd. Cosmet. Toxicol.* 19: 585-605 (1981)

71. De La Iglesia, F.A., and Farber, E., Hypolipidemics carcinogenicity and extrapolation of experimental results for human safety assessments. *Toxicol. Pathol.* 10: 152-170 (1982)

72. Kitagawa, T., Watnabe, R., and Sugano, H., Induction of γ-glutamyl-transpeptidase activity by dietary phenobarbital in "spontaneous" hepatic tumors of C3H mice. *Gann* 71: 536-542 (1980)

73. Williams, G.M., Ohmori, T., Katayama, S., and Rice, J.M., Alteration by phenobarbital of membrane-associated enzymes including gamma-glutamyl-transpeptidase in mouse liver neoplasms. *Carcinogenesis* 1: 813-818 (1980)

74. Ohmori, T., Rice, J.M., and Williams, G.M., Histochemical characteristics of spontaneous and chemically induced hepatocellular neoplasms in mice and the development of neoplasms with γ-glutamyl-transpeptidase activity during phenobarbital exposure. *Histochem.* 13: 85-99 (1981)

75. Pereira, M.A., Herren-Freund, S.L., Britt, A.L., and Khoury, M., Effect of co-administration of phenobarbital on diethylnitrosamine induced gamma-glutamyl-transpeptidase-positive foci and hepatocellular carcinoma. *J. Natl. Cancer Inst.* 72: 741-744 (1984)

76. Scherer, E., Hoffmann, M., Emmelot, P., and Friedrich-Freksa, H., Quantitative study on foci of altered liver cells induced in the rat by a single dose of diethylnitrosamine and partial hepatectomy. *J. Natl. Cancer Inst.* 49: 93-106 (1972)

77. Campbell, H.A., Pitot, H.C., Potter, V.R., and Laishes, B.A., Application of quantitative stereology to the evaluation of enzyme-altered foci in rat liver. *Cancer Res.* 42: 465-472 (1982)

78. Pugh, T.D., King, J.H., Koen, H., Nychka, D., Chover, J., Wahba, G., He, Y., and Goldfarb, S., Reliable stereological method for estimating the number of microscopic hepatocellular foci from their transections. *Cancer Res.* 43: 1261-1268 (1983)

79. Jalanko, H., and Ruoslahti, E., Differential expression of α-fetoprotein and γ-glutamyl-transpeptidase in chemical and spontaneous hepatocarcinogenesis. *Cancer Res.* 39: 3495-3501 (1979)

80. Lipsky, M.M., Hinton, D.E., Klaunig, J.E., Goldblatt, P.J., and Trump, B.F., Gamma-glutamyl-transpeptidase in safrole-induced, presumptive premalignant mouse hepatocytes. *Carcinogenesis* 1: 151-156 (1980)

81. Essigmann, E.M., and Newberne, P.M., Enzymatic alterations in mouse hepatic nodules induced by a chlorinated hydrocarbon pesticide. *Cancer Res.* 41: 2823-2831 (1981)

82. Ruebner, B.H., Gershwin, M.E., Meierhenry, E.F., and Dunn, P., Enzyme histochemical characteristics of spontaneous and induced hepatocellular neoplasms in mice. *Carcinogenesis* 3: 899-903 (1982)

83. Laib, R.J., Brockes, B., Schwaier, A., and Bolt, H.M., Strain and species differences in the induction of ATPase-deficient hepatic foci by diethylnitrosamine. *Cancer Lett.* 15: 145-148 (1982)

84. Pereira, M.A., Herren-Freund, S.L., Britt, A.L., and Khoury, M.M., Effects of strain, sex route of administration and partial hepatectomy on the induction by chemical carcinogens of gamma-glutamyl-transpeptidase foci in rat liver. *Cancer Lett.* 20: 207-214 (1983)

85. Deml, E., Oesterle, D., Wolff, T., and Greim, H., Age-, sex-, and strain-dependent differences in the induction of enzyme-altered islands in rat liver by diethylnitrosamine. *J. Cancer Res. Clin. Oncol.* 100: 125-134 (1981)

86. Hasegawa, T., Tsuda, H., Nakanishi, K., Tatematsu, M., and Ito, N., Route-dependent, organ-specific effects of carcinogens on induction of hyperplastic liver nodules in rats. *Toxicol. Lett.* 14: 229-235 (1982)

87. Herren, S.L., Pereira, M.A., Britt, A.L., and Khoury, M.M., Initiation/promotion assay for chemical carcinogens in rat liver. *Toxicol. Lett.* 12: 143-150 (1982)

88. Imaida, K., Shirai, T., Tatematsu, M., Takano, T., and Ito, N., Dose responses of five hepatocarcinogens for the initiation of rat hepatocarcinogenesis. *Cancer Lett.* 14: 279-283 (1981)

89. Hasegawa, R., Tsuda, H., Ogiso, T., Ohshima, M., and Ito, N., Initiating activities of pyrolysis products of L-lysine and soybean globulin assessed in terms of the induction of γ-glutamyl-transpeptidase-positive foci in rat liver. *Gann* 73: 158-159 (1982)

90. Pereira, M.A., Lin, L.-H.C., Lippitt, J.M., and Herren, S.L., Trihalomethanes as initiators and promoters of carcinogenesis. *Environ. Health Perspect.* 46: 151-156 (1982)

91. Tatematsu, M., Hasegawa, R., Imaida, K., Tsuda, H., and Ito, N., Survey of various chemicals for initiating and promoting activities in a short-term *in vivo* system based on generation of hyperplastic liver nodules in rats. *Carcinogenesis* 4: 381-386 (1983)

92. Mazue, G., Remandet, B., Gouy, D., Berthe, J., Roncucci, R., and Williams, G.M., Limited *in vivo* bioassays on some benzodiazepines: Lack of experimental initiating or promoting effect of the benzodiazepine tranquilizers diazepam, chlorazepate, oxazepam and lorazepam. *Arch. Int. Pharmacodyn. Ther.* 257: 59-65 (1982)

93. Imaida, K., Hirose, M., Ogiso, T., Kurata, Y., and Ito, N., Quantitative analysis of initiating and promoting activities of five mycotoxins in liver carcinogenesis in rats. *Cancer Lett.* 16: 137-143 (1982)

94. Uchida, E., and Hirono, I., Effect of phenobarbital on the development of neoplastic lesions in the liver of cycasin-treated rats. *J. Cancer Res. Clin. Oncol.* 100: 231-238 (1981)

95. Schuppler, J., Damme, J., and Schulte-Hermann, R., Assay of some endogenous and synthetic sex steroids for tumor-initiating activity in rat liver using the Solt-Farber system. *Carcinogenesis* 4: 239-241 (1983)

96. Milks, M.M., Wilt, S.R., Ali, I., Pereira, M.A., and Couri, D., Dibromoethane effects on the induction of γ-glutamyl-transpeptidase positive foci in rat liver. *Arch. Toxicol.* 51: 27-35 (1982)

97. Kitagawa, Y., Pitot, H.C., Miller, E.C., and Miller, J.A., Promotion by dietary phenobarbital of hepatocarcinogenesis by 2-methyl-N,N-dimethyl-4-aminoazobenzene in the rat. *Cancer Res.* 39: 112-115 (1979)

98. Kitagawa, T., and Sugano, H., Enhancing effect of phenobarbital on the development of enzyme-altered islands and hepatocellular carcinomas initiated by 3'-methyl-4-(dimethylamino)azobenzene or diethylnitrosamine. *Gann* 69: 679-687 (1978)

99. Imaida, K., Shirai, T., Tatematsu, M., Takano, T., and Ito, N., Dose responses of five hepatocarcinogens for the initiation of rat hepatocarcinogenesis. *Cancer Lett.* 14: 279-283 (1981)

100. Moore, M.A., Hacker, H.-J., Kunz, H.W., and Bannasch, P., Enhancement of NNM-induced carcinogenesis in the rat liver by phenobarbital: A combined morphological and enzyme histochemical approach. *Carcinogenesis* 4: 473-479 (1983)

101. Moore, M.A., Hacker, H.-J., and Bannasch, P., Phenotypic instability in focal and nodular lesions induced in a short-term system in the rat liver. *Carcinogenesis* 5: 595-603 (1983)

102. Laib, R.J., Stockle, G., Bolt, H.M., and Kunz, W., Vinyl chloride and trichloroethylene comparison of alkylating effects of metabolites and induction of preneoplastic enzyme deficiencies in rat liver. *J. Cancer Res. Clin. Oncol.* 94: 139-147 (1979)

103. Bolt, H.M., Laib, R.J., and Stockle, G., Formation of preneoplastic hepatocellular foci by vinyl bromide in newborn rats. *Arch. Toxicol.* 43: 83-84 (1979)

104. Bolt, H.M., Laib, R.J., and Klein, K.-P., Formation of pre-neoplastic hepatocellular foci by vinyl fluoride in newborn rats. *Arch. Toxicol.* 47: 71-73 (1981)

105. Stockle, G., Laib, R.J., Filser, J.G., and Bolt, H.M., Vinylidene fluoride: Metabolism and induction of preneoplastic hepatic foci in relation to vinyl chloride. *Toxicol. Lett.* 3: 337-342 (1979)

106. Laishes, B.A., and Farber, E., Transfer of viable putative preneoplastic hepatocytes to the livers of syngeneic host rats. *J. Natl. Cancer Inst.* 61: 507-512 (1978)

107. Laishes, B.A., and Rolfe, P.B., Quantitative assessment of liver colony formation and hepatocellular carcinoma incidence in rats receiving intravenous injections of isogeneic liver cells isolated during hepatocarcinogenesis. *Cancer Res.* 40: 4133-4143 (1980)

108. Scherer, E., and Hoffman, M., Probable clonal genesis of cellular islands induced in rat liver by diethylnitrosamine. *Eur. J. Cancer* 7: 369-371 (1971)

109. Emmelot, P., and Scherer, E., Multi-hit kinetics of tumor formation, with special reference to experimental liver and human lung carcinogenesis and some general conclusions. *Cancer Res.* 37: 1702-1708 (1977)

110. Rabes, H.M., Bucher, T., Hartmann, A., Linke, I., and Dunnwald, M., Clonal growth of carcinogen-induced enzyme-deficient preneoplastic cell populations in mouse liver. *Cancer Res.* 42: 3220-3227 (1982)

111. Herren, S.L., and Pereira, M.A., Tumor promotion in rat liver. *Environ. Health Perspect.* 50: 123-129 (1983)

112. Kunz, H.W., Tennekes, H.A., Port, R.E., Schwartz, M., Lorke, D., and Schaude, G., Quantitative aspects of chemical carcinogenesis and tumor promotion in liver. *Environ. Health Perspect.* 50: 113-122 (1983)

113. Rabes, H.M., and Szymkowiak, R., Cell kinetics of hepatocytes during the preneoplastic period of diethylnitrosamine-induced liver carcinogenesis. *Cancer Res.* 39: 1298-1304 (1979)

9

Lung Tumors in Strain A Mice as a Bioassay for Carcinogenicity

Gary D. Stoner

Medical College of Ohio
Toledo, Ohio

Michael B. Shimkin

University of California at San Diego
La Jolla, California

INTRODUCTION

The intent of this report is to describe the basic elements of the strain A mouse lung tumor bioassay and to discuss its strengths and weaknesses. In addition, data on the use of the bioassay for carcinogenicity testing are summarized. The reader is referred to our previous review articles[1,2] for more extensive discussions of the biological characteristics of mouse lung tumors and of the use of the mouse lung tumor bioassay for assessing the carcinogenic potential of specific chemicals.

Background

When compared to other inbred strains, there is general agreement that strain A mice develop the highest incidence of spontaneous lung tumors during their lifetime.[3] At eighteen months of age, the majority of strain A mice will have at least one tumor in their lungs. In contrast, lung tumors are seen less frequently in other mouse strains at the same age.[1,3]

The tumors, commonly referred to as adenomas, are pearly-white, discreet round nodules often situated just below the visceral pleura. They are found throughout the lung; *i.e.*, there is no predilection for side or lobe. After fixation, the tumors can be enumerated either by gross examination or, more accurately, with the use of a dissecting microscope. The histological, morphological, bio-chemical, growth and transplantation characteristics of mouse lung tumors were summarized in detail by Shimkin and Stoner in 1975[1] and by Stoner and Shimkin in 1982.[2] The morphology of adenomas on the lung surface and in histological preparations is illustrated in Figures 1 and 2.

Light and electron microscopic (EM) studies indicate that the majority of lung tumors in strain A mice arise from type 2 cells of the alveolar epithelium.[4-6] However, preliminary EM studies in our laboratory suggest that at least 50% of urethane-induced lung tumors in strain A/J mice arise from Clara cells of the bronchiolar epithelium.[7] Similarly, Kauffman *et al.*[8,9] found that more than 60% of ethylnitrosourea-induced lung tumors in Swiss-Bagg mice were derived from Clara cells. It appears that the cellular origin of lung tumors in strain A mice is an unresolved issue which may require the development of immunological and biochemical markers for cell identification. In this respect, the recent observations of Beer and Malkinson[10] may be useful since they found that glucocorticoid receptors were localized predominately in the nucleus of Clara cell derived tumors but were not seen in the nucleus of type 2 cell derived tumors.

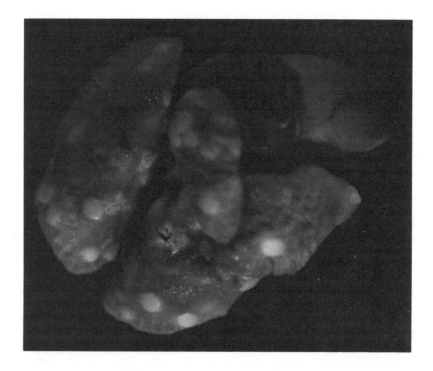

Figure 1: Induced multiple lung tumors in a strain A female mouse 24 weeks after intraperitoneal injection of 1 mg of 3-methylcholanthrene. X 2.5.

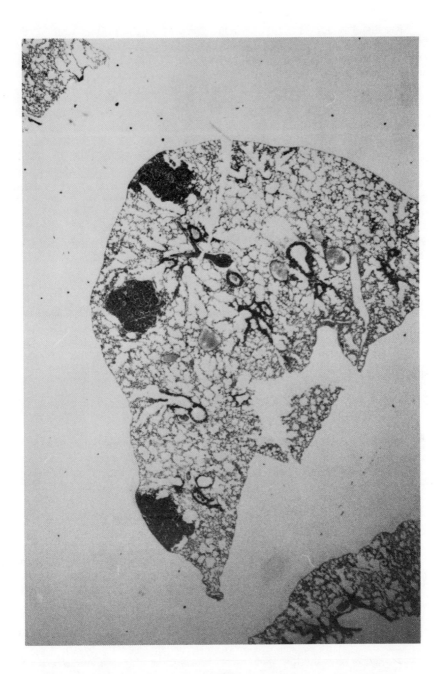

Figure 2: Lung tumors in strain A/J mouse 170 days after intraperitoneal injection of 20 mg of urethane. X 17.

The major determinant for the appearance of lung tumors in strain A mice is the age of the animal. Older animals have a higher frequency of spontaneous lung tumors than do young animals. As shown in Table 1, the age-related incidence of spontaneous lung tumors in strain A mice has not changed appreciably over forty years of experience, indicating that lung tumor susceptibility is a very stable genetic trait.

Table 1: Pulmonary Tumors in Untreated Strain A Mice as a Function of Age

Age (Months)	. Lung Tumor Data: 1940-1942[a] .			. Lung Tumor Data: 1980-1982[b] .		
	Mice (No.)	% Mice with LT	LT/Mouse (Mean No.)	Mice (No.)	% Mice with LT	LT/Mouse (Mean No.)
6	83	7.3	0.06	48	18.8	0.25
7	115	11.3	0.11	24	25.0	0.25
8	127	12.6	0.15	73	42.5	0.49
9	121	24.7	0.28	52	34.6	0.54
10	212	32.1	0.36	94	50.0	0.66
11	106	38.7	0.47	119	47.9	0.60
12	178	40.0	0.58	44	45.5	0.50
13	104	48.0	0.63	24	54.2	0.75
14	132	42.5	0.57	31	64.5	0.94
15	192	67.1	1.06	46	69.6	1.13
16	43	67.5	1.09	73	35.6	1.11
17	50	62.0	1.06	37	70.3	1.35
18	136	77.1	1.43	36	75.0	1.58

[a]Data from Shimkin and Stoner[1]
[b]Unpublished data, Stoner *et al.*
LT = lung tumors

The first description of the induction of lung tumors in mice by carcinogenic agents was that of Murphy and Sturm in 1925.[11] They found an increased incidence of lung tumors following the cutaneous painting of coal tar. Shimkin,[12] and Andervont and Shimkin[13] first used lung tumors induced in strain A mice as a quantitative bioassay for tumorigenic activity of chemicals. They reported that the intravenous administration of 3-methylcholanthrene and other polycyclic hydrocarbons to strain A mice led to a significant increase in the frequency of lung tumors, and the increased frequency was directly related to the dose of carcinogen. Since these reports, numerous chemicals including nitrogen and aniline mustards,[14,15] aziridines,[14,16] carbamates,[16,17] food additives,[18] silylating agents,[19] nitrosamines and nitrosoureas,[20-23] chemotherapeutic drugs,[18] metals,[24] organohalides,[25-27] nucleotide base analogs,[25] aminofluorenes,[1] sulfonic acid derivatives of 1- and 2-naphthylamines,[28] alkylating derivatives of polycyclic aromatic hydrocarbons,[29] aflatoxin B_1,[30] acrylamide,[31] quercetin,[32] vinyl chloride,[33] and nitrotoluenes,[34-36] have been tested for carcinogenic activity by the strain A mouse-lung-tumor-induction technique. In addition, 60 compounds were recently examined for their ability to induce lung tumors in strain A mice and the results from 54 of these were compared to carcinogenesis data from two-year rodent bioassays.[37]

MATERIALS AND METHODS

As indicated above, the strain A mouse lung tumor bioassay has been applied to the testing of several classes of chemicals for carcinogenic activity. Based upon prior experience, a suggested protocol for the assay is as follows:

Animals

The quality of the data developed in the strain A mouse lung tumor bioassay depends, in large part, upon the health status of the animals under study. It is important to use healthy animals previously shown by routine histopathology and serology to be free of pneumonia or other diseases. In reality, however, the majority of strain A mouse colonies are seropositive for one or more of the endogenous mouse viruses, and it is not always possible to eliminate these infections from the colony. Attempts should be made to determine the types of viral infections in the colony since infections with endogenous murine viruses such as Reo-3,[38] Sendai,[39] lactate dehydrogenase virus[40] and Moloney sarcoma virus[41] have been shown to influence the chemical induction of lung adenomas in strain A mice.

To monitor the health status of the mouse colony, we recommend that a random sampling of 0.5% of the animals be harvested every six months and examined as follows:

(1) Complete gross necropsy, tabulating gross lesions and general condition and body weight of each animal.

(2) Histopathological evaluation of formalin-fixed tissues involving all major organs (approximately ten tissues per mouse; one slide per tissue) including tabulation of any lesions that may appear.

(3) Aerobic and anaerobic culture of lung and intestine taken aseptically at necropsy and examination of the tissue for the presence of lung pathogens such as *Streptococcus* and *Staphylococcus* and enteric pathogens such as *Pasteurella* and *Salmonella*.

(4) Fecal examination (both direct smears and fecal flotations) for enteric parasites.

(5) Serological screens for murine viruses such as pneumonitis, Sendai, hepatitis, Reo-3, lymphocytic choriomeningitis, and other endogenous viruses.

For the bioassays, male and female strain A mice, six to eight weeks-old and weighing an average of 18 to 20 grams are randomly distributed among experimental and control groups. The animals are housed in groups of four in plastic boxes on a bedding of ground corn cobs. Cedar wood shavings should not be used as bedding since they contain a terpene compound that induces drug metabolizing enzymes.[42] Commercially available certified diet and water are available *ad libitum*. Hygienic conditions are maintained by twice-weekly changes of the animal cages and water bottles, and cages are sterilized routinely. All chemicals are stored and prepared for injection in a separate room at a distance from the animal quarters.

Chemicals

All chemicals are stored at either 4°C or –20°C (depending upon their stability) in the dark. The chemicals are tested for solubility in deionized doubly-distilled water or in tricaprylin (glycerol trioctanoate). Since some commercial lots of tricaprylin contain toxic aldehydes, it is recommended that the tricaprylin be redistilled. Compounds insoluble in water are injected in tricaprylin. A third vehicle, dimethylsulfoxide (DMSO), is employed for compounds that are insoluble in either water or tricaprylin. The positive carcinogen, urethane, is stored at –20°C in the dark.

All chemicals are weighed out in a chemical fume hood under yellow fluorescent lights. Amber colored bottles stoppered with silicon rubber stoppers are used to protect the chemicals from fluorescent light during the injections. Depending upon their stability, the chemical solutions are either prepared each day before the injections or once per week.

Preliminary Toxicology

For each chemical under test, a maximum tolerated dose (MTD) is determined. Serial 2-fold dilutions (*i.e.*, 100%, 50%, 25%, 12.5%, 6.25%, 3.12%, 1.56%, etc.) of the chemical are injected intraperitoneally (i.p.) into groups of five mice. The MTD for each test chemical is the maximum single dose that all five mice tolerate (survive) for a period of two weeks after receiving six i.p. injections (three injections/week). A holding period of at least two months is recommended for compounds that are potent inhibitors of the immune system and are likely to produce delayed toxicity.

Bioassays

Using the preliminary toxicology as a guide, experimental groups are started for each chemical. Three dose levels are used; the MTD; and 1:2 and 1:5 dilutions of the MTD. There are 30 mice per dose level; 15 males and 15 females. For highly toxic compounds, 50 mice should be used per dose level to insure adequate survival at the termination of the bioassay. The animals are weighed every two weeks during the injections and at monthly intervals thereafter. Each chemical is injected i.p. three times weekly for a total of 24 injections. Fewer injections of the more toxic compounds are administered when in the course of the injection period it becomes apparent that the animals will not tolerate the full 24 injection regimen. With carcinogens such as urethane, a single injection of 2 to 5 mg is sufficient to elicit a significant increase in lung tumors.

Two baseline control groups are maintained in parallel with each series of five chemicals under test. One control group consists of untreated mice (30 animals; 15 males and 15 females) killed along with the treated animals to determine the incidence of spontaneous lung tumors. The other controls (30 animals per group; 15 males and 15 females) receive injections of either water or tricaprylin (vehicle controls).

Positive control groups consist of animals given a single i.p. injection of urethane at two dose levels (ten mg or 20 mg per mouse). Five male and five female mice are used per dose level. Positive controls are used to determine whether the tumor response to urethane is comparable to that observed in previous studies with strain A mice.

In summary, the number of mice used for each series of five chemicals under test is as follows:

Group	No. of Mice
1. Five test chemicals (three doses per chemical; 30 animals per dose)	450
2. Untreated control	30
3. Vehicle control	30
4. Positive control (urethane; two dose levels; ten animals per dose)	20
	530

The bioassays are terminated 16 weeks after the last injection (24-week test). Treated and control animals are killed by cervical dislocation and their lungs removed and fixed in Tellyesniczky's fluid (70% alcohol, 20 parts; formaldehyde, two parts; acetic acid, one part). After fixation for 24 hours, the tumors appear as pearly white nodules that can easily be observed on the surface of the lung. The tumors on each lobe of the lung are counted and recorded while examining the lungs with a dissecting microscope. A few tumors per test chemical and for the controls are taken for histopathological examination to confirm the morphological appearance of adenoma. The lungs are also examined grossly and microscopically for the presence of other abnormalities such as inflammatory reactions and adenomatosis.

Data Evaluation

A compound is considered to be a carcinogen in strain A mice if it induces a significant increase in the lung tumor incidence (*i.e.*, the average number of lung tumors per mouse) when compared to that in the appropriate vehicle control. Lung tumor data in treated and control animals are compared by analysis of variance and Student's *t*-test using the 5% level of significance. Ideally, the tumor response should be dose-related, and positive results in an initial bioassay should be confirmed in a repeat test.

Some investigators have also compared the lung tumor frequency (*i.e.*, the percentage of mice that develop lung tumors) in chemically-treated mice versus the vehicle controls.[32,33] In our experience, this comparison is unnecessary since it usually leads to the same conclusion as that obtained from the analysis of tumor incidence data.

The carcinogenic potency of chemicals tested in the lung tumor bioassay can be compared by determining the dose of each chemical required to produce a minimum carcinogenic response (usually an average number of 0.8 to one adenoma per mouse when compared to vehicle controls). This can be done by plotting the average number of lung tumors versus the log of the molar dose of the chemical. The "carcinogenic index" for each chemical will be the dose at which the response line transects the 0.8 to one tumor per mouse level.[43] This method is applicable only to those chemicals that induce lung tumors in a dose-related manner.

RESULTS

Pulmonary Tumors in Control Mice

Table 2 illustrates representative data obtained in our laboratory during the last two years on the incidence of lung tumors in A/J mice that either received 24 thrice-weekly injections of the two vehicles, water or tricaprylin, or a single injection of urethane (ten mg or 20 mg/mouse), or they were untreated.

Table 2: Pulmonary Tumors in Untreated, Vehicle-Treated and Urethane-Treated Strain A Mice[a]

Treatment	Duration of Experiment (wk)	No. of i.p. Injections	Sex	No. of Animals	Mice with Lung Tumors (%)	No. of Tumors/Mouse
Untreated	24	0	M	121	37	0.40±0.05[b]
			F	134	27	0.33±0.06
Vehicle						
Water	24	24	M	60	22	0.23±0.06
			F	30	30	0.36±0.11
Tricaprylin	24	24	M	160	25	0.31±0.05
			F	85	26	0.33±0.09
Urethane						
10 mg	24	1	M	22	100	13.0±1.55
			F	29	100	11.6±1.18
20 mg	24	1	M	28	100	28.4±1.67
			F	25	100	29.7±1.71

[a]A/J mice were either untreated or received 0.1 ml i.p. injections of water, tricaprylin, or the positive carcinogen, urethane. The animals were killed after a total of 24 weeks and their surface tumors were counted. Data are expressed as mean number of tumors per mouse.
[b]Mean ± S.E.

The incidence of "spontaneous" lung tumors in untreated mice (mean of approximately 0.36 tumor per mouse) usually varies from 0.2 tumor to 0.4 tumor per mouse. Only rarely does the tumor incidence in untreated animals exceed 0.4 tumor per lung. Data from the vehicle controls indicate that the occurrence of lung tumors was not significantly affected by the injections. The tumor response to the positive carcinogen, urethane, was dose related with the production of approximately one tumor to 1.4 tumor per milligram. This response to urethane is somewhat higher than was reported previously; *i.e.*, one tumor per milligram. The lung tumor response to urethane was nearly identical in at least three substrains of strain A; *i.e.*, A/Heston, A/Strong and A/J.[18]

Pulmonary Tumors in Chemically-Treated Mice

Table 3 summarizes data on the majority of chemicals that have been tested for tumorigenic activity by the lung tumor response in strain A mice.

Table 3: Chemicals Tested for Carcinogenic Activity by the Mouse Lung Adenoma Bioassay[37]

Compound	Route of Exposure[a]	Dose (mmol/kg)	Mean No. Lung Tumors per Mouse	Tu[b]	References
Polycyclic Hydrocarbons					
3-Methylcholanthrene	i.p.	0.186	139.0	+	36
	p.o.	0.186	12.0	+	36
	i.v.	0.015	11.0	+	12,13
Benzo(a)pyrene	i.p.	0.400	13.0	+	36
	p.o.	0.400	3.7	+	36
	i.v.	0.400	1.0	+	12,13
Dibenz(a,h)anthracene	i.v.	0.036	31.0	+	12,13
7,12-Dimethylbenz(a)anthracene	i.v.	0.010	1.5	+	29
Benz(a)anthracene	i.v.	0.044	0.2	-	12,13
9-Chloromethylanthracene	i.v.	0.005	0.4	-	29
9-Bromomethylanthracene	i.v.	0.005	1.1	+	29
10-Chloromethyl-9-methylanthracene	i.v.	0.015	3.9	+	29
10-Chloromethyl-9-chloroanthracene	i.v.	0.010	1.9	+	29
9,10-Bis(chloromethyl)anthracene	i.v.	0.004	1.5	+	29
7-Chloromethyl-12-methylbenz(a)-anthracene	i.v.	0.006	9.8	+	29
7-Bromomethyl-12-methylbenz(a)-anthracene	i.v.	0.010	7.8	+	29
7-Chloromethylbenz(a)anthracene	i.v.	0.005	5.7	+	29
7-Bromomethylbenz(a)anthracene	i.v.	0.005	1.2	+	29
7H-Dibenzo(c,g)carbazole	i.v.	0.038	5.7	+	12,13
Dibenz(a,j)aceanthrylene	i.v.	0.036	2.7	+	12,13
Dibenz(a,h)acridine	i.v.	0.036	2.2	+	12,13
8-Methylbenzo(c)phenanthrene	i.v.	0.042	0.7	-	12,13
7-Methylbenzo(a)pyrene	i.v.	0.038	0.6	-	12,13
5-Methoxy-7-propylbenz(a)anthracene	i.v.	0.033	0.1	-	12,13
Carbamates					
Ethyl (urethane)	i.p.	26.93	24.5	+	16

(continued)

Table 3: (continued)

Compound	Route of Exposure[a]	Dose (mmol/kg)	Mean No. Lung Tumors per Mouse	Tub	References
N-Hydroxyethyl	i.p.	22.83	18.6	+	16
Vinyl	i.p.	4.00	4.0	+	17
Allyl	i.p.	0.15	11.3	+	17
N-Cyanoacetylethyl	i.p.	2.75	1.3	+	16
N-Acetylethyl	i.p.	15.37	4.0	+	16
Isopropyl	i.p.	18.30	3.2	+	16
n-Propyl	i.p.	23.27	1.5	+	16
N-Methylnaphthyl	i.p.	24.21	0.8	−	16
N,N-Dimethylolmethoxyethyl	i.p.	1.19	0.7	−	16
Diethyl bicarbamate	i.p.	1.34	0.4	−	16
sec-Butyl	i.p.	1.36	0.3	−	16
n-Hexyl	i.p.	10.24	0.3	−	16
N-Phenylisopropyl	i.p.	18.01	0.3	−	16
Benzyl	i.p.	13.39	0.1	−	16
Phenyl	i.p.	15.87	0.2	−	16
β-Chloroethyl	i.p.	17.50	0.5	−	16
β-Hydroxypropyl	i.p.	19.42	0.4	−	16
n-Butyl	i.p.	20.15	0.2	−	16
Methallyl	i.p.	20.48	0.3	−	16
β-Hydroxyethyl	i.p.	20.85	0.3	−	16
Methyl	i.p.	22.83	0.5	−	16
Aziridines	i.p.	31.95	0.1	−	16
3,4-Dichlorophenyl-N-carbamoyl	i.p.	0.10	1.3	+	16
m-Chlorophenyl-N-carbamoyl	i.p.	1.22	5.0	+	16
Phenyl-N-carbamoyl	i.p.	1.48	2.0	+	16
Cyclohexyl-N-carbamoyl	i.p.	1.43	1.0	+	16
p-Tolyl-N-carbamoyl	i.p.	1.36	0.8	−	16
p-Methoxyphenyl-N-carbamoyl	i.p.	1.25	0.7	−	16
o-Ethoxyphenyl-N-carbamoyl	i.p.	1.17	0.5	−	16

(continued)

Table 3: (continued)

Compound	Route of Exposure[a]	Dose (mmol/kg)	Mean No. Lung Tumors per Mouse	Tu[b]	References
p-Fluorophenyl-N-carbamoyl Bis(1-aziridinyl)morpholino-phosphine sulfide (OPSPA)	i.p.	1.33	0.5	–	16
Tris(1-aziridinyl)phosphine sulfide (Thio-TEPA)	i.p.	0.52	2.0	+	16
2,5-Bis(1-aziridinyl)-3,6-bis(2-meth-oxyethoxy)-*p*-benzoquinone (AZQ)	i.p.	0.11	1.7	+	16
	i.p.	0.09	2.9	+	16
	i.p.	0.15	3.8	+	44
N-Nitroso Compounds					
N-Nitrosodimethylamine	i.p.	0.14	17.47	+	23
	p.o.	0.14	11.36	+	
N-Nitrosodiethylamine	i.p.	1.96	16.0	+	36
	p.o.	1.96	11.0	+	
N-Nitrosodibutylamine	i.p.	7.59	9.8	+	23
	p.o.	7.59	3.2	+	
N-Nitrosonornicotine	i.p.	6.00	1.2	+	21,22
3'-Hydroxy-N-nitrosonornicotine	i.p.	6.00	0.9	+	22
4'-Hydroxy-N-nitrosonornicotine	i.p.	6.00	1.6	+	22
N-Nitrosonornicotine-1-N-oxide	i.p.	6.00	0.8	±	22
4-(Methylnitrosamino)-1-(3-pyridyl)-1-butanone	i.p.	5.50	37.6	+	22
4-(Methylnitrosamino)-1-(3-pyridyl)-butan-1-ol	i.p.	5.50	23.6	+	21,22
4-(Methylnitrosamino)-1-(3-pyridyl)-N-oxide)-1-butanone	i.p.	5.50	3.6	+	21,22
N-Nitrosomethylurea	i.p.	2.91	79.9	+	23
	p.o.	2.91	88.8	+	
N-Nitrosoethylurea	i.p.	0.85	20.1	+	36
	p.o.	0.85	17.4	+	
Nitrogen Mustards					
Uracil mustard	i.p.	0.04	20.3	+	14,18

(continued)

Table 3: (continued)

Compound	Route of Exposure[a]	Dose (mmol/kg)	Mean No. Lung Tumors per Mouse	Tub	References
Nitrogen mustard	i.p.	0.02	2.8	+	14
Melphalan	i.p.	0.06	4.0	+	14
Chloroquine mustard	i.p.	0.04	1.4	+	14
Quinacrine ethyl mustard	i.p.	0.06	1.3	+	14
Benzimidazole mustard	i.p.	0.36	3.6	+	14
Mannitol mustard	i.p.	0.38	2.4	+	14
Chlorambucil mustard	i.p.	0.49	5.1	+	14
Hydroquinone mustard	i.p.	0.43	1.4	+	14
Aniline mustard	i.p.	0.86	5.5	+	14
Cyclophosphamide	i.p.	0.52	1.3	+	14
Naphthylamine mustard	i.p.	4.48	2.0	+	14
Mannitol myleran	i.p.	14.20	3.2	+	14
5-Chloroquine mustard pamoate	i.p.	0.70	0.8	−	14
Quinacrine propyl mustard	i.p.	0.003	0.4	−	14
Quinacrine mustard	i.p.	0.02	0.5	−	14
5-Chloroquine mustard	i.p.	0.02	0.4	−	14
Benzalpurine mustard	i.p.	0.04	0.5	−	14
Chloroquine mustard pamoate	i.p.	0.09	0.7	−	14
Organohalides					
Iodides					
n-Propyl iodide	i.p.	17.6	0.70	±	25
n-Butyl iodide	i.p.	13.1	0.63	±	25
sec-Butyl iodide	i.p.	32.6	0.63	±	25
Isopropyl iodide	i.p.	35.2	0.58	±	25
Methyl iodide	i.p.	0.3	0.55	±	25
Ethyl iodide	i.p.	38.4	0.15	−	25
tert-Butyl iodide	i.p.	2.7	0.42	−	25
Bromides					
Bromoform (tribromomethane)	i.p.	4.3	1.13	+	27

(continued)

Table 3: (continued)

Compound	Route of Exposure[a]	Dose (mmol/kg)	Mean No. Lung Tumors per Mouse	Tub	References
Bromodichloromethane	i.p.	14.6	0.85	–	27
4-Bromodiphenyl ether	i.p.	14.5	0.31	–	27
sec-Butyl bromide	i.p.	43.7	1.15	+	25
2-Bromoethanol	i.p.	1.2	0.79	+	26
tert-Butyl bromide	i.p.	43.7	0.78	+	25
Isobutyl bromide	i.p.	43.7	0.75	+	25
3-Bromopropionic acid	i.p.	3.8	0.53	±	26
1,2-Dibromoethane	i.p.	4.5	1.06	+	23
	p.o.	4.5	0.47	–	
3-Bromopropylamine·HBr	i.p.	5.3	0.56	±	26
Ethyl bromide	i.p.	55.0	0.35	–	25
n-Butyl bromide	i.p.	1.2	0.14	–	25
Ethyl bromoacetate	i.p.	0.4	0.17	–	26
Butyryl bromide	i.p.	1.6	0.45	–	26
Bromomethyl acetate	i.p.	0.4	0.14	–	26
Methyl-2-bromopropionate	i.p.	3.6	0.31	–	26
Methyl bromoacetate	i.p.	0.1	0.29	–	26
3-Bromo-2-butanone	i.p.	0.5	0.40	–	26
Benzoyl bromide	i.p.	10.9	0.27	–	26
Epibromohydrin	i.p.	1.7	0.50	–	26
2-Bromopropionic acid	i.p.	1.9	0.30	–	26
1-Bromo-2-propanol	i.p.	0.8	0.17	–	26
3-Bromo-1-propanol	i.p.	43.0	0.29	–	26
2-Bromoethyl ethyl ether	i.p.	7.7	0.13	–	26
2-Bromobutyric acid	i.p.	1.4	0.53	–	26
2-Bromoethyl acetate	i.p.	2.0	0.46	–	26
Methyl-3-bromopropionate	i.p.	36.0	0.50	–	26
Chlorides					
Chloroform	i.p.	16.2	0.36	–	27
1,2-Dichloroethane	i.p.	24.2	0.75	–	27
1,1,2,2-Tetrachloroethylene	i.p.	57.8	0.50	–	27

(continued)

Table 3: (continued)

Compound	Route of Exposure[a]	Dose (mmol/kg)	Mean No. Lung Tumors per Mouse	Tu[b]	References
Hexachloro-1,3-butadiene	i.p.	0.2	0.68	−	27
2-Chloroethyl ether	i.p.	3.4	0.15	−	27
1-Chlorooctane	i.p.	26.8	0.31	−	27
Dichloromethane	i.p.	32.0	0.94	−	27
Epichlorohydrin	i.p.	26.1	0.67	−	23
	p.o.	26.1	0.41	−	
1,1,2,2-Tetrachloroethane	i.p.	21.4	0.50	−	27
1,1,3,3-Tetrachloroacetone	i.p.	0.6	0.56	−	27
Hexachlorocyclohexane	i.p.	6.1	0.20	−	27
Hexachlorobenzene	i.p.	3.4	0.75	−	27
2-Chloro-N,N-dimethylamine·HCl	i.p.	12.5	1.30	+	26
sec-Butyl chloride	i.p.	35.0	1.20	+	25
tert-Butyl chloride	i.p.	65.0	1.00	+	25
3-Chlorobutyric acid	i.p.	9.6	0.89	+	26
3-Chloropropionic acid	i.p.	6.7	0.90	+	26
4-Chloro-1-butanol	i.p.	33.6	0.70	+	26
Ethyl chloroacetate	i.p.	24.0	0.61	±	26
n-Butyl chloride	i.p.	65.0	0.31	−	25
Benzyl chloride	i.p.	11.8	0.5	−	25
1-Chloromethylnaphthalene	i.p.	1.4	0.47	−	25
1-Chloro-2-propanol	i.p.	50.8	0.56	−	26
2-Chloroethyl acetate	i.p.	12.0	0.63	−	26
Isobutyryl chloride	i.p.	4.1	0.46	−	26
Methyl chloroacetate	i.p.	8.6	0.15	−	26
2,4,6-Trichlorophenol	i.p.	6.1	0.23	−	23
	p.o.	6.1	0.18	−	
Metal salts					
Lead(II) subacetate	i.p.	0.19	1.47	+	24
Nickelous(II) acetate	i.p.	1.45	1.26	+	24
Manganous sulfate	i.p.	3.91	1.20	+	24

(continued)

Table 3: (continued)

Compound	Route of Exposure[a]	Dose (mmol/kg)	Mean No. Lung Tumors per Mouse	Tub	References
Molybdenum(III) trioxide	i.p.	32.99	1.13	+	24
Iron(II) 2,4-pentanedione	i.p.	2.95	0.60	-	24
Vanadium (III) 2,4-pentanedione	i.p.	0.34	0.79	-	24
Zinc(II) acetate	i.p.	1.64	0.78	-	24
Cupric(III) acetate	i.p.	0.99	0.56	-	24
Cobalt(III) acetate	i.p.	2.01	0.79	-	24
Chromium(III) sulfate	i.p.	6.12	0.63	-	24
Calcium(II) acetate	i.p.	7.59	0.58	-	24
Stannous chloride	i.p.	6.33	0.50	-	24
Cadmium(II) acetate	i.p.	0.05	0.40	-	24
Food additives					
Acetoin	i.p.	681.82	0.44	-	18
Aldehyde C-10	i.p.	13.78	0.38	-	18
Aldehyde C-16	i.p.	10.43	0.38	-	18
n-Amyl alcohol	i.p.	68.18	0.13	-	18
Anethole	i.p.	81.08	0.86	-	18
Butylated hydroxyanisole	i.p.	33.33	0.33	-	18
Butylated hydroxytoluene	i.p.	27.27	0.31	-	18
d-Camphor	i.p.	118.42	0.21	-	18
d-Carvone	i.p.	40.00	0.44	-	18
l-Carvone	i.p.	40.00	0.08	-	18
Cineole	i.p.	77.92	0.27	-	18
Cinnamyl alcohol	i.p.	52.24	0.70	-	18
Cinnamyl aldehyde	i.p.	30.30	0.89	-	18
Cinnamyl anthranilate	i.p.	47.43	2.69	+	18
Diacetyl	i.p.	97.67	0.89	-	18
1-Dodecanol	i.p.	64.52	0.23	-	18
3-Ethoxy-4-hydroxybenzaldehyde	i.p.	10.84	0.1	-	18
Ethyl acetate	i.p.	204.54	0.33	-	18
Ethyl formate	i.p.	162.16	0.36	-	18

(continued)

Table 3: (continued)

Compound	Route of Exposure[a]	Dose (mmol/kg)	Mean No. Lung Tumors per Mouse	Tub	References
α-Irone	i.p.	46.61	0.33	−	18
d-Limonene	i.p.	176.47	0.27	−	18
Linalool	i.p.	19.48	0.27	−	18
Linalyl acetate	i.p.	122.45	0.19	−	18
Menthol	i.p.	12.82	0.62	−	18
Menthone	i.p.	30.84	0.82	−	18
Methyl anthranilate	i.p.	74.17	0.32	−	18
Methyl salicylate	i.p.	78.95	0.39	−	18
Monosodium glutamate	i.p.	213.02	0.50	−	18
Nerolin	i.p.	69.77	0.42	−	18
Octyl alcohol	i.p.	92.31	0.36	−	18
Phenylethyl acetate	i.p.	36.59	0.08	−	18
Piperidine	i.p.	11.18	0.29	−	18
Propyl gallate	i.p.	11.32	0.25	−	18
Saccharin	i.p.	426.23	0.67	−	18
Safrole	i.p.	27.78	0.31	−	18
Santoquin	i.p.	55.30	0.27	−	18
α-Terpineol	i.p.	62.34	0.17	−	18
β-Terpineol	i.p.	62.34	0.35	−	18
Thymol	i.p.	40.0	0.40	−	18
Tributyrin	i.p.	198.68	0.91	−	18
Vanillin	i.p.	118.42	0.27	−	18
Chemotherapeutic drugs					
Estradiol mustard	i.p.	2.01	4.95	+	18
Phenesterin	i.p.	18.61	3.90	+	18
Mannitol myleran	i.p.	0.38	2.40	+	14
Isophosphamide	i.p.	5.00	1.83	+	18
β-Deoxythioguanosine	i.p.	0.58	1.00	+	18
Imidazole mustard	i.p.	5.34	1.00	+	18
1-Propanol-3,3'-iminodimethane-sulfonate	i.p.	3.37	1.00	+	18

(continued)

Table 3: (continued)

Compound	Route of Exposure[a]	Dose (mmol/kg)	Mean No. Lung Tumors per Mouse	Tub	References
Dapsone	i.p.	5.29	0.87	+	18
Dibenzyline	i.p.	0.29	0.79	±	18
Pyrimethamine	i.p.	0.50	0.78	±	18
5-Azacytidine	i.p.	0.37	0.73	±	18
Phenformin	i.p.	7.32	0.53	−	18
Phenazopyridine	i.p.	6.20	0.50	−	18
ICRF-159	i.p.	9.33	0.53	−	18
Emetine	i.p.	0.38	0.50	−	18
Tolbutamide	i.p.	177.58	0.45	−	18
Adriamycin	i.p.	0.07	0.40	−	18
Acronycine	i.p.	8.10	0.300	−	18
Myleran	i.p.	24.39	0.300	−	18
Silylating agents					
Trimethylchlorosilane	i.p.	9.17	1.79	+	19
N-Acetylimidazole	i.p.	0.91	1.75	+	19
N-(Trimethylsilyl)imidazole	i.p.	7.14	1.50	+	19
1-Ethyl-3-*p*-tolyltriazene	i.p.	0.61	1.50	+	19
N,O-Bis-(trimethylsilyl)-acetamide	i.p.	4.93	1.15	+	19
1,3-Bis(chloromethyl)-1,1,3,3-tetra-methyldisilazane	i.p.	0.87	1.00	+	19
Hexamethyldisilazane	i.p.	6.25	0.60	−	19
tert-Butyldimethylchlorosilane	i.p.	6.62	0.59	−	19
N-Trimethylsilylacetamide	i.p.	0.76	0.53	−	19
N-Methyl-N-trimethylsilyltrifluoro-acetamide	i.p.	1.00	0.45	−	19
Nitrotoluenes and derivatives					
2,3-Dinitrotoluene	i.p.	16.5	0.22	−	23
2,4-Dinitrotoluene	i.p.	16.5	0.28	−	34
	p.o.	32.9	0.27	−	36

(continued)

Table 3: (continued)

Compound	Route of Exposure[a]	Dose (mmol/kg)	Mean No. Lung Tumors per Mouse	Tu[b]	References
2,5-Dinitrotoluene	i.p.	16.5	0.50	−	23
2,6-Dinitrotoluene	i.p.	16.5	0.40	−	35
	p.o.	32.9	0.53	−	35,36
3,4-Dinitrotoluene	i.p.	17.8	0.22	−	23
3,5-Dinitrotoluene	i.p.	12.4	0.64	−	23
2,4-Diaminotoluene	i.p.	6.15	0.28	−	23
	p.o.	6.15	0.36	−	23
2,6-Diaminotoluene	i.p.	3.10	0.78	+	23
	p.o.	3.10	0.59	−	23
Naphthylamines and derivatives					
1-Naphthylamine	i.p.	8.39	0.20	−	28
1-Naphthylamine-4-sulfonic acid	i.p.	97.00	0.20	−	28
1-Naphthylamine-5-sulfonic acid	i.p.	99.58	0.25	−	28
1-Naphthylamine-7-sulfonic acid	i.p.	31.12	0.46	−	28
1-Naphthylamine-8-sulfonic acid	i.p.	99.58	0.53	−	28
2-Naphthylamine	i.p.	41.96	1.38	+	28
2-Naphthylamine-5-sulfonic acid	i.p.	269.00	0.41	−	28
2-Naphthylamine-8-sulfonic acid	i.p.	80.72	0.88	+	28
2-Naphthylamine-6,8-disulfonic acid	i.p.	24.75	0.70	+	28
Miscellaneous chemicals					
Acrylamide	i.p.	10.14	2.2	+	31
2-Acetylaminofluorene	i.p.	27.00	2.3	+	1
N-Hydroxy-2-acetylaminofluorene	i.p.	25.00	1.9	+	1

(continued)

Table 3: (continued)

Compound	Route of Exposure[a]	Dose (mmol/kg)	Mean No. Lung Tumors per Mouse	Tu[b]	References
Aflatoxin B$_1$	i.p.	0.48	24.5	+	30,23
	p.o.	0.48	13.1	+	23
2-Amino-5-azotoluene	i.p.	18.70	4.1	+	1
Azaserine	i.p.	0.87	14.7	+	23
	p.o.	0.87	0.6	−	
Azobenzene	i.p.	1.65	0.3	−	23
	p.o.	1.65	0.4	−	
Bis(chloromethyl) ether	inhal.	25.87	2.9	+	89
Bromodeoxyuridine	i.p.	0.16	0.4	−	25
Diepoxybutane	i.p.	2.23	1.5	+	14
Diepoxypiperazine	i.p.	0.97	0.8	−	14
Diglycidyltriethylene glycol	i.p.	27.50	1.2	+	14
1,2-Dimethylhydrazine	i.p.	1.80	7.4	+	23
	p.o.	1.80	26.6	+	
1,4-Dioxane	i.p.	136.30	0.5	−	23
	p.o.	272.70	0.4	−	
Epoxypropidine	i.p.	0.20	0.6	−	14
Fluorodeoxyuridine	i.p.	0.20	0.3	−	25
N-[4-(5-Nitro-2-furyl)-2-thiazolyl]-formamide (FANFT)	i.p.	3.10	0.3	−	23
	p.o.	3.10	0.2	−	
Iododeoxyuridine	i.p.	0.14	0.4	−	25
Methylmethane sulfonate	i.p.	2.70	0.5	−	23
	p.o.	2.70	0.5	−	
1-Nitropyrene	i.p.	6.40	1.25	+	23
β-Propiolactone	i.p.	8.33	0.4	−	23
	p.o.	8.33	0.5	−	

[a] i.v. = intravenously; i.p. = intraperitoneally; p.o. = orally; inhal. = inhalation
[b] Tu = Tumorigenicity

As indicated, the compounds were administered by different routes, although the i.p. route was the most common. For brevity, only the data from the dose that gave the highest tumor response are given. Not included in the table are several of the 60 compounds recently evaluated for carcinogenic activity in strain A mice for comparison with their tumorigenic potential in two-year carcinogenesis bioassays.[37]

Polycyclic hydrocarbons. Fifteen of 20 polycyclic hydrocarbons (PAH) produced a significant increase in the lung tumor response relative to controls. On a molar dose basis, 7-chloromethyl-12-methylbenz(a)anthracene and 7-chloromethylbenz(a)anthracene were the most potent PAH in the lung tumor assay. Both compounds were more active than their brominated analogs. 3-Methylcholanthrene and dibenzo(a,h)anthracene had approximately equal activity for lung tumor production. Benzo(a)pyrene, 7,12-dimethylbenz(a)anthracene, 9-bromomethylanthracene, 10-chloromethyl-9-methylanthracene, 10-chloromethyl-9-chloroanthracene, 9,10-bis(chloromethyl)anthracene, 7*H*-dibenzo(c,g)carbazole, dibenz(a,j)aceanthrylene and dibenz(a,h)acridine were less active. A marginal response was produced by 8-methylbenzo(c)phenanthrene and 7-methylbenzo(a)pyrene. Benz(a)anthracene, 9-chloromethylanthracene, and 5-methoxy-7-propylbenz(a)anthracene were negative for lung tumor induction. On a molar dose basis, 3-methylcholanthrene was approximately ten times more active when administered either i.p. or intravenously (i.v.) than when given orally (p.o.). Similarly, benzo(a)pyrene was significantly more active following either i.p. or i.v. administration than when given p.o.

Carbamates. Twenty-two carbamates were tested for lung tumor induction, and seven compounds were active.[16,17] On a molar dose basis, vinyl carbamate was the most active carbamate in the assay. Ethyl carbamate and N-hydroxyethylcarbamate were of approximately equal activity. The methyl ester was entirely negative, indicating that minor changes in chemical structure (such as the removal of a methyl group from ethyl carbamate) can have a marked influence on carcinogenicity. A marginal response was obtained with *n*-propyl- and N-methylnaphthylcarbamate. In general, the PAH are more potent as inducers of lung tumors than the carbamates.

Aziridines. Seven of the 11 aziridine compounds were positive for lung tumor production in strain A mice.[16] These include two drugs used in chemotherapy, OPSPA [bis(1-aziridinyl)morpholino-phosphine sulfide] and Thio-TEPA [tris(1-aziridinyl)phosphine sulfide], and one potential antineoplastic drug, AZQ [2,5-bis(1-aziridinyl)-3,6-bis(2-methoxyethoxy)-*p*-benzoquinone]. It is noteworthy that the lung tumor response to the AZQ in 1983[44] was nearly identical to that obtained in 1969.[16] The aziridines include chemicals that are more active than most carbamates, but less active than the polycyclic hydrocarbons.

N-nitroso compounds. Twelve N-nitroso compounds have been examined for their ability to induce lung tumors in strain A mice and all were active.[20-23] On a molar dose basis, N-nitrosodimethylamine was the most active compound of the series, and it was 14 times more potent than N-nitrosodiethylamine. The tobacco-specific nitrosamines, N-nitrosonornicotine (NNN) and 4-(methylnitrosamino)-1-(3-pyridyl)-1-butanone (NNK) and their metabolites were examined for lung tumor induction by Hecht *et al.*[21] and Castonguay *et al.*[22] NNK was approximately 35 times more active than NNN. Similarly, the metabolites of NNK were more potent as inducers of lung tumors than were those of NNN. Metabolic studies using cultured strain A mouse peripheral lung tissues indicated that both NNK and NNN were metabolized by α-carbon hydroxylation. N-Nitrosomethyl-urea and N-nitrosoethylurea were of similar potency for lung tumor induction when administered either i.p. or p.o.

Nitrogen mustards. The nitrogen mustards include several compounds used as chemotherapeutic agents in disseminated neoplasms in man. Uracil mustard was found to be the most active, with nitrogen mustard and melphalan in the same order of activity as the more active polycyclic hydrocarbons.[14]

Organohalide compounds. Data for the organohalide compounds were taken from four studies: Poirier *et al.*,[25] Theiss *et al.*,[26,27] and Stoner *et al.*[23] Some of the chemicals are contaminants in drinking waters in the United States.[27] In the four studies, different mean tumor values were obtained for the vehicle controls. Therefore, some compounds such as methyl iodide and *n*-propyl iodide were marginally active when eliciting responses as low as 0.55 tumors to 0.70 tumors per mouse, and other compounds such as hexachlorobenzene, dichloromethane and bromodichloromethane were negative when producing responses as high as 0.75 tumor to 0.94 tumor per mouse. As discussed by Poirier *et al.*,[25] the re-sults with the organohalides indicated that carcinogenicity was related to the structure of the compound. Usually, chemicals with primary structures did not produce a significant increase in the lung tumor response when compared to controls, whereas those with secondary or tertiary structures were positive. How-ever, there were exceptions; for example, the primary halide, methyl iodide was positive, whereas *tert*-butyl iodide was negative. On a molar dose basis, the most active alkyl halide was methyl iodide. Bromoform (tribromomethane) and 1,2-dibromoethane were equally active for lung tumor induction. It is important to note that 1,2-dibromoethane was carcinogenic by the i.p. route, but not when given p.o.

Seven of the organohalides were carcinogenic in other experimental systems yet were negative for lung tumor production in strain A mice. Chloroform,[45] tetrachloroethylene,[46] 2-chloroethyl ether,[47] and hexachlorocyclohexane[48] are all hepatotoxins that elicit a carcinogenic effect primarily on the liver. Benzyl chloride[49] and ethyl bromoacetate[50] produced sarcomas on subcutaneous injec-tion into animals. Epichlorohydrin produced tumors in the nasal turbinates of rats.[51]

Metals. The i.p. administration of lead (II) subacetate, nickelous (II) ace-tate, manganous sulfate and molybdenum (III) trioxide led to a significant in-crease in the lung tumor response in A mice.[24] The activity of nickelous acetate and lead subacetate might have been expected since these compounds have been shown to produce tumors in other systems. Moreover, nickel is thought to be carcinogenic for the nasal cavity, paranasal sinuses and lung of man.[52] The car-cinogenic activities of manganese or molybdenum are not well documented. However, manganous chloride has been shown to hasten the appearance of lym-phosarcoma in mice.[53] Metals that were negative for lung adenoma production in strain A mice but positive in other experimental systems are cadmium, chro-mium, cobalt, iron and zinc.[54,55]

The effect of metals administered either in the drinking water or in the diet on the lung adenoma response in Swiss mice was investigated by Schroeder and

his associates.[56-59] Chromium, lead, cadmium, nickel, titanium, arsenic, germanium, tin, vanadium, selenium, tellurium, zirconium, antimony, and niobium as
well as fluoride did not increase the frequency of lung tumors during the lifetime
of the animals.

Food additives. Forty-one food additives were tested for lung tumor induction in strain A mice.[18] These compounds were selected from the GRAS
(generally recognized as safe for human consumption) list either randomly or because they contained double bonds, keto groups, several methoxy groups on a
benzene ring, or other structures similar to those of known carcinogens. Cinnamyl anthranilate was the only food additive that produced a significant increase in the lung tumor response relative to tricaprylin controls. The carcinogenicity of cinnamyl anthranilate may have been due to the interaction of both
the cinnamyl and anthranilic acid moieties since cinnamyl alcohol, cinnamyl aldehyde and methyl anthranilate were negative. A publication by Ward *et al.*[60] reported that cinnamyl anthranilate induced liver tumors in mice.

Several possible food constituents found by others to be carcinogenic in
other bioassay systems were negative for lung tumor induction in strain A mice.
Subcutaneous injection of safrole and santoquin into neonatal Swiss mice resulted in liver hepatomas and a slight, but not statistically significant, increase in
pulmonary adenomas.[61] Safrole has also produced hepatocellular carcinomas
when fed to CD1 mice and CD rats; the 1'-hydroxy form is more active and appears to be the proximate carcinogen.[62] Saccharin was also negative for lung
tumor induction in A mice but has been reported to be carcinogenic for mouse
and rat bladder.[63,64] In addition, saccharin exhibited promoting activity for carcinogen-initiated tumors in the rat liver[65] and bladder.[66]

Chemotherapeutic drugs. The chemotherapeutic agents listed in Table 3
were tested for lung tumor production by Shimkin *et al.*[14] and Stoner *et al.*[18]
The carcinogenic responses obtained with several of these agents were not unexpected since they are capable of alkylating DNA. On a molar dose basis, uracil mustard (listed under the nitrogen mustards) was considerably more active
than either imidazole mustard or estradiol mustard. The enhanced activity of
uracil mustard can most logically be attributed to its role as an analog of uracil
and its probable incorporation into RNA.[67]

Shimkin *et al.*[14] reported that mannitol Myleran was carcinogenic by lung
tumor induction in A mice. However, Myleran was negative at a ten-fold higher
dose than that used for mannitol Myleran.[18] Since the activity of mannitol
Myleran is probably due to the Myleran moiety, the negative result for Myleran
was unexpected, and the compound should be re-tested.

Silylating agents. Reactive silylating agents are used extensively in many
laboratories to introduce a trimethylsilyl group into otherwise nonvolatile molecules, thus rendering them volatile. Stoner *et al.*[19] found that six of ten silylating compounds were positive for lung tumor production in strain A mice. Because of their alkylating ability, this was not a surprising result.

It is difficult to assign definitive structure-activity correlations with the
silylating agents. However, compounds in which the trimethylsilyl group was
attached only to an amide or amino nitrogen were generally inactive (hexa-
methyldisilazane, N-methyl-N-trimethylsilyltrifluoroacetamide, N-trimethylsilyl-

acetamide). If a chlorine was attached to the trimethylsilyl moiety (trimethyl-chlorosilane), the compound was active. Replacing the methyl group in the tri-methylsilyl moiety by the hindered *tert*-butyl group led to loss of activity (*tert*-butyldimethylchlorosilane). The activity of 1-ethyl-3-tolyltriazene was expected since it is an analog of some triazenes which Druckrey *et al.*[68] found to be potent and selective carcinogens.

Nitrotoluenes and derivatives. Six dinitrotoluenes and 2,4-diaminotoluene were negative for tumorigenic potential in strain A/J mice.[34,36] 2,6-Diaminotoluene was marginally active when given i.p. and negative following p.o. administration.

The lung tumor data for the dinitrotoluenes and the diaminotoluenes are at variance with the results of other bioassays. 2,4-Dinitrotoluene was tested for carcinogenicity in rats and mice with both positive[69] and negative[34,70] results. 2,6-Dinitrotoluene induces both gamma-glutamyl transpeptidase-positive foci[71] and unscheduled DNA synthesis[72] in rat liver, and a recent report[73] appears to confirm the hepatocarcinogenicity of this compound in the rat. 2,4-Diamino-toluene is a hepatocarcinogen in the rat[74,75] and in female mice.[76] In contrast, 2,6-diaminotoluene was not carcinogenic in other mouse studies or in rats.[77]

Naphthylamines and derivatives. Theiss *et al.*[28] tested various sulfonic acid derivatives of 1-naphthylamine and 2-naphthylamine by the pulmonary adenoma bioassay to determine if this class of compounds, used as intermediates in the dye-stuff industry, possesses tumorigenic activity. Neither 1-naphthylamine nor the four sulfonic acid derivatives of 1-naphthylamine induced lung tumors in strain A mice. 2-Naphthylamine and two of the three sulfonic acid derivatives of 2-naphthylamine; *i.e.*, 2-naphthylamine-8-sulfonic acid and 2-naphthylamine-6,8-disulfonic acid, produced statistically significant lung tumor responses at comparable doses.

The mouse lung tumor data for the napthylamines are in close accord with the results of other carcinogenicity tests. 2-Naphthylamine is a potent animal carcinogen, producing bladder cancer in hamsters,[78] dogs[79,80] and monkeys,[81] as well as hepatomas[82] in mice. This chemical is also a bladder carcinogen in humans.[83,84] 2-Naphthylamino-1-sulfonic acid, a sulfonic acid derivative of 2-naph-thylamine, was not carcinogenic for BALB/c mice when administered in the diet at 2,500 ppm to 10,000 ppm for 66 weeks.[85] 1-Naphthylamine appears to be much less potent than 2-naphthylamine, since it was not tumorigenic in hamsters,[78] and gave inconclusive or negative results when tested in mice[86] and dogs.[80,87,88] Occupational exposure to 1-naphthylamine has been associated with bladder cancer in humans,[83,89] but in each case the 1-naphthylamine contained 4% to 10% 2-naphthylamine.

Miscellaneous chemicals. Four carcinogenic chemicals; *i.e.*, 2-amino-5-azotoluene, 2-acetylaminofluorene, N-hydroxy-2-acetylaminofluorene, and afla-toxin B_1, whose predominant biological effect is hepatotoxicity and hepato-carcinogenicity in the rat, were positive for lung tumor induction in strain A mice.[1,30] Aflatoxin B_1 was the most active of the four in producing lung tumors and on a molar dose basis was about ten times as active as urethane. Amino-azotoluene was intermediate in activity, and the aminofluorene compounds the least active.

Azaserine, a pancreatic carcinogen,[90] was positive for lung tumor induction in strain A mice when given i.p., but not after p.o. administration. In contrast, the colon carcinogen, 1,2-dimethylhydrazine,[91] was approximately four times more active following p.o. administration than when given i.p. Leong et al.[92] reported the production of lung tumors in strain A mice by the chronic inhalation of bis(chloromethyl) ether. Diepoxybutane and diglycidyltriethylene glycol produced a significant increase in the lung tumor response and both diepoxypiperazine and epoxypropidine were negative.[14]

The three nucleotide base analogs, fluorodeoxyuridine, bromodeoxyuridine and iododeoxyuridine, were found to be without significant carcinogenic activity for mouse lung. Previous studies have reported that neither bromodeoxyuridine nor iododeoxyuridine possess significant carcinogenic activity.[93] The carcinogens azobenzene,[94] 1,4-dioxane,[95] FANFT [N-[4-(5-nitro-2-furyl)-2-thiazolyl-formamide],[96] methylmethanesulfonate,[97] and β-propiolactone[98] were inactive for lung tumor induction at the dose levels tested.[23]

Acrylamide, a potent neurotoxin,[99] and 1-nitropyrene, a combustion product in diesel engines,[100] have recently been observed by our laboratory (Medical College of Ohio) to induce a significant increase in the lung tumor response in A/J mice.[23,31] Acrylamide was also found to induce tumors in the skin of female Sencar mice,[31] and nitropyrene induced mammary tumors in CD rats.[101]

Relative Carcinogenicity of Selected Compounds

Table 4 illustrates the use of the method of Zweifel[43] (see Materials and Methods section) to estimate the relative potency of some of the positive compounds, selected from Table 3, as inducers of lung adenomas in strain A mice. Among the compounds tested to date, 7-chloromethyl-12-methylbenz(a)anthracene is the most potent inducer of lung tumors. Uracil mustard, dibenz(a,h)-anthracene and 3-methylcholanthrene are of approximately equal activity with 1 μmol/kg required to induce an average of one lung tumor per mouse. When compared to 3-methylcholanthrene, the other polycyclic hydrocarbons, 7,12-di-methylbenz(a)anthracene, 7-bromomethyl-12-methylbenz(a)anthracene, dibenz-(a,h)acridine, and benzo(a)pyrene, were one-seventh, one-thirteenth, one-eighteenth and one-thirty-first as active, respectively, for lung tumor induction. Aflatoxin B_1, a very potent inducer of liver tumors in rats, was less active than 3-methylcholanthrene, but more active than benzo(a)pyrene. The other two hepatocarcinogens, 2-acetylaminofluorene and N-hydroxy-2-acetylaminofluorene were weakly active for lung tumor production in mice. 2-Naphthylamine, a potent bladder carcinogen, was the least active compound tested.

Comparison of Lung Tumor Data with Results from Two-Year Rodent Bioassays

Maronpot et al.[37] recently summarized data from two laboratories on the ability of 54 chemicals to induce lung tumors in strain A mice. The purpose was to compare mouse lung tumor data with results from two-year rodent bioassays. The results of this comparison (Table 5) indicate a significant disparity between the lung tumor bioassay and two-year rodent bioassays. According to Maronpot et al.[37] the strain A mouse system correctly predicted the carcinogenicity or lack thereof for 20 (37%) of the 54 chemicals. There were $^7/_{16}$ (44%) "false positives" and $^{27}/_{38}$ (71%) "false negatives." Of the 27 chemicals with "false negative" strain A test results, 14 were carcinogenic in rat and mouse in two-year bioassays,

Table 4: Relative Carcinogenic Activity of Selected Chemicals for Lung Tumor Production in Strain A Mice[a]

Compound	Total Dose (μmol/kg)	Mice with LT/ No. of Mice	Mean No. of LT/Mouse	Dose for 1 LT[b] Response (μmol/kg)
7-Chloromethyl-12-methylbenz(a)-anthracene	6	5/5	9.8	0.6
Uracil mustard	38	30/30	20.3	1
Dibenz(a,h)anthracene	36	10/10	31.0	1
3-Methylcholanthrene	186	31/31	140.0	1
7,12-Dimethylbenz(a)anthracene	10	6/6	1.5	7
Nitrogen mustard	20	36/38	2.8	7
N-Nitrosodimethylamine	140	15/15	17.5	8
Triethylene melamine	25	24/28	26.0	8
7-Bromomethyl-12-methylbenz(a)-anthracene	100	6/6	7.8	13
Vinyl carbamate	150	15/15	11.3	13
Dibenz(a,h)acridine	36	11/12	2.0	18
Aflatoxin B$_1$	480	20/20	24.5	20
Benzo(a)pyrene	400	32/32	13.0	31
Aziridinylbenzoquinone	90	24/28	2.9	31
N-Nitrosomethylurea	2,190	23/23	79.9	36
N-Nitrosoethylurea	850	31/31	20.1	42
Azaserine	870	31/31	14.7	59
3,4-Dichlorophenyl-N-carbamoyl aziridine	101	12/15	1.3	85
N-Nitrosodiethylamine	1,960	28/28	16.0	123
Lead(II)subacetate	190	11/15	1.5	127
Thio-TEPA	499	16/20	1.5	143
4-(Methylnitrosamino)-1-(3-pyridyl)-1-butanone (NNK)	5,500	23/23	37.6	146
Estradiol mustard	2,028	19/19	4.9	179
1,2-Dimethylhydrazine	1,800[c]	32/32	7.4	243
	1,800[d]	29/29	26.6	68

(continued)

Table 4: (continued)

Compound	Total Dose (μmol/kg)	Mice with LT/ No. of Mice	Mean No. of LT/Mouse	Dose for 1 LT[b] Response (μmol/kg)
Cyclophosphamide	520	20/27	1.3	400
1-Ethyl-3-*p*-tolyl-triazene	610	16/19	1.5	407
5-Azacytidine	370	6/11	0.73	507
Methyl iodide	300	5/11	0.55	545
Dibutylnitrosamine	7,590	32/32	9.8	774
Nickelous(II) acetate	1,450	12/19	1.3	1,115
Diepoxybutane	2,230	14/19	1.5	1,487
2-Bromoethanol	1,200	n.a.[e]	0.79	1,519
Ethyl carbamate (urethane)	26,933	12/12	24.5	1,963
N-Acetylethyl carbamate	18,203	15/16	3.2	2,371
Manganous sulfate	3,910	12/18	1.2	3,258
Bromoform	4,300	n.a.[e]	1.1	3,909
2,6-Diaminotoluene	3,100	17/29	0.78	3,974
1,2-Dibromoethane	4,500	21/32	1.1	4,091
2-Amino-5-azotoluene	18,700	15/15	4.1	4,560
Acrylamide	10,140	27/30	2.2	4,609
N-Nitrosonornicotine	6,000	16/24	1.2	5,000
1-Nitropyrene	6,400	22/28	1.25	5,120
Trimethylchlorosilane	9,200	11/14	1.8	5,350
2-Acetylaminofluorene	27,000	20/21	2.3	11,739
N-Hydroxy-2-acetylaminofluorene	25,000	16/19	1.9	13,158
Cinnamyl anthranilate	47,000	11/15	2.4	19,800
Isopropyl carbamate	23,275	8/10	1.5	26,300
2-Naphthylamine	41,960	n.a.[e]	1.4	29,971

[a] Data taken from Shimkin and Stoner,[1] Stoner and Shimkin,[2] and Stoner et al.[23]
[b] LT = lung tumor
[c] Dose given i.p.
[d] Dose given p.o.
[e] n.a. = data not available

eight were carcinogenic in rats only, and five were carcinogenic in mice only. In addition, there was a lack of consistency in the strain A lung tumor bioassay results in the two laboratories.

Table 5: Comparative Data on Carcinogenicity of Chemicals in Strain A
Mouse Lung Tumor Bioassay and Two-Year Rodent Bioassay

Chemicals Positive in Two-Year Bioassay and Pulmonary Tumor Bioassay	Chemicals Positive in Two-Year Bioassay and Negative in Pulmonary Tumor Bioassay
Aromatic Amines	
3-Amino-9-ethylcarbazole·HCl	2-Aminoanthraquinone
4-Amino-2-nitrophenol	3-Amino-4-ethoxyacetanilide
2-Nitro-*p*-phenylenediamine	4-Chloro-*m*-phenylenediamine
5-Nitro-*o*-toluidine	*m*-Cresidine
	p-Cresidine
	Direct black 38
	Direct blue 6
	Direct brown 95
	4,4'-Methylenebis-(N,N'-dimethyl-aniline)
	1,5-Naphthalenediamine
	5-Nitro-*o*-anisidine
	p-Nitrosodiphenylamine
	Phenazopyridine·HCl
Aliphatic Chlorides	
3-Chloromethylpyridine·HCl	Aldrin
Sulfallate	1,1,2,2-Tetrachloroethane
	Tetrachloroethylene
	Toxaphene
Miscellaneous	
Captan	Cupferron
N,N'-Dicyclohexyl thiourea	3,3'-Dimethoxybenzidine-4,4'-diisocyanate
2,4-Dinitrotoluene	2,5-Dithiobiurea
Hydrazobenzene	6-Nitrobenzimidazole
5-Nitroacenaphthalene	Nitrofen
	Pivalolactone
	p-Quinone dioxime
	Selenium disulfide
	1,1,3-Trimethyl-2-thiourea
Chemicals Negative in Two-Year Bioassay and Positive in Pulmonary Tumor Bioassay	Chemicals Negative in Two-Year Bioassay and Pulmonary Tumor Bioassay
Aromatic Amines	
Anthranilic acid	*p*-Anisidine
4'-(Chloroacetyl)acetanilide	Chloropropamide
p-Phenylenediamine·HCl	2,4-Dimethoxyaniline
	N-(1-Naphthyl)ethylenediamine
	4-Nitro-*o*-phenylenediamine
	Sulfisoxazole
	2,5-Toluenediamine sulfate

(continued)

Table 5: (continued)

Chemicals Negative in Two-Year Bioassay and Positive in Pulmonary Tumor Bioassay	Chemicals Negative in Two-Year Bioassay and Pulmonary Tumor Bioassay
Miscellaneous	
Diazinon	Tolbutamide
Parathion	3-Sulfolene
Triphenyltin hydroxide	
L-Tryptophan	

Data taken from the report of Maronpot *et al.*[37]

DISCUSSION

This report describes the basic protocol of the strain A mouse lung tumor bioassay and provides summary data on its application for the testing of several classes of chemicals for carcinogenic activity. Most compounds that were tested for carcinogenic activity by the lung tumor bioassay are shown in Tables 3 and 5. Omitted from the tables were studies with crude mixtures of chemicals such as tobacco tar, coal tar, and extracts from diesel engine emissions, and of compounds for which there were insufficient quantitative data; *i.e.*, the data were not expressed in terms of the average number of lung tumors per mouse. For example, vinyl chloride, given by inhalation, induces a significant increase in the lung tumor frequency among strain A mice,[33] but no tumor incidence data were given. In addition, this report does not summarize the extensive data on the effects of promoters (*e.g.*, butylated hydroxytoluene[102]) and inhibitors (*e.g.*, butylated hydroxyanisole[103]) of carcinogenesis, and of co-carcinogens (*e.g.*, saccharin[104]) on the lung tumor response.

The major criterion for a positive carcinogenic response in the lung tumor assay is a statistically significant increase in the average number of lung tumors in chemically treated mice *versus* the vehicle-injected controls. Generally, when 30 mice are used per concentration of test chemical, levels of statistical significance ($p = <0.05$) may be reached when a mean of 0.7 tumors to 0.8 tumors per mouse is observed as compared to a mean of 0.2 lung tumors to 0.3 lung tumors among the controls at the age of eight to nine months. However, as indicated in Table 3, some compounds were positive when inducing a mean of 0.5 tumors to 0.6 tumors per mouse because the vehicle-control data were lower than a mean of 0.2 tumors to 0.3 tumors per mouse. These should be considered very marginal responses. In fact, in our experience with the assay, chemicals should be considered positive if the following conditions are met: (a) The mean number of lung tumors in the test animals is significantly increased, preferably to one or more per mouse; (b) there is a dose-response relationship; (c) the mean number of lung tumors in the vehicle-injected and untreated controls is approximately the anticipated number for untreated mice of the same age; and (d) for marginally active compounds, positive results in an initial test are repeatable in a second test.

At least two factors can interfere with the development of a dose-response relationship in the lung tumor assay: (a) If the test chemical is highly toxic at the maximum tolerated dose, then the tumor response to this dose is frequently lower than the response at the second dose level. In addition, toxicity at the highest dose can lead to delayed mortality and too few survivors from which to obtain reliable data. Therefore, three dose levels are essential to provide at least two groups from which to obtain data toward a dose-response relationship; and (b) weakly active chemicals often do not induce lung tumors in a dose-related manner. As stated above, for these chemicals it is necessary to verify results from an initial test in a second bioassay.

Lung tumors can be induced in strain A mice when chemicals are given by several routes; *i.e.*, intraperitoneally, subcutaneously, orally, intravenously, by inhalation, and when painted on the skin. In general, the tumor response to i.p. administered chemicals is equal to or higher than by any other route because the dose exposure of the animals is best assured. This appears to be particularly true for lipid soluble chemicals. For example, 3-methylcholanthrene and benzo(a)pyrene were significantly more active when administered in tricaprylin by the i.p. route as compared to p.o. (Table 3). Pharmacologic studies showed that more of the 3-methylcholanthrene reached the lung after i.p. administration, and the compound persisted in the lungs for longer periods of time.[36] On the other hand, the water-soluble compound, urethane, is equally active when given either i.p. or p.o. (Table 3). The route of administration has an important bearing on the carcinogenic potential of both azaserine and 2,6-diaminotoluene; both compounds were active when given i.p. and negative after p.o. administration (Table 3). Among the chemicals tested, only 1,2-dimethylhydrazine was more active when given by the p.o. route as compared to i.p.

The lack of congruity between the results of the strain A mouse lung tumor bioassay and the two-year rodent bioassays is, perhaps, not too surprising. Several of the chemicals found positive in the two-year rodent bioassays are hepatocarcinogens, and it has been known for years that several potent hepatocarcinogens in the rat; *e.g.*, aflatoxin B_1, acetylaminofluorene and N-hydroxyacetylaminofluorene, are more weakly active for lung tumor production in mice[1] (*see* Table 4). On the other hand, the lung tumor bioassay is very sensitive to the polycyclic hydrocarbons (Table 4) and many of the PAH do not induce liver tumors unless the test animals are partially hepatectomized. Studies of the pharmacokinetics of distribution and metabolism of carcinogens in the liver and lung should be undertaken in efforts to explain differences in their potency in the two organs. In an effort to develop a mouse strain with a wide range of susceptibility to both lung and liver carcinogens, our laboratory is currently evaluating the susceptibility of a hybrid strain, derived by crossing A/J mice (high lung tumor incidence) with C3H mice (high liver tumor incidence), to carcinogens. Preliminary data indicate that the hybrid develops both lung and liver tumors in response to diethylnitrosamine within six months after administration of the carcinogen.[23]

Two additional criticisms of the lung tumor bioassay are that the adenoma is a benign tumor, has no human neoplastic equivalent, and that the numerical increase and earlier appearance of the tumor merely accelerate a process already present in the animal rather than being a truly inductive process. In answer to these criticisms, it should be recognized that some adenomas progress to adenocarcinomas with invasion of the surrounding lung if the mice are maintained for sufficient periods (18 to 24 months) after administration of the carcinogen, and a small percentage of the adenocarcinomas metastasize to other organ sites. Therefore, at least some of the adenomas do not exhibit the behavioral characteristics of benign tumors. In addition, some alveologenic carcinomas in man are derived from type 2 alveolar epithelial cells and are similar in morphology to adenocarcinomas of the mouse lung. Regarding the second criticism; *i.e.*, the question of induction *versus* acceleration of lung tumors, the administration of a carcinogen such as methylcholanthrene at a dose of one mg per mouse can lead to the production of a mean of 40 lung adenomas per mouse within six months or less. We have never observed more than an average of 0.2 lung tumor to 0.5 lung tumor per mouse in controls at six months, or one to two tumors per mouse in controls at 18 to 20 months. Moreover, histological examination of the lungs of control mice at six to 18 months does not reveal evidence of numerous foci of small, developing tumors. Therefore, it is likely that the production of lung adenomas in strain A mice by carcinogenic agents is an inductive rather than an accelerative process.

In our opinion, the strain A mouse lung tumor bioassay deserves further investigation in the following areas: (a) There is very little information on the distribution and metabolism of carcinogens in the whole lung and in specific lung cell types such as the type 2 alveolar epithelial cells. Studies should be undertaken to provide more information in this area; (b) The lung adenoma bioassay should be examined further for its ability to detect promoting agents; (c) The assay should be used for quantitative studies of the potential inhibitory, additive or synergistic effects of administering more than one chemical to the test animal. This seems particularly relevant in view of the fact that humans are constantly exposed to a large number of environmental chemicals.

Acknowledgements

We thank Academic Press, Inc., Mary Ann Liebert, Inc., and Plenum Press, Inc., for permission to reproduce portions of the lung tumor data presented in this chapter. Carcinogenesis bioassays of the nitrotoluene compounds and 1-nitropyrene were supported by the U.S. Army Medical Research and Development Command.

REFERENCES

1. Shimkin, M.B., and Stoner, G.D., Lung tumors in mice: Application to carcinogenesis bioassay. *Adv. Cancer Res.* 21: 1-58 (1975)
2. Stoner, G.D., and Shimkin, M.B., Strain A mouse lung tumor bioassay. *J. Amer. Coll. Toxicol.* 1: 145-169 (1982)
3. Shimkin, M.B., Pulmonary tumors in experimental animals. *Adv. Cancer Res.* 3: 223-267 (1955)
4. Brooks, R.E., Pulmonary adenoma of strain A mice: An electron microscopic study. *J. Natl. Cancer Inst.* 41: 719-742 (1968)
5. Svoboda, D.J., Ultrastructure of pulmonary adenomas in mice. *Cancer Res.* 22: 1197-1201 (1962)

6. Witschi, H., and Haschek, W.M., Cells of origin of lung tumors in mice. *J. Natl. Cancer Inst.* 70: 991 (1983)
7. Gunning, W.T., III, Stoner, G.D., Malkinson, A.M., and Goldblatt, P.J., Cellular origin of urethane-induced lung tumors in strain A mice. (in press)
8. Kauffman, S.L., Alexander, L., and Sass, L., Histologic and ultrastructural features of the Clara cell adenoma of the mouse lung. *Lab Invest.* 40: 708-716 (1979)
9. Kauffman, S.L., Histogenesis of the papillary Clara cell adenoma. *Am. J. Pathol.* 103: 174-180 (1981)
10. Beer, D.S., and Malkinson, A.M., (personal communication)
11. Murphy, J.B., and Sturm, E., Pulmonary tumors in mice following the cutaneous application of coal tar. *J. Exp. Med.* 42: 693-700 (1925)
12. Shimkin, M.B., Induced pulmonary tumors in mice. II. Reaction of lungs of strain A mice to carcinogenic hydrocarbons. *Arch. Pathol.* 29: 239-255 (1940)
13. Andervont, H.B., and Shimkin, M.B., Biologic testing of carcinogens. II. Pulmonary-tumor-induction-technique. *J. Natl. Cancer Inst.* 1: 225-239 (1941)
14. Shimkin, M.B., Weisburger, J.H., Weisburger, E.K., Gubareff, N., and Suntzeff, V., Bioassay of 29 alkylating chemicals by the pulmonary-tumor response in strain A mice. *J. Natl. Cancer. Inst.* 36: 915-935 (1966)
15. Leo, A., Panthananickal, A., and Hansch, C., A comparison of mutagenic and carcinogenic activities of aniline mustards. *J. Med. Chem.* 24: 859-864 (1981)
16. Shimkin, M.B., Weider, R., McDonough, M., Fishbein, L., and Swern, D., Lung tumor response in strain A mice as a quantitative bioassay of carcinogenic activity of some carbamates and aziridines. *Cancer Res.* 29: 2184-2190 (1969)
17. Dahl, G.A., Miller, E.C., and Miller, J.A., Comparative carcinogenicities and mutagenicities of vinyl carbamate, ethyl carbamate, and ethyl N-hydroxy carbamate. *Cancer Res.* 40: 1194-1203 (1980)
18. Stoner, G.D., Shimkin, M.B., Kniazeff, A.J., Weisburger, J.H., Weisburger, E.K., and Gori, G.B., Test for carcinogenicity of food additives and chemotherapeutic agents by the pulmonary tumor response in strain A mice. *Cancer Res.* 33: 3069-3085 (1973)
19. Stoner, G.D., Weisburger, E.K., and Shimkin, M.B., Tumor response in strain A mice exposed to silylating compounds used for gas-liquid chromatography. *J. Natl. Cancer Inst.* 54: 495-497 (1975)
20. Mirvish, S.S., Cardesa, A., Wallcave, L., and Shubik, P., Induction of mouse lung adenomas by amines or ureas plus nitrite and by N-nitroso compounds: Effect of ascorbic acid, gallic acid, thiocyanate, and caffeine. *J. Natl. Cancer Inst.* 55: 633-636 (1975)
21. Hecht, S.S., Chi-hong, B.C., Hirota, N., Ornaf, R.M., Tso, T.O., and Hoffmann, D., Tobacco-specific nitrosamines: Formation from nicotine *in vitro* and during tobacco curing and carcinogenicity in strain A mice. *J. Natl. Cancer Inst.* 60:819-824 (1978)
22. Castonguay, A., Lin, D., Stoner, G.D., Radok, P., Furuya, K., Hecht, S.S., Schut, H.A.J., and Klaunig, J.E., Comparative carcinogenicity in A/J mice and metabolism by cultured mouse peripheral lung of N'-nitrosonornicotine, 4-(methylnitrosamino)-1-(3-pyridyl)-1-butanone, and their analogues. *Cancer Res.* 43: 1223-1229 (1983)
23. Stoner, G.D., Greisiger, E., and Ash, D., (unpublished observations)

24. Stoner, G.D., Shimkin, M.B., Troxell, M.C., Thompson, T.L., and Terry, L.S., Test for carcinogenicity of metallic compounds by the pulmonary tumor response in strain A mice. *Cancer Res.* 36: 1744-1747 (1976)

25. Poirier, L.A., Stoner, G.D., and Shimkin, M.B., Bioassay of alkyl halides and nucleotide base analogs by pulmonary tumor response in strain A mice. *Cancer Res.* 35: 1411-1415 (1975)

26. Theiss, J.C., Shimkin, M.B., and Poirier, L.A., Induction of pulmonary adenomas in strain A mice by substituted organohalides. *Cancer Res.* 39: 391-395 (1979)

27. Theiss, J.C., Stoner, G.D., Shimkin, M.B., and Weisburger, E.K., Test for carcinogenicity of organic contaminants of United States drinking waters by pulmonary tumor response in strain A mice. *Cancer Res.* 37: 2717-2720 (1977)

28. Theiss, J.C., Shimkin, M.B., and Weisburger, E.K., Pulmonary adenoma response of strain A mice to sulfonic acid derivatives of 1- and 2-naphthylamines. *J. Natl. Cancer Inst.* 67: 1299-1302 (1981)

29. Peck, R.M., Tan, T.K., and Peck, E.B., Pulmonary carcinogenesis by derivatives of polynuclear aromatic alkylating agents. *Cancer Res.* 36: 2423-2427 (1976)

30. Weider, R., Wogan, G.N., and Shimkin, M.B., Pulmonary tumors in strain A mice given injections of aflatoxin B_1. *J. Natl. Cancer Inst.* 40: 1195-1197 (1968)

31. Bull, R.J., Robinson, M., Laurie, R.D., Stoner, G.D., Griesiger, E., Meier, J.R., and Stober, J., Carcinogenic effects of acrylamide in Sencar and A/J mice. *Cancer Res.* 44: 107-111 (1984)

32. Hosaka, S., and Hirono, I., Carcinogenicity test of quercetin by pulmonary-adenoma bioassay in strain A mice. *Gann* 72: 327-328 (1981)

33. Hehir, R.M., McNamara, B.P., McLaughlin, Jr., J., Willigan, D.A., Bierbower, G., and Hardisty, J.F., Cancer induction following single and multiple exposures to a constant amount of vinyl chloride monomer. *Environ. Health Perspect.* 41: 63-72 (1981)

34. Schut, H.A.J., Loeb, T.R., and Stoner, G.D., Distribution, elimination, and test for carcinogenicity of 2,4-dinitrotoluene in strain A mice. *Toxicol. Appl. Pharmacol.* 64: 213-220 (1982)

35. Schut, H.A.J., Loeb, T.T., Grimes, L.A., and Stoner, G.D., Distribution, elimination, and test for carcinogenicity of 2,6-dinitrotoluene after intraperitoneal and oral administration to strain A mice. *J. Toxicol. Environ. Health* 12: 659-670 (1983)

36. Stoner, G.D., Greisiger, E.A., Schut, H.A.J., Pereira, M.A., Loeb, T.R., Klaunig, J.E., and Branstetter, D.G., A comparison of the lung adenoma response in strain A/J mice after intraperitoneal and oral administration of carcinogens *Toxicol. Appl. Pharmacol.* 72: 313-323 (1984)

37. Maronpot, R.R., Witschi, H.P., Smith, L.H., and McCoy, J.L., Recent experience with the strain A mouse pulmonary adenoma bioassay. *Environ. Sci. Res.* 27: 341-349 (1983)

38. Theiss, J.C., Stoner, G.D., and Kniazeff, A.J., Effect of reovirus infection on pulmonary tumor response to urethane in strain A mice. *J. Natl. Cancer Inst.* 61: 131-134 (1978)

39. Peck, R.M., Eaton, G.J., Peck, E.B., and Litwin, S., Influence of Sendai virus on carcinogenesis in strain A mice. *Lab. Animal Sci.* 33: 154-156 (1983)

40. Theiss, J.C., Shimkin, M.B., Stoner, G.D., Kniazeff, A.J., and Hoppenstand, R.D., Effect of lactate dehydrogenase virus on chemically induced mouse lung tumorigenesis. *Cancer Res.* 40: 64-66 (1980)

41. Stoner, G.D., Kniazeff, A.J., Shimkin, M.B., and Hoppenstand, R.D., Suppression of chemically induced pulmonary tumors by treatment of strain A mice with murine sarcoma virus. *J. Natl. Cancer Inst.* 53: 493–498 (1974)

42. Malkinson, A.M., Prevention of butylated hydroxytoluene-induced lung damage in mice by cedar terpene administration. *Toxicol. Appl. Pharmacol.* 49: 551–560 (1979)

43. Zweifel, J.R., Use of the likelihood principle for the determination of carcinogenic activity in pulmonary tumor assays. *J. Natl. Cancer Inst.* 36: 937–946 (1966)

44. Stoner, G.D., McGuire, E.J., Heifetz, C.L., and Iglesia, F.A. de la (in preparation)

45. National Cancer Institute, *Report on the Carcinogenesis Bioassay of Chloroform.* Bethesda, MD (Mar. 1, 1976)

46. Kylin, B., Istuan, S., and Yllner, S., Hepatotoxicity of inhaled trichloroethylene and tetrachloroethylene: Long-term exposure. *Acta Pharmacol. Toxicol.* 22: 379–385 (1965)

47. Innes, J.R.M., Ulland, B.M., Valerio, M.G., Petrucelli, L., Fishbein, L., Hart, E.R., Pallotta, A.J., Bates, R.R., Falk, H.L., Gart, J.J., Mitchell, I., Klein, M., and Peters, J., Bioassay of pesticides and industrial chemicals for tumorigenicity in mice: A preliminary note. *J. Natl. Cancer Inst.* 42: 1101–1104 (1969)

48. Nagaski, H., Tomii, S., Mega, T., Marugami, M., and Ito, N., Development of hepatomas in mice treated with benzene hexachloride. *Gann* 62: 431–434 (1971)

49. Druckrey, H., Kruse, H., Preusmann, R., Ivankovic, S., and Landschutz, C., Cancerogene alkylierende Substanzen. III. Alkyl-halogenide, -sulfate, -sulfonate and ringgespannte Heterocyclen. *Z. Krebsforsch* 74: 241–273 (1970)

50. Van Duuren, B.L., Goldschmidt, B.M., Katz, C., Seidman, I., and Paul, J.S. Carcinogenic activity of alkylating agents. *J. Natl. Cancer Inst.* 53: 695–700 (1974)

51. Laskin, S., Sellakumar, A.R., Kuschner, M., Nelson, N., Mendola, S.L., Rusch, G.M., Katz, G.V., Dulak, N.C., and Albert, R.F., Inhalation carcinogenicity of epichlorohydrin in noninbred Sprague-Dawley rats. *J. Natl. Cancer Inst.* 65: 751–757 (1980)

52. Heuper, W.C., Carcinogens in the human environment. *Arch. Pathol.* 71: 237–267 (1971)

53. DiPaolo, J.A., The potentiation of lymphosarcomas in mice by manganous chloride. *Fed. Proc.* 23: 393 (1964)

54. Furst, A., and Haro, R.T., A survey of metal carcinogenesis. *Prog. Exptl. Tumor Res.* 12: 102–133 (1969)

55. Sunderman, F.W., Jr., Metal carcinogenesis in experimental animals. *Fd. Cosmetics Toxicol.* 9: 105–120 (1971)

56. Schroeder, H.A., Balassa, J.J., and Vinton, W.H., Jr., Chromium, lead, cadmium, nickel and titanium in mice: Effect on mortality, tumors and tissue levels. *J. Nutr.* 83: 239–250 (1964)

57. Schroeder, H.A., and Mitchener, M., Selenium and tellurium in mice. *Arch. Environ. Health* 24: 66–71 (1972)

58. Kanisawa, M., and Schroeder, H.A., Life-time studies on the effects of arsenic, germanium, tin, vanadium on spontaneous tumors in mice. *Cancer Res.* 27: 1192–1195 (1967)

59. Kanisawa, M., and Schroeder, H.A., Life time studies on the effects of trace elements on spontaneous tumors in mice and rats. *Cancer Res.* 29: 892-895 (1969)

60. Ward, J.M., Griesemer, R.A., and Weisburger, E.K., The mouse liver as an endpoint in carcinogenesis tests. *Toxicol. Appl. Pharmacol.* 51: 389-397 (1980)

61. Epstein, S.S., Fujii, K., Andrea, J., and Mantel, N., Carcinogenicity testing of selected food additives by parenteral administration to infant Swiss mice. *Toxicol. Appl. Pharmacol.* 16: 321-334 (1970)

62. Borchert, P., Miller, J.A., Miller, E.C., and Shires, T.K., 1'-Hydroxysafrole, a proximate carcinogenic metabolite of safrole in the rat and mouse. *Cancer Res.* 33: 590-600 (1973)

63. Bryan, G.T., Erturk, E., and Yoshida, O., Production of urinary bladder carcinomas in mice by sodium saccharin. *Science* 168: 1238-1240 (1970)

64. Munro, I.C., and Arnold, D.L., in: *Health and Sugar Substitutes* (B. Guggenheim, ed.), pp 76-81, Karger, Basel (1978)

65. Pereira, M.A., Herren, S.L., and Britt, A.L., Effect of dibutylnitrosamine and saccharin on glutamyl transpeptidase positive foci and liver cancer. *Environ. Health Perspect.* 50: 169-176 (1983)

66. Cohen, S.M., Masayuki, A., Jacobs, J.B., and Friedell, G.H., Promoting effect of saccharin and DL-tryptophan in urinary bladder carcinogenesis. *Cancer Res.* 39: 1207-1217 (1979)

67. Abell, C.W., Falk, H.L., Shimkin, M.B., Weisburger, E.K., Weisburger, J.H., and Gubareff, N., Uracil mustard: A potent inducer of lung tumors in mice. *Science* 147: 1443-1445 (1965)

68. Druckrey, H.S., Ivankovic, S., and Preussmann, R., Neurotrope carcinogene Wirkung von Phenyldimethyltriazen an Ratten. *Naturwissenschaften* 54: 171 (1967)

69. Ellis, H.V., Hagensen, J.H., Hodgson, J.R., Minor, J.L., Hong, C.B., Ellis, E.R., Girvin, J.D., Helton, D.O., Herndon, B.L., and Lee, C-C., *Mammalian Toxicity of Munitions Compounds*: Phase III. *Effects of Lifetime Exposure*. I. *2,4-Dinitrotoluene*. Report ADAO 77692. Midwest Research Institute, Kansas City, MO (1979)

70. U.S. Department of Health, Education and Welfare, *Bioassay of 2,4-Dinitrotoluene for Possible Carcinogenicity*. DHEW Publication No. (NIH) 78-1304. Public Health Service, National Institutes of Health, Washington, DC (1977)

71. Leonard, T.B., and Popp, J.A., Investigation of the carcinogenic initiating potential of dinitrotoluene: Structure-activity study. *Proc. Am. Assn. Cancer Res.* 22: 82 (1981)

72. Mirsalis, J.C., and Butterworth, B.E., Induction of unscheduled DNA synthesis in rat hepatocytes following *in vivo* treatment with dinitrotoluene. *Carcinogenesis* 3: 241-245 (1982)

73. Popp, J.A., and Leonard, T.B., Hepatocarcinogenicity of 2,6-dinitrotoluene (DNT). *Proc. Am. Assn. Cancer Res.* 24: 91 (1983)

74. Ito, N., Hiasa, Y., Konishi, Y., and Marugami, M., The development of carcinoma in liver of rats treated with m-toluenediamine and the synergistic and antagonistic effects with other chemicals. *Cancer Res.* 29: 1137-1145 (1969)

75. Cardy, R.H., Carcinogenicity and chronic toxicity of 2,4-toluenediamine in F-344 rats. *J. Natl. Cancer Inst.* 62: 1107-1116 (1979)

76. U.S. Department of Health, Education and Welfare, *Bioassay of 2,4-Di-aminotoluene for Possible Carcinogenicity*, DHEW Publication No. (NIH) 79-1718. Public Health Service, National Institutes of Health, Washington, DC (1978)
77. National Cancer Institute (USA), *Bioassay of 2,6-Diaminotoluene for Possible Carcinogenicity. Carcinogenesis Technical Report Series*, No. 200 (1980)
78. Saffiotti, U., Cefis, F., Montesano, R., and Sellakumar, A.R., in: *Bladder Cancer, A Symposium* (W. Deichmann and K.F. Lampe, eds.), pp 129, Aesculapius, Birmingham, Alabama (1967)
79. Conzelman, G.M., Jr., and Moulten, J.E., Dose-response relationships of the bladder tumorigen 2-naphthylamine: A study in beagle dogs. *J. Natl. Cancer Inst.* 49: 193-205 (1972)
80. Purchase, I.F.H., Kalinowski, A.E., Ishmael, J., Wilson, J., Gore, C.W., and Chart, I.S., Lifetime carcinogenicity study of 1- and 2-naphthylamine in dogs. *Br. J. Cancer* 44: 892-901 (1982)
81. Conzelman, G.M., Jr., Moulten, J.E., Flanders, L.E. III, Springer, K., and Crowt, D.W., Induction of transitional cell carcinomas of the urinary bladder in monkeys fed 2-naphthylamine. *J. Natl. Cancer Inst.* 42: 825-836 (1969)
82. Bonser, G.M., Clayson, D.B., Jull, J.W., and Pyrah, L.N., The carcinogenic properties of 2-amino-1-naphthol hydrochloride and its parent amine 2-naphthylamine. *Br. J. Cancer* 6: 412-424 (1952)
83. Case, R.A., Hosker, M.E., McDonald, D.B., and Pearson, J.T., Tumours of the urinary bladder in workmen engaged in the manufacture and use of certain dyestuff intermediates in the British chemical industry. I. The role of aniline, benzidine, alpha-naphthylamine and beta-naphthylamine. *Br. J. Ind. Med.* 11: 75-104 (1954)
84. Mancuso, T.F., and El-Attar, A.A., Cohort study of workers exposed to beta-naphthylamine and benzidine. *J. Occup. Med.* 9: 277-285 (1967)
85. Della Porta, G., and Dragani, T.A., Non-carcinogenicity in mice of a sulfonic acid derivative of 2-naphthylamine. *Carcinogenesis* 3: 647-649 (1982)
86. Radomski, J.L., Brill, E., Deichmann, W.B., and Glass, E.M., Carcinogenicity testing of N-hydroxyl and other oxidation and decomposition products of 1- and 2-naphthylamine. *Cancer Res.* 31: 1461-1467 (1971)
87. Bonser, G.M., Clayson, D.B., and Jull, J.W., Some aspects of the experimental induction of tumours of the bladder. *Br. Med. Bull.* 14: 146-152 (1958)
88. Radomski, J.L., Deichmann, W.B., Altman, N.H., and Radomski, T., Failure of pure 1-naphthylamine to induce bladder tumors in dogs. *Cancer Res.* 40: 3537-3539 (1980)
89. Gehrmann, G.H., Foulger, J.H., and Fleming, A.J., in: *Proceedings of the Ninth International Congress on Industrial Medicine*, pp 472, Wright, Bristol (1949)
90. Longnecker, D.S., and Curphey, T.J., Adenocarcinoma of the pancreas in azaserine-treated rats. *Cancer Res.* 35: 2249-2258 (1975)
91. Evans, J.T., Hauschka, T.S., and Mittelman, A.J., Differential susceptibility of four mouse strains to induction of multiple large bowel neoplasms by 1,2-dimethylhydrazine. *J. Natl. Cancer Inst.* 52: 999-1000 (1974)
92. Leong, B.K.J., MacFarland, H.N., and Reese, W.H., Jr., Induction of lung adenomas by chronic inhalation of bis(chloromethyl) ether. *Arch. Environ. Health* 22: 663-666 (1971)

93. Hadidian, Z., Frederickson, T.N., Weisburger, E.K., Weisburger, J.H., Glass, R.M., and Mantel, N., Tests for chemical carcinogens. Report on the activity of aromatic amines, nitrosamines, quinolines, nitroalkanes, amides, epoxides, aziridines, and purine antimetabolites. *J. Natl. Cancer Inst.* 41: 9895-10036 (1968)

94. Innes, J.R.M., *Evaluation of carcinogenic, teratogenic and mutagenic activities of selected pesticides and industrial chemicals. Vol. 1, Carcinogenic study.* Bionetics Research Labs. Inc., Bethesda, National Technical Information Service, U.S. Department of Commerce (1968)

95. Kociba, R.J., McCollister, S.B., Park, C., Torkelson, T.R., and Gehring, P.J., 1,4-Dioxane. I. Results of a 2-year ingestion study in rats. *Toxicol. Appl. Pharmacol.* 30: 275-286 (1974)

96. Erturk, E., Cohen, S.M., and Bryan, G.T., Urinary bladder carcinogenicity of N-[4-(5-nitro-2-furyl)-2-thiazolyl]formamide in female Swiss mice. *Cancer Res.* 30: 1309-1311 (1970)

97. Clapp, N.K., Craig, A.W., and Toya, R.E., Sr., Oncogenicity by methylmethane sulfonate in male RF mice. *Science* 161: 913-914 (1968)

98. Van Duuren, B.L., Langseth, L., Orris, L., Baden, M., and Kuschner, M., Carcinogenicity of epoxides, lactones, and peroxy compounds. V. Subcutaneous injection in rats. *J. Natl. Cancer Inst.* 39: 1213-1217 (1967)

99. Teal, J.J., and Evans, H.L., Behavioral effects of acrylamide in the mouse. *Toxicol. Appl. Pharmacol.* 63: 470-480 (1982)

100. Newton, D.L., Erickson, M.D., Tomer, K.B., Pellizzari, E.D., and Gentry, P., Identification of nitroaromatics in diesel exhaust particulate using gas chromatography/negative ion chemical ionization mass spectrometry and other techniques. *Environ. Sci. Technol.* 16: 206-213 (1982)

101. Hirose, M., Lee, M-S., Vaught, J.B., Wang, C.V., and King, C.M., Carcinogenicity and metabolic activation of 1-nitropyrene. *Proc. Am. Assn. Cancer Res.* 24: 83 (1983)

102. Witschi, H.P., Hakkinen, P.J., and Kerrer, J.P., Modification of lung tumor development in A/J mice. *Toxicol.* 21: 37-45 (1981)

103. Wattenberg, L.W., Inhibition of chemical carcinogenesis. *J. Natl. Cancer Inst.* 60: 11-18 (1978)

104. Theiss, J.C., Arnold, L.J., and Shimkin, M.B., Effect of commercial saccharin preparations on urethane-induced lung tumorigenesis in strain A mice. *Cancer Res.* 40: 4322-4324 (1980)

10

Tumorigenesis of the Rat Mammary Gland

David L. McCormick
Richard C. Moon

I.I.T. Research Institute
Chicago, Illinois

INTRODUCTION

The induction of adenocarcinomas in the mammary glands of the female rat provides a limited test system which is a useful adjunct to long-term animal bioassays for carcinogenic activity. A number of attributes of this model contribute to its utility for carcinogen screening. Mammary cancers can be induced in rats by a wide variety of chemical and physical agents, including radiation (neutrons, x-rays, gamma rays) and chemical carcinogens of diverse structure (polycyclic aromatic hydrocarbons, N-nitroso compounds, hydroxamic acids). A single exposure to the test agent generally is sufficient for the induction of tumors. Induced tumors are similar to human mammary tumors with respect to both hormone dependence[1] and histology.[2] The superficial location of mammary tumors permits their detection by palpation, thus allowing the determination of tumor latent period without extensive serial sacrifice. Finally, dose-response parameters for the induction of mammary tumors by several classes of carcinogens have been defined.

In this chapter, the use of the rat mammary cancer model will be discussed with respect to its utility in carcinogen testing. In the first section of the chapter, methodology for screening compounds for activity as mammary carcinogens will be described. In the second section, attributes, limitations and possible modifications of the test system will be discussed. Finally, a brief review of the literature will describe the range of compounds which have been found to have carcinogenic activity in this model system.

METHODOLOGY FOR SCREENING OF COMPOUNDS AS MAMMARY CARCINOGENS

Experimental Animals

Strain. Successful induction of mammary tumors has been reported in a wide variety of rat strains, including outbred Sprague-Dawley and Wistar rats, and inbred Lewis, F344, Long-Evans, Wistar-Furth, and ACI rats. The Sprague-Dawley rat appears to be the animal of choice for the purposes of screening for mammary carcinogens, although the use of other strains may provide advantages under certain experimental conditions.

The Sprague-Dawley rat is by far the most widely used and has a number of qualities which make it a desirable model for carcinogenesis studies. This rat is widely available, is a generally healthy animal with a lifespan of over two years, and is susceptible to the induction of mammary tumors by a variety of chemical and physical agents. The Sprague-Dawley rat is considered to be a "high responder" strain for mammary carcinogenesis, *i.e.*, tumors can be induced with doses of carcinogen which elicit either a quantitatively smaller or no tumorigenic response in less sensitive strains such as F344 or Long-Evans.[3]

Although the Sprague-Dawley rat has the desirable sensitivity to the induction of mammary cancer, and a significant amount of literature exists concerning mammary carcinogenesis in this strain, two caveats regarding the use of these rats should be noted. First, dose-response may vary substantially among Sprague-Dawley rats obtained from different sources. Second, the Sprague-Dawley rat develops a relatively high incidence of spontaneous mammary tumors with increasing age.[4,5] Although these tumors are predominantly benign fibroadenomas, spontaneous adenocarcinomas do occur in rats older than one year. The presence of such spontaneous lesions may complicate interpretation of experimental data should a group of rats exposed to a test agent develop mammary cancers in low incidence with a long latent period.

Age. Studies conducted in a number of laboratories have demonstrated a peak in the susceptibility of the rat mammary gland to the induction of cancer when administration of the carcinogen is to young adult rats (50 to 70 days of age).[6-8] Prepubertal rats (age 25 to 30 days) exposed to mammary carcinogens such as 7,12-dimethylbenz(a)anthracene (DMBA) show a significantly lower incidence of mammary cancer than 50 day old rats; similarly, sensitivity to induction of mammary cancer declines with increasing age past approximately 70 days.[6] For this reason, assays for mammary carcinogenic activity ideally should involve administration of the test compound to 50 day old rats. While induction of tumors can also be achieved in younger or older rats, their lessened sensitivity to mammary carcinogenesis increases the likelihood of a false negative response.

Dao[9] has demonstrated that changes in the mammary gland itself, rather than in the host, are responsible for the peak sensitivity to induction of cancer observed in 50 to 70 day old rats. In this study, tumor incidence was greater in the mammary glands of rats exposed to DMBA at age 56 days and subsequently transplanted into isologous 56 or 120 day old rats than in glands taken from rats exposed to DMBA at age 120 days and transplanted into 56 or 120 day old hosts.

Several age-related changes occur in the mammary glands, changes which may form the mechanistic basis for the differential sensitivity to induction of mammary cancer seen in rats of different ages. Nagasawa and Yanai[10] have reported that mammary cell division, as measured by uptake of ^{3}H-thymidine, is maximal in 50 day old rats and shows a progressive decline with age past 70 days. Similar data have been reported by Russo and Russo[11] and Sinha and Dao.[7] Age-related alterations in mammary gland morphology have also been documented. Hadfield and Young[12] reported in 1956 that the mammary gland in the young adult mouse is characterized by the presence of numerous "terminal clubs," parenchymal structures having a relatively high level of cellular proliferation in comparison to the rest of the gland. This rapid proliferation is followed by differentiation of the terminal clubs into acini and lobules, parenchymal structures with less proliferative capacity.[12] A similar situation exists in the rat mammary gland. The Russos have identified a parenchymal structure, the terminal end bud (TEB), which has the highest ^{3}H-thymidine labelling index of any structure in the rat mammary gland. The TEB is found in much higher multiplicity in 50 day old rats than in older rats, and it has been suggested that this structure is the most sensitive target for chemical carcinogens.[11]

Although changes in mammary parenchymal cell kinetics appear to be the most likely basis for age-related changes in tumor response, other possible mammary gland-mediated mechanisms have been suggested. Greiner *et al.*[13] have reported a peak in inducible aryl hydrocarbon hydroxylase (AHH) activity in mammary parenchymal cells isolated from 50 day old rats, with a decline in inducible AHH activity with age that roughly parallels age-related changes in tumor response. Furthermore, Tay and Russo[14,15] noted that DNA repair was less effective in primary mammary epithelial cell cultures obtained from young (45 to 55 day old) rats than from older (145 to 155 day old) rats. These data suggest that, in addition to having increased rates of cell division in the mammary gland, young rats may metabolize procarcinogens to active metabolites in the mammary glands more effectively, and repair carcinogen-induced DNA damage less effectively than do older rats; either of these factors could result in an increased cancer response.

It should be noted that Nagasawa and Yanai,[10] among others, were unable to correlate age-related changes in mammary tumor response with circulating levels of prolactin or other hormones.

Reproductive status. All screening assays for carcinogenic activity in the rat mammary gland should employ virgin females as experimental animals. Virgin rats are significantly more sensitive to induction of mammary tumors than are rats which have undergone a full term pregnancy; a second full term pregnancy appears to reduce induction of tumors still further.[16] The higher sensitivity to mammary carcinogenesis of the virgin rat has been attributed to the state of differentiation of the mammary gland at the time of administration of the carcinogen.[11] The hormones of pregnancy cause differentiation of structures which are sensitive to mammary carcinogenesis (*i.e.*, terminal end buds) into dense lobuloalveolar structures which are less sensitive to carcinogenesis. Following parturition, these lobuloalveolar structures involute, but do not return completely to the pre-pregnancy stage of differentiation. Thus, while the virgin gland contains numerous terminal end buds and alveolar buds, mammary glands of parous rats contain primarily alveolar buds and lobules without the sensitive terminal end bud structures.[11]

As previously stated, the terminal end bud is the mammary structure with the highest rate of cell division, as determined by ^{3}H-thymidine labelling index. Consistent with this is the observation that mammary glands obtained from old parous rats have significantly reduced labelling indices when compared to old virgin or young virgin rats.[11] Similarly, parous rats show a lower level of carcinogen binding to mammary cell DNA,[15,16] and a higher level of DNA repair in mammary epithelial cells than do virgin rats.[14,15] These factors may all contribute to the reduced susceptibility of the parous rat to mammary carcinogenesis. Because sensitivity to induction of tumors is clearly an important factor in the choice of a relevant animal model, the use of virgin rats for mammary carcinogenesis screening is indicated.

Administration of Test Compounds

Several routes of administration have been demonstrated to be of use in the induction of mammary cancers in rats. Most experimental studies of mammary carcinogenesis have used either intragastric or intravenous administration of test compounds; however, successful induction of mammary cancers has also been achieved with subcutaneous injection or direct application of the carcinogen to the mammary fat pad.

In experiments using polycyclic aromatic hydrocarbons such as DMBA, benzo(a)pyrene [B(a)P], or 3-methylcholanthrene (3-MC), the carcinogen ordinarily is dissolved in a vehicle such as corn oil, sesame oil, or trioctanoin and administered by gavage. Administration by gavage is performed without anesthesia using a syringe equipped with either a feeding needle or a soft rubber catheter. Standard procedure is to administer the compound in a total volume of 1.0 ml; however, should solubility limit the concentration of dissolved material, a volume of up to 3 ml can be tolerated by a 50 day old rat. To eliminate the influence of stomach contents on carcinogen absorption, intragastric administration of test agents should follow an overnight fast. Administration of carcinogen to rats which have not been fasted can markedly increase variability in animal response, and will ordinarily reduce carcinoma multiplicity and increase cancer latent period in comparison to fasted rats receiving the same dose.

Intravenous (i.v.) administration of the carcinogen has been used primarily with water soluble compounds such as the nitrosamides, but can also be used for lipid emulsions of fat soluble compounds. Intravenous administration of test agents results in the exposure of the mammary gland prior to a pass through the liver. This may be the route of choice for administration of potentially direct acting agents. Obviously, fasting of animals is not required prior to intravenous administration of a test agent.

In our laboratory, we have found administration via the jugular vein to be the least difficult and most reproducible route for intravenous administration of mammary carcinogens, although injections into the tail vein have been used in other laboratories. Immediately prior to administration, the test compound is dissolved in sterile phosphate-buffered saline or other suitable vehicle. For the i.v. administration animals are anesthetized with ether, an incision is made to expose the jugular vein, and the injection is performed. Normal injection volume is 0.4 ml carcinogen solution per 100 g body weight. Following administration of the test compound, the incision is approximated with wound clips. Wound clips are removed approximately seven days after administration of the carcinogen.

Observation of Animals

Palpation to monitor the appearance of the mammary tumors should begin a maximum of four weeks following administration of the test compound, and should continue weekly or semiweekly for the duration of the study. Routine palpation of rats can be performed without anesthesia, since this procedure causes little or no discomfort to the animals. During palpation, particular attention should be paid to the cervical-thoracic chains of mammary glands which surround the forepaws: the majority of chemically-induced tumors arise in these glands rather than in the abdominal-inguinal glands,[17] and with careful palpation, tumors can be detected at a diameter of 2 mm or smaller.

When a tumor is detected, its location should be noted on a map for future reference. Identification of tumors is important for several reasons. First, at necropsy each tumor should be identified in order to correlate histological classification with time of appearance. Secondly, not all palpable masses in the mammary region are actually mammary tumors: enlarged lymph nodes, epidermal cysts, milkpools, and salivary or preputial glands may be mistaken for tumors, and these errors in palpation can be detected at necropsy or via histopathological evaluation. Finally, induced mammary cancers in rats do occasionally undergo spontaneous regression;[18] notation of the location of a palpable mass will aid in determining whether the mass regressed completely or merely to a non-palpable size.

A highly potent mammary carcinogen such as DMBA or N-methyl-N-nitrosourea (MNU) will induce tumors after very short latent periods; the first tumors induced by high doses of either of these agents will become palpable 4 to 6 weeks after administration of the carcinogen.[6,19] By contrast, however, the first tumor induced by a less potent mammary carcinogen such as B(a)P may have a latent period of more than nine months.[20] Thus, conduct of a screening study for only six months may not be adequate to assess the activity of a test compound as a mammary carcinogen.

It shoud be noted that no consistent pattern is evident in mammary tumor growth, nor is the rate of growth of a palpable mammary tumor necessarily related to its latency. Tumors with long latent periods can grow rapidly, while the size of a lesion which became palpable early in a study may remain static for long periods.[2] Indeed, a single animal may bear several tumors with widely varying growth rates: one or two palpable lesions may grow rapidly while others remain static or actually regress.

Necropsy and Histopathology

At the termination of the study, sections of all palpable and non-palpable mammary tumors should be taken for histopathological analysis. Transillumination of the skin in the mammary regions can be of great help in locating non-palpable lesions. Histopathological classification of mammary tumors is extremely important in assessment of carcinogenicity, because the ratio of malignant to benign mammary lesions can vary by chemical and by dose of the same chemical.

Benign lesions (fibroadenomas, adenomas, fibromas) can frequently be detected during palpation by their soft, rubbery consistency. By contrast, mammary carcinomas tend to exhibit a much firmer lesion, albeit one that is not infrequently accompanied by central necrosis. However, because a relatively high percentage of mammary tumors are of mixed histological type, palpation alone is not an adequate predictor of tumor histology. Furthermore, it is very useful to obtain multiple sections of large mammary tumors, since the histology of large lesions may show considerable intratumoral variability.

Routine histopathological processing and staining with hematoxylin and eosin are generally adequate for mammary tumors. The predominant tumor type is an adenocarcinoma, with or without papillary characteristics, and mixed adeno-carcinoma/fibroadenomas are fairly common. Although metastases to the lung, spleen and kidney have been reported for certain classes of carcinogens, such as nitrosamides,[19,21] they are infrequent occurrences. A useful discussion of tumor pathology in the rat mammary gland has been presented by Young and Hallowes.[2]

CHARACTERISTICS OF THE RAT MAMMARY CARCINOMA MODEL SYSTEM

Attributes and Limitations

The rat mammary adenocarcinoma model system has a number of attributes which make it a useful limited bioassay of carcinogenic potency. Perhaps most important of these attributes is the fact that mammary cancers can be induced in female Sprague-Dawley rats by a wide variety of chemical and physical agents: structurally unrelated compounds such as the polycyclic aromatic hydrocarbon, DMBA, and the nitrosamide, MNU, are both potent mammary carcinogens. Although it has not been demonstrated that the activity of various classes of carcinogens in the induction of mammary tumors necessarily parallels their activity in other test systems, the broad spectrum of chemicals with mammary carcinogenic activity indicates that the utility of this test system is not limited to compounds of any one chemical class. Conversely, weak or non-carcinogens such as benz(a)anthracene and phenanthrene appear to have little or no activity as mammary oncogens.[22]

A second attribute of the mammary model system is that tumors can ordinarily be induced with a single intravenous or intragastric dose, rather than by chronic dietary administration of the test agent. This single dose protocol allows for precise determination not only of administered dose, but also of tumor latent period. Additional advantages of a single dose model are that less test compound is required for an assay than would be required for dietary administration, and potential problems of animal room contamination and exposure of personnel to hazardous substances are minimized.

Induced mammary tumors are predominantly of epithelial origin (adenocarcinomas and papillary carcinomas), although an occasional mammary sarcoma is observed. Since the vast majority of clinically significant human tumors are of epithelial origin, the induction of an epithelial lesion in this model system is an advantage. Furthermore, induced rat mammary carcinomas bear many histological similarities to human breast carcinomas.[2] Certain physiologic characteristics of chemically-induced rat mammary cancers, such as hormone dependence[1] and modulation by pregnancy and lactation[16] also parallel the human situation.

The superficial location of the rat mammary glands allows the detection of tumors by palpation, thus permitting accurate determination of tumor latent period without serial sacrifice necessitating the use of a large number of animals. In addition, because each animal possesses six pairs of glands, multiple discrete lesions may be detected; this yields data concerning tumor multiplicity as well as incidence and latent period, data which can be used in the assessment of carcinogenic potency.

A final attribute of this model system is the existence of established dose-response relationships for carcinogens of several different classes. The availability of established rat mammary carcinogens for use as a positive control in assays for mammary carcinogenesis may facilitate data interpretation.

Although this model system does have a variety of attributes as previously discussed, certain limitations of the system should be mentioned. Probably the most important of these limitations is the occurrence of spontaneous mammary tumors in older animals. Lifetime studies conducted in our and other laboratories have noted incidences of mammary tumors of up to 50% to 60% in untreated groups of Sprague-Dawley rats.[4,5,19] In terms of multiplicity, benign tumors (fibroadenomas and adenomas) are the predominant tumor type, although spontaneous mammary cancer has been observed in up to approximately 25% of rats older than two years. The presence of such a high incidence of spontaneous tumors can be of significant consequence when interpreting studies involving compounds of weak or equivocal carcinogenic activity: is a tumor, particularly a benign tumor, which appeared in a treated animal at 700 days of age an effect of exposure to the test chemical, or is it due to a "background" incidence of such lesions in the population? However, spontaneous tumors become of significance only if the assay period extends beyond six to nine months.

A second limiting factor is the possibility that a compound may induce mammary cancer not as a result of its direct action on the mammary gland, but as a secondary effect due to the induction of tumors or toxicity in another organ. For instance, Furth *et al.* have reported that chronic administration of estrogens can induce prolactin-secreting pituitary tumors in rats.[23] Shellabarger and colleagues[24,25] have produced mammary cancers in ACI rats by subcutaneous implantation of a cholesterol pellet containing the synthetic estrogen diethylstilbestrol (DES). The dose-response for mammary tumor induction parallels that for the induction of pituitary tumors and hyperprolactinemia by DES,[25] suggesting that the carcinogenic effect of this agent in the mammary gland is an indirect one, mediated via the induction of a pituitary tumor. Although the same effect apparently does not occur in Sprague-Dawley rats,[24] its existence in any rat mammary tumor system should suggest caution in the determination of carcinogenic mechanism: an agent which appears to be a potent mammary carcinogen may be exerting its effect via influences on the pituitary, ovaries, or other extra-mammary site.

Because administration of test compounds in this animal model is systemic, the potential exists for the induction of tumors in non-target organs. Should treatment with a test agent result in the rapid induction of mammary tumors, such non-mammary tumor induction will most likely be incidental. However, administration of agents which are not potent mammary carcinogens, or of low doses of compounds with mammary carcinogenic activity, may induce significant oncogenesis in non-mammary sites. The influence of such induction of non-mammary tumors on patterns of mammary tumorigenesis has not been studied systematically, but could dramatically alter patterns of mammary cancer response. It appears that production of non-mammary tumors occurs infrequently with polycyclic aromatic hydrocarbons, but may be a routine occurrence with various N-nitroso compounds.[19,26]

A final limitation of this tumor system is one that is common to many rodent carcinogenesis test systems, namely, absence of tumor metastases. Local invasion and metastases have been observed with tumors induced by MNU, although metastasis is an infrequent occurrence.[19] To our knowledge, evidence of metastasis of mammary cancers induced by polycyclic aromatic hydrocarbons is lacking.

Possible Modifications

The basic mammary carcinogenesis protocol as described above should provide a reasonable mechanism for the identification of agents which merit further study in long-term animal bioassays for carcinogenicity. However, several modifications of this assay system can be utilized in the attempt to increase the sensitivity of the test system; such modifications may allow the detection of agents with very weak carcinogenic activity in the mammary gland.

In the basic protocol, animals are fed a standard laboratory chow diet, containing approximately 5% fat by weight. Induction of tumors can be increased slightly by feeding a semi-purified diet containing 5% fat.[3] Although the mechanism by which the semi-purified diet increases cancer response is unknown, it has been postulated that the presence of natural inhibitors of carcinogenicity in the chow diet and their absence in the semi-purified diet may be involved. In addition, due to periodic changes in the composition of chow diets, inter-experiment variability in dose-response patterns may be minimized with the use of a semi-purified diet.

A much larger increase in mammary cancer response can be induced by increasing the fat content of the experimental diet from the normal 5% to 20% or 25% by weight.[27] This increased fat content, while far in excess of the nutritional requirements of the rat, more closely simulates the fat content of the human diet in Western societies. A significant correlation between consumption of fat and incidence of breast cancer has been found in human populations.[28] Similarly, rats exposed to a carcinogen and then fed a diet containing 10% or 20% fat show a significantly increased response to a given dose of carcinogen than do rats fed a diet containing 0.5% or 5% fat.[29] This increased response is characterized by increased incidence of mammary cancer and multiplicity, with a decreased tumor latent period in comparison to animals fed the lower fat regimen.

The mechanism by which high fat diets enhance mammary carcinogenesis remains an area of controversy. Although conflicting data have been reported, current evidence indicates that feeding a high fat diet does not act via an elevation of serum prolactin levels.[30] Similarly, while a variety of mechanisms involving prostaglandins, lipid peroxidation, and immune function have been presented, none can be identified at this time as the predominant route by which dietary fat stimulates the induction of cancer.

A second method by which mammary cancer response may be increased is via surgical procedures or administration of drugs which will increase circulating levels of estrogens or prolactin; conversely, endocrine ablation or administration of antihormones will decrease cancer response.[31] As with high fat diets, such manipulations will increase the incidence of cancer and multiplicity while decreasing latent period. Current evidence suggests that prolactin has direct effects on the rat mammary gland, while the effects of estrogens may be mediated by influences on prolactin synthesis or release in the pituitary, or by alterations of prolactin binding in the target tissue.[31]

Although increasing dietary fat content or hormonal manipulation may increase the incidence and multiplicity of induced tumors, the possibility exists that a similar enhancement of "spontaneous" tumorigenesis will occur.[32] Such an enhancement may not influence studies where the agent induces tumors with a relatively short latent period. However, in the case of a compound inducing few mammary tumors which become palpable only after a long latent period, any such stimulation of "spontaneous" tumorigenesis may complicate data interpretation.

A final modification of the test system which may address such problems would be the use of a rat strain other than the Sprague-Dawley. Although Sprague-Dawley rats are generally considered to be most sensitive to induction of tumors, this strain develops a high incidence of spontaneous tumors. In addition, tumors induced in Sprague-Dawley rats by some classes of compounds, particularly polycyclic aromatic hydrocarbons, may be predominantly benign fibroadenomas rather than adenocarcinomas. The use of strains of rats with lower rates of spontaneous appearance of tumor, and a higher malignant to benign tumor ratio, may be called for in some instances.

In response to chemical carcinogens such as DMBA, the Lewis rat develops adenocarcinomas almost exclusively, while Sprague-Dawley rats develop both adenocarcinomas and fibroadenomas in high multiplicity.[33] This lack of chemical induction of benign tumors in Lewis rats, when coupled with a spontaneous tumor response which is somewhat lower than that seen with the Sprague-Dawley strain, may make the use of Lewis rats beneficial in long-term assays with compounds of equivocal potency as mammary carcinogens. It should be noted, however, that in response to x-rays, tumorigenesis in Lewis rats resembles that in Sprague-Dawley rats in that malignant and benign mammary tumors are induced in both strains.[33] The reason for the differential response of Lewis rats to chemical and physical carcinogens is not known.

Perhaps due to its great sensitivity to induction of mammary tumors, the Sprague-Dawley rat shows less enhancement of carcinogenesis in response to increased dietary fat than do strains such as F344 and Long-Evans.[3] For this reason, induction of cancer by a weak carcinogen may be enhanced to a relatively greater extent by dietary or pharmacologic manipulation in F344 rats than in Sprague-Dawley rats. This greater enhancement of chemical carcinogenesis in F344 rats may obviate the potential problem of fat enhancement of "spontaneous" tumorigenesis in Sprague-Dawley rats, as discussed above. It should be noted, however, that the Sprague-Dawley rats are significantly more sensitive to mammary carcinogenesis than are F344 or Long-Evans rats, and appear to be slightly more sensitive than Lewis rats. Therefore, with the possible exception of long-term mammary carcinogenesis studies in which one may wish to attempt to increase the induced cancer response while avoiding the appearance of large numbers of induced benign or spontaneous tumors, the Sprague-Dawley rat remains the strain of choice for mammary carcinogenicity bioassays.

CHEMICAL AND PHYSICAL AGENTS WITH CARCINOGENIC ACTIVITY IN THE RAT MAMMARY GLAND

The chemical induction of mammary cancers in rats has been studied for more than 40 years. The earliest studies, conducted independently by Bielschowsky[34] and Shay and colleagues[35] examined the carcinogenic effects of N-acetyl-2-aminofluorene and 3-MC. In these and other studies conducted in the 1940's and 1950's, administration of carcinogen was chronic or subchronic in nature. In a now classic series of papers published between 1959 and 1962, Huggins reported that mammary cancers could be induced in rats by a single intragastric or intravenous administration of any of several polycyclic aromatic hydrocarbons.[1,6,21] It is this single dose model of induction of mammary cancer, often called the Huggins model, which has been the basis for much of the mammary carcinogenesis research over the past two decades.

Polycyclic Aromatic Hydrocarbons (PAH's)

Huggins tested a variety of PAH's for carcinogenic activity, finding DMBA to be the most potent.[22] Although DMBA was highly active in induction of mammary cancer, benz(a)anthracene had no carcinogenic activity in this model system, and the 7- and 12-monomethylbenz(a)anthracenes were of relatively low potency as mammary carcinogens. A similar situation was reported by Huggins with respect to phenanthrene: although the parent compound was inactive, 2-aminophenanthrene was highly potent as a mammary carcinogen.[22]

Subsequent to these early studies, a number of investigators have examined dose-response characteristics for induction of mammary tumors by PAH's. An intragastric instillation of 20 mg DMBA appears to be the most effective dose level for induction of mammary cancer; doses of DMBA above 20 mg are acutely toxic, inducing deaths due to massive necrosis in the adrenal cortex,[36] while doses below 20 mg result in decreases in carcinoma incidence and multiplicity. The generally accepted dose-time response parameters for DMBA are that administration of a single intragastric dose of 20 mg to 50 day old, virgin, female Sprague-Dawley rats will induce a near 100% incidence of mammary cancer in approximately 100 days. Non-mammary tumors induced by DMBA are observed infrequently, usually occurring in the ear duct.[2]

By comparison to the high potency of DMBA in induction of mammary cancer, intragastric administration of B(a)P induces mammary cancers in lower incidence with a much longer latent period. McCormick[20] noted a minimum latent period of approximately 35 weeks for induction of mammary cancer in rats treated with 100 mg B(a)P, with an incidence of cancer of approximately 70% at 650 days. In parallel studies conducted using DMBA and B(a)P as mammary carcinogens, a 100 mg dose of B(a)P was found to be equivalent to a dose of approximately 2 mg DMBA.[20] Similar data concerning the relatively low potency of B(a)P as a mammary carcinogen has been reported by Sydnor *et al.*[37]

3-MC appears to be intermediate between DMBA and B(a)P in potency as a mammary carcinogen: Huggins reported that a 100% incidence of mammary cancer can be induced with a single intragastric dose of 100 mg 3-MC.[6] In this study, 100 mg 3-MC was found to be approximately as active as a dose of 15 mg DMBA in terms of final incidence of cancer, tumor multiplicity, and latent period.

Aromatic Amides and Derivatives

The carcinogenicity of N-acetyl-2-aminofluorene (2-AAF) in the rat mammary gland was first described by Bielschowsky in 1944.[34] Huggins and colleagues found that 2-AAF had significant carcinogenic activity in the single dose mammary carcinogenesis model; the activity of an intragastric dose of 100 mg 2-AAF was similar to that of 10 mg 3-MC.[6]

Since these early studies, a number of aromatic amide derivatives (arylhydroxamic acids) have been shown to have carcinogenic activity in the rat mammary gland.[38,39] However, due to the highly reactive nature of the arylhydroxamic acids, induction of tumors with these agents has been achieved via topical application or local injection rather than intragastric or intravenous administration. A comparative study by Allaben *et al.*[39] found N-hydroxy-N-acetyl-2-aminofluorene to be the most potent of these compounds when administered by local injection; when the acetyl moiety was replaced by a formyl or propionyl group, carcinogenicity was reduced.

Nitrosamides

The nitrosamides, MNU and N-ethyl-N-nitrosourea (ENU), are two of the more potent mammary carcinogens in the rat. Administration of a single dose of either of these compounds by any of a number of routes (MNU: intravenous, subcutaneous; ENU: intraperitoneal) results in the rapid induction of mammary cancers without acute toxicity in treated animals.[19,26] On a weight basis, MNU appears to be as active as DMBA in inducing mammary cancer. Although the histological and physiologic characteristics of MNU-induced mammary cancers resemble tumors induced by DMBA, the MNU-induced lesions have the additional, although infrequent, capacity to invade locally and metastasize to distant sites.[19]

Administration of MNU to female rats, as originally described by Gullino[40] and subsequently modified to a single dose model in our laboratory,[19] provides a model for mammary carcinogenesis which is currently being investigated as intensively as the DMBA model. The MNU model has the advantage of a direct acting carcinogen with a short half-life at physiologic pH;[41] similar dose-response characteristics have been reported for intravenous and subcutaneous administration of MNU.[42] Metastases, although infrequent, have been observed in the lung, liver, and kidney of MNU-treated animals.[19,21] By contrast, tumor metastases have not been reported for the DMBA model. In addition, MNU appears to induce a higher ratio of adenocarcinomas to fibroadenomas in Sprague-Dawley rats than does DMBA.[19] The ENU model is less well characterized than the MNU model, although the incidence, latency, and hormone dependence of ENU-induced mammary cancers[26] appear to resemble those of lesions induced by MNU. Induction of mammary cancer by other members of this class of compounds has not been reported.

One limitation of induction of mammary cancer by nitrosamides is their lack of absolute target organ specificity at low doses. Although high doses of MNU induce mammary tumors almost exclusively, lower doses induce primary epithelial tumors of the kidney and lung, and sarcomas of a variety of abdominal organs in addition to mammary tumors.[19] Similarly, induction by ENU of renal sarcomas, neural tumors, and lymphomas occurs in addition to carcinogenesis in the mammary gland.[26]

Ethyl Methanesulfonate

Recent reports by Ueo *et al.*[43,44] indicate that oral administration of ethyl methanesulfonate can induce a high incidence of mammary cancers in rats. By contrast, methyl methanesulfonate appears to lack this mammary carcinogenic activity. As was seen with lower doses of MNU, administration of ethyl methane-sulfonate induces tumors at extra mammary sites (sarcomas of kidney and uterus) in addition to mammary cancers.

Radiation

The induction of rat mammary carcinomas by radiation has been studied extensively. Shellabarger and colleagues have reported the induction of mammary tumors in Sprague-Dawley rats following single exposures to neutrons, x-rays, or ^{60}Co gamma rays.[45,46] In general, exposure to radiation produced a tumor response which could be defined as a forward shift in the spontaneous incidence curve;[45] a similar effect of weak mammary carcinogens [*i.e.*, B(a)P] has been noted.[47] However, several differences between induction of rat mammary cancer by radiation and chemicals have been reported. Administration of DMBA or other chemical carcinogens results in the preferential induction of mammary cancers in the cervical-thoracic as opposed to the abdominal-inguinal mammary chains;[17] by contrast, no such preferential induction of tumors in the cervical-thoracic mammary glands is observed following exposure to x-rays.[48] In addition, radiation-induced mammary carcinogenesis does not appear to be age-dependent in virgin females, nor is it altered by pregnancy and lactation, findings in direct opposition to the situation observed in rats exposed to chemical carcinogens.[49] The reasons for such differences in chemically-induced and radiation-induced mammary carcinogenesis are unknown; however, the lack of effect of age and parity on radiation carcinogenesis suggests that this process may exhibit a qualitatively different response to alterations in cell kinetics or tissue differentiation in the mammary gland than does the induction of mammary carcinogenesis by chemicals.

REFERENCES

1. Huggins, C., Briziarelli, G., and Sutton, H., Jr., Rapid induction of mammary carcinoma in the rat and the influence of hormones on the tumors. *J. Exp. Med.* 109: 25-41 (1959)

2. Young, S., and Hallowes, R.C., in: *Pathology of Tumours in Laboratory Animals* (V.S. Turusov, ed.), Vol. 1–Tumours of the Rat, part 1, pp 31–74, International Agency for Research on Cancer, Lyon (1973)

3. Chan, P.C., and Dao, T.L., Enhancement of mammary carcinogenesis by a high fat diet in Fischer, Long-Evans, and Sprague-Dawley rats. *Cancer Res.* 41: 164–167 (1981)

4. Noble, R.L., and Cutts, J.H., Mammary tumors of the rat: a review. *Cancer Res.* 19: 1125–1139 (1959)

5. Okada, M., Takeuchi, J., Sobue, M., Kataoka, K., Inagaki, Y., Shigemura, M., and Chiba, T., Characteristics of 106 spontaneous mammary tumours appearing in Sprague-Dawley female rats. *Br. J. Cancer* 43: 689–695 (1981)

6. Huggins, C., Grand, L.C., and Brillantes, F.P., Mammary cancer induced by a single feeding of polynuclear hydrocarbons, and its suppression. *Nature* 189: 204–207 (1961)

7. Sinha, D.K., and Dao, T.L., Induction of mammary tumors in aging rats by 7,12-dimethylbenz(a)anthracene: role of DNA synthesis during carcinogenesis. *J. Natl. Cancer Inst.* 64: 519–521 (1980)

8. Nagasawa, H., Yanai, R., and Taniguchi, H., Importance of mammary gland DNA synthesis on carcinogen-induced mammary tumorigenesis in rats. *Cancer Res.* 36: 2223–2226 (1976)

9. Dao, T.L., Mammary cancer induction by 7,12-dimethylbenz(a)anthracene: relation to age. *Science* 165: 810–811 (1969)

10. Nagasawa, H., and Yanai, R., Brief Communication: Frequency of mammary cell division in relation to age: its significance in the induction of mammary tumors by carcinogen in rats. *J. Natl. Cancer Inst.* 52: 609–610 (1974)

11. Russo, J., and Russo, I.H., DNA labelling index and structure of the rat mammary gland as determinants of its susceptibility to carcinogenesis. *J. Natl. Cancer Inst.* 61: 1451–1459 (1978)

12. Hadfield, G., and Young, J.S., The mammotrophic potency of human urine. *Br. J. Cancer* 10: 145–168 (1956)

13. Greiner, J.W., Bryan, A.H., Malan-Shibley, L.B., and Janss, D.H., Aryl hydrocarbon hydroxylase and epoxide hydratase activities: age effects in mammary epithelial cells of Sprague-Dawley rats. *J. Natl. Cancer Inst.* 64: 1127–1133 (1980)

14. Tay, L.K., and Russo, J., Formation and removal of 7,12-dimethylbenz(a)-anthracene-nucleic acid adducts in rat mammary epithelial cells with different susceptibility to carcinogenesis. *Carcinogenesis* 2: 1327–1333 (1981)

15. Tay, L.K., and Russo, J., 7,12-Dimethylbenz(a)anthracene-induced DNA binding and repair synthesis in susceptible and nonsusceptible mammary epithelial cells in culture. *J. Natl. Cancer Inst.* 67: 155–161 (1981)

16. Moon, R.C., in: *Banbury Report 8: Hormones and Breast Cancer* (M.C. Pike, P.K. Siiteri, and C.W. Welsch, eds.), pp 353–364, Cold Spring Harbor Laboratory, Cold Spring Harbor, New York (1981)

17. Torgersen, O., Regional distribution of DMBA-induced mammary tumours in the rat. *Acta Path. Microbiol. Scand. Sect. A.* 83: 639–644 (1975)

18. Young, S., and Cowan, D.M., Spontaneous regression of induced mammary tumours in rats. *Br. J. Cancer* 17: 85–89 (1963)

19. McCormick, D.L., Adamowski, C.B., Fiks, A., and Moon, R.C., Lifetime dose-response relationships for mammary tumor induction by a single administration of N-methyl-N-nitrosourea. *Cancer Res.* 41: 1690–1694 (1981)

20. McCormick, D.L., Influence of retinyl acetate administration schedule on inhibition of rat mammary carcinogenesis. Ph.D dissertation, New York University (1979)

21. Moon, R.C., Grubbs, C.J., Sporn, M.B., and Goodman, D.G., Retinyl acetate inhibits mammary carcinogenesis induced by N-methyl-N-nitrosourea. *Nature* 267: 620-621 (1977)

22. Huggins, C., and Yang, N.C., Induction and extinction of mammary cancer. *Science* 137: 257-262 (1962)

23. Furth, J., Clifton, K.H., Gadsden, E.L., and Buffett, R.F., Dependent and autonomous mammotropic pituitary tumors in rats: their somatotropic features. *Cancer Res.* 16: 608-616 (1956)

24. Shellabarger, C.J., Stone, J.P., and Holtzman, S., Rat differences in mammary tumor induction with estrogen and neutron radiation. *J. Natl. Cancer Inst.* 61: 1505-1508 (1978)

25. Stone, J.P., Holtzman, S., and Shellabarger, C.J., Synergistic interactions of various doses of diethylstilbestrol and x-irradiation on mammary neoplasia in female ACI rats. *Cancer Res.* 40: 3966-3972 (1980)

26. Stoica, G., Koestner, A., and Capen, C.C., Characterization of N-ethyl-N-nitrosourea-induced mammary tumors in the rat. *Am. J. Pathol.* 110: 161-169 (1983)

27. Carroll, K.K., and Khor, H.T., Effects of dietary fat and dose level of 7,12-dimethylbenz(a)anthracene on mammary tumor incidence in rats. *Cancer Res.* 30: 2260-2264 (1970)

28. Carroll, K.K., and Khor, H.T., Dietary fat in relation to tumorigenesis. *Prog. Biochem. Pharmacol.* 10: 308-353 (1975)

29. Carroll, K.K., and Khor, H.T., Effects of level and type of dietary fat on incidence of mammary tumors induced in female Sprague-Dawley rats by 7,12-dimethylbenz(a)anthracene. *Lipids* 6: 415-420 (1971)

30. Ip, C., Yip, P., and Bernardis, L.L., Role of prolactin in the promotion of dimethylbenz(a)anthracene-induced mammary tumors by dietary fat. *Cancer Res.* 40: 374-378 (1980)

31. Welsch, C.W., and Nagasawa, H., Prolactin and murine mammary tumorigenesis: a review. *Cancer Res.* 37: 951-963 (1977)

32. Benson, J., Lev, M., and Grand, C.G., Enhancement of mammary fibroadenomas in the female rat by a high fat diet. *Cancer Res.* 16: 135-138 (1956)

33. Shellabarger, C.J., Mammary neoplastic response of Lewis and Sprague-Dawley female rats to 7,12-dimethylbenz(a)anthracene or x-ray. *Cancer Res.* 32: 883-885 (1972)

34. Bielschowsky, F., Distant tumours produced by 2-amino- and 2-acetyl-amino-fluorene. *Brit. J. Exp. Pathol.* 25: 1-4 (1944)

35. Shay, H., Aegerter, E.A., Gruenstein, M., and Komarov, S.A., Development of adenocarcinoma of the breast in the Wistar rat following the gastric instillation of methylcholanthrene. *J. Natl. Cancer. Inst.* 10: 255-270 (1949)

36. Huggins, C., and Morii, S., Selective adrenal necrosis and apoplexy induced by 7,12-dimethylbenz(a)anthracene. *J. Exp. Med.* 114: 741-760 (1961)

37. Sydnor, K.L., Allen, C., and Higgins, B., Effect of an aqueous extract of cigarette smoke condensate on benzo(a)pyrene-induced sarcoma and body weight in the rat. *J. Natl. Cancer Inst.* 48: 893-909 (1972)

38. Malejka-Giganti, D., Gutmann, H.R., and Rydell, R.E., Mammary carcinogenesis in the rat by topical application of fluorenylhydroxamic acids. *Cancer Res.* 33: 2489-2497 (1973)

39. Allaben, W.T., Weeks, C.E., Weis, C.C., Burger, G.T., and King, C.M., Rat mammary gland carcinogenesis after local injection of N-hydroxy-N-acyl-2-aminofluorenes: relationship to metabolic activation. *Carcinogenesis* 3: 233-240 (1982)
40. Gullino, P.M., Pettigrew, H.M., and Grantham, F.H., N-Nitrosomethylurea as mammary gland carcinogen in rats. *J. Natl. Cancer Inst.* 54: 401-414 (1975)
41. Druckrey, H., Preussmann, R., Ivankovic, S., and Schmahl, D., Organotrope carcinogene Wirkungen bei 65 verschiedenen N-Nitroso-Verbindungen an BD-Ratten *Z. Krebsforsch* 69: 103-201 (1967)
42. Thompson, H.J., and Meeker, L.D., Induction of mammary gland carcinomas by the subcutaneous injection of 1-methyl-1-nitrosourea. *Cancer Res.* 43: 1628-1629 (1983)
43. Ueo, H., Ryosaburo, T., Yamagami, H., Nakano, S., Okeda, T., and Sakikibara, K., High incidence of rat mammary carcinoma by oral administration of ethyl methanesulphonate. *Cancer Lett.* 7: 79-84 (1979)
44. Ueo, H., Takaki, R., Yamagami, H., and Sugimachi, K., Mammary carcinoma induced by oral administration of ethyl methanesulphonate. Determination of some of the parameters affecting tumor induction. *Carcinogenesis* 2: 1223-1228 (1981)
45. Shellabarger, C.J., Chmelevsky, D., and Kellerer, A.M., Induction of mammary neoplasms in the Sprague-Dawley rat by 430-KeV neutrons and x-rays. *J. Natl. Cancer Inst.* 821-833 (1980)
46. Shellabarger, C.J., Bond, V.P., Aponte, G.E., and Cronkite, E.P., Results of fractionation and protraction of total-body radiation on rat mammary neoplasia. *Cancer Res.* 26: 509-513 (1966)
47. Burns, F.J., and McCormick, D.L., Unpublished observations.
48. Shellabarger, C.J., in: *Biology of Radiation Carcinogenesis* (J.M. Yuhas, R.W. Tennant, and J.D. Regan, eds.), pp 31-43, Raven Press, New York (1976)
49. Holtzman, S., Stone, J.P. and Shellabarger, C.J., Radiation-induced mammary carcinogenesis in virgin, pregnant, lactating and post lactating rats. *Cancer Res.* 42: 50-53 (1982)

11

SENCAR Mouse Skin Tumorigenesis

Thomas J. Slaga

The University of Texas System Cancer Center
Science Park–Research Division
Smithville, Texas

Stephen Nesnow

U.S. Environmental Protection Agency
Research Triangle Park, North Carolina

INTRODUCTION

In order to better understand the SENCAR mouse skin tumorigenesis model, it is necessary to first discuss some important aspects of the induction of skin tumors in mice in general. It is well known that skin tumors (*e.g.*, papillomas, keratoacanthomas, and squamous cell carcinomas) can be induced in mice by the sequential application of a subthreshold dose of a carcinogen (initiation stage) followed by repetitive treatment with a non-carcinogenic tumor promoter (promotion stage). The initiation stage requires only a single application of either a direct or an indirect carcinogen at a subthreshold dose and is essentially irreversible, while the promotion stage is brought about by repetitive treatments after initiation and is initially reversible, later becoming irreversible.[1] This system can be used not only to determine the tumor-initiating and promoting activities of a compound, but if the agent is given repeatedly by itself, one can also determine if it is a complete carcinogen, *i.e.*, if it has both tumor initiating and promoting activities. In addition, if the agent is given concurrently with a known complete carcinogen or a tumor initiator one can also determine if the agent has co-carcinogenic or co-initiating activity. Likewise, if the agent is given concurrently with a known tumor promoter one can determine if the agent has co-promoting or anti-promoting activity. Furthermore, as in most carcinogenic systems, skin carcinogens may have additive or synergistic effects. This system has provided an important model not only for studying carcinogenesis and for bio-assaying carcinogenic agents, but also for the study of modifiers of carcinogenesis. The major disadvantage of the skin system is that some carcinogens are tissue specific.

Figure 1 summarizes schematically both complete and two-stage carcinogenesis in mouse skin. A single large dose of a carcinogen such as 7,12-dimethylbenz(a)anthracene (DMBA) is capable of inducing skin tumors in mice. Papillomas and some keratoacanthomas occur after a relatively short latent period (ten to 20 weeks); squamous cell carcinomas develop after a much longer period (20 to 60 weeks). If this dose is decreased, it becomes necessary to administer DMBA repeatedly in order to induce tumors. If progressively reduced, a subthreshold dose of DMBA is reached that does not give rise to tumors over the lifespan of the mouse.[2] If either croton oil or a phorbol ester such as 12-O-tetradecanoylphorbol-13-acetate (TPA) is subsequently applied repetitively to the backs of mice previously given a single subthreshold dose of DMBA for initiation, multiple papillomas and some keratoacanthomas will appear after a short latent period followed by squamous cell carcinomas after a much longer period. The repetitive application of the promoter without initiation by DMBA, in general either does not give rise to tumors or produces only a few, but never in a dose-response relationship.[3] If mice receive a subthreshold dose of a carcinogen such as DMBA as the initiator, there is a very good dose-response using TPA as the promoter.[3] Likewise, there is a very good dose-response with benzo(a)pyrene [B(a)P] or DMBA as tumor initiators when the dose of a promoter is held constant.[4] The order of treatments of the initiator and promoter is also important. If repetitive applications of the promoter are administered before initiation, no tumors will develop.

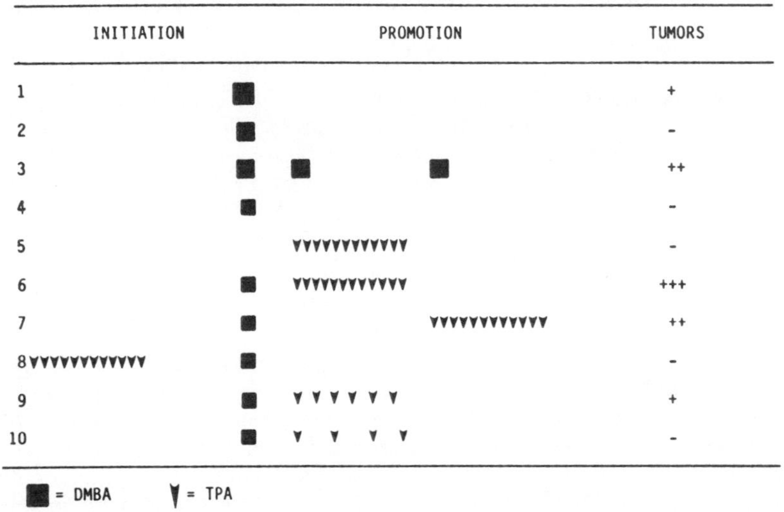

	INITIATION	PROMOTION	TUMORS
1	■		+
2	■		-
3	■ ■	■	++
4	■		-
5		ＶＶＶＶＶＶＶＶＶＶＶＶＶ	-
6	■	ＶＶＶＶＶＶＶＶＶＶＶＶ	+++
7	■	ＶＶＶＶＶＶＶＶＶＶＶＶ	++
8	ＶＶＶＶＶＶＶＶＶＶＶＶ ■		-
9	■	Ｖ Ｖ Ｖ Ｖ Ｖ Ｖ	+
10	■	Ｖ Ｖ Ｖ Ｖ	-

■ = DMBA   Ｖ = TPA

Figure 1: A schematic diagram of complete and two-stage skin carcinogenesis.

The real hallmark of the two-stage carcinogenesis system in mouse skin is the irreversibility of tumor initiation. A lapse of up to one year between the application of the initiator and the beginning of the promoter treatment provides a tumor response similar to that observed when the promoter is given only one week following initiation.[2] Unlike the initiation stage, the promotion stage is reversible, requiring a certain frequency of application in order to induce tumors.[2,5]

In general, mice are more sensitive than rats and hamsters to skin carcinogenesis by either the complete carcinogenesis protocol or by the initiation-promotion protocol.[5] The complete carcinogenesis protocol in mice gives rise to a low number of papillomas and keratoacanthomas followed by a moderate incidence of squamous cell carcinomas. Both the complete carcinogenesis and initiation-promotion protocols in rats give rise to basal cell carcinomas and very few papillomas and squamous cell carcinomas. The complete carcinogenesis protocol in hamsters produces mainly squamous cell carcinomas and some melanomas, whereas the initiation-promotion protocol produces primarily melanomas.

COMPLETE *vs* TWO-STAGE SKIN CARCINOGENESIS

Under appropriate test conditions, skin carcinogens show skin tumor initiating activity.[4,5] In a two-stage mouse skin system, initiation is the only stage that requires the presence of the carcinogen, and the measured carcinogenic potency of a chemical reflects its capacity for tumor initiation. There is both a good qualitative and quantitative correlation in mouse skin between the complete carcinogenic and tumor-initiating activities of several chemical carcinogens (Table 1). This is true when one considers the number of papillomas per mouse at early times (ten to 20 weeks) or the final incidence of carcinomas after tumor initiation.

Table 1: Comparison of Complete Carcinogenesis and Initiation of Carcinogenicity in Mouse Skin

| Compound | . . . . Relative Potency* . . . . | |
	Complete Carcinogenesis, Carcinomas	Initiation, Papillomas
7,12-Dimethylbenz(a)anthracene	100	100
3-Methylcholanthrene	50	50
Benzo(a)pyrene	30	30
2-Hydroxybenzo(a)pyrene	30	30
7-Bromomethyl-12-methylbenz-(a)anthracene	20	20
Benzo(a)pyrene-7,8-oxide	20	20
Dibenz(a,h)anthracene	20	20
Benz(a)anthracene	5	5
Dibenz(a,c)anthracene	0	3
Pyrene	0	0
Benzo(a)pyrene-4,5-oxide	0	0
Anthracene	0	0

*Relative potency was determined from dose-response data. 7,12-Dimethylbenz(a)anthracene was given a maximum value of 100.[5]

A carcinogen lacking promoting ability may not be detected when tested as a complete carcinogen. In confirmation, a number of chemical compounds have tumor-initiating activity but lack complete carcinogenic activity;[4] these are listed in Table 2. Due to these considerations, we feel that it is important to test a compound as a tumor initiator as well as a complete carcinogen.

Table 2: Agents That Are Possible Pure Initiators of Carcinogenicity in Mouse Skin*

Benzo(a)pyrene-7,8-diol-9,10-epoxide
N-Methyl-N'-nitro-N-nitrosoguanidine
Benz(a)anthracene-3,4-diol-1,2-epoxide
Benz(a)anthracene
Dibenz(a,c)anthracene
Chrysene
Urethane
Triethylenemelamine

*Reviewed in reference 5

Table 3: Polycyclic Aromatic Hydrocarbons, Derivatives and Metabolites That Are Positive as Initiators of Skin Carcinogenicity and/or Carcinogens*

1. Over 100 polycyclic aromatic hydrocarbons, derivatives and metabolites have been found to be positive as initiators of skin carcinogenicity and/or carcinogens.

2. Examples of polycyclic aromatic hydrocarbons that are moderate to strong initiators of skin carcinogenicity and/or carcinogens:

   7,12-Dimethylbenz(a)anthracene
   3-Methylcholanthrene
   Benzo(a)pyrene
   7-Methylbenz(a)anthracene
   5-Methylchrysene
   Dibenz(a,h)anthracene
   Dibenzo(a,h)pyrene
   Dibenzo(a,i)pyrene
   Dibenzo(a,e)pyrene
   Benzo(o)phenanthrene
   Dibenzo(a,j)anthracene
   Benzo(c)chrysene
   Benzo(g,h,i)perylene
   Dibenzo(a,c)naphthacene
   11-Methylcyclopenta(a)phenanthren-17-one

*Source of data is reference 5

Polycyclic aromatic hydrocarbons (PAH) are one of the major classes of chemical carcinogens that have skin tumor initiating and/or complete carcinogenic activity on mouse skin and have been studied extensively in this system. As summarized in Table 3, over 100 PAH's, PAH derivatives, and PAH metabolites are known to be mouse skin tumor initiators and/or complete carcinogens.[4,5] In addition, the mouse skin tumorigenesis bioassay system has identified many potential carcinogens other than PAH's (Table 4). These chemicals represent a wide

Table 4: Chemicals Other than Polycyclic Aromatic Hydrocarbons That Are Positive as Initiators of Skin Carcinogenicity and/or Carcinogens*

Class	Chemical
Aldehyde	Malonaldehyde
Aziridine	2-Hydroxy-1-ethylaziridine
Carbamate	Urethane Vinyl carbamate N-Butyl-N-nitrosourethane
Epoxide, diepoxide	Glycidaldehyde 1,2,3,4-Diepoxybutane 1,2,4,5-Diepoxypentane 1,2,6,7-Diepoxyhexane Chloroethylene oxide 1,2-Epoxybutyronitrile
Haloalkylether	Bis(chloromethyl)ether 1,1-Dichloromethyl methyl ether Chloromethyl methyl ether
Haloaromatic	2,3,4,5-Tetrachloronitrobenzene 2,3,4,6-Tetrachloronitrobenzene 2,3,5,6-Tetrachloronitrobenzene Pentachloronitrobenzene
Haloalkyl ketone, acid	Chloroacetone 3-Bromopropionic acid
Hydroxylamine	N-Acetoxy-4-acetamidobiphenyl N-Acetoxy-2-acetamidofluorene N-Hydroxy-2-aminonaphthalene N-Acetoxy-N-acetamidophenanthrene N-(4-Methoxy)benzoyloxypiperidine N-(4-Nitro)benzoyloxypiperidine N-Acetoxy-2-acetamidostilbene
Lactone	Propiolactone
Multifunctional	Triethylenemelamine 4-Nitroquinoline-N-oxide
Natural products	Aflatoxin B_1 Sterigmatocystin
Nitrosamide	N-Methyl-N'-nitro-N-nitrosoguanidine
Sulfonate	Allyl methylsulfonate
Sultone	1,3-Propanesultone
Urea	N-Nitrosomethylurea N-Nitrosoethylurea

*Reviewed in reference 6

variety of structural classes including: aldehyde, carbamate, epoxide, haloalkylether, haloaromatic, haloalkylketone, hydroxylamine, lactone, nitrosamide, sulfonate, sultone, and urea. This list of 32 chemicals includes such well-known carcinogens as aflatoxin B_1, bis(chloromethyl) ether, chloromethyl methyl ether, urethane, N-acetoxy-2-acetamidofluorene, β-propiolactone, N-methyl-N'-nitro-N-nitrosoguanidine, 1,3-propanesultone, N-nitrosomethylurea, triethylenemelamine, and 4-nitroquinoline-N-oxide. In addition to the response in the mouse skin bioassay to compounds other than PAH's, chemicals which cause tumors in the respiratory tract of animals can also be detected (Table 5). Of 11 known animal respiratory carcinogens, the mouse skin tumorigenesis system has to this date detected polycyclic aromatic hydrocarbons, quinolines, and carbamates. Of 11 highly suspect occupational respiratory carcinogens, the mouse skin system has detected chloromethyl ethers and coke oven emissions. This indicates that the mouse skin bioassay has a broad spectrum capability for detecting agents that are dermal as well as nondermal carcinogens.

Table 5: Response of Carcinogens in Humans, Animals, and Mouse Skin

	Occupational Respiratory Carcinogen*	Animal Respiratory Carcinogen*	Mouse Skin Tumorigen**
Arsenic	+		
Asbestos	+	+	
Beryllium	+	+	
Carbamates		+	+
Chloromethyl ethers	+	+	+
Chromium	+		
Coke oven	+		+
Isopropyl oil	+		
MBOCA	+	+	
Mustard gas	+	+	
Nickel	+	+	
Nitrosamines		+	
Polycyclic aromatics		+	+
Quinolines		+	+
Vinyl chloride	+	+	

*Reviewed in reference 7
**Reviewed in reference 8

A diversity of chemical agents act as skin tumor promoters.[3] Following the diterpenes (phorbol esters), indole alkaloids (teleocidin and lyngbyatoxin), and a polyacetate (aplysiatoxin), the most potent tumor promoters known of the compounds listed in Table 6 are chrysarobin and anthralin. Van Duuren and Goldschmidt[9] have reported a fairly extensive structure-activity study with anthralin and derivatives. Likewise, Boutwell and Bosch[10] have reported a structure-activity study of a number of phenolic compounds that are weak promoters in comparison to the phorbol esters and anthralin. Although several other compounds listed in Table 6 have moderate to weak activity as tumor promoters, no extensive structure-activity studies have been performed with these.

Benzo(e)pyrene and benzoyl peroxide also are relatively good tumor promoters.[11,12] In addition, Scribner and Scribner[13] reported that the moderate complete carcinogenic activity of 7-bromomethylbenz(a)anthracene was due to its strong promoting activity and weak initiating activity. Also shown in Table 6 are free radical generating compounds such as benzoyl peroxide which are good skin tumor promoters. These agents can be considered "cleaner" promoters than TPA in that they have not been found to have skin tumor initiating or complete carcinogenic activity.[12]

Table 6: Promoters of Skin Carcinogenicity*

Promoters	Potency
Croton oil	Strong
Certain phorbol esters in croton oil	Strong
Some synthetic phorbol esters	Strong
Certain euphorbia latices	Strong
7-Bromomethylbenz(a)anthracene	Strong
Indole alkaloids (teleocidin and lyngbyatoxin)	Strong
Polyacetates (aplysiatoxin)	Strong
Chrysarobin and anthralin	Moderate
Extracts of unburned tobacco	Moderate
Tobacco smoke condensate	Moderate
1-Fluoro-2,4-dinitrobenzene	Moderate
Benzo(e)pyrene	Moderate
Benzoyl peroxide	Moderate
Lauroyl peroxide	Moderate
Certain fatty acids and fatty acid methyl esters	Weak
Certain long-chain alkanes	Weak
A number of phenolic compounds	Weak
Surface active agents (sodium lauryl sulfate, Tween 60)	Weak
Citrus oils	Weak
Iodoacetic acid	Weak

*Reviewed in reference 5

SENCAR MOUSE SKIN TUMORIGENESIS MODEL

Derivation

The SENCAR stock of mice was selectively bred for sensitivity to skin tumor induction in two-stage tumorigenesis. Consequently, the SENCAR mouse is extremely sensitive in two-stage carcinogenesis and coincidentally is sensitive to complete carcinogens. The SENCAR mouse was derived from crossing Charles River CD-1 mice with skin-tumor sensitive mice (STS) and selecting for sensitivity to DMBA-TPA two-stage carcinogenesis for eight generations starting with the F_1 cross, as originally described by Boutwell.[2] Figure 2 outlines the method used by Boutwell to select for the STS mice. A similar selection procedure was used by Boutwell and coworkers to derive the SENCAR mice as outlined in Figure 3. In both cases, the mice developing the earliest and the most papillomas after initiation-promotion treatment were selected for each breeding.

Comparison to Other Stocks and Strains of Mice

The SENCAR mice are between ten and twenty times more sensitive to DMBA tumor initiation than the CD-1 mice (Table 7). However, as shown in Table 8, they are only between three and five times more sensitive to B(a)P tumor initiation than the CD-1 mice.[14] In addition, the SENCAR mice are two to three times more sensitive to TPA promotion than the CD-1 mice.[14]

Although there exist several stocks and strains of mice that have been used in skin tumor induction experiments, very little dose-response data are available and there are very few comparative studies on the relative sensitivity, except for SENCAR and C57BL/6 mice. There is an even greater difference in the sensitiv-

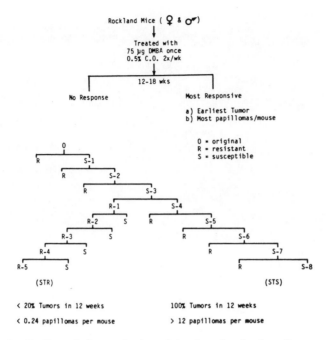

Figure 2: Outline of the method used in the selective breeding experiments for skin tumor sensitive (STS) and resistant (STR) mice (Boutwell[2]).

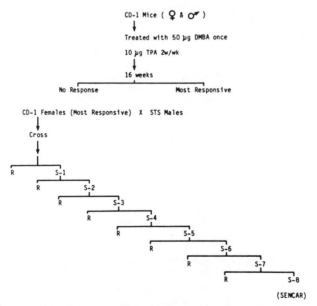

Figure 3: Outline of the method used in the selective breeding experiments for SENCAR mice (outbreeding).

Table 7: Comparison of the Tumor-Initiating Activity of DMBA in SENCAR *vs* CD-1 Mice*

Each experimental group is an average of three experiments containing 30 mice per experiment. DMBA was applied topically once and followed seven days later by twice weekly promoting applications of 8.5 nmol of TPA**

Mice	DMBA (Dose, nmol)	Number of Papillomas per Mouse at 15 Weeks	Number of Mice with Papillomas at 15 Weeks	Number of Papillomas per Mouse at 25 Weeks	Percent of Mice with Papillomas at 25 Weeks
SENCAR	100	22.0	100	24.0	100
SENCAR	10	6.4	100	7.0	100
SENCAR	1	3.2	90	3.8	95
SENCAR	0.1	0.3	15	0.6	20
SENCAR	0.0***	0	0	0.1	10
CD-1	100	4.8	75	5.6	90
CD-1	10	2.2	60	3.0	72
CD-1	1	0	0	0.2	10
CD-1	0.1	0	0	0	0
CD-1	0.0***	0	0	0.2	10

*Data taken from reference 5
**The maximum percent standard deviation for all groups was 15%
***TPA only group; the mice received twice weekly applications of 8.5 nmol of TPA for 25 weeks

Table 8: Comparison of the Tumor-Initiating Activity of B(a)P in SENCAR *vs* CD-1 Mice*

The maximum percent standard deviation for all groups was 18%.

Mice	DMBA (Dose, nmol)	Number of Papillomas per Mouse at 15 Weeks	Number of Mice with Papillomas at 15 Weeks	Number of Papillomas per Mouse at 25 Weeks	Percent of Mice with Papillomas at 25 Weeks
SENCAR	200	7.6	100	8.2	100
SENCAR	100	3.4	78	3.8	80
SENCAR	50	1.4	56	1.6	60
SENCAR	10	0.6	36	0.9	42
SENCAR	0**	0	0	0.1	10
CD-1	200	1.4	56	3.8	72
CD-1	100	1.0	44	1.8	58
CD-1	50	0.5	36	0.7	40
CD-1	10	0	0	0.1	10
CD-1	0**	0	0	0.1	10

*Data taken from reference 5
**TPA only groups; the mice received twice weekly applications of 8.5 nmol of TPA for 25 weeks

ity to two-stage skin carcinogenesis between SENCAR and C57BL/6 mice than between the SENCAR and CD-1 mice. C57BL/6 mice are very refractory to two-stage skin carcinogenesis by B(a)P-TPA. As shown in Table 9, even high initiating doses of B(a)P (1,600 nmoles) and high promoting doses of TPA (10 μg) are quite ineffective in causing skin tumors in C57BL/6 mice. However, C57BL/6 mice do respond to complete carcinogenesis by B(a)P and, in this regard, they appear to be slightly more sensitive than the SENCAR mice.[15] This unequal susceptibility to complete and two-stage carcinogenesis within a stock or strain of mice strongly suggests that the promotional phases of complete and two-stage carcinogenesis are dissimilar. In addition, differences in sensitivity to initiation and promotion between mice may be due to alterations in the promotional phase of two-stage carcinogenesis. In this regard, we have recently found that benzoyl peroxide is an effective promoter in C57BL/6 and SENCAR mice,[15] but for some reason, TPA is not an effective promoter in C57BL/6 mice.

Table 9: Initiation-Promotion in SENCAR and C57BL/6 Mice*

1. Repetitive applications of various dose levels of TPA for 52 weeks without initiation in SENCAR mice will give a low level of papillomas (5% to 20%) and carcinomas (<15%) but does not show a dose response relationship. Benzoyl peroxide gives less than 5% tumors in similar experiments.

2. Repetitive applications of various dose levels of TPA or benzoyl peroxide after initiation in SENCAR mice will give a dose-response in terms of papillomas (early) and carcinomas (late).

3. Repetitive applications of various dose levels of TPA or benzoyl peroxide for 52 weeks without initiation in C57BL/6 mice did not give any tumors.

4. Repetitive applications of various dose levels of TPA after initiation in C57BL/6 mice gave a very low level of papillomas (<5%) and carcinomas (<10%). In this experiment B(a)P doses of 50 to 1,600 nmols were used to initiate the mice.

5. Repetitive applications of benzoyl peroxide after initiation in C57BL/6 mice gave a 45% carcinoma incidence.

*See reference 15

Carcinogens and/or Initiators Used in SENCAR Mice

Although not all of the various chemicals listed in Tables 3 and 4 have been assayed in SENCAR mice or in any other strain or stock of mice, one of the largest data bases of carcinogens and/or initiators is presently available for the SENCAR mouse model. All the carcinogens and/or initiators that have been tested in both the CD-1 and SENCAR mice were positive in both stocks. The major difference was the increased sensitivity and shorter latent period until tumor development in the SENCAR mice. As was the case in CD-1 mice, DMBA and B(a)P show a good dose-response relationship in SENCAR mice (Table 10). In addition, a good correlation exists between the number of papillomas per mouse at 15 weeks and the final carcinoma incidence at 50 weeks. The percent of mice with papillomas also has a reasonable correlation but the dose-response is very narrow (Table 10).

Table 10: Dose Response Studies on the Ability of DMBA and B(a)P to
Initiate Skin Tumors in SENCAR Mice*

The mice were treated one week after initiation with twice weekly
applications of 5 µg of TPA

Initiator	Dose (nmols)	Number of Papillomas per Mouse at 15 Weeks	Percent of Mice with Papillomas at 15 Weeks	Percent of Mice with Carcinomas at 50 Weeks
DMBA	100	22.9	100	100
DMBA	10	6.8	100	40
DMBA	1	3.2	93	22
DMBA	0.1	0.5	20	5
B(a)P	200	7.5	100	55
B(a)P	100	3.2	78	30
B(a)P	50	1.4	60	18

*Data taken from reference 5

Most of the carcinogenic PAH's metabolites and derivatives summarized in
Table 3 have been tested in the SENCAR mouse skin tumorigenesis model.[16-37]
Besides the PAH's some other chemical carcinogens are positive in a dose-response relationship as skin carcinogens and/or initiators in the SENCAR mouse,
such as sterigmatocystin, urethane, 1,3-propanesultone, 4-nitroquinoline-N-ox-
ide, N-methyl-N'-nitro-N-nitrosoguanidine (MNNG), N-nitrosoethylurea (ENU),
N-nitrosomethylurea, epichlorohydrin, and 2-naphthylamine (Slaga and co-
workers, unpublished data). In this regard, both MNNG and ENU were very potent skin carcinogens and tumor initiators which suggests that these compounds
will be useful direct-acting carcinogens in the skin model (Slaga and Nesnow, unpublished data). Several other chemicals (*e.g.*, dimethylnitrosamine, dimethylhydrazine, acetylaminofluorene and 4-aminobiphenyl) which are carcinogens in
certain tissues have been extensively studied in SENCAR mouse skin and were
negative (Slaga and co-workers, unpublished data). A possible explanation may
be the lack of metabolic activation of these compounds in the skin. In addition,
several controversial compounds, such as chloroform and malonaldehyde, were
also negative in the SENCAR mouse skin tumorigenesis model (Slaga and co-
workers, unpublished data).

Besides pure chemicals, a number of environmentally important complex
mixtures have also been extensively studied for skin carcinogenic and/or tumor
initiating activity in the SENCAR mouse.[8,38-42] Table 11 summarizes the complex mixtures tested and their activity as mouse skin carcinogens and/or tumor
initiators. Of the complex mixtures tested, coke oven main and roofing tar had
both strong carcinogenic and tumor-initiating activity for skin, whereas the
Nissan diesel exhaust sample was only a strong tumor initiator.

Promoters Used in SENCAR Mice

As in the case with carcinogens and/or tumor initiators, not all of the various tumor promoters listed in Table 6 have been assayed in SENCAR mice. As
shown in Table 12, a good dose-response relationship exists for TPA skin tumor

Table 11: Environmentally Important Complex Mixtures Tested
in the SENCAR Mouse Skin Tumorigenesis Model*

	Initiators of Carcinogenicity	Complete Carcinogenesis	Promoters of Carcinogenicity
Extracts of Olds diesel exhaust condensate	+**	NT***	NT
Extracts of Nissan diesel exhaust condensate	+	–	–
Extracts of V.W. Rabbit diesel exhaust condensate	+**	NT	NT
Extracts of Caterpillar diesel exhaust condensate	–	NT	NT
Extracts of Mustang gasoline catalyst exhaust condensate	+**	NT	NT
Extracts of topside coke oven	+	NT	NT
Extracts of coke oven main	+	+	+
Extracts of roofing tar	+	+	+
Extracts of cigarette smoke condensate	–	NT	NT
Diesel fuel	–	–	+†
B(a)P (control)	+	+	+
TPA (control)	–	±	+

*See references 8, 38–42 for details
**These were weakly positive
***NT; not tested
†Slaga and co-workers, unpublished data

Table 12: Dose-Response Studies on the Ability of TPA to Promote
Carcinogenicity After DMBA Initiation*

The mice were initiated with 10 nmols of DMBA and promoted one
week later with various dose levels of TPA

Promoter	Dose (μg)	Time to First Papilloma (weeks)	Number of Papillomas per Mouse at 15 Weeks	Percent of Mice with Papillomas at 15 Weeks	Percent of Mice with Carcinomas at 50 Weeks
TPA	10	8	3.0	100	32
TPA	5	6	7.2	100	46
TPA	2	7	6.5	100	45
TPA	1	8	3.6	80	25
TPA	0.1	11	0.4	5	8

*See reference 5 for details

promotion after DMBA initiation, considering either the number of papillomas per mouse at 15 weeks or the percent of mice with squamous cell carcinomas at 50 weeks. The repetitive application of the promoter, TPA, without initiation by DMBA in general gives a few tumors, but a dose-response relationship has never been noted (Table 13). The maximum response observed after 50 weeks of treatment with TPA was a 22% incidence of mice with papillomas and 5% with carcinomas.

Table 13: Dose-Response Studies on the Ability of TPA to Act
as a Complete Carcinogen in SENCAR Mice*

TPA Dose (μg)	Number of Papillomas per Mouse at 50 Weeks	Percent of Mice with Papillomas at 50 Weeks	Percent of Mice with Carcinomas at 50 Weeks
0	0	0	0
1	0.09	8	0
2	0.07	7	0
4	0.20	22	5
6	0.15	12	0

*The mice (80 per group) were treated twice weekly with various dose levels of TPA

Unlike the initiation phase, the promotion stage is reversible, requiring a certain frequency of applications in order to induce tumors. Table 14 compares the promoting activity of various doses of TPA when given either three times, two times or one time per week. In general, as the frequency of application of TPA decreases, the promoting activity also decreases. It should be pointed out, however, that one application per week of TPA after initiation by 20 nmoles of DMBA is still fairly effective for promotion. However, even high doses of TPA given once every two weeks or once every three weeks, are ineffective in the promotion stage.[5]

Table 14: Comparison of the Frequency of Application and Dose of TPA
on Promotion of Carcinogenicity in Skin*

DMBA Initiation (Dose, nmols)	TPA (Dose, μg)	Frequency of Application**	Papillomas per Mouse at 16 Weeks	Percent of Mice with Papillomas at 16 Weeks
10	1	3	7.8	100
10	1	2	3.6	80
10	2	2	6.5	100
10	5	2	10.2	100
10	10	2	4.6	100
10	0.5	1	1.0	40
10	1	1	1.8	66
10	2	1	3.2	74
10	3	1	4.3	78
10	4	1	5.1	82
10	5	1	6.4	86
20	1	1	4.2	76
20	2	1	6.0	96
20	4	1	9.0	100

*30 female SENCAR mice were used for each group. Slaga *et al.*, unpublished results
**Number of applications per week

Several other phorbol ester tumor promoters have been assayed in SENCAR mice. Phorbol 12,13-dibutyrate and 12-deoxyphorbol-13-decanoate both show a good dose-response relationship (Slaga and co-workers, unpublished data). Although 4-O-methyl-TPA is generally not considered a tumor promoter, it does have some promoting activity at doses greater than 200 μg per application. 12-O-Retinylphorbol-13-acetate also had tumor promoting activity for skin, but less than TPA. In general, mezerein can be considered a weak skin tumor promoter in SENCAR mice.[5]

Besides the phorbol esters, a number of other chemicals have skin tumor promoting activity in SENCAR mice, including teleocidin, retinoic acid, benzoyl peroxide, lauryl peroxide, cumene peroxide, decanoyl peroxide, cumene hydroperoxide, tertiary butyl-hydroperoxide, butylated hydroxytoluene-hydroperoxide, 1-fluoro-2,4-dinitrobenzene, benzo(e)pyrene, anthralin and chrysarobin (references 3, 5, and 12, and Slaga and co-workers, unpublished data). A number of chemicals which were negative or very weak as skin tumor promoters in SENCAR mice were hydrogen peroxide, hydroquinone, butylated hydroxyanisole, butylated hydroxytoluene, calcium ionophore A23187, chloroquine, Quaboin, chlorpromazine, epichlorohydrin, chloroform, malonaldehyde, phenanthrene, 2-aminoanthracene, 1-aminoanthracene, phenanthrenequinone, and 2,3,7,8-tetrachlorodibenzo-*p*-dioxin (Slaga and co-workers, unpublished data).

In terms of complex mixtures, diesel fuel had moderate skin tumor promoting activity, but it was negative as a carcinogen in SENCAR mice (Slaga, and co-workers unpublished data). As shown in Table 11, several complex mixtures such as roofing tar and coke oven main have promoting activity, but they also are complete carcinogens.[41]

Experimental Protocol

SENCAR mice can be obtained commercially from either the Oak Ridge Research Institute in Oak Ridge, Tennessee or Harlan Sprague Dawley, Indianapolis, Indiana. In addition, a new inbred strain of Super SENCAR can be obtained from the Oak Ridge Research Institute. Although male SENCAR mice, in general, are slightly more sensitive than female mice, we prefer to use female mice because they can be housed together without the extensive fighting which is common among male mice. Because the hair of mice is in a non-growing phase between seven and nine weeks of age, mice of this age are commonly used at the beginning of a tumor experiment. The dorsal surface is shaved with surgical clippers at least two days before the first application of a carcinogen or tumor initiator. Although some investigators shave the mice repeatedly, we find very consistent results after only one initial shaving. Generally, 30 mice per group are sufficient to obtain statistically significant results.[41] Five or ten mice are housed in plastic cages with corn cob chips for bedding and they are allowed food and water *ad libitum*. Yellow lights are used and are set for a 12 hours on and 12 hours off cycle. The temperature is maintained at 22°C-23°C with at least ten changes of air per hour. The mice are weighed once every two weeks in order to determine if the protocol is affecting their normal growth.

Formation of skin tumor is recorded weekly, and papillomas >2 mm in diameter and carcinomas are included in the cumulative total if they persist for one week or longer. The number of mice with tumors, the number of mice surviving, and the total number of tumors are determined and recorded weekly. At six months, the number of papillomas per surviving animal are recorded for statistical purposes. Carcinomas are statistically analyzed after 12 months of treatment, and the tumors are histologically verified at the termination of the experiment or when animals die during the treatment period.

The major protocols used are complete carcinogenesis, tumor initiation and tumor promotion. For the complete carcinogenesis protocol, the mice are treated once a week for at least 52 weeks. For lipid soluble compounds, acetone and tetrahydrofuran are commonly used as solvents. For water-soluble compounds, a combination of acetone and water or acetone and dimethylsulfoxide (DMSO) is used in order to facilitate spreading and penetration of the compounds. All solutions of test compounds are made up immediately before use. In determining the tumor initiating activity of a compound, a single topical treatment is generally used and tumor promotion is started either one or two weeks after initiation. Although TPA is a widely used promoter, it is recommended that either benzoyl peroxide or chrysarobin be used as the promoter since TPA is subject to degradation by esterases. The tumor promoters are given topically either twice or once a week.

The skin tumor initiating activity of B(a)P in acetone, benzene or tetrahydrofuran (THF) was found to be very similar. However, the reactive metabolite of B(a)P, B(a)P-diol-epoxide, has very little activity as a skin tumor initiator when applied in acetone.[5] The effectiveness of the various solvents for B(a)P-diol-epoxide was as follows: THF > benzene > acetone. In these experiments, the THF used was redistilled over lithium aluminum hydride and stored over sodium wire, the benzene was of spectroquality and treated with lead wire, and the acetone used was of spectroquality.[5] In later experiments we found that the B(a)P-diol-epoxide was active as an initiator if applied in dry acetone: DMSO (3:1). However, the acetone and DMSO are very difficult to keep water-free and consequently with time are not very effective solvents. In addition, reactive carcinogens are more effective as initiators when given repetitively for a week or two.

DMBA, B(a)P and 3-methylcholanthrene (3-MC) are potent skin tumor initiators when given either topically or intraperitoneally; however, they are more effective when given topically. In general, lipid soluble carcinogens and reactive carcinogens are more effective when given topically as skin tumor initiators. Epichlorohydrin, 2-naphthylamine and 2-acetylaminofluorene are weak skin tumor initiators when given either topically or intraperitoneally but are slightly more effective when given intraperitoneally (Slaga and Daniels, unpublished data). In general, carcinogens that are water-soluble are more effective as initiators of skin carcinogenicity when given intraperitoneally. Besides the poor penetration of water-soluble compounds into the skin, metabolism of some carcinogens by internal organs may be an important factor in their greater tumor-initiating activity for skin when given intraperitoneally.

When determining the tumor-promoting activity of a compound, repetitive treatment either once or twice a week is necessary after tumor initiation. Either DMBA (a pro-carcinogen) or MNNG (a direct carcinogen) are recommended as the tumor initiators because of the large data base available on these compounds.

The solvent vehicle is very important when determining skin tumor-promoting activity. Acetone is the best solvent for applying TPA, benzoyl peroxide and chrysarobin to the skin. The promoting activity of TPA is decreased by approximately 50% when applied topically in 0.2 ml of ethanol. If TPA is applied in 0.2 ml of a mixture of ethanol:acetone (1:1), there is no difference in tumor response compared to the use of acetone as a solvent. The promoting activity of 1 μg of TPA is decreased by more than 99% and that of 5 μg of TPA is decreased by 79% when applied topically in 0.2 ml of DMSO. Even when 1 μg of TPA is applied in 0.2 ml mixture of acetone:DMSO (6:1), the promoting activity is decreased by 71%. The reason(s) for the decreased promoting activity of TPA in ethanol and DMSO is currently not known.[5]

As previously discussed, compounds can also be assayed for co-carcinogenic, co-initiating, and co-promoting activities. In these cases, the test agent is given simultaneously with either the carcinogen, tumor initiator or tumor promoter. In addition, as will be discussed later, the SENCAR mouse skin model can be used to determine if a compound has anti-carcinogenic, anti-initiating activity and anti-promoting activity. The important consideration when determining the above activities is that the tumorigenic response must produce approximately a 50% response in order to increase significantly or decrease the response by the test compound.

TWO-STAGE PROMOTION IN SENCAR MICE

Slaga *et al.*[43,44] have recently found that skin tumor promotion can be operationally and mechanistically further divided into at least two stages. This was established when they noted that mezerein induced many of the cellular events in a fashion similar to TPA, but mezerein was a weak or nonpromoting agent. They rationalized that TPA must be inducing some additional cellular event(s) that mezerein could not do so effectively. As a test, they initiated mice, gave a limited treatment of TPA that would not promote tumors, and then treated the mice repetitively with mezerein. This two-stage promotion protocol was a very effective means of inducing tumors and both stages of promotion showed a good dose-response relationship.[4,43,44] It should be emphasized that only one application of a first-stage promoter is required and that this stage is irreversible for four to six weeks.[4] Besides TPA and 12-deoxyphorbol-13-decanoate, which are known tumor promoters, non-tumor-promoters such as 4-O-methyl-TPA, calcium ionophore A23187, and hydrogen peroxide, as well as wounding are effective stage I tumor promoters.[4] The second stage of tumor promotion is initially reversible but later becomes irreversible. A number of weak or non-promoting agents, such as mezerein and 12-deoxyphorbol-13-2,4,5-decatrienoate, are effective second-stage promoters.[4]

TUMOR PROGRESSION IN SENCAR MICE

The initiation-promotion protocol, either by single stage promotion or by two-stage promotion, induces a large number of benign papillomas followed by a few malignant squamous cell carcinomas compared to the total number of papillomas.[3,4] A complete carcinogenesis protocol (repetitive applications of a carcinogen) induces a low level of papillomas followed by a large number of carcinomas.[3,4] Although the initiation-promotion protocol is less effective than the complete carcinogenesis protocol in causing carcinomas, the initiation-promotion protocol allows one to critically examine the differences in papillomas and carcinomas as well as to study the factors involved in the progression of papillomas to carcinomas. Klein-Szanto and co-workers[45] have found that all squamous cell carcinomas lack several differentiation proteins such as high molecular weight keratins (60,000 to 62,000) and filaggrin, but they are positive for gamma glutamyltransferase (GGT) whereas a similar condition exists in only about 20% of the papillomas generated by an initiation-promotion protocol. These conditions appear to be very late responses. Slaga (unpublished results) has found that if papillomas are treated only once with an initiating dose of MNNG the conversion of papillomas to carcinomas is significantly increased, possibly by a genetic mechanism. This type of treatment (initiation-promotion-initiation) gives a carcinoma response similar to complete carcinogenesis, *i.e.*, giving a carcinogen such as DMBA or MNNG repetitively which probably supplies initiating and promoting influences continuously.

ANTICARCINOGENS

Although preventing the exposure of man to carcinogens is theoretically the best way to reduce cancer incidence, such an approach is not always practical for obvious reasons. Therefore, alternative means of modifying the process of carcinogenesis in man must be found. Since carcinogenesis is a prolonged multistage process, a variety of approaches may be considered toward the inhibition of either the initiation or the promotion phases. Table 15 summarizes various general classes of chemicals used to inhibit the process of chemical carcinogenesis, initiation and/or promotion.[3,4]

Table 15: General Classes of Chemicals That Inhibit Chemical Carcinogenesis*

> Antioxidants and free radical scavenging agents
> Vitamins
> Protease inhibitors
> Retinoids
> Flavones
> Anti-inflammatory steroids
> Certain noncarcinogenic PAH and environmental contaminants
> Polyamine synthesis inhibitors
> Prostaglandin synthesis inhibitors
> Chemicals that alter cyclic nucleotide levels

*Reviewed in reference 4

Using the two-stage skin tumorigenesis system, one can specifically study the effects of potential inhibitors on both the initiation and the promotion phases.[3,4] Studies have been performed on many compounds that have the capacity to inhibit the initiation phase by either: (1) alteration of the metabolism of the carcinogen (decreased activation and/or increased detoxification), (2) scavenging of active molecular species of carcinogens to prevent their reaching critical target sites in the cells, or (3) competitive inhibition. In addition, there have been a number of studies on compounds that inhibit promotion or the progression of cancer by altering the state of differentiation, by inhibiting the promoter-induced cellular proliferation or by preventing gene activation by promoters.

CONCLUSION

The SENCAR mouse skin tumorigenesis model has one of the largest data bases for skin carcinogens, tumor initiators, tumor promoters, and anticarcinogens (anti-initiators and anti-promoters). It gives excellent dose-responses with both pure substances and complex mixtures. The two-stage tumorigenesis protocol can be considered a reliable and relatively short-term bioassay for carcinogens and promoters. This model has also been very important for investigating the mechanism of action of carcinogens, promoters, and anticarcinogens.

Acknowledgements

The research was supported by Public Service grants CA 34890, CA 34962 and CA 34521 from the National Cancer Institute.

REFERENCES

1. Slaga, T.J., in: *Carcinogenesis* (T.J. Slaga, ed.), Vol. 5, pp 285, Raven Press, New York (1979)
2. Boutwell, R.K., Some biological aspects of skin carcinogenesis. *Progr. Exptl. Tumor Res.* 4: 207-250 (1964)
3. Slaga, T.J., Overview of tumor promotion in animals. *Environ. Health Perspect.* 50: 3-14 (1983)
4. Slaga, T.J., Fischer, S.M., Weeks, C.E., Klein-Szanto, A.J.P., and Reiners, J.J., Studies on the mechanisms involved in multistage carcinogenesis in mouse skin. *J. Cellular Biochem.* 18: 99-119 (1982)
5. Slaga, T.J., and Fischer, S.M., Strain differences and solvent effects in mouse skin carcinogenesis experiments using carcinogens, tumor initiators and promoters. *Prog. Exp. Tumor Res.* 26: 85-109 (1983)
6. Slaga, T.J., in: *Mechanisms of Tumor Promotion* (T.J. Slaga, ed.), pp 189-196, CRC Press, Boca Raton (1983)
7. Frank, A.L., in: *Pathogenesis and Therapy of Lung Cancer* (C.C. Harris, ed.), pp 25-51, Marcel Dekker, Inc., New York (1978)
8. Nesnow, S., Triplett, L.L., and Slaga, T.J., in: *Proc. EPA Second Symposium on Application of Short-Term Bioassays in the Analysis of Complex Environmental Mixtures*, II. (M.D. Waters, S.S. Sandhu, J.L. Huisingh, L. Claxton, and S. Nesnow, eds.), pp 277-297, Plenum Publishing Co. (1981)
9. Van Duuren, B.L., and Goldschmidt, B.M., in: *Carcinogenesis*, Mechanisms of Tumor Promotion and Cocarcinogenesis (T.J., Slaga, A. Sivak, and R.K. Boutwell, eds.), Vol. 2, pp 491-507, Raven Press, New York (1978)
10. Boutwell, R.K., and Bosch, D.K., Tumor promoting action of phenol and related compounds for mouse skin. *Cancer Res.* 19: 413-419 (1959)

11. DiGiovanni, J., Slaga, T.J., Berry, D.L., and Juchau, M.R., in: *Carcinogenesis*, (T.J. Slaga, ed.), Vol. 1, p 145, Raven Press, New York (1979)
12. Slaga, T.J., Klein-Szanto, A.J.P., Triplett, L.L., Yotti, L.P., and Trosko, J.E., Skin tumor promoting activity of benzoyl peroxide, a widely used free radical generating compound. *Science* 213: 1023-1025 (1981)
13. Scribner, N.K., and Scribner, J.D., Separation of initiating and promoting effects of the skin carcinogen 7-bromomethylbenz(a)-anthracene. *Carcinogenesis* 1: 97-100 (1980)
14. DiGiovanni, J., Slaga, T.J., and Boutwell, R.K., Comparison of the tumor-initiating activity of 7,12-dimethylbenz(a)anthracene and benzo(a)pyrene in female SENCAR and CD-1 mice. *Carcinogenesis* 1: 381-389 (1980)
15. Reiners, Jr., J.J., Nesnow, S., and Slaga, T.J., Murine susceptibility to two-stage skin carcinogenesis is influenced by the agent used for promotion. *Carcinogenesis* (In press)
16. Slaga, T.J., Bracken, W.M., Dresner, S., Levin, W., Yagi, H., Jerina, D.M., and Conney, A.H., Skin tumor initiating activities of benzo(a)pyrene (BP) and various BP phenols. *Cancer Res.* 38: 678-681 (1978)
17. Slaga, T.J., Bracken, W.M., Viaje, A., Berry, D.L., Fischer, S.M., and Miller, D.R., The role of 6-hydroxymethylation in benzo(a)pyrene skin tumor initiation. *J. Natl. Cancer Inst.* 61: 451-455 (1978)
18. Slaga, T.J., Bracken, W.M., Viaje, A., Berry, D.L., Fischer, S.M., Miller, D.R., Levin, W., Conney, A.H., Yagi, H., and Jerina, D.M., in: *Carcinogenesis* (R.I. Freudenthal and O.W. Jones, eds.), Vol. 3, pp 371-382, Raven Press, New York (1978)
19. Slaga, T.J., Huberman, E., Selkirk, J.K., Harvey, R., and Bracken, W.M., Carcinogenicity and mutagenicity of benz(a)anthracene diols and diol-epoxides. *Cancer Res.* 38: 1699-1704 (1978)
20. Slaga, T.J., Bracken, W.M., Gleason, G., Levin, W., Yagi, H., Jerina, D.M. and Conney, A.H., Marked differences in the skin tumor-initiating activities of the optical enantiomers of the diastereomeric benzo(a)pyrene 7,8-diol-9,10-epoxides. *Cancer Res.* 39: 67-71 (1979)
21. Huberman, E., DiGiovanni, J., and Slaga, T.J., Carcinogenicity and mutagenicity of various fluoro derivatives of 7,12-dimethylbenz(a)anthracene. *Cancer Res.* 39: 411-414 (1979)
22. Slaga, T.J., Gleason, G.L., DiGiovanni, J., Berry, D.L., Juchau, M.R., and Harvey, R.G., Tumor initiating activities of various derivatives of benz(a)-anthracene and 7,12-dimethylbenz(a)anthracene in mouse skin. Proc. III International Battelle Conference on Polycyclic Aromatic Hydrocarbons. *Ann Arbor Press* 1: 753-764 (1979)
23. Slaga, T.J., Huberman, E., DiGiovanni, J., and Gleason, G., The importance of the "bay region" diol-epoxide in 7,12-dimethylbenz(a)anthracene skin tumor initiation and mutagenesis. *Cancer Lett.* 6: 213-220 (1979)
24. Slaga, T.J., Becker, L., Bracken, W.M., and Weeks, C.E., The effects of weak or non-carcinogenic polycyclic hydrocarbons on 7,12-dimethylbenz(a)-anthracene and benzo(a)pyrene skin tumor initiation. *Cancer Lett.* 7: 51-59 (1979)
25. Slaga, T.J., Gleason, G.L., DiGiovanni, J., and Harvey, R.G., The potent tumor initiating activity of the bay region 3,4-dihydrodiol of 7,12-dimethyl-benz(a)anthracene in mouse skin. *Cancer Res.* 39: 1934-1936 (1979)
26. Slaga, T.J., Gleason, G.L., and Hardin, L., Comparison of the skin tumor initiating activity of 3-methylcholanthrene and 3,11-dimethylcholanthrene in mice. *Cancer Lett.* 7: 39-43 (1979)

27. Slaga, T.J., Iyer, R.P., Lyga, W., Secrist, A., Daub, G.H., and Harvey, R.G., Comparison of the skin tumor-initiating activities of dihydrodiols, diol epoxides, and methylated derivatives of various polycyclic aromatic hydrocarbons. *Proc. Fourth International Symposium of Polynuclear Aromatic Hydrocarbons,* pp 753–769, Battelle Press, Columbus, Ohio (1980)

28. Slaga, T.J., Gleason, G.L., Mills, G., Ewald, L., Fu, P.P., Lee, H.M., and Harvey, R.G., Comparison of the skin tumor-initiating activities of dihydrodiols and diol-epoxides of various polycyclic aromatic hydrocarbons. *Cancer Res.* 40: 1981–1984 (1980)

29. Iyer, R.P., Lyga, W., Secrist, A., Daub, G.H., and Slaga, T.J., Comparative tumor-initiating activity of methylated benzo(a)pyrene derivatives in mouse skin. *Cancer Res.* 40: 1073–1076 (1980)

30. Levine, W., Buening, M.K., Woods, A.W., Slaga, T.J., Jerina, D.M., and Conney, A.H., An enantiomeric interaction in the metabolism and tumorigenicity of (+)- and (-)-benzo(a)pyrene 7,8-oxide. *J. Biol. Chem.* 255: 9067–9074 (1980)

31. Hennings, H., Devor, D., Wenk, M.L., Slaga, T.J., Former, B., Colburn, N.H., Bowden, G.T., Elgjo, K., and Yuspa, S.H., Comparison of two-stage epidermal carcinogenesis initiated by 7,12-dimethylbenz(a)anthracene or N-methyl-N'-nitro-N-nitrosoguanidine in newborn and adult SENCAR and BALB/c mice. *Cancer Res.* 41: 773–779 (1981)

32. DiGiovanni, J., and Slaga, T.J., Effects of benzo(e)pyrene and dibenz(a,c)-anthracene on the skin tumor initiating activity of polycyclic aromatic hydrocarbons. *Proc. Fifth International Symposium on Polynuclear Aromatic Hydrocarbons.* pp 17–31, Battelle Press, Columbus, Ohio (1981)

33. DiGiovanni, J., Rymer, J., Slaga, T.J., and Boutwell, R.K., Anticarcinogenic and cocarcinogenic effects on benzo(a)pyrene and dibenz(a,c)anthracene on skin tumor initiation by polycyclic hydrocarbons. *Carcinogenesis* 3: 371–375 (1982)

34. Wood, A.W., Levin, W., Chang, R.L., Conney, A.H., Slaga, T.J., O'Malley, R., Newman, M.S., Buhler, D.R., and Jerina, D.M., Mouse skin tumor-initiating activity of 5-, 7-, and 12-methyl and fluorine substituted benzo-(a)anthracenes. *J. Natl. Cancer Inst.* 69: 725–728 (1982)

35. DiGiovanni, J., Diamond, L., Singer, J.M., Daniels, F.B., Witiak, D.T., and Slaga, T.J., Tumor-initiating activity of 4-fluoro-7,12-dimethylbenz(a)-anthracene and 1,2,3,4-tetrahydro-7,12-dimethylbenz(a)anthracene in female SENCAR mice. *Carcinogenesis* 3: 651–655 (1982)

36. Raveh, D., Slaga, T.J., and Huberman, E., Cell-mediated mutagenesis and tumor initiating activity of the ubiquitous polycyclic hydrocarbon, cyclopenta(c,d)pyrene. *Carcinogenesis* 3: 763–766 (1982)

37. Buhler, D.R., Unlu, F., Thakker, D.R., Slaga, T.J., Newman, M.S., Levin, W., Conney, A.H., and Jerina, D.M., Metabolism and tumorigenicity of 7-, 8-, 9-, and 10-fluorobenzo(a)pyrene. *Cancer Res.* 42: 4779–4783 (1982)

38. Slaga, T.J., Triplett, L.L., and Nesnow, S., Mutagenic and carcinogenic potency of extracts of diesel and related environmental emissions: Two stage carcinogenesis in skin tumor sensitive mice. *Environ. Intl.* 5: 417–423 (1981)

39. Slaga, T.J., Fischer, S.M., Triplett, L.L., and Nesnow, S., Comparison of complete carcinogenesis and tumor initiation and promotion in mouse skin. The induction of papillomas by tumor initiation-promotion—a reliable short term assay. *J. Environ. Pathol. Toxicol.* 26: 83–99 (1981)

40. Nesnow, S., Triplett, L.L., and Slaga, T.J., Comparative tumor-initiating activity of complex mixtures on SENCAR mouse skin. *J. Natl. Cancer Inst.* 68: 829–834 (1982)

41. Nesnow, S., Triplett, L.L., and Slaga, T.J., Mouse skin tumor initiation-promotion and complete carcinogenesis bioassays: Mechanisms and biological activities of emission samples. *Environ. Health Perspect.* 47: 255-268 (1983)

42. Nesnow, S., Triplett, L.L., and Slaga, T.J., in: *Proc. EPA Second Symposium on Application of Short-Term Bioassays in the Analysis of Complex Environmental Mixtures*, III, (M.D. Waters, S.S. Sandhu, J. Lewtas, L. Claxton, N. Chernoff and S. Nesnow, eds.), pp 367-390, Plenum Publishing Co., New York, (1983)

43. Slaga, T.J., Fischer, S.M., Nelson, K., and Gleason, G.L., Studies on the mechanism of skin tumor promotion: Evidence for several stages in promotion. *Proc. Natl. Acad. Sci. U.S.A.* 77: 3659-3663 (1980)

44. Slaga, T.J., Klein-Szanto, A.J.P., Fischer, S.M., Nelson, K., and Major, S., Studies on the mechanism of action of anti-tumor promoting agents: Specificity in two-stage promotion. *Proc. Natl. Acad. Sci. U.S.A.* 77: 2251-2254 (1980)

45. Klein-Szanto, A.J.P., Nelson, R.G., Shah, Y., and Slaga, T.J., Simultaneous appearance of keratin modifications and GGT activity as indications of tumor progression in skin papillomas. *J. Natl. Cancer Inst.* 70: 161-168 (1983)

Part V

Long-Term Animal Bioassays

12

Design of a Long-Term Animal Bioassay for Carcinogenicity

Thomas E. Hamm, Jr.*

Chemical Industry Institute of Toxicology
Research Triangle Park, North Carolina

INTRODUCTION

Many references provide information about the design of bioassays for carcinogenicity and there are several good reviews.[1-3] The design of a bioassay should be approached in the same manner used for the design of any experiment. First, the purpose of the study should be formulated. If the purpose is routine toxicological screening then "the objective of a long-term oncogenicity study is to observe test animals for a major portion of their life span for the development of neoplastic lesions during or after exposure to various doses of a test substance by an appropriate route of administration".[1] Even this general objective places several constraints (test animals, life span, various doses, appropriate route) on experimental design. Other objectives constrain the experimental design further. For example, if the study is conducted for submission to a regulatory agency, then the design must meet or exceed the testing protocol requirements of that agency. Although requirements vary, attempts have been made to standardize agency requirements for bioassays in the United States[4] and worldwide.[5]

Experience obtained in the National Cancer Institute (NCI) Bioassay Program prompted the proposal of the following essential features of a bioassay for carcinogenicity: "(1) Sensitive and reliable animal test system; (2) Optimal exposure conditions to reveal a carcinogenic response; (3) Elimination of all extraneous factors that might influence the conduct of the test and the interpretation of the results; (4) In-depth pathology examination to detect the minute as well as the more obvious carcinogenic changes; and (5) Complete documentation

---

*Present address: Stanford University, Stanford, California

of all data to allow those responsible for interpretation of human relevance to make the best judgments possible."[3]

Bioassays for carcinogenicity may also be designed to study the mechanisms of carcinogenesis. An important initial decision that must be made in the design of a bioassay is the allocation of resources. There are basically three choices: (1) A screening bioassay designed to determine only if the compound is carcinogenic; (2) A complete bioassay designed to provide time to tumor, dose response, and mechanistic data; or (3) A compromise between the two. A compromise protocol should usually be considered since the complete bioassay is wasteful of resources when the compound is negative and the screening bioassay provides limited information when the compound is positive. Regardless of the design that is used other studies should be designed to provide more information about compounds that are found to be positive for carcinogenicity in the bioassay.

THE DESIGN OF THE "STANDARD" BIOASSAY

The following is a summary of the standard bioassay for carcinogenicity design currently used at the Chemical Industry Institute of Toxicology (CIIT). This design is used as a basis for discussing the final testing protocol which is modified to fit the chemical to be studied.

(1) Both sexes of the F-344 rat and B6C3F1 mouse are used and the animals are approximately six to eight weeks old at the start of the bioassay.

(2) Four groups are used—control, maximum tolerated dose, and two intermediate doses. The route of exposure mimics, if possible, the route of human exposure. The exposure period is 24 months. The grade of chemical (purity) is the same as that to which humans are usually exposed.

(3) The animals are weighed weekly for the first 12 weeks and then every two weeks for the remainder of the study. The animals are observed twice daily, seven days/week, to find dead, moribund, or clinically abnormal animals. Detailed clinical observations are recorded during the scheduled weighings.

(4) A minimum of 70 animals per sex per species per dose group are used. All animals that die during the study, as well as ten animals per sex per dose group at 15 months, and all surviving animals at 24 months are subjected to a detailed necropsy and histopathologic examination. Four additional animals are included in each group to be used as sentinels to detect disease problems. Blood is collected by cardiac puncture from all animals at necropsy for appropriate clinical pathology tests.

Except for the use of an additional dose group and a 15-month interim necropsy this design is a "screening" bioassay design.

FACTORS TO BE CONSIDERED WHEN DESIGNING A BIOASSAY

Test Substance

An early step in a bioassay for carcinogenicity is to select a chemical to test. The selection of test chemicals should be done carefully since a bioassay currently costs between 0.5 and 1.5 million dollars and takes a minimum of three to four years to complete. The chemical selection process used by the NCI prior to 1977 has been published.[3] At CIIT we select chemicals that are high volume chemicals to which substantial numbers of people are exposed. A thorough review of the literature is done on each chemical prior to the design of the bioassay. This review is prepared by a multidisciplinary review group composed of doctoral level scientific staff and is published as a Current Status Report (*e.g.*, reference 6). The purpose of these reviews is to identify and evaluate previously published studies and to determine what further testing and research are needed.

The next decision that must be made is the source and purity of the compound that will be tested. Since most compounds are mixtures and/or contain some impurities, the significance of those impurities on the bioassay must be considered. Usually very little data on the potential carcinogenicity of the impurities are known. The bioassay should use the chemical of the same purity as that to which humans are exposed. If the impure compound is found to be carcinogenic, then further studies should be designed to determine whether the pure compound, the impurities, or the mixture is the carcinogen (*e.g.*, reference 7).

The chemical should be analyzed on arrival and at intervals during the study to establish the composition of the substance actually being tested. Results of these analyses should be in the report of the bioassay.

Dosage

The number of dose groups and the dose for each group are critical decisions. Munro[8] and the Food Safety Council[9] have published discussions on the selection of the high dose. It is generally accepted that the highest dose should be the maximum tolerated dose (MTD).[2] The MTD is the highest dose that can be given that does not cause a significant decrease in survival from effects other than carcinogenicity. The MTD is chosen based on published information as well as acute, 14 day, 90 day, and metabolism studies, as needed, in the same species, strain, and sex of animals by the same route of chemical administration. In the absence of other signs of toxicity, a decrease in body weight gain can be used to define an MTD. The ideal MTD should cause no more than a 10% reduction in body weight gain. If no lesions or decrease in body weight gain are found, but the metabolism studies show that the compound is absorbed, then the dosages are selected to be as high as possible. In inhalation studies the limiting factor is the available oxygen which should not be below 18% by volume under normal atmospheric pressure or the test agent will act as an asphyxiant.[10] Other factors such as the explosive concentration of the chemical should also be considered. In feeding studies the chemical should not exceed 5% of the diet to avoid altering the nutritive balance of the diet. (*See* chapter 19 for information about the testing of inert substances.) The MTD is used deliberately to bias the bioassay towards determining if the test substance has any carcinogenic potential. If compounds are found to be carcinogenic under the test conditions then studies should be conducted to determine the mechanism of carcinogenicity including the possibility that the use of the MTD may have resulted in an abnormal pathway which would not occur at lower doses.

National Cancer Institute bioassays were designed as screening bioassays using only three dose groups; MTD, ½ MTD and control. This approach was designed to provide information about the carcinogenicity of a compound at the MTD but did not always produce a dose response or a no effect concentration, both being important for interpretation of positive studies. Multiple doses give a better opportunity to obtain a dose near the MTD, a dose response and a dose where no carcinogenicity occurs, but greatly increase the cost. A reasonable compromise is to have 4 groups: a control group, a MTD group, and two intermediate groups. We select the low dose to be close to the threshold limit value (TLV) for those chemicals that have TLV's.[10] In general, the lowest dose should not be lower than 10% of the highest dose.[1] The mid dose is selected to be intermediate between the low dose and the MTD on a log scale. If a vehicle is used, a vehicle-treated control group should be included. If the toxicity of the vehicle is unknown an additional untreated control group should be considered. Positive controls are usually not included in bioassays since the use of a known positive chemical creates problems of safety and cross contamination.

Route

Nearly all toxic chemicals gain entry to the body by ingestion, inhalation or percutaneous absorption. If possible, the route of administration used for a carcinogenesis bioassay should be similar to the route by which humans are usually exposed to the chemical. Other routes may be used for special reasons. For example, gavage gives a more accurate measure of dosage and minimizes chemical contamination of the facility with the chemical. However, it is a very artificial dosage route. Weisburger and Weisburger[11] and Page[3] have discussed in detail the advantages and disadvantages of each route of exposure. Regardless of the route chosen, studies should be conducted to determine the similarities and differences between chemical exposure by the chosen route and the route of human exposure. The route of exposure may partially determine the number of days of treatment each weeek. Dosed water or feed are usually provided seven days a week while inhalation, gavage, and dermal doses are usually administered five days a week. If the test substance is administered in food or water, the consumption of food or water should be measured weekly the first 13 weeks and at least monthly for the rest of the study. Although it is desirable to measure food and water consumption regardless of the route of exposure, these measurements are very labor intensive and are not very accurate.

Animal Selection

The occurrence of tumors increases with age in all species. Rodents are the only mammalian species with short enough lifespans to make it practical to conduct a bioassay which includes most of the lifespan. The majority of carcinogen bioassays have been conducted using mice or rats, but several have used hamsters.[12] Copies of technical reports of National Cancer Institute/National Toxicology Program bioassays can be obtained from the Public Information Office, National Toxicology Program, P.O. Box 12233, Research Triangle Park, NC 27709. The B6C3F1 mouse and the F-344 rat are currently the most commonly used rodents in bioassays for carcinogenicity. Since the F-344 rat is an inbred rat and the B6C3F1 mouse is a cross of two inbred strains of mice, they both have a minimum of genetic variability. This is an advantage since they tend to exhibit a more uniform response to a chemical. However, the genetic homogeneity is also a disadvantage since these animals may react to a chemical in a manner unlike humans or even unlike other rats and mice. Other species, strains or other stocks of rodents may be used but the considerable historical data base available for the B6C3F1 mouse and F-344 rat facilitates interpretation of experiments using these strains. Repeated use of the same strains or stocks allows an individual laboratory the opportunity to develop its own historical control data base over time. The strain or stock of animal used should be correctly identified, using standardized nomenclature, in all publications of the data.[13-15] Both sexes should be used since sex differences in response to chemical carcinogens are common.[16,17]

Duration of Exposure

Treatment should be started in young animals to assure that the animals are treated for most of their expected life span. Six to eight week old animals are usually used to allow time for weaning, shipping, acclimation, health quality studies, and randomization. In some protocols the treatment of the animals is started *in utero* or soon after birth since the susceptibility of some organs to certain carcinogens is greater at these times.[18,19] When a chemical is shown to be carcinogenic in the fetus or neonate, studies should be done to determine if the carcinogenic effect is also found in animals whose exposure is started at six to eight weeks. A multigenerational study should be considered if information on exposure from conception to death is needed. Prenatal and multigenerational tests are not recommended for routine bioassay screens for carcinogenicity.[2]

At CIIT, mice and rats are dosed for twenty-four months. Some investigators advocate eighteen months for mice and hamsters.[2] A carcinogenicity study should not be continued beyond week 130 of age for rats, 120 for mice, and 100 for hamsters.[2] If the exposure period is stopped before necropsy then it is recommended that treatment should continue to at least week 104 of age for rats, week 96 for mice, and week 80 for hamsters.[2] A bioassay is not considered adequate if the mortality in the control or low dose group is above 50% before week 104 for rats, week 96 for mice or week 80 for hamsters.[2] The cause of any mortality should be determined and evaluated as a potential contributing factor to the results of the bioassay.

Number of Animals

The number of animals used is a compromise between the limited possibility of detecting a carcinogenic response with a small number of animals and the cost of large bioassays. Fifty animals/sex/species/group is generally accepted as the minimum adequate number of animals needed.[2] At CIIT, we use 74 animals/sex/species/group to provide 10 animals for a 15 month necropsy, four sentinel animals for animal health studies throughout the bioassay, and 60 animals for a 24 month necropsy (hoping to have as many animals survive to 24 months as possible). The actual numbers of animals needed to make a decision on a marginal or negative bioassay depend on the tumor type, its incidence in the treated groups, and the incidence of the tumor in the concurrent and historical control animals so that no general rules can be given. Larger numbers of animals should be considered in certain situations. If time to appearance of tumor and tumor progression data are needed, then multiple interim necropsies should be considered. The original CIIT bioassay protocol had interim necropsies of 10 animals/sex/species/group at 6, 12 and 18 months. This significantly increased the work and cost of the bioassay and was of limited value in negative bioassays. In laboratories that do only a small number of bioassays an increased control population should be considered to provide a larger contemporary control animal data base to be used in interpreting bioassays. In some cases bioassays designed to consider only particular sites using very large numbers of animals must be used to answer fully the question of the carcinogenic properties of a particular chemical.

Animal Husbandry

Several excellent sources of general information on the use of laboratory rodents are available and should be used as a basis for an animal care program.[20-22] The following will summarize important considerations for the design of bioassays. A detailed description of animal husbandry procedures at CIIT has been published.[23]

Genetic monitoring. Animals should be monitored genetically prior to the start of a long-term bioassay to assure that they are the proper strain or stock. Methods for genetic monitoring have been published.[24-27] This service is now available commercially. Results of this monitoring should be included in the publication from the bioassay.

Health quality. Recent conferences have included discussions of the effects of health quality on bioassays.[28-30] Since the effects of infectious agents may invalidate a bioassay or make interpretation difficult, the use of animals carrying infectious agents should be minimized. In addition, a sentinel program should be used to determine the health quality of the animals prior to and during the bioassay. Since 1979, the National Cancer Institute/National Toxicology Program has used a program designed to provide viral titer information at 6, 12, 18, and 24 months on all bioassays.[31] The CIIT program is designed to provide monthly serology data so that decisions can be made during the study.[23] The sera remaining after the clinical pathology determinations have been done can be frozen and stored for future analysis if needed. Health quality monitoring results should be included in the report of the bioassay.

Feed. Diet is an important variable in toxicology studies[32] and the need for a well-defined diet has been emphasized.[33,34] A committee of the American Institute of Nutrition (AIN) was formed in 1973 to develop recommendations on nutritional guidelines for devising diets which could be used for rats and mice in long-term toxicology, carcinogenicity, and aging studies. Their report[35] defined the types of experimental diets and described recommended diets. The first type of diet defined by the committee was the cereal based diet, also known as the unrefined diet or non-purified diet. These terms were applied to diets composed predominantly of unrefined plant and animal materials which also may contain added vitamins and minerals. There are two types of cereal based diets, the "closed formula" and the "open formula." The "closed formula" diet is a diet for which the manufacturers do not disclose the exact composition. Purina Lab Chows and Wayne Laboratory animal diets are two commonly used closed formula diets. An "open formula" diet is a diet whose precise composition is published and these diets must always be assembled exactly as specified. NIH-07[36] and NIH-31 are the most commonly used open formula rodent diets. The AIN committee and other committees[2,28,33,34,37] have recommended that the NIH-07 open formula diet be used for bioassays. The National Institutes of Health has used this diet since 1972, the National Cancer Institute/National Toxicology Program has been using NIH-07 for all bioassays since 1979 and CIIT has been using it for all bioassays since 1981. If an autoclavable open formula diet is required, NIH-31 is a frequent choice. Precautions should be taken to avoid adversely affecting the nutrient composition or physical properties of the diet during autoclaving.[21]

The other type of diet discussed by the AIN committee was the purified diet. These diets are composed primarily of commercially refined proteins, carbohydrates, and fat with added mineral and vitamin mixtures. A new purified diet, AIN-76™ was proposed. Problems with this diet prompted the publication of changes in the formulation.[38] The new formulation, AIN-76a, still caused problems such as hepatic lipidosis,[39,40] kidney mineralization[41] and effects on metabolism by gut flora.[42] Therefore purified diets as currently formulated are unacceptable for long-term bioassays.

See reference 21 for a discussion of the shipment, handling, and the storage of feeds. Feed should be used within 90 days of manufacture. Each new batch of feed should be analyzed for nutrient value (our feed is assayed for protein, fat, fiber, ash, calcium, phosphorus, thiamine, vitamin A, and carotene) and contaminants (our feed is assayed for aflatoxins, nitrosamines, arsenic, cadmium, lead, mercury, selenium, nitrate, nitrite, standard plate count, total coliform bacteria, *Escherichia coli*, butylated hydroxyanisole (BHA), butylated hydroxytoluene (BHT), α-, β-, γ- (lindane), and Δ-hexachlorocyclohexane, heptachlor, aldrin, heptachlor epoxide, DDT and related chlorinated hydrocarbon residues, mirex, methoxychlor, dieldrin, endrin, telodrin, chlordane, toxaphene, estimated polychlorinated biphenyls (PCB's), ronnel, ethion, trithion, diazinon, methyl parathion, ethyl parathion, malathion, endosulfan I, endosulfan II, and endosulfan sulfate). Various organizations have published lists of permissible concentrations of contaminants in animal diets.[21,43] The type of feed, manufacturer, and results of the feed analysis should be included in the publication resulting from the bioassay results.

Water. Based on the lack of published information, the potential effect of chemical contamination of the water apparently has been given little attention. The Environmental Protection Agency has reported extensive chemical contamination of both raw and treated water in various areas of the United States,[44] and a recent review of the problem has been published.[45] Acidification of drinking water has been shown to affect selected biologic phenomena in male mice,[46] hyperchlorination of drinking water has been shown to depress the activity of macrophages in mice,[47] and variation in water quality has been reported to cause reproductive failure in female mice.[48] The system for producing purified water for laboratory animals as used at CIIT is one way to minimize water contaminants.[49] Water should be monitored for contaminants[49] and the results included in the report of the bioassay data.

Temperature and humidity. Temperature and humidity are important variables in animal experimentation.[21,22,50] Temperature should be maintained with a minimum of variability within the thermoneutral zone for each species (about 68° to 75°F and 50% to 60% relative humidity for rats and mice). In the CIIT facility we attempt to maintain temperature at 70° ± 2°F (with alarms at 65°F and 75°F) and humidity at 50% ± 10% (with alarms at 40% and 60%) in the animal cages. Alarms should be monitored 24 hours/day and any deviations in temperature and humidity promptly corrected. Emergency systems to maintain light, temperature, and humidity in the animal rooms during power failures should be available and tested monthly under full load. Data on temperature and humidity should also be included in the publication from the bioassay.

Lighting. A large number of biologic responses are on a circadian cycle[51] and these cycles can be affected by the lighting used in the animal rooms. We use 12 hours of light followed by 12 hours of darkness controlled by an automatic timer that is checked daily. Hamsters reportedly need a 14 hour light and 10 hour dark cycle.[52] The photoperiod used and any deviations should be reported.

The current recommendation for lighting intensity in the room is 75 to 125 ft-candles.[20] Light can cause eye lesions in albino rats[53] and this should be considered when designing experiments. Cages should be rotated so that all animals spend equal amounts of time in all parts of the rack. The intensity of light should be the minimum of lumens consistent with good study practices; a two-stage light cycle which allows the light to be decreased for the animals and increased when needed for animal care has been proposed.[28]

Caging. Animals exposed by inhalation should be housed in stainless steel wire mesh cages and chemical distribution studies should be done to guarantee that the type of cage does not affect exposure to the test chemical. Animals exposed by other routes should be housed in solid cages that are designed to contain the chemical. Plastic cages with filter tops and bedding are commonly used. A review on bedding for rodents has been published recently.[54] Disposable cages that are incinerated after use are expensive but simplify handling dangerous chemicals. The use of filter tops increases carbon dioxide, humidity, ammonia and temperature in the cage.[55,56] Cages should be changed at intervals which minimize the concentration of ammonia in the cage. The current TLV for ammonia, 25 ppm,[10] should not be exceeded. Dalhamn[57] reported that concentrations of ammonia as low as three ppm cause ciliastasis in the rat trachea. Heat-treated hardwood chip bedding manufactured for animal use should be used since cedar wood or soft wood beddings contain compounds that affect hepatic microsomal enzymes.[58,59] To minimize inhalation or ingestion of the bedding, wire floorwalks that suspend the animals above the bedding may be used.[60] Autoclaving hardwood chip bedding eliminates the potential for transmission of disease from potential pathogenic organisms in the bedding and reduces generation of ammonia.[61] In our program cages containing autoclaved bedding are changed twice per week which keeps concentrations of ammonia below five ppm. Regardless of cage type, animals should be given adequate space that meets or exceeds the recommendations in the *Guide for Care and Use of Laboratory Animals.*[20]

The decision must be made to house the animals individually or in groups. Individual housing has the possible disadvantage of producing "isolation stress" with its potential impact on drug response.[62] However, fighting among group housed animals also produces a great deal of stress. Individual housing has the advantages that identification of the animals is faster and easier and fighting and cannibalism are eliminated. In dosed-feed or dosed-water studies individual housing is required if the individual dose to each animal needs to be determined. If group housing is chosen, the groups should not be changed as animals die to avoid increased fighting associated with the reestablishment of dominance hierarchies. Cages should be rotated in the rack to assure that all animals stay in each location on the rack for an equal amount of time. The type and size of the cage, the population density and the type and treatment of the bedding should be included in the report of the bioassay.

Sanitation. The animals should not be exposed to any chemical except the test chemical. No paint, insecticide, deodorant, disinfectant, soap or chemicals of any kind should be used in the animal rooms (or in the facility if fumes will enter the rooms) while animals are present to avoid potential effects on the animals. Scrubbing with hot water alone usually will effectively clean animal rooms. In addition, soaps or chemicals should not be used in the cage washing equipment unless prior studies demonstrated they are needed. In a study in our facility, cages were not cleaner (measured as microbial and fluorescein contamination after washing) when soap was used in the cage washing equipment. Contamination between groups or of other experiments with the test chemical must be avoided. Bioassay animals should be housed in a room that does not contain other experiments. Control animals should be housed in the same room as test animals and adequately managed to avoid contact with the test chemical.

Randomization

After successfully obtaining the needed animals and their passing the genetic monitoring and health quality testing, the final step before starting the experiment is to randomize the animals throughout the treatment groups. Some randomization procedures stratify the animals accounting for litter, age or body weight differences. When using animals from a commercial vender it is difficult to allow for litter and age since all animals were removed from their mothers on the same day and grouped by sex. Therefore, the weaning age of the animals varies by up to seven days and no record is kept of which animals were litter mates. Body weight of young rodents is determined by litter size and age. Another method for randomization allows for equal body weights in each of the dose groups. This procedure has the advantage that each group starts at the same weight which simplifies comparing body weight gain curves. Body weights taken before the second week of acclimatization are inaccurate because of body weight loss caused by the stresses of shipment. The weight variation in each group should not exceed ± 20% of the mean weight for the group.[1] There are two main methods for eliminating very heavy and very light animals. One is to order a narrow weight range letting the supplier eliminate the heavy and light animals and the other is to eliminate the extreme weight range animals prior to the final randomization.

Clinical Observations

Collection of weighing and clinical observation data throughout the study is desirable. However, these procedures are very labor intensive and less than weekly weighings are usually done after the initial 12 week period. The list of clinical observations used at CIIT is presented in Table 1. In addition to detailed examinations, the animals should be observed twice daily seven days/week to find dead, moribund, or clinically abnormal animals. Daily observations become increasingly important as the study progresses. The daily observations should be thorough enough to minimize loss of animals caused by autolysis. If animals are group housed, debilitated animals should be individually housed as soon as they are identified to avoid loss caused by cannibalism. Since neoplasia increases with age and metastasis increases with the age of the tumor, the sacrifice of animals should not be overly rigorous. Animals with large or ulcerated tumors or clinical abnormalities that are painful should be necropsied to minimize further suffering of the animal.

Necropsy

In the standard CIIT protocol, ten animals are necropsied at 15 months providing information about long-term toxicity which is less complicated by aging effects than in older animals. Sixty animals are available to attempt to have 50 animals for necropsy at 24 months. Complete pathology methods are discussed in Chapter 16.

Clinical pathology tests. The clinical pathology tests from the standard CIIT protocol are listed in Table 2. Additional tests are scheduled based on the expected effects of the chemical. Tests are done on all the animals at scheduled necropsies. If desired, a randomly selected group of approximately 20 animals can be used for clinical pathology tests at 24 months. Serum from the remaining animals should be stored and examined as required. Blood samples should be taken from animals at necropsy only to avoid any effect of blood loss on the bioassay. If blood is needed at other time periods extra animals should be dosed with the chemical and killed for blood at the required time. The results of the clinical pathology tests should be included in the published report of the bioassay.

Organ weights. Brain, liver, and kidney are routinely weighed. Other organs are selected based on the expected effects of the chemical. Organ weights are compared to control as absolute organ weight, organ weight to body weight ratio and organ weight to brain weight ratio. The results should be in the report of the bioassay data.

Histopathology. Table 3 contains the list of tissues collected for a basic bioassay. The lungs and urinary bladder should be inflated with fixative to facilitate interpretation. All tissues from high dose and control animals killed or dying prior to 21 months are examined. Only tissues found to be target sites for toxicity in the high dose group and gross lesions are examined in the mid and low dose groups. Histopathology on all high dose and control animals killed or dying after 21 months is done on liver, kidneys, lung, brain, pituitary gland, pancreas, heart, stomach, urinary bladder, spleen, thyroid and parathyroid glands, testis (ovary), epididymis (uterus), prostate, seminal vesicles, mandibular lymph node, larynx, trachea and five sections of the nasal passages. Additional tissues may be examined based on the results of the 15 month necropsy. Results of the histopathological examinations should be included in the report of the bioassay data.

Table 1: Master List of Clinical Observations Used at CIIT

Normal
  No significant observations

Dead
  1) Found dead
  2) Sacrificed moribund
  3) Accidental trauma

Cage conditions
  1) Diarrhea present
  2) Diminished feces
  3) Abnormal feces
  4) Vomitus present
  5) Blood/exudates

Total body
  1) Emaciated
  2) Dehydrated
  3) Decomposed
  4) Cannibalism
  5) Obese
  6) Limb laceration
  7) Tail laceration

Hair/Skin
  1) Alopecia
  2) Cyanotic
  3) Jaundiced
  4) Erythematous
  5) Edema
  6) Dermatosis

Food/Water intake
  1) Enter free text

Eyes
  1) Discharge
  2) Lacrimation
  3) Corneal lesion
  4) Dilated pupils
  5) Contracted pupils
  6) Corneal opacity
  7) Eyes squinted

Ears/Nares
  1) Edema
  2) Laceration
  3) Discharge

Oral cavity/Dental
  1) Bleeding gums
  2) Inflamed gums
  3) Loose teeth
  4) Abscessed teeth
  5) Overgrown teeth
  6) Oral growths
  7) Foul mouth odor
  8) Malocclusion

Respiration
  1) Cough
  2) Frothing
  3) Apnea
  4) Labored respiration
  5) Wheezing
  6) Congestion

Behavioral/Activity
  1) Aggressive
  2) Hyperexcitable
  3) Lethargic
  4) Comatose
  5) Hyperactivity
  6) Ataxia
  7) Paralysis
  8) Convulsions
  9) Limping

Ano-Genital
  1) Enter free text

Palpable masses
  1) Superficial
  2) Subcutaneous

*Each observation or an observation not on the list can be defined
  using a free text description

Table 2: Clinical Pathology Tests Done for a Basic Bioassay at CIIT

Blood Cell Studies	Serum Chemistries
White blood cell total count	Albumin
White blood cell differential counts	Alkaline phosphatase
Hemoglobin	SGPT
Hematocrit	SGOT
RBC volume	Bilirubin total
RBC hemoglobin	Blood urea nitrogen
Mean corpuscular hemoglobin concentration	calcium

Table 3: Tissues Collected for a Basic Bioassay at CIIT

Adrenal glands	Aorta	Bone, femur	Bone marrow
Brain	Bone, sternum	Carcass	Cecum
Colon	Cervix	Duodenum	Ear canal
Epididymis	Esophagus	Eyes & optic nerve	Harderian gland
Heart	Ileum	Jejunum	Kidney
Liver	Mand. lymph nodes	Mese. lymph nodes	Lungs
Larynx	Mammary glands	Nose/Turbinates	Oviducts
Ovaries	Pancreas	Pituitary gland	Prostate
Parathyroid	Spinal chord	Salivary gland	Skin
Skeletal muscle	Sciatic nerve	Spleen	Stomach
Seminal vesicle	Testes	Thyroid glands	Thymus
Tongue	Trachea	Urinary bladder	Uterus
Vagina	Gross lesion	Zymbals gland	

Quality Assurance

Methods for quality assurance of bioassays should be considered during the design of the bioassay. Such methods have been published.[63,64] When a bioassay is done at a contract laboratory, a comprehensive independent third party audit should be considered. Results of the quality assurance audits should be included in the report of the bioassay.

Safety

Chemicals are tested in a bioassay for carcinogenicity to determine if they are animal carcinogens. Therefore, the chemical should be contained and exposure to humans working in the facility minimized. Chemical safety is a complex problem. Several references are available which may help in the design of an effective program.[65-70]

CONCLUSION

This chapter has been an attempt to present the author's opinion of the current consensus of the scientific community concerning the design of bioassays for carcinogenicity. Many aspects of bioassay design are controversial, especially the use of the B6C3F1 mouse and the use of the maximum tolerated dose. A complete discussion of bioassay design including varying viewpoints has been published.[71] Bioassay design should not be done without reference to how the statistical evaluation will be conducted (Chapter 17).

REFERENCES

1. United States Environmental Protection Agency, *Guideline HG-Chronic-Onco Health Effects Test Guidelines*, Report # EPA 560/6-82-001, Office of Pesticides and Toxic Substances (1982)
2. International Agency for Research on Cancer, Report 1, Basic Requirements for Long-Term Assays for Carcinogenicity. *IARC Monographs*, Supplement #2, 21-83 (1980)
3. Page, N.P., in: *Modern Toxicology* (H. Kraybill, and M. Mehlman, eds.), Vol. 3, pp 87-171, Wiley & Sons, New York (1977)
4. Interagency Regulatory Liaison Group, Scientific bases for identification of potential carcinogens and estimations of risks. *J. Natl. Cancer Inst.* 63: 241-268 (1979)
5. Organization for Economic Cooperation and Development, *Guidelines for Testing Chemicals*, Section 4, Health Effects, Paris, France (1981)
6. Beauchamp, R.O., Jr., Irons, R.D., Rickert, D.E., Couch, D.B., and Hamm, T.E., Jr., A critical review of the literature on nitrobenzene toxicity. *CRC Crit. Rev. Toxicol.* 11: 33-84 (1982)
7. Popp, J.A., and Leonard, T.B., The use of *in vivo* hepatic initiation promotion systems in understanding the hepatocarcinogenesis of technical grade dinitrotoluene. *Toxicol. Pathol.* 10: 190-196 (1982)
8. Munro, I.C., Considerations in chronic toxicity testing: The chemical, the dose, the design. *J. Environ. Pathol. Toxicol.* 1: 183-187 (1977)
9. Food Safety Council, Chronic toxicity testing, proposed system for food safety assessment. *Fd. Cosmet. Toxicol.* 16: 97-108 (1978)
10. American Conference of Governmental Industrial Hygienists, *Documentation of the Threshold Limit Values for Chemical Substances in the Workroom Environment*, Cincinnati, Ohio (1982)
11. Weisburger, J.H., and Weisburger, E.K., in: *Methods in Cancer Research* (H. Busch, ed.), Vol. 1, pp 307-398, Academic Press, New York (1967)
12. Sher, S.P., Tumors in control hamsters, rats, and mice: Literature tabulation. *CRC Crit. Rev. Toxicol.* 10: 49-79 (1982)
13. Staats, J., Standardized nomenclature for inbred strains of mice: Fifth listing. *Cancer Res.* 32: 1609-1646 (1972)
14. Festing, M., and Staats, J., Standardized nomenclature for inbred strains of rats. *Transplantation* 16: 221-245 (1973)
15. Institute of Laboratory Animal Resources, *International Standardized Nomenclature for Outbred Stocks of Laboratory Animals*, National Research Council, Washington, DC (1972)
16. Hamm, T.E., Jr., in: *Current Perspectives in Mouse Liver Neoplasia* (J.A. Popp, ed.), Hemisphere Publishing Corp., Washington, DC (1984)
17. Hamm, T.E., Jr., in: *Application of Biological Markers to Carcinogen Testing*, (H.A. Milman, and S. Sell, eds.), Plenum Publishing Corp., New York (1983)
18. Rice, J.M., Carcinogenesis: A late effect of irreversible toxic damage during development. *J. Environ. Health Perspect.* 18: 133-139 (1971)
19. Rice, J.M., in: *National Cancer Institute Monographs* 51: 1-282 (1979)

20. United States Department of Health, Education and Welfare, *Guide for the Care and Use of Laboratory Animals*, Publication No. (NIH) 78-23, ILAR, National Research Council, Washington, DC (1978)
21. Institute of Laboratory Animal Resources, *Long-Term Holding of Laboratory Rodents*, National Research Council, Washington, DC (1976)
22. Institute of Laboratory Animal Resources, *Laboratory Animal Housing*, National Research Council, Washington, DC (1978)
23. Hamm, T.E., Jr., Raynor, T.H., and Sherrill, M.S., in: *Complications of Viral and Mycoplasmal Infections in Rodents to Toxicology Research and Testing* (T.E. Hamm, Jr., ed.), Hemisphere Publishing Corporation, Washington, DC (1984)
24. Hedrich, H.A., in: *The Mouse in Biomedical Research* (H.L. Foster *et al.*, eds.), pp 159-173 (1981)
25. Hoffman, H.A., Smith, K.T., Crowell, J.S., Nomura, T., and Tomita, T., in: *Proceeding of the 7th ICLAS Symposium* (A. Spiegel, S. Erichsen, and H.A. Solleveld, eds.), (Utrecht, 1979), Gustav Fisher Verlag, Stuttgart (1980)
26. Festing, M.F.W., Genetic contamination of laboratory animal colonies: An increasingly serious problem. *ILAR News* 25: 6-10 (1982)
27. Festing, M.F.W., *Inbred Strains in Biomedical Research*, the MacMillan Company, London (1979)
28. Hamm, T.E., Jr., in: *Proceedings of a Workshop on the Optimal Use of Facilities for Carcinogenicity/Toxicity Testing.* NTP/NCI Carcinogenesis Testing Program, Boiling Springs, Pennsylvania (1980)
29. Hamm, T.E., Jr. (ed.), *Complications of Viral and Mycoplasma Infections in Rodents to Toxicology Research and Testing*, Washington, DC: Hemisphere Publishing Corporation (1984)
30 Hamm, T.E., Jr., in: *Proceedings of the Fifth Charles River Symposium, Biomedical Research: The Importance of Laboratory Animal Genetics, Health and the Environment*, Academic Press, New York (1984)
31. Boorman, G.A., Hickman, R., Davis, G., Rhodes, L., White, N.W., Griffin, T., Mayo, J., and Hamm, T.E., Jr., in: *Complications of Viral and Mycoplasmal Infections in Rodents to Toxicology Research and Testing* (T.E. Hamm, Jr., ed.), Hemisphere Publishing Corp., Washington, DC (1984)
32. Wise, A., Interaction of diet and toxicity—the future role of purified diet in toxicological research. *Arch. Toxicol.* 50: 287-299 (1982)
33. Newberne, P.M., Bieri, J.G., Briggs, G.M., and Nesheim, M.C., *Control of Diets in Laboratory Animal Experimentation*, Institute of Laboratory Animal Resources, Assembly of Life Sciences, National Research Council, National Academy of Sciences, Washington, DC (1978)
34. Coates, M., Workshop on laboratory animal nutrition. *ICLAS Bulletin* 50: 4-11 (1982)
35. Report of the American Institute of Nutrition Ad Hoc Committee on Standards for Nutritional Studies. *J. Nutr.* 107: 1340-1348 (1977)
36. Knapka, J.J., Smith, K.P., and Judge, F.J., Effects of open and closed formula rations on the performance of three strains of laboratory mice. *Lab. Animal Sci.* 24: 480-487 (1974)
37. National Cancer Institute, *Guidelines for Carcinogen Bioassay in Small Rodents*, National Cancer Institute Carcinogenesis Technical Report Series No. 1 (1976)
38. Bieri, J.G., Second report of the ad hoc committee on standards for nutritional studies. *J. Nutr.* 110: 1726 (1980)

39. Medinsky, M.A., Popp, J.A., Hamm, T.E., Jr., and Dent, J.G., Development of hepatic lesions in male Fischer-344 rats fed AIN-76A purified diet. *Toxicol. Appl. Pharmacol.* 62: 111-120 (1982)
40. Hamm, T.E., Jr., Raynor, T., and Caviston, T., Unsuitability of the AIN-76A diet for male F-344 and CD rats and improvement by substituting starch for sucrose. *Lab. Animal Sci.* 32: 414-415 (1982)
41. Nguyen, H.T., and Woodard, T.C., Intranephronic calcinosis in rats. *Am. J. Path.* 100: 39-55 (1980)
42. deBethizy, J.D., Sherrill, J.M., Rickert, D.E., and Hamm, T.E., Jr., Effects of pectin-containing diets on the hepatic macromolecular covalent binding of 2,6-dinitro-(^{3}H)toluene in Fischer-344 rats. *Toxicol. Appl. Pharmacol.* 69: 369-376 (1983)
43. Toxic Substances Control Act Test Rules, Proposed Health Effects Test Standards. *Fed. Register* 44(91): 27334-27374 (1979)
44. Symons, J.M., Bellar, J.A., Carswell, J.K., Kropp, K.L., Robeck, G.G., Seeger, D.R., Slocum, C.J., Smith, B.L., and Stevens, A.A., National organics reconnaisance survey for halogenated organics in drinking water. *J. Am. Water Works Assoc.* 67: 634-637 (1975)
45. Pye, V.I., and Patrick, R., Ground water contamination in the United States. *Science* 221: 713-718 (1983)
46. Hall, J.E., White, W.J., and Lang, L.M., Acidification of drinking water: Its effects on selected biologic phenomena in male mice. *Lab. Animal Sci.* 30: 643-651 (1980)
47. Fidler, I.J., Depression of macrophages in mice drinking hyperchlorinated water. *Nature* 270: 735-736 (1977)
48. McKinney, J.D., Maurer, R.R., Hass, J.R., Thomas, R.O., in: *Identification and Analysis of Organic Pollutants in Water* (K. Lawrence, ed.), pp 417-432, Ann Arbor Science, Michigan (1977)
49. Raynor, T.H., White, E.L., Cheplen, J.M., Sherrill, J.M., and Hamm, T.E., Jr., An evaluation of a water purification system for use in animal facilities. *Lab. Animals* 18 (1984)
50. Clough, G., Environmental effects on animals used in biomedical research. *Biol. Rev.* 57: 487-523 (1982)
51. Lindsey, J.R., Conner, M.W., and Baker, H.J., in: *Laboratory Housing*, pp 31-43, National Academy of Sciences, Washington, DC (1978)
52. Schwarz, B.D., and Gevall, A.A., Influence of photoperiod and neonatally administered androgen on estrous cycles and behavior in hamsters. *Biol. Reprod.* 21: 1115-1124 (1979)
53. Lai, Y.L., Jacoby, R.O., and Jonas, A.M., Age related and light associated retinal changes in Fischer rats. *Invest. Ophthalmol. Visual Sci.* 17: 634-638 (1978)
54. Kraft, L.M., The manufacture, shipping and receiving and quality control of rodent bedding materials. *Lab. Animal Sci.* 30: 366-376 (1980)
55. Serrano, L.J., Carbon dioxide, and ammonia in mouse cages: Effect of cage cover, population and activity. *Lab. Animal Sci.* 21: 75-85 (1971)
56. Simmons, M.L., Robie, D.M., Jones, J.B., and Serrano, L.J., Effect of a filter cover on temperature and humidity in a mouse cage. *Lab. Animals.* 2: 113-120 (1968)
57. Dalhamn, T., Mucous flow and ciliary activity in the trachea of healthy rats and rats exposed to respiratory irritant gases (SO_2, H_3N, HCHO): A functional and morphologic (light microscopic and electron microscopic) study, with special reference to technique. *ACTA Physiol. Scand.* 36 (Suppl. 123): 1-161 (1956)

58. Ferguson, H.C., Effect of red cedar chip bedding on the hexobarbital and pentobarbital sleep time. *J. Pharm. Sci.* 55: 1142-1148 (1966)

59. Vessell, E.S., Induction of drug metabolizing enzymes in liver microsomes of mice and rats by softwood bedding. *Science* 157: 1057-1058 (1967)

60. Raynor, T.H., Steinhagen, W.H., and Hamm, T.E., Jr., Differences in the microenvironment of a polycarbonate caging system: Bedding vs. raised wire floors. *Lab. Animals* 17: 85-89 (1983)

61. Gale, G.R., and Smith, A.B., Ureolytic and urease-activating properties of commercial laboratory bedding. *Lab. Animal Sci.* 31: 56-58 (1981)

62. Baer, H., Long-term isolation stress and its effects on drug response in rodents. *Lab. Animal Sci.* 21: 341-349 (1971)

63. Gralla, E.J. (ed.), *Scientific Considerations in Monitoring and Evaluating Toxicological Research*, Washington, DC: Hemisphere Publishing Corp. (1981)

64. Douglas, J.F., Hamm, T.E., Jr., Jameson, C.W., Mahar, H., Stinson, S., and Whitmire, C.E., *Monitoring Guidelines for the Conduct of Carcinogen Bioassays*, USDHEW Publication Number (NIH) 80-1774 (1980)

65. Sansone, E.B., and Losikoff, A.M., Contamination from feeding volatile test chemicals. *Toxicol. Appl. Pharmacol.* 46: 703-708 (1978)

66. Sansone, E.B., and Fox, J.G., Potential chemical contamination in animal feeding studies: Evaluation of wire and solid bottom caging systems and gelled feed. *Lab. Animal Sci.* 27: 457-465 (1977)

67. Sansone, E.B., Losikoff, A.M., and Pendleton, A., Sources and dissemination of contamination in material handling operations. *J. Amer. Ind. Hyg. Assoc.* 38: 433-442 (1977)

68. Sansone, E.B., and Losikoff, A.M., Potential contamination from feeding test chemicals in carcinogen bioassay research: Evaluation of single- and double-corridor animal housing facilities. *Toxicol. Appl. Pharmacol.* 50: 115-121 (1979)

69. Cockerell, G.L., Gilmartin, J.E., Albern, W.F., Losikoff, A.M., and Sansone, E.B., Design and testing of a biocontainment system for chemical carcinogens. *J. Toxicol. Environ. Hlth.* 7: 1-7 (1981)

70. Fox, J.G., and Newberne, P.M., Environmental safety and chemical hazards in animal research. *Lab. Animals* Nov.-Dec., 35-51 (1979); and Jan.-Feb., 24-61 (1980)

71. Occupational Safety and Health Administration, Identification Classification and Regulation of Potential Occupational Carcinogens, *Fed. Register* 45: 5002-5296 (1980)

13

Conduct of Long-Term Animal Bioassays

J. David Prejean

Southern Research Institute
Birmingham, Alabama

INTRODUCTION

There are numerous articles and monographs in current literature written on conducting a long-term rodent bioassay study.[1-9] Each document provides extensive detail and discussion concerning the various individual elements that make up these studies—experimental design, personnel requirements and responsibilities, animal care and treatment, data collection and analysis and, of course, reporting. There is little need, therefore, to reiterate what has already been covered in some detail.

What has not been done, however, is to provide a linear flow to describe the step-by-step sequence of actions designed to produce a well organized, smoothly functioning, high quality study. This chapter will, therefore, provide that organization.

The first step in conducting a long-term rodent bioassay is subdividing the study into a series of logical phases. For instance, we normally have four phases we consider critical.

- Preliminary planning
- Initiation
- Execution (In-life activities)
- Completion

Each of these phases is of equal importance in producing a quality study; however, more problems have been created by inadequate preliminary planning than by any other factor. Emphasis will therefore be placed on this phase.

PRELIMINARY PLANNING

A study usually begins with the general experimental design. Once this information is available, it is carefully reviewed to determine whether there are enough data to begin formalized planning. This involves using the data provided to answer the following questions:

(1) What is the chemical to be tested?

(2) Is the chemical hazardous?

(3) What is the proposed route of administration?

(4) What is the frequency of dosing?

(5) How long will the study last?

(6) When should the study start?

(7) What species is to be used for the evaluation?

(8) How many animals are to be involved?

(9) What are the housing requirements?

(10) What type of in-life data will be collected (weights, clinical signs, clinical chemistry/hematology profiles, etc.) and at what frequency?

(11) What are the requirements for dosage analysis and bulk chemical reanalysis? Are procedures available?

(12) What are the requirements for dosage formulation? Is a procedure available?

(13) What are the histopathology requirements?

(14) What type(s) of report(s) is to be prepared? What is the deadline for final report submission?

With the answers to these questions, it can then be determined whether the available laboratory space, expertise of personnel and equipment on hand are sufficient to warrant initiation of preliminary planning. This assessment is the first critical decision and requires an unbiased evaluation of the laboratory's true capabilities. It's much better to say no at this point than to say yes, start the study, and then fail. With the latter situation, everyone loses.

Once it has been established that the facilities and capabilities are compatible with the study design, the first phase of preliminary planning can begin. General plans are made. Each of the major events in the study is laid out on a master study schedule. The first item considered is the start date. Normally, there is a range in which to operate. If a bioassay for carcinogenicity is conducted by a contract toxicology laboratory, a number of events must take place between signing the contract and starting the study. At least a two-week leeway should be given prior to the start of quarantine. This allows time to order the animals, obtain the test chemical, arrange for additional animal housing, validate the dosage formulation and dosage analysis procedures, validate the bulk chemical reanalysis procedure and complete and submit the protocol for conducting the study to the sponsor for final approval.

Based on the selected tentative start date, the terminal sacrifice period, the histology laboratory processing period and the pathology evaluation period can then be established. The necropsy/histopathology requirements for this study are then compared to requirements for other studies already scheduled. Adjustments are made so that sufficient necropsy, histology and pathology personnel are available to perform their functions in a timely manner. Whatever changes are necessary to accommodate the histopathology are translated into a revised start date.

At this point, it is extremely important to realize that it is relatively easy to start a chronic study, even one of fairly extensive size. For instance, with relatively little planning, two studies can be started every week until no more study rooms are available. The standard daily/weekly/monthly activities, such as collecting clinical observations, dosing, etc., can also be maintained with relatively little effort. It is an entirely different matter, however, to perform all of the tasks associated with terminating a study in a timely manner. Only a limited number of necropsies can be completed each day; only so many slides can be produced; and most important, a pathologist can provide a quality evaluation on only a limited number of tissues. Too, the efficient functioning of a laboratory is dependent upon establishing a reasonably standard workload so that a nucleus of well-trained personnel can be maintained and effectively utilized at all times. Thus, in scheduling the start of a study, it is imperative that the "rate-limiting steps" and the general impact on the daily workload be taken into consideration.

After this preliminary general scheduling has been satisfactorily completed—the projected start date meets the sponsor's deadlines, and the "rate-limiting steps" have been integrated into the master study schedule—it is time to begin the specific preliminary planning phase. It is here that each of the major events in the experimental design is scheduled. Probably the most efficient way to do this is to use a standard protocol format for the type of study to be conducted and simply fill in the blanks. Although protocol formats differ from sponsor to sponsor—and it is best to use one that is acceptable to the sponsor of that particular study—all formats are basically the same. The data are merely arranged in different ways or statements are made concerning subjects such as "Test Article Characterization," etc., using different words. One should keep in mind that some activities require rigid scheduling (*i.e.*, start date, necropsy, pathology evaluation, final report submission, etc.), whereas others are planned within general time frames and offer a reasonable degree of flexibility even after the study has been initiated. Most interim activities such as clinical chemistry profiles, serial sacrifices, etc., fall into this category of flexible scheduling (*e.g.*, months 3, 6 and 15).

It is also expedient at this time to run a literature search on the chemical to be evaluated. The sponsor probably has already done this and has taken all known factors into consideration in the experimental design; however, the more the test laboratory knows about the test material, the more effectively the evaluation techniques can be utilized.

Information to complete the preliminary planning is provided in answers to the 14 questions covered in the experimental design. Additional information should also be available from the literature search. During this phase of preliminary planning, great care should be given to understanding why the chemical is to be evaluated, exactly how the sponsor has planned for the evaluation to be performed, and how the study described in the protocol responds to these factors. It is better to take extra time at this point than to move ahead rapidly and encounter problems that could easily have been avoided. This is emphasized only because there is great temptation to start a study too quickly just because the sponsor has a short deadline.

Additional steps beyond those mentioned above include:

(1) Checking with suppliers to see if the proper animals and the specified feed are available at the proper time;

(2) Verifying that sufficient caging, racks, and feeders are available;

(3) Verifying that qualified laboratory personnel are available to provide animal care and test chemical administration and to collect in-life data;

(4) Verifying that the chemical laboratory anticipates no problems with the formulation, dose analysis or chemical reanalysis procedures and that the proper instrumentation is on hand or readily available;

(5) Verifying that all clinical pathology procedures requested are available;

(6) Verifying that the quality assurance unit can handle the audit requirements (particularly the protocol review);

(7) Checking with the sponsor to see if the necessary quantity of test chemical will be available at the proper time; and

(8) Calculating the final estimated costs to perform the study and supplying this information to the sponsor.

Obviously, the exact sequencing of the events included under "preliminary scheduling" will vary depending on the sponsor, the exact nature of the study requested, and the capabilities and expertise available within each laboratory. Every item mentioned, however, must be addressed in order to maximize the probability of a successful study.

INITIATION

Depending on how the opportunity arose to perform the study, the time frame between preliminary preparations and the initiation of the study may be lengthy or very short (true with industrial contracts). If the time frame is lengthy, it may be necessary to repeat a number of the preliminary planning requirements to assure that the original scheduling is still valid. Once this has been accomplished, specific preparations can begin for initiating the study. As with preliminary planning, starting a study requires that a number of very important steps be taken prior to the dosing of the first animal, which marks the end of this phase. These can be broken down into the following subcategories: protocol and final scheduling, chemical, animals, animal housing and maintenance, laboratory procedures and data handling, quarantine, randomization and finally, initial dosing.

Protocol/Final Scheduling

First, the official study protocol and study schedule(s) are prepared. This means establishing firm dates for all study activities including:

(1) Start date for quarantine;

(2) Date of health check;

(3) Date of randomization;

(4) Date of first dosing;

(5) Date of first dosage formulation and subsequent scheduling thereafter (usually a specified weekday, Monday through Friday, on a once per week or once per two weeks basis);

(6) Date of first dosage analysis and subsequent scheduling (an example of one way this schedule can be prepared is shown in Table 1);

(7) Date of first chemical reanalysis and subsequent scheduling (an example of one way this schedule can be prepared is shown in Table 2);

(8) Date of first clinical chemistry/hematology analyses and the scheduling of subsequent analyses (normally the initial prestudy baseline data is scheduled for a specific date. All subsequent analyses are usually scheduled by "week of study." This provides some leeway in the advanced scheduling of this particular activity.);

(9) Dates of other interim procedures such as serial sacrifices (normally scheduled by the week of study or by the month of study);

(10) Dates of weighings and clinical observations (usually scheduled by day of week for once per week and by day of week and week of month for once per month or once per four weeks);

(11) Date of last dosing;

(12) Date of start of necropsy; and

(13) Date that the final report is due.

Table 1: Sample of a Dosage Analysis Schedule

Dosage Analysis Schedule for XXXX
July, 1983–August, 1983

Chemical	Dose Level or Concentration (ppm)	Date of Mixing* (month and day)	
		July	August
XXXX	435	7,14,21,28	4,11,18,25
	871	7,14,21,28	4,11,18,25
	218	7,14,21,28	4,11,18,25
	326	7,14,21,28	4,11,18,25
	435	7,14,21,28	4,11,18,25
	653	7,14,21,28	4,11,18,25

*Underline denotes day of analysis

Table 2: Sample of a Chemical Reanalysis Schedule

Chemical Reanalysis Schedule
November, 1983–January, 1984

Chemical	Batch	11/83	12/83	1/84
X	03			*
XX	01	*		
XXX	06	*		
XXXX	02		*	
XXXXX	01			*

*Denotes scheduled reanalysis

Dates, however, are not the only items included in the protocol, but close attention to dates in relation to other laboratory plans provides a sound base on which to operate for the next two years. Details concerning the elements involved in a good protocol are presented in Chapter 12 of this book.

There are a number of items that must be completed prior to dosing the first animal other than completion of the protocol. Most can be accomplished concurrently with protocol preparation. Included are:

Chemical

(1) Calculating and informing the sponsor of the amount of test chemical that will be required along with the date the shipment should arrive at the laboratory;

(2) Receiving the test chemical;

(3) Using the dose formulation procedure to mix the established mixtures;

(4) Analyzing dosage mixtures to establish that the analytical procedure works properly in the ranges selected and that the mixing procedure works properly at the dosages selected; and

(5) Reanalyzing the bulk chemical to establish that it is the proper substance and the prescribed purity.

Animals

(1) Ordering the proper animals to use on the study. Animals should be pathogen- and virus-free and shipped in filtered shipping crates. A microbiological/serological profile should be requested from the supplier;

(2) Receiving the animals in good physical condition.

Animal Housing and Maintenance

(1) Ascertaining that the proper caging, racks, etc., are available at the laboratory or are readily available from a supplier;

(2) Obtaining cages, etc., from suppliers if ordering is necessary;

(3) Ordering the proper feed and projecting future requirements to maintain the study;

(4) Obtaining the feed.

Laboratory Procedures and Data Handling

(1) Assuring that the proper structure for the efficient systematic handling of the data is in place;

(2) Reviewing the protocol with all professional staff, supervisors and technical staff associated with conducting the study;

(3) Ascertaining that all required Standard Operating Procedures (SOPs) are up to date and available to the proper personnel.

Quarantine

(1) Paying careful attention to the general appearance and health of the animals while uncrating and during the quarantine period;

(2) Sometime prior to randomization, sacrificing several animals of each sex and species and examining all internal organs grossly for abnormalities. Histopathology may be required. At this time, the animals should also be carefully checked for external and internal parasites (pinworms, tapeworms, etc.). A blood sample for bacteriological and serological testing can also be obtained at this point.

(3) Assuring that the food, water, temperature, room lighting and humidity are the same as those to be used in the chronic study. Group housing, however, should be used regardless. Thus, if the watering systems at the animal supplier and laboratory are different, the less intelligent animals can learn to drink by copying the more intelligent ones.

(4) Handling the animals during quarantine at least once a day, particularly if they are to be dosed by gavage or painting on the skin.

Randomization

The final step prior to dosing the first animal involves randomization into the proper test groups. Randomization is probably best performed on the day prior to first dosing, although this may vary depending on the requirements of the specific study. Regardless of the exact procedure, several items should be taken into consideration during the process—average group weights, unique animal identification, appropriate cage labeling and cage and rack configurations.

The randomization procedure should be designed so that the final weights of the test groups differ by no more than approximately five grams for rats and hamsters and two grams for mice. In other words, the average weights of the groups should all be close although it is not absolutely necessary that they be exactly the same.

Each animal in the study must be uniquely identified at randomization. Ear tags are fine for individually housed animals but are not very good if group housing is used. Ear marks (punch and notch) are also satisfactory for individually housed animals but are again not very satisfactory for group housed ones particularly for male mice. Ear marks also have a tendency to disappear with time and remarking is normally required once or twice during the study. Toe clipping may be the best all-around method for uniquely identifying an animal. One possible method, which is recommended by the National Toxicology Program, is presented in Figure 1.

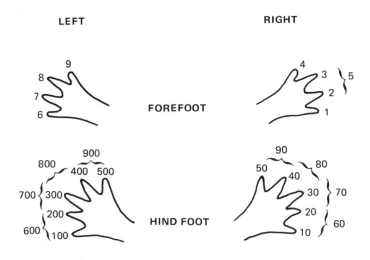

Figure 1: Example of individual animal identification using toe clips.

Cage labeling is also an important consideration, especially since cages and racks are normally rotated during the course of the study. As with animal identification, different systems are acceptable. The exact system used will depend on how the animals are housed (individually or by group), how the cages are arranged on the rack and obviously, upon individual laboratory preferences. The inclusion of several items on these labels, however, is important and helpful: The chemical name or identification number, the dose level, the cage number and the identification number(s) of the animal(s) housed within the cage. In addition, it is helpful to color code the cages by dose level and then color code the various dosing containers to help preclude misdosing. One way is to use a colored dot on the cage label and a similar dot on the dosing container. Further, it is extremely helpful to assign the chemical a color code as it arrives in the facility. For example, a combination of three colors could be used. These colors, as horizontal or vertical stripes, are then placed on all bulk chemical containers, dose formulation containers, animal cages and on the doors to the animal rooms. Again, this procedure helps eliminate misdosing.

The final consideration during randomization should be the cage and rack configuration. Since it is now routine to rotate both the cages and racks during a study, usually once every two weeks, it is imperative that some careful thought be given to the placement of dose groups on a rack. A vertical configuration is normally preferable to a horizontal one. With the vertical plan, cages can move from the top of the rack to the bottom and vice versa. Some horizontal variation is also obtained since multiple verticle columns are usually required to house a chronic study. If group housing is used, consideration must be given at the out-set regarding how animals that require individual housing will be handled. If sentinels are to be used for screening for disease, their positioning should also be considered. Finally, once the initial cage and rack configurations are set, rotation schedules should be prepared so that the system can function smoothly without the need for hurried preparation of a new configuration each time the cages and racks are due for rotation.

First Dosing

The completion of first dosing marks the end of the initiation of the study. At this point, there should be few complications, expecially if the design has been properly translated into the protocol, SOPs and schedules. One or two con-siderations do require a brief mention, however. If animal weights are to be used in the dosing process (*e.g.*, gavage), a decision should be made concerning when the weights will be used. For example, if the weights are taken in the morning, are they used in dosing the animals on that day or on the next? In a two-year study, the decision is probably not critical but consistency is necessary.

It is also necessary to consider the time of day that the animals will be dosed. For dosed-feed studies, it obviously should make little difference but for gavage and skin painting studies, the time of day could be an important factor. Regardless, dosing at a specific period of the day on a consistent basis is necessary.

EXECUTION (IN-LIFE ACTIVITIES)

If all of the preceding suggestions and requirements (along with any others not mentioned) have been properly addressed, conducting the in-life phase of the study should be the easiest part. In general, the study director should be able to spend the time where it is most desirable—reviewing the data, observing the conduct of the various aspects of the study at first hand and monitoring the bud-get. Usually, regardless of how carefully the protocol and activity schedules have been prepared, there will always be problems that require attention; these should be minor, however.

Although the protocol and schedules prepared prior to the start of the study should be sufficient notice for most activities, it is wise to prepare monthly schedules that summarize each of the critical activities. Dosage analysis schedules should therefore be prepared on a monthly basis and submitted to the analytical chemistry laboratory, as should chemical reanalysis schedules. As is evident from a sample dosage analysis schedule presented in Table 1, this activity is scheduled on a daily basis. Chemical reanalysis is normally scheduled on a monthly basis as shown by the example in Table 2. Most other laboratory activities should also be formally scheduled once a month. Figure 2 shows an example of a weighing schedule and Figure 3 an example of a cage and rack rotation schedule. Copies of all interim schedules should also be provided to the Quality Assurance Unit.

NOVEMBER 1983

		1 STUDY XXXX	2 STUDY XX	3	4	5
6	7	8	9	10	11 STUDY X	12
13	14 STUDY XXX	15	16	17	18	19
20	21	22	23	24	25	26
27	28	29 STUDY XXXX	30 STUDY XX			

Figure 2: Example of a periodic animal weighing schedule.

NOVEMBER 1983

		1 STUDY XXX	2 STUDY X	3	4	5
6	7 STUDY XX	8	9	10	11 STUDY XXXX	12
13	14	15 STUDY XXX	16 STUDY X	17	18	19
20	21 STUDY XX	22	23	24	25 STUDY XXXX	26
27	28	29 STUDY XXX	30 STUDY X			

Figure 3: Example of a cage and rack rotation schedule.

Results of the various study activities—body weight averages, average food/water consumption, dosage analysis results, clinical observations, survival data, etc.—are normally available on either a same day or next day basis and should be reviewed almost immediately. In addition to the standard information available on a study, it can also be advantageous to have other important data such as gavage accidents or dosing errors tracked and summarized on a weekly basis. Animals housed alone on studies requiring group housing is another parameter that is important to follow.

COMPLETION

Activities associated with the completion of the study phase should have been well laid out in the protocol and final study schedule. As with other critical activities, however, it is good to provide insurance. For that reason, beginning approximately three months prior to the terminal sacrifice date, all activities associated with the completion of the study should be reevaluated and the schedule and available personnel reverified. This should be repeated at the start of the next two months so that nothing unexpected can easily upset the plans.

Completion of the study can be subdivided into necropsy and associated activities, histopathologic processing of the tissues, microscopic evaluation of the tissues, preparation of the final report, including the contributing scientists' reports, submission and acceptance of the final report and finally, the archiving of all study data and specimens. Most of these activities occur on a concurrent basis.

Necropsy

The scheduling of necropsy activities on a daily basis becomes necessary approximately three to four weeks prior to the initiation of this event. Consideration must be given to the following items:

(1) Are there any other activities, such as clinical chemistry/hematology profiles or bacteriological/serological profiles, that must be scheduled into the necropsy sequence? This invariably complicates matters, especially if mice are involved and the maximum amount of blood (or serum or plasma) is needed.

(2) How many animals are remaining on the study and how many days are available to complete the necropsy?

(3) How many prosectors are available during the necropsy period? It may well be necessary to make certain reassignments in order to house a staff of sufficient size to complete the task.

(4) How many necropsy stations are available at any one time?

(5) Is the designated pathologist aware of the proposed schedule and available?

Once the above questions are answered, specific plans can be made. For most chronic studies, necropsies should be completed within seven calendar days from the start; however, the shorter the time frame the better. While seven days is the maximum, a more realistic time frame is five days. If the number of animals remaining on study is multiplied by the number of hours it takes to perform the necropsy, the projected total hours for necropsy can be obtained. Dividing this by the estimated number of hours that the necropsy area can be manned each day and then dividing by the estimated number of prosectors available to man the stations, will give a reasonably good estimate of the length of time (in days) it will take to complete the necropsy. One additional point should be kept in mind. It takes just as much pathology time to supervise the necropsy of one animal as it does five if five animals are necropsied at the same time. Pathology time is valuable and every effort should be made to use it effectively. In other words, the prosector stations should be fully manned during a terminal sacrifice.

Although each laboratory will obviously have its own procedures (SOPs, etc.) for conducting the necropsy, one or two points are worth emphasizing. Animal identification should be verified at each step along the way, especially if the animal or animal tissues are passed from one technician to another. Labeling on the necropsy forms, blood sample vials (if used), blood smears (if used) and wet tissue containers should be verified in the same manner. Finally, someone should match the necropsy forms and wet tissue labels and review the necropsy forms for completeness and legibility.

For convenience, it might be wise to maintain a special record of all necropsy activity on a study-by-study, dose-by-dose basis. An example is provided in Table 3. This record is kept in addition to any computer records that might also be maintained.

Table 3: Example of a Sacrifice Schedule for Chemicals on Test

Month	Group Number	Species	Phase	Chemical	First Day of Scheduled Sacrifice	Group
August	1	Rats	Subchronic	XXX	8/9/83	All
	2	Rats	Subchronic	XXX	8/23/83	All
September	3	Mice	Chronic	X	9/19/83	All
October	4	Rats	Chronic	X	10/3/83	All
	5	Rats	Chronic	XXXXX	10/11/83	All
	6	Mice	Chronic	XXXXX	10/25/83	All

Histologic Processing

Histologic processing also requires that significant attention be paid to scheduling. As with necropsy, the number of animals to be processed, the approximate number of tissues from each animal (translated into the number of slides), the number of available histotechnicians and, of course, the number of weeks allowed for this activity are all important in developing and monitoring the schedule. In developing the schedules, one should remember that histology production rates will directly affect the effectiveness of the pathology evaluation. Thus, it is necessary to plan carefully the expected workload for this study in conjunction with scheduled workloads from other studies and also with unscheduled workloads (*i.e.*, interim deaths) so as to provide a steady supply of processed tissues for microscopic evaluation. It is absolutely necessary that the identification of each animal be confirmed by comparing the identifying material in the wet tissue bag (*e.g.*, ears or feet with appropriate marking, ear tags, etc.) with the header information on the necropsy record. This process should be extended to checking the identification on the trimmed tissue with that shown on the necropsy record. Further checks should be made when the tissues are embedded, when they are placed on pencil labeled slides for staining, and when the cover slips and final paper labels are placed on the slides.

Histology technicians should be cautioned to record any additional abnormalities they observe as well as any missing or extra tissues. All tissues specified in the protocol should be found or listed as missing.

Prior to the submission of the processed tissues to the pathologist, the laboratory supervisor should review the slides for air bubbles, torn tissue, knife marks, etc., which may make a recut necessary. It is preferable to catch problems in the laboratory rather than leave them to the pathologist. In addition to checking the slides for quality, the supervisor should also check to see that all gross lesions have been processed and that the slide labels are accurate.

Microscopic Evaluation

Although each step in performing a long-term bioassay study is of obvious importance, the microscopic evaluation is probably the most important. It is this information upon which the decision concerning the carcinogenicity (and/or toxicity) of a test chemical in the test species is based. Because of the importance of these data, a great deal of emphasis has been placed on it, especially in the areas of quality, consistency and accuracy. Complicating this portion of the study, is the fact that the time remaining before submission of the final report is growing short and any delays encountered in histology only compound themselves during the microscopic evaluation. Also, the satisfactory completion of this phase of the study rests on one person—the pathologist.

As with histologic processing, the initial step in the pathologic evaluation process is the correlation of slide labels with animal identification information on the necropsy/histology forms. Normally, the order in which a pathologist reviews the slides on a particular study is a matter of choice. Some prefer to evaluate the controls first. Others like to start with the high dose. As for the end product, it probably really doesn't matter. What does matter is that each tissue be carefully examined for lesions and abnormalities. Whether they are the result of age or are chemically-related is really immaterial at this point.

In all likelihood, the pathologist will have to review all of the tissues from the animals which died early in order to obtain a complete picture of dose-related effects and produce the required consistency in diagnoses. The pathologist should also be careful to address each gross lesion recorded at necropsy or during histologic processing.

Reporting

This phase of the bioassay study actually began with the preparation of the study protocol. Regardless of how the records were maintained and the data were collected and analyzed (by hand or by computer), the process has been continuous. Thus, by the time of terminal sacrifice, most of the in-life data should have already been reduced to tables, charts and summaries so that work can begin immediately on the "Methods and Materials Section" of the report.

Exact time tables for summarizing the data and preparing the final report will vary depending on personnel and organizational structure. As a rule of thumb, the final report should be submitted to the sponsor no later than six months after the last animal is sacrificed. It is, therefore, necessary to plan carefully and execute efficiently. Milestone schedules are very helpful but they are only schedules and are subject to change. One should not wait until the day the contributing scientist's report for chemistry is due to check on its status. People are busy and forget. Report deadlines are met because there is someone tracking and pushing, not because reasonable deadlines for submission have been set.

The preceding recommendations, along with those supplied in the chapter on experimental design and the information included in the numerous articles and monographs available in the literature, should provide a sound basis upon which to plan, start, conduct and terminate a successful long-term animal bioassay.

One final bit of advice, however, is paramount in avoiding the consequences suffered by several toxicology laboratories in recent years. There are no perfect long-term studies—mistakes do happen. When they do, be honest. It is easier (and smarter) in the long run to admit a mistake when it is made than to have someone else discover it at a later date.

REFERENCES

1. Berenblum, I. (ed.), *Carcinogenicity Testing*. UICC Technical Report Series, No. 2, Geneva: International Union Against Cancer (1969)
2. Food and Drug Administration, Advisory Committee on Protocols for Safety Evaluation: Panel on Carcinogenesis Report on Cancer Testing in the Safety Evaluation of Food Additives and Pesticides. *Toxicol. Appl. Pharmacol.* 20: 419–438 (1971)
3. Food Safety Council, Chronic Toxicity Testing. Proposed System for Food Safety Assessment. *Fd. Cosmet. Toxicol.* 16, Suppl. 2, 97–108 (1978)
4. Sontag, J.M., Page, N.P. and Saffioti, U., *Guidelines for Carcinogen Bioassay in Small Rodents* (National Cancer Institute Carcinogenesis Technical Report Series No. 1), DHEW Publication No. NIH 76–801, Washington: DHEW (1976)
5. National Toxicology Program, *General Statement of Work for Conduct of Acute, Fourteen Repeated Dose, 90-Day Subchronic, and 2-Year Chronic Studies in Rodents*, Research Triangle Park: National Institute of Environmental Health Sciences (1982)
6. Krewski, D., Clayson, D., Collins, B. and Munro, I.C., Toxicological procedures for assessing the carcinogenic potential of agricultural chemicals. *Basic Life Sci.* 21: 461–497 (1982)
7. International Agency for Research on Cancer, *Long-term and Short-term Screening Assays for Carcinogens: A Critical Appraisal*. IARC Monographs on the Evaluation of the Carcinogenic Risk of Chemicals to Human, Supplement 2, Lyon: IARC (1980)
8. Interagency Regulatory Liaison Group, Scientific basis for identification of potential carcinogens and estimation of risks. *J. Natl. Cancer Inst.* 63: 241–268 (1979)
9. Munro, I.C., Consideration in chronic toxicity testing: The chemical, the dose, the design. *J. Natl. Cancer Inst.* 61: 183–197 (1977)

14

Selection and Use of the B6C3F1 Mouse and F344 Rat in Long-Term Bioassays for Carcinogenicity

Dawn G. Goodman

PATHCO Inc.
Potomac, Maryland

Gary A. Boorman

National Institute of Environmental Health Sciences
National Institutes of Health
Research Triangle Park, North Carolina

John D. Strandberg

Johns Hopkins University
Baltimore, Maryland

INTRODUCTION

Animals have long been used as models for human disease and for predicting potential risks or hazards for humans. In ancient Babylonia, animals were sacrificed and their entrails examined in the practice of divination both for medical and other crises. Galen, a physician in Roman times, dissected Barbary apes to learn anatomy.[1] In more recent times, animals have been used to study infectious diseases, such as tuberculosis and rabies. Studies included new and more accurate methods of diagnosis, and elucidation of the pathogenesis and treatment or cure of the disease. Currently, animals are used extensively in basic and applied biomedical research and in safety testing of new drugs, environmental and occupational toxins, pesticides, and food additives as well as in assessing the efficacy of new drugs. In the last fifty years, animals have been used more and more in experimental oncology, as models for specific types of cancer, in the study of basic mechanisms of carcinogenesis, and in studies for carcinogenicity to determine the potential of various chemical, physical and infectious agents to cause cancer.

The use of animals in these ways is often questioned by the general public. Some responses to this question include: (1) It is undesirable to use humans as experimental subjects for possible harmful studies when other means exist to determine potential risk to humans; (2) animals and humans have many of the same responses to injury, whether induced by physical, chemical or infectious agents; (3) animals have long been used in a variety of toxicity tests and in many cases have been found to be excellent predictors of human toxicity; and (4) most known human carcinogens are also animal carcinogens [2,3] (Tables 1 and 2). The fact that several chemicals were found to be carcinogenic in animals before they were determined to be carcinogenic in humans suggests that extrapolation from animal studies to humans is both feasible and relevant.

There are a number of characteristics which should be considered when selecting an animal species for chronic toxicity/carcinogenicity studies.[6-8] These include: (1) Availability of extensive data on incidences of natural diseases, including spontaneous tumor rates; (2) low spontaneous tumor rates; (3) sensitivity to a wide variety of chemicals; (4) comparable metabolism of test chemical between the animal species used and humans; (5) knowledge of good husbandry practices; (6) relatively short life span; (7) size of the animal; (8) hardiness of the animal; (9) cost of maintaining the animals; (10) ease of breeding; (11) ease in handling; (12) availability; and (13) availability of inbred strains which have less variation in the incidence of background lesions than random bred animals.

Many animal species have been used in long term toxicity/carcinogenicity studies including rats, mice, hamsters, dogs, nonhuman primates, rabbits and fish. However, from a practical point of view, rodents, primarily rats and mice, are usually considered the most appropriate species for routine carcinogenicity and toxicity studies as they have many of the characteristics enumerated above. Frequently, hamsters are used as a third test species.

Some of the more common strains and stocks of rats used in carcinogenicity studies are the inbred F344 (Fischer) and OM (Osborne-Mendel) rat and the random bred Sprague-Dawley, Wistar and, to a lesser extent, Long-Evans (LE) and Holtzman stocks.[7] For each of these strains and stocks there are varying amounts of published data on natural diseases and spontaneous tumor rates.[9-31] Strains and stocks of mice frequently used include the Swiss and related stocks, the inbred BALB/c strain, and the (C57B1/6N x C3H/HeN)F_1 or B6C3F1 hybrid. Spontaneous age-associated lesions have been documented in these strains and stocks.[17,20,21,25,32-38]

SELECTION OF THE B6C3F1 MOUSE AND F344 RAT FOR CARCINO-GENICITY STUDIES

The selection of a species and strain for toxicological testing is based on available current data, and is a compromise between the known advantages and disadvantages of the species and strains in question. The selection of the hybrid B6C3F1 mouse and F344 rat by the National Cancer Institute (NCI) and their

Table 1: Known Chemical Carcinogens in Humans; Comparison with Animal Data[a]

Chemical	Human Target Organ(s)	Animal(s) Tested	Animal Target Organ(s)
Aflatoxin	Liver	Rat, mouse, duck, nonhuman primates, fish	Liver, stomach, colon, kidney, lung, local
4-Aminobiphenyl	Urinary bladder	Mouse, rabbit, rat, dog	Urinary bladder, liver, mammary gland, intestine
Arsenic	Skin, lung, liver	Inadequate tests[a,b] in mice, rat, dog	
Asbestos	Lung, pleura, gastro-intestinal tract	Mouse, rat, hamster, rabbit	Lung, pleura, local
Benzene	Hematopoietic system	Mouse, rat[c]	Zymbal gland, oral cavity, skin, hematopoietic system, lung, Harderian gland, preputial gland, ovary, mammary gland
Benzidine	Urinary bladder	Mouse, rat, dog, hamster	Liver, urinary bladder, Zymbal's gland, colon
Bis(chloromethyl) ether	Lung	Mouse, rat	Lung, nasal cavity, skin, local
Chloroamphenicol	Hematopoietic system	No adequate tests	
Chloromethyl methyl ether	Lung	Mouse, rat	Skin, lung, local
Cyclophosphamide	Urinary bladder	Mouse, rat	Hematopoietic system, lung, urinary bladder, mammary gland, multiple sites

(continued)

Table 1: (continued)

Chemical	Human Target Organ(s)	Animal(s) Tested	Animal Target Organ(s)
Diethyl-stilbestrol	Uterus, vagina	Mouse, rat, hamster, nonhuman primate	Mammary gland, uterus, vagina, testis, hematopoietic system, kidney, urinary bladder, pituitary
Isopropyl oils	Nasal cavity, larynx	No adequate tests	
Melphalan	Hematopoietic system	Mouse, rat	Skin, lung, hematopoietic system, local
Mustard gas	Lung, larynx	Mouse	Lung, mammary, local
2-Naphthylamine	Urinary bladder	Mouse, nonhuman primate, dog	Urinary bladder, liver, lung
N,N-Bis(2-chloro-ethyl)-2-naph-thylamine	Urinary bladder	Mouse, rat	Lung, local
Oxymetholone	Liver	No adequate tests	
Phenacetin	Kidney	No adequate tests	
Phenytoin	Hematopoietic system	Mouse	Hematopoietic system
Vinyl chloride	Liver, lung, brain	Mouse, rat	Liver, lung, blood vessels, mammary gland, Zymbal's gland, kidney

[a]Taken from references 2 and 3
[b]Taken from reference 4
[c]Taken from reference 5

Table 2: Industrial Processes Associated with Carcinogenic Effects in Humans; Comparison with Animal Data*

Chemical	Human Target Organ(s)	Animal(s) Tested	Animal Target Organ(s)
Auramine manufacture	Urinary bladder	Mouse, rat	Liver, intestine, site of application
Cadmium-using industries	Prostate, lung	Rat	Testis, site of application
Chromium (chromate production)	Lung, nasal cavities	Mouse, rat	Lung, site of application
Hematite mining	Lung	Mouse, hamster, rat, guinea pig	Negative
Nickel refining	Nasal cavity, lung	Rat, mouse, hamster	Lung, site of application
Soot, tars, oils	Lung, skin (scrotum)	Mouse, rabbit	Skin

*Taken from references 2 and 3

continued use by the National Toxicology Program (NTP) is no exception. The NCI awarded its first contract for a carcinogen bioassay in 1962[39] with moderate growth of testing during the 1960s. The National Cancer Act of 1971 provided a rapid influx of financial support for carcinogen testing, resulting in a greatly expanded program. It was at this time that a decision was made to standardize the tests as much as possible. To diminish interspecies variation, it was decided that essentially all test guidelines and protocols would require at least two species.[39,40] Even at that time, cost was a major consideration leading to selection of smaller rodents. The mouse was a natural choice because of its small size, ease of care, relatively short life span, and the fact that it had been widely used in research as an animal model for chemical carcinogenesis. The rat is second to the mouse in importance and use as a research animal. It has found especially wide utilization in toxicology testing and was a logical choice for the second species to be used in the NCI testing program. A factor against selecting the guinea pig may have been its inability to metabolize the aromatic amine 2-acetylaminofluorene (AAF) to the carcinogenic metabolite as occurs in rat, mouse, hamster, dog, cat, and man.[39,41]

Selection of the B6C3F1 Mouse

The strain of mouse preferable for carcinogenicity testing was a highly controversial issue.[39] The Food and Drug Administration (FDA) advisory committee[42] and Canadian Ministry of Health and Welfare[43] recommended outbred mice while Shimkin[44] and others[45] supported the use of inbred strains. The argument for inbred strains was that genetic homogeneity, and known and uniform behavioral, biochemical and developmental attributes would allow the investigator to carry out experiments with greatly reduced variables. Smaller numbers of animals could be used and there would still be good reproducibility between studies.[45] The principal argument against inbred strains was loss of genetic variability including the possibility of deletion of some essential characteristic necessary for detection of a carcinogen. In addition, some experimental evidence indicated that homozygous individuals adapted less well to minor environmental agents.[45] The use of F_1 hybrids from two inbred strains offered advantages to proponents advocating either outbred animals or inbred strains. The hybrid has genetic uniformity while still having greater genetic diversity than inbred strains, and the hybrid is generally hardier than inbred strains.[45]

Early in the NCI bioassay program several strains of mice were used including strain A mice, random bred CD-1 HaM/ICR mice, and two F_1 hybrid strains of mice, the (C57BL/6 x C3H/Anf)F_1 strain (B6C3F1) and the (C57BL/6 x AKR)F_1 strain.[46] The F_1 hybrids were used in a large scale study by Innes *et al.*[47] to detect the possible carcinogenicity of pesticides and industrial chemicals. This program involved 20,000 mice exposed to 127 different chemicals for 18 months. Two different F_1 hybrids were used for all studies and thus were available for direct comparison. Female C57BL/6 mice were mated with C3H/Anf or AKR males to produce the (C57BL/6 x C3H/Anf)F_1 or (C57BL/6 x AKR)F_1 hybrid, respectively. Eighty-nine of the test chemicals were considered negative for carcinogenicity in both sexes of both hybrid strains and a further 20 chemicals gave equivocal results that would require further study. Eleven chemicals were reported to be positive and seven additional chemicals known to be carcinogens had been included as positive controls.

The F_1 hybrids differed in their responses to chemicals that were considered known carcinogens. Both the B6C3F$_1$ male and female mice had significantly elevated incidences of liver tumors for six of seven positive control compounds with a different compound being negative for each sex (Table 3). Thus, all seven positive controls produced an elevated incidence of liver tumors in male and/or female B6C3F1 mice. This was not true for the other F_1 hybrid where males were positive for four of seven studies and females for three of seven studies; two of seven positive control compounds did not cause an elevated tumor incidence for either sex. This specific issue was not dealt with in the discussion of this study.

Table 3: Liver Tumors in Mice[a]

Mouse	Incidence in Negative Controls (%)[b]	... Positive Controls ...		.Experimental Chemicals.	
		Studies Positive[c]	Overall Incidence (%)	Studies Positive	Overall Incidence (%)
(C57BL/6 x C3H/Anf)F$_1$					
Males	8/79 (10%)	6/7	71/123 (58%)	8/11	104/185 (56%)
Females	0/87 (–)	6/7	59/122 (48%)	9/11	57/193 (30%)
(C57BL/6 x AKR)F$_1$					
Males	5/90 (6%)	4/7	53/124 (43%)	10/11	103/190 (54%)
Females	1/82 (1%)	3/7	41/115 (36%)	3/11	25/187 (13%)

[a]Taken from reference 47
[b]Incidence = mice with hepatomas/total mice necropsied (%)
[c]Positive studies = number of studies where hepatoma incidence was significant at 0.01 level/total studies

The Innes study was probably instrumental in the eventual selection of the B6C3F1 mouse by the NCI testing program.[48] In addition, the B6C3F1 mouse was found to be hardy, easy to breed, disease resistant, and had a low spontaneous tumor incidence at most sites with up to 75% survival at 18 months. Only the hepatocellular tumors in male mice were considered to exceed 10%.[47] The CD-1 HaM/ICR mouse which had also been used early in the NCI bioassay program had a relatively short life span coupled with a high incidence of spontaneous tumors.[49] The strain A mouse develops a high incidence of lung tumors at an early age. Thus, neither of these strains was considered suitable for long-term bioassays and the B6C3F1 mouse became the strain of choice.

Current National Toxicology Program (NTP) studies use the B6C3F1 mouse almost exclusively. The animals have been demonstrated to retain the characteristics responsible for their original selection. The relatively high incidence of hepatocellular tumors, particularly in males, has been thought by some to be a drawback to the use of this strain. An important factor in the continued use of this hybrid is the extensive historical data base available in the literature.[17,38] Thus, this strain is becoming more widely used for toxicity and carcinogenicity evaluation.

Selection of the F344 Rat

Early in the NCI bioassay program, the F344 and OM rat strains were the most widely used along with the Sprague-Dawley stock and to a lesser extent, Charles River (CR) Wistar stock.[39] The F344 rat was apparently eventually selected as the main test strain because of its small size, vigor, good survival and relative disease resistance compared to other strains.[46] The fact that it was an inbred strain was probably also important in its selection for the NCI testing program. The high incidence of interstitial cell tumors of the testicle was recognized at that time and was felt not to detract significantly from its usefulness as a general test animal.[39] In contrast to the B6C3F1 mouse which has been used almost exclusively from early in the NCI Carcinogen Testing Program, the switch to using the F344 rat exclusively occurred in the mid-1970s. The F344 rat continues to be used in the NTP testing program despite several disadvantages. The almost universal occurrence of testicular tumors limits its usefulness for long-term studies where male reproductive organs might be the target. Similarly, the presence of mononuclear cell leukemia is quite high, but usually appears only in the last few months of a two year study.

ORIGIN OF THE B6C3F1 MOUSE AND F344 RAT

As mentioned previously, the B6C3F1 mouse is properly designated (C57BL/6 x C3H/HeN)F_1 and is the F_1 hybrid of two inbred strains, the C57BL/6 and the C3H/Anf. The F344 rat is an inbred strain of rat. These strains are maintained at the National Institutes of Health (NIH) Genetic Resource in the Veterinary Research Branch (VRB). They are also available from commercial breeders as is the B6C3F1 hybrid. In order to minimize genetic drift, the production colonies for the F344 rat and the parent inbred strains for the B6C3F1 mouse are rederived from the NIH Foundation Colony stock on a regular basis for the NTP studies.

Origin of the B6C3F1 Mouse

The female parent for the B6C3F1 mouse is from the C57BL/6 strain. This strain was originated by Dr. Little in 1921, from the brother-sister mating of female 57 to male 52; both animals were from Miss Abby Lathrop's stock.[37] A black subline of the strain developed from this mating was maintained with subline 6 separated prior to 1937. Subline 6 was given to Dr. Fekete and then to Dr. Hall. Dr. Hall gave the C57BL/6 strain to Jackson Laboratories in 1948. The C57BL/6 was obtained by NIH in 1951 and now is designated as C57BL/6N.[20]

The male parent for the B6C3F1 is from the C3H strain. The C3H strain originated with Dr. Strong from a cross of a Bagg albino female and a DBA male in 1920. A litter of four females and two males was sent to Dr. Andervont in 1930 who, in turn, gave the strain to Dr. Heston in 1941. The C3H strain was obtained by NIH from Dr. Heston in 1951 and was designated as C3H/HeN. When this strain was established behind the specific pathogen free (SPF) barrier facility, two groups of C3H/HeN mice were obtained, one with and one without the mammary tumor virus (MTV). The MTV is transmitted vertically through the milk; thus, when the C3H/HeN strain was caesarean derived in the barrier facility, the resulting offspring did not carry the MTV. This strain is designated C3H/HeN-MTV⁻. The C3H/HeN-MTV⁺ strain was established behind the barrier by inoculating newly caesarean derived mice with purified MTV. The C3H/HeN-MTV⁻ strain is periodically rederived from the C3H/HeN-MTV⁺ strain to maintain genetic homogeneity.[20] The C3H/HeN-MTV⁻ strain is used to provide the male parent for the B6C3F1 currently used by NTP and its proper designation is (C57BL/6 x C3H/HeN-MTV⁻)F$_1$. Thus, the B6C3F1 used in NTP studies does not carry MTV.[20] It should be noted, however, that B6C3F1 mice obtained from other sources may be derived from C3H mice carrying MTV. There is some evidence such mice may have titers to MTV.[50]

Origin of the F344 Rat

The current F344 rat strain appears to have originated from a colony of rats started at the Columbia University Institute for Cancer Research by Drs. Curtis, Dunning, and Bullock. The initial stocks were purchased from seven different breeders including Fischer, August, Marshall, and others; subsequent inbreeding of each stock led to the formation of several strains including the F344 strain.[45,48] The strain was given to Dr. Heston in 1949 and to NIH by Dr. Heston in 1951. Its current strain designation is F344/N.[13,20]

CHARACTERISTICS OF THE B6C3F1 HYBRID MOUSE

The B6C3F1 hybrid is a brown mouse. Adult males weigh 40 grams to 45 grams and females weigh 35 grams to 40 grams. B6C3F1 mice are good breeders and produce large litters. They have good longevity with around 75% to 80% surviving to two years.[48]

The B6C3F1 mouse has been used for about ten years, primarily in carcinogenicity studies, and there are extensive data on the incidences of spontaneous neoplasms although much less information is available regarding nonneoplastic lesions.[17,33,38,47] Although such data are available, each laboratory should develop its own historical data base since necropsy protocols, tissue sampling techniques and diagnostic criteria vary between laboratories, thus profoundly affecting tumor incidence. Currently, there are little historical data available for nonneoplastic lesions of the B6C3F1 mouse. Nomenclature and diagnostic criteria are even less well standardized for nontumor pathology, and great care should be taken when comparing data between laboratories. With increasing emphasis on toxic lesions, an historical control data base for nonneoplastic lesions is necessary for toxicity evaluations.

Neoplasms with an incidence of 1% or more in untreated B6C3F1 mice are listed in Table 4. The figures in this table are from the most recently reported NTP historical control data.[17] The NTP historical controls are derived from studies conducted for NTP at various contract testing laboratories and include only untreated control animals. The pathology portion of these bioassays undergoes an extensive review under the auspices of the NTP (*see* Chapter 16).[51,52] Because of these reviews and numerous pathology workshops, the terminology, at least for neoplastic lesions, is generally consistent throughout the NTP Carcinogenesis Testing Program even though different pathologists perform the histopathologic evaluation on the individual control groups.

Common Spontaneous Neoplasms

The most common tumors include hepatocellular neoplasms, lymphomas, and alveolar/bronchiolar tumors of the lung. These tumors are rarely observed in animals less than one year of age, with few being seen prior to 18 months. After 18 months, the incidence for all types of tumors increases rapidly.[33,38] The common neoplasms are discussed below.

Hepatocellular neoplasms. Hepatocellular neoplasms are the most common tumors in B6C3F1 mice, particularly in males, where the combined incidence of adenomas and carcinomas ranges from 16% to 58% in untreated controls, with an average of 31% (Table 4). These tumors are uncommon in animals less than 18 months old; however, the incidence increases dramatically after that time. Most of these tumors are hepatocellular carcinomas. Hepatocellular tumors are often observed grossly and are described as tan, yellow or mottled, firm masses either raised above the surface of the liver or pedunculated. Adenomas usually have smooth or circumscribed borders whereas carcinomas tend to have irregular or nodular margins. Hepatocellular tumors are usually solitary in untreated animals but are often multiple when induced.

At microscopic examination, hepatocellular adenomas in mice may be composed of cells with eosinophilic, basophilic or vacuolated cytoplasm. In untreated B6C3F1 mice, the most common histologic types seen are basophilic or mixed basophilic-vacuolated tumors. Adenomas are generally solid nodules of closely packed cells with inapparent sinusoids. They are sharply demarcated from and compress adjacent parenchyma (Figure 1). In basophilic tumors, the cells are smaller than normal hepatocytes with basophilic granular cytoplasm and prominent central vesicular nuclei. In some tumors, fatty change or cytoplasmic vacuolization is prominent (vacuolar type). In occasional tumors the cells are larger than usual with abundant, eosinophilic, faintly granular cytoplasm (eosinophilic type). Bile ducts are usually absent; when present, they are commonly

Table 4: Common Primary Neoplasms in B6C3F1 Mice[a,b]

	Male			Female		
	Number of Tumors (%)	Standard Deviation, %	Range, %	Number of Tumors (%)	Standard Deviation, %	Range, %
Circulatory system	2343[d]			2486[d]		
Hemangioma	34 (1.5)	3.3	0–16	39 (1.6)	1.9	0–6
Hemangiosarcoma	64 (2.7)	2.6	0–10	48 (1.9)	2.3	0.8
Digestive system	2334[c]			2469[c]		
Liver						
Hepatocellular adenoma	240 (10.3)	5.5	0–24	98 (4.0)	3.9	0–18
Hepatocellular carcinoma	498 (21.3)	6.9	8–36	101 (4.1)	3.0	0–15
Total	725 (31.1)	7.5	16–58	196 (7.9)	4.6	0–20
Endocrine system						
Anterior pituitary	1903[c]			2051[c]		
Adenoma	11 (0.6)	1.5	0–6	163 (7.9)	8.5	0–32
Carcinoma	1 (0.1)	0.3	0–2	8 (0.4)	0.9	0–5
Adrenal	2240[c]			2306[c]		
Cortical adenoma	53 (2.4)	3.0	0–15	7 (0.3)	1.1	0–4
Cortical carcinoma	3 (0.1)	0.6	0–4	1 (<0.1)	0.3	0–2
Pheochromocytoma	28 (1.2)	1.9	0–6	16 (0.7)	1.2	0–4
Pheochromocytoma, malignant	2 (0.1)	0.4	0–2	0	–	–
Thyroid	2178[c]			2203[c]		
Follicular cell adenoma	22 (1.0)	1.6	0–6	40 (1.8)	2.1	0–9
Follicular cell carcinoma	5 (0.2)	0.6	0–2	6 (0.3)	1.5	0–10
Hematopoietic system	2343[d]			2486[d]		
Lymphoma/leukemia	297 (12.7)	7.3	2–32	677 (27.2)	9.9	8–62

(continued)

Table 4: (continued)

	Male			Female		
	Number of Tumors (%)	Standard Deviation, %	Range, %	Number of Tumors (%)	Standard Deviation, %	Range, %
Integumentary system	2343[d]			2486[d]		
Fibroma/neurofibroma	28 (1.2)	2.7	0-12	1 (<0.1)	0.6	0-4
Sarcoma (all types)	106	–	0-19	38	–	0-10
Reproductive system						
Mammary gland	2343[d]			2486[d]		
Adenoma	0	–	–	8 (0.3)	1.1	0-6
Carcinoma	0	–	–	40 (1.6)	2.3	0-12
Respiratory system						
Lung	2328[c]			2388[c]		
Alveolar/bronchiolar adenoma	282 (12.1)	6.7	0-28	131 (5.5)	3.6	0-14
Alveolar/bronchiolar carcinoma	119 (5.1)	4.3	0-18	47 (2.0)	2.3	0-8
Special sense organs						
Harderian gland	2343[d]			2486[d]		
Adenoma	50 (2.1)	2.8	0-12	32 (1.3)	1.7	0-6
Carcinoma	1 (0.1)	0.4	0-2	1 (<0.1)	0.3	0-2

[a]Tumors with an incidence of 1% or greater in one or both sexes
[b]Taken from Reference 17
[c]Number of tissues examined histopathologically
[d]Number of animals necropsied

near the edge as though entrapped. At present, there is no evidence that there is any difference in biologic behavior of these morphologic types. Several reports suggest that induced and spontaneous hepatocellular neoplasms may have different morphologic patterns.[53-57]

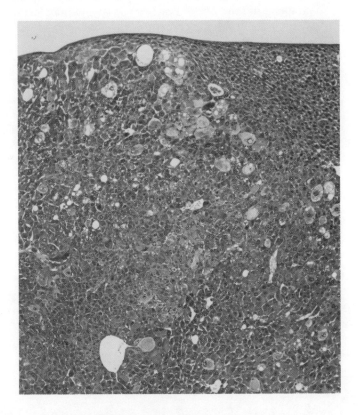

Figure 1: Hepatocellular adenoma from a female mouse with compression of adjacent normal hepatic tissue. Tumor cells are large, irregular in size and arrangement, and focally degenerate. 160X; H&E.

Hepatocellular carcinomas are usually large and can possess several architectural patterns, including solid, trabecular and glandular (Figure 2). The cell types seen are the same as in hepatocellular adenomas; in some well differentiated tumors they may closely resemble normal hepatocytes. Most carcinomas have some areas of trabecular arrangement. This consists of hepatic cords and plates many cells thick with a random pattern often ending abruptly in a dilated sinusoid (Figure 3). Occasionally, small spaces surrounded by hepatocytes and resembling acini are present. Sinusoids are often dilated and hemorrhage, thrombosis and necrosis of adjacent hepatocytes are common in larger tumors. In some tumors, there may be a relatively small focus of trabecular pattern in a large solid tumor otherwise resembling an adenoma, thus suggesting that some adenomas may give rise to carcinomas. In some apparently solid tumors, a trabecular pattern can often be discerned by careful observation, noting the relative positions of the sinusoidal lining cells and the number of intervening tumor cells. In other solid tumors, cells may be very pleomorphic and bizarre. Anaplastic tumors are uncommon as are those with glandular differentiation. Metastases occasionally occur, primarily to the lung (Figure 4), and are usually associated with the larger tumors which have a trabecular pattern.

Lymphoreticular neoplasms. Tumors of the lymphoid system are also commonly observed in both male and female B6C3F1 mice, particularly in females. In females, these range in incidence from 8% to 62% with a mean of 27%; the rate in males is approximately half that in females. The most common histologic type is a pleomorphic lymphoma (Figure 5). Synonyms include follicular cell lymphoma,[58] reticulum cell sarcoma, type B,[59,60] or mixed lymphoma. The mesenteric lymph nodes, Peyer's patches or spleen are the most common sites, with secondary involvement of the liver. Leukemia (malignant cells in the peripheral blood) may occur late in the disease accompanied by solid tumors elsewhere in the body. These tumors originate from B-cells, arising from cells of the germinal follicles,[58] hence the term follicular cell lymphoma.

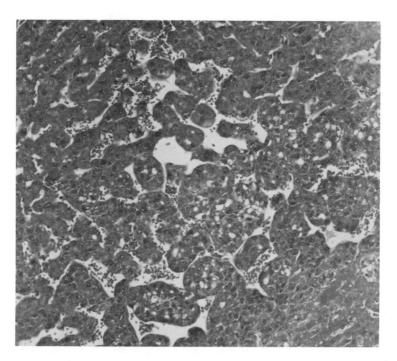

Figure 2: Hepatocellular carcinomas from a 312 day female mouse. Neoplastic hepatocytes form irregular cords separated by irregular vascular channels. 170X; H&E.

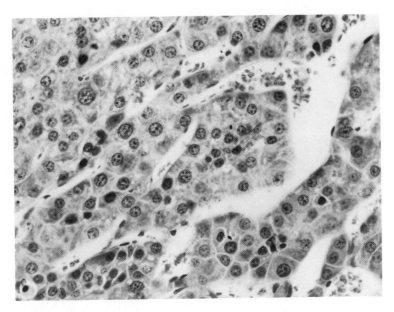

Figure 3: Hepatocellular carcinoma from a mouse. The hepatic cords are many cell layers thick. There is a large cord in the center ending abruptly in a dilated sinusoid. 330X; H&E stain.

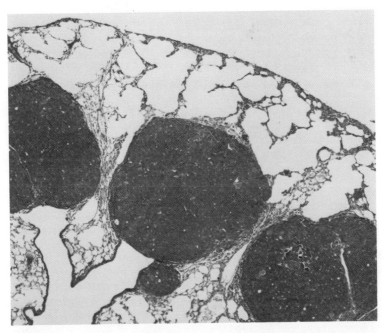

Figure 4: Pulmonary metastases of the hepatocellular carcinoma shown in Figure 2. Large nodules of tumor replace and compress the normal pulmonary structures. 60X; H&E.

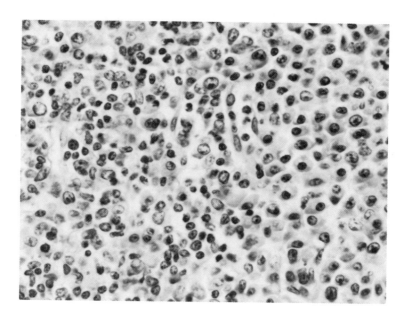

Figure 5: Pleomorphic lymphoma in a lymph node from a mouse. The neoplasm is characterized by a mixed cell population including reticular cells, epitheloid cells, lymphocytes and plasma cells. 540X; H&E.

Pleomorphic lymphomas frequently have a nodular appearance both grossly and microscopically. In the spleen, neoplastic cells are limited primarily to the white pulp, forming large nodules which eventually replace the entire spleen. In lymph nodes, the tumors are usually seen in the cortex but may eventually efface the node.

These lymphomas are composed of a pleomorphic or mixed cell population including large pale epithelioid cells with abundant cytoplasm and prominent vesicular nuclei; reticular cells with large nuclei, prominent nucleoli and scant cytoplasm; small and large lymphocytes, and plasma cells. The lymphocytes and plasma cells are often histologically normal although they may occasionally appear atypical. The cellular composition of tumors may vary between animals and from site to site within an individual. In its early stages, this tumor may be mistaken for an inflammatory process due to its pleomorphic nature; however, it follows a progressive course and no underlying cause, such as a chronic infection, can be found.

Alveolar/bronchiolar neoplasms. Alveolar/bronchiolar (A/B) tumors of the lung are also frequently seen in the B6C3F1 mouse, particularly in males. A/B tumors are twice as common in males as in females (Table 4) and adenomas are observed twice as often as carcinomas in both sexes. In males, adenomas range in incidence from 0% to 28% with a mean of 12%. A/B neoplasms were originally thought to arise from alveolar type II epithelial cells.[61,62] Recently it has been reported that some may be of Clara cell origin.[63]

Alveolar/bronchiolar neoplasms are grossly seen as spherical, firm white masses elevating the pleural surface. Those designated as adenomas tend to be solitary lesions, usually less than 2 mm in diameter, while carcinomas are larger, multinodular and sometimes multifocal. Histologically, adenomas are well circumscribed, although not encapsulated, masses coi posed of cuboidal to low columnar cells with amphophilic cytoplasm and vesicular nuclei resting on a delicate connective stroma which may be thrown into papillary fronds or tubular formations (Figure 6). Near the periphery of the nodule, the neoplastic cells appear to follow pre-existing alveolar septa. The larger carcinomas are similar morphologically, and there tends to be piling up of the epithelium resulting in many cell layers or solid sheets of cells. Both cellular morphology and architectural patterns are more pleomorphic in malignant lesions, and hemorrhage, focal necrosis and fibrosis are sometimes present. The tumor margins are not well circumscribed, and they often extend into the adjacent lung parenchyma. Metastases, although uncommon, are generally intrapulmonary with multiple small foci of neoplastic cells scattered throughout the lung. Occasionally, there is widespread extrapulmonary dissemination, most commonly to the pleura. Particularly when metastatic or transplanted, these tumors can develop a sarcomatous histologic pattern. It should be noted that some investigators consider all A/B neoplasms to be malignant[62] since there is progression from hyperplasia to large transplantable tumors. There appears to be a spectrum from alveolar cell hyperplasia to adenoma to carcinoma and the distinctions between each are not always clear-cut.

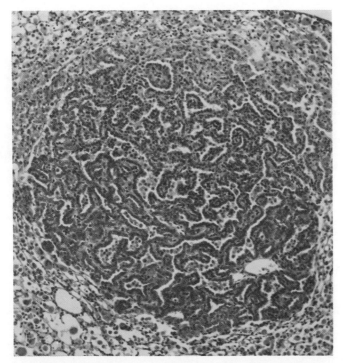

Figure 6: Bronchopulmonary adenoma merges with and compresses the surrounding pulmonary alveoli. The alveoli contain pigment-laden macrophages. Aged mouse. 105X; H&E.

Common Age-Associated Lesions

The incidences of nonneoplastic lesions in the B6C3F1 mouse are not as well documented as the neoplastic lesions. Common age-associated lesions have often not been recorded in the past unless unusually severe. In addition, there is frequently great variability in terminology between pathologists to describe the same lesion. Some of the more common lesions include adrenal subcapsular cell hyperplasia, ovarian cysts, cystic endometrial hyperplasia of the uterus, mineralization in the brain, and mild chronic inflammation of the kidney.[33,38]

Subcapsular cell hyperplasia of the adrenal gland (Figure 7) is common in aged mice, particularly females, of many strains, including the B6C3F1 mouse.[64,65] There is a focal or diffuse proliferation of spindle cells originating beneath the capsule of the adrenal gland. This involves the zona glomerulosa and may extend downwards into the cortex, forming triangular lesions with the apex directed toward the medulla. The spindle cells are referred to as type A cells and are oval to fusiform with elliptical nuclei and scant basophilic or amphophilic cytoplasm. These cells have recently been demonstrated by electron microscopy to represent adrenal cortical cells.[66] Occasionally, another cell type (type B) is found either as single cells scattered among the spindle cells or in small nests surrounded by type A cells. Type B cells are large round to polygonal cells with abundant pale eosinophilic, faintly granular or clear, vacuolated cytoplasm and round, usually central, vesicular nuclei.

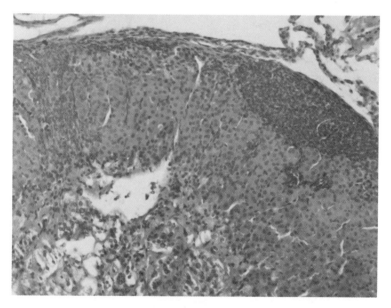

Figure 7: Subcapsular cell hyperplasia in the adrenal of an adult mouse. The small hyperplastic cells extend from the capsule into the cortex in several areas. 160X; H&E.

Ovarian cysts are common in female B6C3F1 mice, with a reported incidence of 11%[33,38] although the actual incidence, as noted earlier, may be higher.
While many of these cysts appear to be follicular in origin, it is often difficult to
determine their origin as the adjacent ovarian stroma is usually atrophic. Thus,
they may have risen from paraovarian structures as well. Pigment laden cells are
often present in the ovarian stroma. These cells have abundant, foamy, pale yellow cytoplasm which is acid fast and is thus a form of the aging pigment, lipofuscin.

Cystic endometrial hyperplasia of the uterus (Figure 8) is extremely common in B6C3F1 female mice with an incidence greater than 35%.[33,38] Diagnoses
of uterine cysts or hydrometra often represent components or variants of this
lesion. There is proliferation of the endometrial glands with marked dilatation
resulting in cyst formation. The cystic glands are usually lined by high cuboidal
to columnar epithelium. Eosinophilic secretion is often present. In severe cases,
when the uterine lumen is obliterated by cysts, the lining epithelium may be
flattened or squamous and secondary infection may occur.

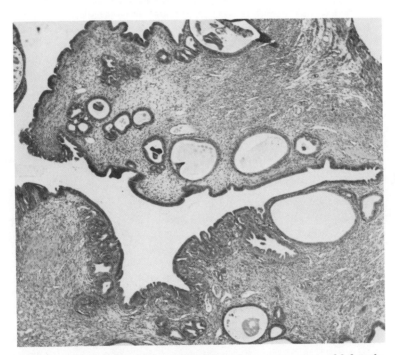

Figure 8: Cystic endometrial hyperplasia from a two year old female
mouse. The illustration shows the irregular proliferation of endometrial
stroma and cystic glandular elements. 40X; H&E.

Common Induced Tumors

In the NCI/NTP carcinogenesis program over 200 chemicals have been tested and final reports have been published. In the B6C3F1 mouse, a positive carcinogenic response has been observed in more than 20 different organs (Table 5)[67] with a number of chemicals being positive in more than one organ. The most common site was the liver, which was positive for more than a quarter of the chemicals. The next most common sites included lung, lymphoreticular system, and vascular system. The first three sites, *i.e.*, liver, lung and lymphoreticular system, are also common sites of development of spontaneous tumors in the B6C3F1 mouse. Thus, great care must be exercised in evaluating the significance of these tumors in treated animals. Not only the incidences reported in control *versus* treated animals, but the historical tumor rate must be considered and, even more importantly, the range of incidences seen, particularly at the laboratory conducting the study. It is known that diet, housing, and other environmental factors may influence tumor incidence, particularly of the liver.[68-70] Decreased latency and multiplicity of tumors of a single cell type in treated animals *versus* controls should also be considered in determining carcinogenicity of a chemical. The morphology and behavior of most induced tumors resemble those of their spontaneous counterparts; however, they may also be more anaplastic or of a morphologic type uncommon in untreated animals. Liver, lung and lymphoreticular tumors have been described above under spontaneous tumors. Vascular tumors of the blood vessels, hemangiomas and hemangiosarcomas, have also been induced frequently in mice. These induced tumors occur at a variety of sites, most commonly subcutis, liver and mesentery.[71] Vascular tumors in untreated animals are also found in these sites. A few chemicals have induced vascular tumors at unusual sites. 1,3-Butadiene was associated with hemangiomas and hemangiosarcomas of the heart,[72] and propylene oxide inhalation was associated with vascular tumors of the nasal cavity.[73]

CHARACTERISTICS OF THE F344 RAT

The F344 rat is a small albino rat. Adult males weigh about 400 grams to 450 grams and females weigh about 300 grams. F344 rats are good breeders and produce large litters. They have 70% to 80% survival at two years. Median survival is 29 to 30 months, and a few animals survive longer than 36 months.[11,13,23,26,48]

The F344 rat has been used for a number of years in toxicity and carcinogenicity studies and a great deal of data are available on the incidences of age-associated lesions, including tumor rates.[9,11,15,17,19,20,22,23,25,26,30] Neoplasms with an incidence of 1% or more in untreated F344 rats are listed in Table 6. The data in this table are from the most current NTP historical control data.[17] The derivation of the data is described in the section on the B6C3F1 mouse.

Common Spontaneous Neoplasms

The most common tumors observed in two year studies include interstitial cell tumors of the testis, anterior pituitary tumors, mammary tumors and mononuclear cell leukemia (Table 6). Although these neoplasms are occasionally seen in animals less than 18 months of age, their incidences increase dramatically after 18 months.[15]

Table 5: Number of Chemicals Tested by NCI/NTP Inducing Neoplasms at Specific Sites[a,b,c]

	F344 Rat	B6C3F1 Mouse
Integumentary system		
Skin	4	4
Subcutaneous tissue	5	1
Special sense organs		
Zymbal's gland	7	1
Harderian gland	–	2
Reproductive system		
Mammary gland	9	5
Ovary	–	1
Uterus	4	3
Seminal vesicle	–	1
Preputial/clitoral gland	5	–
Respiratory system		
Nasal cavity	3	3
Lung	2	8
Digestive system		
Oral cavity	1	–
Forestomach	5	8
Intestine	4	1
Liver	21	57
Pancreas	1	–
Hematopoietic system		
Spleen	6	–
Lymphoma/leukemia	3	8
Circulatory system		
Blood vessels	3	9
Heart	–	2
Urinary system		
Kidney	8	2
Urinary bladder	12	2
Endocrine system		
Adrenal gland	2	1
Thyroid	8	6
All other systems		
Body cavities	6	1

[a]Total of 215 chemicals reviewed
[b]Some chemicals positive at multiple sites
[c]Taken from references 14 and 32

Solleveld *et al.*[26] recently reported life span data for both male and female F344 rats. The incidences of the common tumors seen at two years continued to increase after this time. In addition, tumors of the endocrine system, uterus and subcutaneous connective tissue also increased dramatically. The spectrum of tumor types seen in older animals was comparable to that in animals killed at two years.

Interstitial cell tumors of the testis. Interstitial cell tumors of the testis are the single most common spontaneous tumor type, with an incidence ranging between 59% and 98% at two years (Table 6). Such a high incidence makes it virtually impossible in chronic studies to detect a toxic or carcinogenic effect at this site. This is a major drawback to the use of the F344 rat. Recently, Turek

Table 6: Common Primary Neoplasms in Untreated F344 Rats[a,b]

	Male			Female		
	Number of Tumors (%)	Standard Deviation, %	Range, %	Number of Tumors (%)	Standard Deviation, %	Range, %
Digestive system						
Liver	2306[c]			2356[c]		
Neoplastic nodule	78 (3.4)	3.5	0–12	71 (3.0)	3.0	0–12
Hepatocellular carcinoma	18 (0.8)	1.1	0–4	4 (0.2)	0.7	0–4
Total	96 (4.2)	3.9	0–14	75 (3.1)	3.2	0–12
Endocrine system						
Anterior pituitary	2158[c]			2262[c]		
Adenoma	468 (21.7)	11.7	2–52	995 (44.0)	11.4	18–70
Carcinoma	51 (2.4)	3.0	0–11	80 (3.5)	4.7	0–19
Adrenal	2280[c]			2338[c]		
Cortical adenoma	27 (1.2)	1.3	0–4	74 (3.2)	4.0	0–24
Cortical carcinoma	5 (0.2)	0.6	0–2	7 (0.3)	0.7	0–2
Pheochromocytoma	388 (17.0)	9.2	6–41	81 (3.5)	3.0	0–16
Pheochromocytoma, malignant	23 (1.0)	1.4	0–6	11 (0.5)	1.0	0–4
Thyroid	2230[c]			2265[c]		
C-cell adenoma	114 (5.1)	4.4	0–18	111 (4.9)	4.1	0–13
C-cell carcinoma	84 (3.8)	3.3	0–12	81 (3.6)	3.0	0–12
Follicular cell adenoma	22 (1.0)	1.4	0–5	10 (0.4)	1.0	0–4
Follicular cell carcinoma	17 (0.8)	1.4	0–7	10 (0.4)	0.9	0–2
Pancreatic islets	2226[c]			2303[c]		
Adenoma	84 (3.8)	3.6	0–12	18 (0.8)	1.5	0–7
Carcinoma	46 (2.1)	2.3	0–9	6 (0.3)	0.8	0–4
Hematopoietic system	2320[d]			2370[d]		
Lymphoma/leukemia	699 (30.1)	10.5	10–54	448 (18.9)	7.0	6–38
Integumentary system	2320[d]			2370[d]		
Squamous cell papilloma	29 (1.2)	1.7	0–5	6 (0.3)	0.7	0–2

(continued)

Table 6: (continued)

	Male			Female		
	Number of Tumors (%)	Standard Deviation, %	Range, %	Number of Tumors (%)	Standard Deviation, %	Range, %
Squamous cell carcinoma	20 (0.9)	1.3	0–4	15 (0.6)	1.2	0–4
Fibroma/neurofibroma	107 (4.6)	3.2	0–12	34 (1.4)	1.5	0–4
Sarcoma (all types)	37 (1.6)	–	0–4	27 (1.1)	–	0–2
Reproductive system						
Mammary gland	2320[d]			2370[d]		
Fibroadenoma	51 (2.2)	2.0	0–8	572 (24.1)	10.1	2–44
Carcinoma	6 (0.3)	0.7	0–2	48 (2.0)	2.4	0–8
Preputial/clitoral gland	2320[d]			2370[d]		
Adenoma	50 (2.2)	3.4	0–16	28 (1.2)	1.8	0–6
Carcinoma	63 (2.7)	3.0	0–11	46 (1.9)	2.7	0–12
Testis	2285[c]					
Interstitial cell tumor	2002 (87.6)	8.9	59–98	0	–	–
Uterus				2318[c]		
Endometrial stromal polyps	0	–	–	424 (18.3)	8.1	4–37
Endometrial stromal sarcoma	0	–	–	25 (1.1)	1.7	0–6
Respiratory system	2305[c]			2354[c]		
Lung						
Alveolar/bronchiolar adenoma	35 (1.5)	2.1	0–6	18 (0.8)	1.4	0–6
Alveolar/bronchiolar carcinoma	20 (0.9)	1.6	0–6	9 (0.4)	0.9	0–4
Body cavities	2320[d]			2370[d]		
Mesothelioma	53 (2.3)	1.7	0–8	1 (<0.1)	0.3	0–2

[a] Tumors with an incidence of 1% or greater in one or both sexes
[b] Taken from Reference 17
[c] Number of tissues examined histopathologically
[d] Number of animals necropsied

and Desjardins[74] have shown that tumor development is preceded by nodular hyperplasia of interstitial cells which can be seen as early as 12 months of age. As this becomes extensive, there is also atrophy of the epithelium of the seminiferous tubules. Interstitial tumors are grossly yellow, discrete, tend to be spherical and are often multiple and/or bilateral. Microscopically, the tumor cells resemble normal Leydig (interstitial) cells, being uniform polyhedral cells with abundant eosinophilic, finely vacuolated cytoplasm with round central to slightly eccentric vesicular nuclei. Frequently, around the periphery there are small basophilic cells with scant cytoplasm which form bands within the tumor (Figure 9). These are thought to be reserve cells. The tumors compress adjacent testicular tissue which is usually atrophic. In large neoplasms, there are frequently hemorrhage and necrosis. Other testicular neoplasms have not been reported in the F344 rat.[30,75]

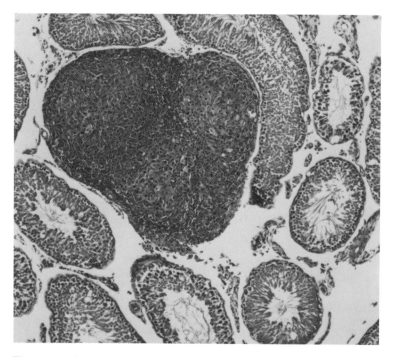

Figure 9: This section of testis from a 29 month old F344 rat contains a small interstitial cell tumor surrounded by atrophic seminiferous tubules. 85X.

Anterior pituitary neoplasms. Neoplasms of the anterior pituitary, as in most strains of rat, are also extremely common, particularly in females, with a wide range in the incidence rate in control groups (Table 6). A positive carcinogenic response at this site, especially in females, would be difficult to detect.

Most of these neoplasms are probably chromophobe adenomas. The cell type is usually not designated since special stains are not routinely used. However, when such stains are used, most tumors are of chromophobe origin. In rats, this type of tumor is often associated with prolactin production. A variety of mammary gland lesions, particularly fibroadenomas and cystic ducts, is frequently seen in animals bearing chromophobe adenomas.[76] However, Van Zwieten[77] was unable to show a statistical relationship between the occurrence of pituitary tumors and mammary carcinomas in the WAG/Riig and Sprague-Dawley rats.

Mammary gland neoplasms. Mammary neoplasms, primarily fibroadenomas, are common in female F344 rats (Table 6). Although the incidence of these tumors is relatively high, a carcinogenic effect can be detected in the F344 rat (Table 5).[78] This is often manifested by a marked increase in the number of adenocarcinomas with a similar or decreased incidence of fibroadenomas when compared to controls. Macroscopically, fibroadenomas are firm, well-circumscribed, lobulated, subcutaneous masses located on the ventral thorax and abdomen. They may become quite large, even impairing the mobility of the animal, but they rarely ulcerate. Fibroadenomas are composed of variable amounts of glandular and fibrous connective tissue (Figure 10), the latter often forming concentric whorls around individual acini. These tumors originate in the terminal ductules and lobules of the mammary gland, and this lobular pattern is often retained in the tumors. Cysts are often present within these tumors as well. The epithelium is usually one to two cell layers thick (Figure 11); secretory activity is variable. Mitotic activity is rare. Carcinomas which are much less common than fibroadenomas, are composed primarily of epithelial cells which form nests, acini, tubular or papillary structures. There is pleomorphism, anaplasia and piling up of the epithelium which also often has a high mitotic index. These tumors are fairly well circumscribed with only moderate local invasion. They may metastasize late in the course of the disease, but many animals die from other causes before this occurs.

Mononuclear cell leukemia. Another very common neoplasm in both males and females is the so-called "Fischer rat leukemia." Synonyms for this disease include monocytic leukemia, myelomonocytic leukemia, large granular lymphocyte (LGL) leukemia, and mononuclear cell leukemia (Table 6); the last is the term currently used by the NTP.[9,25,79-84]

Gross splenic enlargement is the most consistent finding. Hepatomegaly is frequently observed; lymphadenopathy and involvement of other visceral organs are variable. Histologically, the splenic pulp is consistently involved, the cellular proliferation apparently beginning in the marginal zone and involving the red pulp. The entire spleen is eventually involved. Early in the course of the disease, neoplastic cells are usually found in the liver sinusoids, first appearing in scattered foci that must be distinguished from foci of extramedullary hematopoiesis. The leukemic cells are often lined up in a row within the sinusoid rather than in small clusters as is often the case with extramedullary hematopoiesis. As the disease progresses, there is extensive involvement of the liver (Figure 12) with spread to pulmonary alveolar capillaries, lymph nodes, bone marrow and, to a lesser extent, other organs. In tissue sections the cells are large and round with oval, indented or folded nuclei with a moderate amount of faintly eosinophilic cytoplasm with indistinct borders. Other common microscopic findings are hepato-

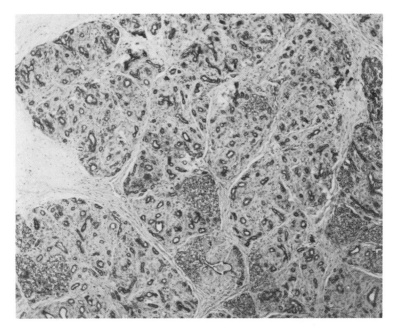

Figure 10: This small mammary fibroadenoma is composed of small lobules of ductular and stromal elements of variable cellularity. Aged rat. 45X; H&E.

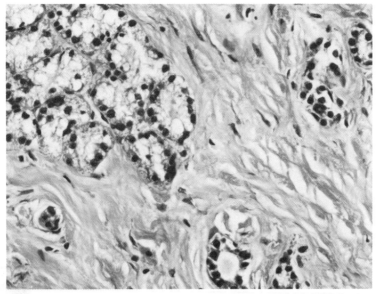

Figure 11: Fibroadenoma of the mammary gland from a F344 rat. The tumor is composed of both glandular elements and fibrous connective tissue. 350X; H&E.

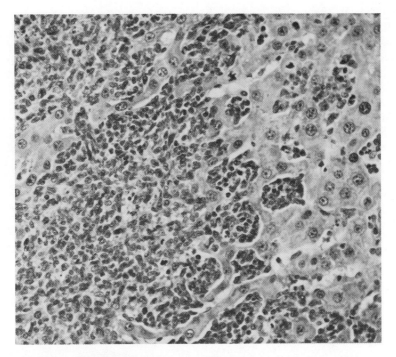

Figure 12: This section of liver from an aged male F344 rat illustrates invasion of hepatic sinusoids by neoplastic lymphoid cells ("Fischer rat leukemia"). 280X; H&E.

cellular degeneration and necrosis with secondary hypertrophy and hyperplasia, extramedullary hematopoiesis and erythrophagocytosis in the spleen, liver and lymph nodes, and bone marrow hyperplasia.

In the later stages of the disease, an immune-mediated hemolytic anemia often develops with a concomitant regenerative response.[83] Thrombocytopenia, elevated serum bilirubin, lactate dehydrogenase, alkaline phosphatase, alanine aminotransferase, aspartate aminotransferase, hemoglobinuria, urine urobilinogen, as well as bilirubinuria are common terminally.[82] Leukemia also occurs late in the disease with leukocyte counts up to 180,000 mm^3 with 20% to 90% being neoplastic cells. These cells are 12 μm to 20 μm in diameter with a high nucleus to cytoplasm ratio. The nucleus is usually round or indented, eccentrically located with coarse chromatin and occasional nucleoli. Cytoplasm is abundant and blue with azurophilic-granules when stained with Wright-Giemsa strains. Periodic-acid Schiff and oil red 0 stains are negative. A variety of histochemical studies are also negative, including alkaline phosphatase, esterase and peroxidase. Recently, the granules have been reported to be lysosomes containing β-glucuronidase and acid phosphatase.[84] Until recently, a specific classification of the cell involved had not been made. Ward and Reynolds[84] have reported that the neoplastic cell is a large granular lymphocyte.

Common Age-Associated Lesions

Some nonneoplastic lesions commonly seen in older F344 rats include chronic progressive nephropathy, basophilic foci of the liver, bile duct hyperplasia and cardiomyopathy.[11,15,29,85] Accurate incidences of these lesions are not well documented since these lesions are often not reported when mild and are considered to be "normal background" by many pathologists.

Chronic progressive nephropathy of a mild-to-moderate degree is commonly seen in aged F344 rats of both sexes, although it tends to be more severe in males than in females. This lesion consists of thickened glomerular basement membranes occasionally resulting in sclerosis of the glomerular tuft, dilatation of tubules with atrophy of the epithelium, protein casts in the tubular lumens, thickening of the tubular basement membranes, tubular epithelial hyperplasia (regenerative), and interstitial fibrosis with lymphocytic and plasma cell infiltrates (Figure 13). On occasion, golden-brown pigment (hemosiderin) can be seen in the tubular epithelial cells.

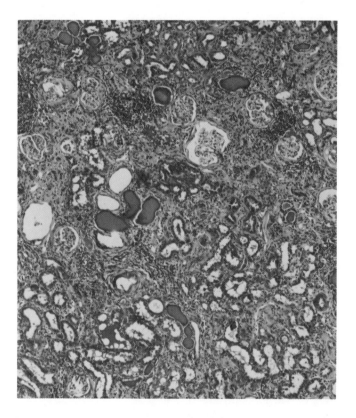

Figure 13: The chronic renal disease of aged F344 rats is a complex entity with glomerular scarring, interstitial inflammation and eosinophilic tubular casts. 65X; H&E.

Basophilic foci occur frequently in the liver of old F344 rats, particularly females. The lesion consists of foci of altered hepatocytes which are smaller than normal hepatocytes with basophilic cytoplasm. There is usually an increased number of cells per unit area within the focus, resulting in a somewhat distorted, tortuous cord pattern. The cells at the periphery of the focus blend into the surrounding parenchyma with no evidence of compression. These foci are similar to those described by Squire and Levitt.[86]

Bile duct hyperplasia (Figure 14) is also seen in the liver of aged F344 rats. This consists of clusters of tubular structures lined by low cuboidal cells with round central or basally located nuclei and a small amount of pale eosinophilic cytoplasm. These structures are surrounded by variable amounts of dense collagenous stroma. A mild lymphocytic infiltrate may also be present.

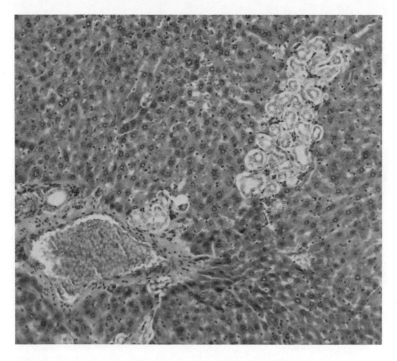

Figure 14: Bile duct hyperplasia is common in the liver of older animals. Male F344 rat, 24 months. 140X; H&E.

Cardiomyopathy (chronic degenerative myocarditis) is a common age-associated lesion increasing in incidence and severity with age. It can be seen to a mild degree in a few animals less than six months of age. It is most common and most severe, however, in animals over 18 months of age. This lesion is most frequently observed in the papillary muscles and wall of the left ventricle. Other parts of the heart may also be involved but with less frequency. Microscopically, there is degeneration and atrophy of the myocytes with fibrosis isolating and replacing myocytes (Figure 15). Inflammatory infiltrates are usually absent or minimal. When present, they consist primarily of lymphocytes and macrophages. Even severely affected rats rarely show clinical signs associated with cardiomyopathy. Some rats do have thrombosis of the left atrium. The relationship of this lesion, if any, to the cardiomyopathy is unknown.

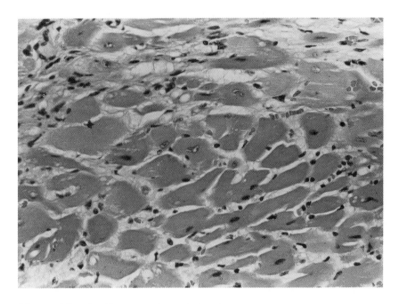

Figure 15: Cardiomyopathy of the heart in an aged F344 rat. The myocytes in the center of the photograph are swollen and more eosinophilic. At the periphery, there is atrophy of myocytes with a small amount of fibrosis. A few lymphocytes are scattered between the muscle fibers. H&E stain.

Common Induced Neoplasms

As described for the B6C3F1 mouse, more than 200 chemicals have been tested for carcinogenicity by NCI/NTP. In all, some 20 separate tissue sites in the rat have shown a positive carcinogenic response (Table 5). A number of chemicals were positive at more than one site. The most common site affected was the liver; other common sites include urinary bladder and mammary gland (Table 5).[67] These neoplasms are described below except for mammary tumors which have been previously described.

Hepatocellular neoplasms. Liver tumors in rats have been well described in the literature.[14,25,29,86,87] The term "neoplastic nodule" is used for nonmalignant neoplastic lesions in the liver in rats. The term originated from a workshop on hepatocellular lesions in rats held in 1975[86] and was used to reflect the biologic behavior of these lesions, *i.e.*, that these lesions are neoplasms and some have the *potential* to progress to malignant neoplasms. Neoplastic nodules are morphologically comparable to hepatocellular adenomas in other species. Microscopically, neoplastic nodules may be divided into eosinophilic, basophilic, clear cell or mixed, based on the morphology of the cells comprising the neoplasm. Basophilic neoplastic nodules are probably the most frequently observed as spontaneous age-associated tumors. These nodules are composed of basophilic cells with granular cytoplasm, and are generally somewhat smaller than surrounding hepatocytes. There is distinct compression of adjacent parenchyma along at least part of the border of the nodule. Cells within the nodule are arranged in irregular, distorted cords, one or two cell layers thick, which are perpendicular to hepatic cords in the adjacent parenchyma, at least in some areas. Angiectasis within the nodule may be present. Portal triads are occasionally observed within the nodule, usually located near the periphery as though entrapped. Eosinophilic or clear cell neoplastic nodules are similar to the basophilic nodules except for the size and tinctorial properties of the neoplastic cells. In both types the cells are larger than normal hepatocytes with abundant cytoplasm which is either eosinophilic or clear with a ground glass appearance. The latter are uncommon as spontaneous lesions but have been induced by a number of chemicals.

Hepatocellular carcinomas have many of the same histologic features as neoplastic nodules, particularly the more well differentiated ones. They are generally larger than neoplastic nodules and exhibit a trabecular pattern in at least a portion of the tumor. In these areas, the cords or plates are several cell layers thick and often end abruptly, projecting into sinusoids. In trabecular carcinomas, this pattern predominates. There are also large dilated sinusoids and hemorrhage and necrosis are common. Occasionally, glandular patterns may be present within the tumor, suggesting bile duct origin; however, areas of obvious hepatocellular carcinoma are generally present with transitions between the two patterns. Trabecular hepatocellular carcinomas are the most likely to metastasize. Occasionally, hepatocellular carcinomas may be very bizarre and anaplastic.

The recognition of precancerous lesions in the rat liver and the progression of neoplastic nodules to hepatocellular carcinomas is an area of controversy.[88-90] It has been shown that liver nodules induced in the rat by a known carcinogenic regimen will disappear through a process of remodeling when the stimulus is removed.[88] However, despite remodeling the hepatocytes within this area continue to express a new antigen[89] and may well represent the progeny of initiated cells. This is an important issue in evaluating the results of carcinogenicity studies and is the subject of much research.

Urinary bladder neoplasms. The urinary bladder seems to be a fairly common site of induced tumors in the F344 rat, at least in the NCI/NTP studies. This predilection may be a function of the type of chemicals tested, a number of which are aromatic dyes[14,78,91] or the compound or a metabolite may be excreted in the urine. The tumors range from transitional cell neoplasms, either papillomas or carcinomas, to transitional cell neoplasms with squamous metaplasia, to squamous cell neoplasms, predominantly carcinomas. Induced tumors tend to be multifocal, and within a single bladder several different types of lesions, both hyperplastic and neoplastic may be seen. Occasionally, mesenchymal tumors, usually of smooth muscle origin, may be induced in addition to the epithelial tumors. For critical evaluation of the urinary bladder, the bladder should be distended with fixative at necropsy. This will minimize folding artifacts due to contraction of the bladder. In addition, viewing the intact, distended bladder over a strong light source (transillumination) will often highlight even small lesions which might otherwise be missed.

In rats treated with a bladder carcinogen, a spectrum of lesions may be observed, from hyperplasia to metaplasia to benign and malignant neoplasia. There is usually focal or diffuse hyperplasia of the urothelium, where the number of cell layers is markedly increased, *i.e.*, from one to three layers in the normal distended bladder to ten or more. In addition, there may be proliferation, either upward in the lumen or downward into the submucosa resulting in fingerlike projections into the submucosa, still surrounded by a basement membrane. In the latter case, nests of cells in the submucosa or plaque-like lesions may be found, some of which are so extensive that the term endophytic or inverted papilloma may be used. Most transitional cell papillomas are of the more traditional type, being arborized projections consisting of a core of delicate connective tissue covered by well differentiated transitional cell epithelium. These lesions should be carefully examined to insure that there is no invasion of the connective tissue stalk. Transitional cell carcinomas have evidence of submucosal invasion which is often seen primarily in the stalk of the papillary lesion. Many carcinomas are well differentiated and such local invasion is the main criterion for diagnosis. In other cases, dysplasia and atypia may also be present. Metastases are uncommon.

In any of the lesions described above, squamous metaplasia may be present. In some cases, squamous differentiation is so extensive that the neoplasm is classified as a squamous cell papilloma or carcinoma. Squamous cell carcinomas tend to be more invasive and metastatic than transitional cell carcinomas.

In summary, the F344 rat is characterized by high incidences of interstitial cell tumors of the testes, mononuclear cell leukemia, pituitary neoplasms and mammary gland tumors. These tumors increase in incidence with age, being most commonly observed after 18 months of age.[15] In other respects, it has a moderate background of degenerative and neoplastic diseases not unlike other rat strains. It also responds to a wide variety of chemical carcinogens.

COMPARISON OF CARCINOGENIC RESPONSES BETWEEN STRAINS AND SPECIES

In selecting species and strains for carcinogenicity studies the question arises as to whether a specific strain or species may react to a chemical in an aberrant fashion. This is one of the reasons that most carcinogenicity studies are routinely performed in at least two species. Many chemicals are carcinogenic in more than one species.[2,3,78] Interestingly, although there is fairly good correlation for a positive response when multiple species are tested, there is often a very different target organ response, *i.e.*, liver may be the target organ in one species and urinary bladder in another (Tables 1 and 2). The question also arises as to whether one strain of a given species reacts similarly to all other strains of the same species. It is a difficult question to answer. A number of chemicals have been tested in a variety of species and strains of the same species. These tests, however, have usually been conducted at different times and in different laboratories. It is difficult to compare tests done in different laboratories since dose, route of exposure, necropsy protocols and even diagnostic criteria vary between laboratories.

There have been a few studies conducted which compare directly the B6C3F1 mouse with other strains or stocks of mice and the F344 rat with other strains or stocks of rats. These are discussed in the following sections. In referring to the types of animals used, no attempt was made to differentiate between inbred strains and random bred stocks unless the citation made such distinctions. Since many inbred strains have been derived from random bred stocks,[45] the nomenclature in the literature is often confusing unless the standardized nomenclature for inbred strains of mice[37] or rats[13] or for random bred stocks of rats and mice[20] is used.

Comparison of the B6C3F1 Mouse with Other Strains

An important consideration is whether the B6C3F1 mouse responds to toxicants and carcinogens in the same way as do other species and mouse strains. A number of review articles regarding carcinogenicity in multiple species[2,3,78,91,92] suggest that chemicals that cause cancer in other species often cause cancer in the mouse. A few studies have been conducted in which the response of the B6C3F1 mouse is compared with other strains. In a large study by Innes *et al.,*[47] the B6C3F1 mouse (both sexes) had a higher significant increase in hepatocellular neoplasms following exposure to known carcinogens than did the (C57BL/6 x AKR) F_1 hybrid. Two positive control chemicals also caused lung tumors in both sexes of both F_1 hybrids while the other five chemicals did not cause pulmonary tumors in either sex of the hybrids. The one exception was dihydrosafrole which caused increased pulmonary tumors in female B6C3F1 mice only. Thus, both hybrids had a similar response to the induction of pulmonary tumors by a known carcinogen. Eleven experimental pesticides and industrial chemicals were judged to be carcinogens in this study. Eight of 11 caused hepatocellular neoplasms in male B6C3F1 mice, nine of 11 caused liver tumors in the male C57BL x AKR hybrid and also in the female B6C3F1 hybrid. However, only three compounds caused increased hepatocellular neoplasms in the female C57BL x AKR hybrid. This study would suggest that the B6C3F1 mouse responded more consistently with increased hepatocellular neoplasms than did the other hybrid. Further, there was better agreement between the sexes in the B6C3F1 mouse.

When both outbred Swiss mice and B6C3F1 mice were exposed to vinyl chloride, which has been shown to cause hemangiosarcomas in a variety of species, including man, each responded in a similar manner with increased incidence of hemangiosarcomas in multiple organs.[71] This is an example of the animal model, including the B6C3F1 mouse, responding to a carcinogen in a manner similar to humans.

The NTP program conducted a skin painting study with 7,12-dimethylbenz[a]anthracene (DMBA) and 12-O-tetradecanoyl phorbol-13-acetate (TPA) in both the B6C3F1 hybrid and Swiss-Webster stock. Both responded in a similar, although not identical, fashion to these compounds.[93] The most striking difference was the occurrence of hyperplasias of melanocytes and pigmented tumors in some of the B6C3F1 mice as opposed to none in the Swiss mouse. The B6C3F1 mouse is an agouti (brown) mouse whereas the Swiss mouse is an albino.

Thirteen substituted benzenediamines (SBD) were tested for carcinogenicity in B6C3F1 mice and F344 rats while two were tested in Swiss mice and Sprague-Dawley rats.[94] The liver was a target in both strains of mice and, in both, females were more often observed to have a significant increase in hepatocellular neoplasms than males. This is interesting since males have a higher historical incidence of liver tumors, and their use has been criticized for being overly sensitive to the induction of liver tumors. This study, while limited, suggests that the B6C3F1 mouse responds in a similar fashion to the outbred Swiss mouse to SBD carcinogenesis.

Thus, several studies indicate that the response of the B6C3F1 mouse to toxic chemicals is not unique but similar to that of other mouse strains.

Comparison of the F344 Rat with Other Rat Strains

Many early references to selection of the F344 rat mention size as one of the advantages of this strain. In a comparison of Long-Evans, Sprague-Dawley and F344 rats, it was noted that the F344 rat did not become excessively obese with age (24 months, mean body fat 15%, range 8% to 18%) in contrast to the Sprague-Dawley rat which becomes obese by 24 months (mean body fat 24%, range 13% to 30%).[95]

A disadvantage of the F344 rat is progressive renal disease which is as, or more, severe than that of other common rat strains and stocks. In a two year study to compare results of chemical exposure to different inbred strains, the NCI Carcinogen Testing Program used ACI, August, F344, Marshall and OM rats. Since the studies were conducted in the same laboratory over a similar time period, it was possible to compare spontaneous renal disease in control rats of these various strains. All kidneys were reviewed by the same pathologist and scored for the presence and severity of renal disease. Renal lesions were minimal in male and female August rats and in female OM rats; minimal to mild in male and female Marshall and ACI rats and female F344 rats and mild to moderate in male OM and F344 rats.[96] The ACI and Marshall strains had an additional disadvantage since both strains have a high spontaneous incidence of hydronephrosis. The ACI strain is also characterized by unilateral renal agenesis (up to 20%)[97] and extensive mineralization in the pelvic region.[96]

To compare strain responses to important industrial chemicals, NCI tested trichloroethylene and tetrachloroethylene in several strains of rats.[98,99] For each chemical, the rats used were tested under comparable conditions. Trichloroethylene was tested in OM, August, F344, Marshall, and ACI rats. Tetrachloroethylene was tested in F344, Long-Evans, Wistar, and Sherman rats. Neither of these compounds was carcinogenic in any strain of rat in these studies. However, both compounds produced the same toxic lesion in both sexes and in all eight strains of rats, *i.e.*, cytomegaly of the renal tubular epithelium, particularly at the corticomedullary junction. The lesion was quite striking and was characterized by both nuclear and cytoplasmic hypertrophy. The enlarged cells were pleomorphic and occasionally cytologically bizarre. This lesion was superimposed upon the chronic nephropathy.

F344 rats had a qualitative toxic response to dietary nitrilotriacetic acid and trisodium nitrilotriacetate, similar to that seen in CR Sprague-Dawley rats. While the CR Sprague-Dawley rats consumed more compound per kg body weight per day, both had decreased weight gain, crystalluria and hematuria.[100]

Studies have been done to compare the response of various rat strains and stocks to potential carcinogens. Among the first were Dunning *et al.*[101] who compared the response of four strains of rats, August 990, AxC 9935, Fischer 344, and Copenhagen 2331 to subcutaneous implants of estrone and to diethylstilbestrol (DES)/cholesterol implants. Briefly, this study indicated that, in the order listed, August, AxC and Fischer male rats were susceptible to both DES, and to a lesser degree, estrone induction of mammary tumors. There was considerably more strain variation among August, AxC and Fischer 344 females. Copenhagen rats of both sexes were resistant to the induction of mammary tumor by either compound, but stones and tumors of the urinary bladder could be induced with either one or two estrone pellets. Similar bladder lesions were induced in male August rats by one estrone pellet, and in AxC males and Fischer females by two pellets; AxC females developed a few bladder calculi with two estrone pellets. Female Copenhagen rats also developed adrenal tumors, as did male August rats. August, and to a lesser extent, Copenhagen rats had poor survival rates when treated with estrone compared to the Fischer and AxC rats.

Pamukcu *et al.*[102] reported that both F344 and Sprague-Dawley female rats appeared equally responsive to induction of urinary bladder and intestinal tumors by bracken fern. Berman *et al.*[103] administered a single intraperitoneal injection of methyl (acetoxymethyl) nitrosamine to five week old male and female Sprague-Dawley, Buffalo (BUF), or F344 rats. Treated animals of each strain developed a large number of intestinal tumors. The histological features were the same in all strains and in both sexes. In this study the F344 rat did not appear to differ qualitatively from other strains when exposed to a known intestinal carcinogen, but the number of tumors induced appeared to vary by sex and strain of rat (Table 7). The F344 rats had fewer induced tumors than the Sprague-Dawley animals but more than the BUF strain. In all three strains the females appeared less sensitive than the males.

Table 7: Life Span and Intestinal Tumor Frequencies[a]

Strain	Age at Death (mo.)	No. Rats with Small Intestinal Tumors/Rats	No. Rats with Large Intestinal Tumors/Rats	Total Tumors/ Rats with Tumors
SD				
Male	15	25/29	9/29	70/26
Female	16.1	25/30	3/30	41/25
F344				
Male	14.7	22/28	4/28	53/23
Female	17.2	4/28	1/28	8/5
Buffalo				
Male	16.0	6/26	2/26	10/7
Female	16.1	3/27	0/27	4/3

[a]Taken from reference 103

Reuber[104] evaluated the susceptibility of males of four rat strains (Marshall, Buffalo, ACI, and Fischer) to development of liver lesions following administration of N-2-fluorenyldiacetamide. Marshall rats were relatively resistant, whereas the F344 were most susceptible to hepatocarcinogenesis; the Buffalo and ACI animals were both moderate in their response.

When subtoxic doses of azaserine, a known pancreatic carcinogen, were given to outbred Wistar rats and inbred W/LEW and F344 rats, atypical acinar cell nodules (AACN) of the pancreas were induced. These AACN were found in 90% of the outbred Wistar, 100% of the W/LEW rats, but in only 10% of the F344 rats. Thus, the inbred F344 rat was much less responsive than the other stocks and strains tested. In addition, in both inbred and outbred rats studied, females appeared less responsive than males.[105]

Weisburger *et al.*[106] studied the response of male Sprague-Dawley and F344 rats to 1,4-bis(4-fluorophenyl)-2-propynyl-N-cyclooctyl carbamate. Both strains developed Zymbal's gland tumors at low doses. F344 rats developed lymphomas at lower doses than Sprague-Dawley rats; only Sprague-Dawley rats developed mammary tumors. F344 rats in this study had poorer survival rates than the Sprague-Dawley rats.

When 2-ethyl-N-nitrosourea (ENU) was injected neonatally into Wistar/Furth (WF), Long Evans (LE), WF/LE (F1), or F344, all strains developed 97% to 100% incidence of tumors of the central nervous system. In the peripheral nervous system (PNS), however, only the LE was highly susceptible and the F344 and WF developed a lower tumor incidence. The authors stated that the differences in susceptibility of the PNS in different strains may be due to population of target cells, rate of development or capacity for elimination repair of the PNS.[107]

Strain differences in susceptibility for chemical carcinogenesis have also been noted for the urinary bladder. With a known carcinogen, N-butyl-N-(4-hydroxybutyl) nitrosamine (BBN), greatest susceptibility to bladder cancer was found in the ACI strain of rats followed in decreasing order by Wistar, Sprague-Dawley and Lewis rats.[108] Sodium saccharin, shown to act as a promoter, induced hyperplasia, papillomas and carcinomas in the bladder of ACI rats by 52 weeks, but only slight changes were observed by scanning electron microscopy in Wistar and F344 rats exposed to similar treatment. Sprague-Dawley rats appeared completely resistant, and changes were not found by either light or scanning electron microscopy.[109] In this study, mice, hamsters and guinea pigs were also resistant to the effects of sodium saccharin. For compounds such as BBN, differences in metabolic pathways for activation to the proximate carcinogen might account for species and strain differences, however, sodium saccharin does not appear to be metabolized and thus other factors must play a role in differential host susceptibility.[109] Lijinsky and Taylor[110] administered nitrosomethyldodecylamine by gavage in olive oil solution to male and female Sprague-Dawley and F344 rats which were also injected subcutaneously with a suspension of urinary bladder tissue. There was no clear evidence of carcinogenicity in the transplants, but there was 100% incidence of tumors in the host bladder. The F344 rats died earlier with transitional cell carcinomas than the Sprague-Dawley rats suggesting that the F344 rat may be more sensitive. Since only 24 Sprague-Dawley rats and 12 F344 rats were used in the study, however, the findings were not conclusive.

Sunderman[111] reviewed data on the carcinogenicity of nickel subsulfide in rats and other species. Studies with nickel are generally conducted by injection of the compound directly into the test site. Several rat strains were evaluated for susceptibility to tumor induction by intrarenal injection. Long Evans rats were resistant and Fischer rats, NIH Black rats and Wistar-Lewis exhibited increasing susceptibility in that order. Males and females of each strain were comparable in susceptibility.

In general, it appears that F344 rats respond to most carcinogens in a fashion qualitatively similar to other rat strains, but that quantitatively the response may be quite different. However, it is difficult to predict in advance which strain will be the most sensitive to a given carcinogen. Female rats seem to be less sensitive than males of the same strain to many carcinogens although the reverse is occasionally true.

Comparison of the B6C3F1 Mouse and F344 Rat with Other Species

In chemical carcinogenicity testing, species differences in response to chemicals are very likely. For this reason, unknown chemicals are usually tested in two or more species. Both similarities and differences in the response of rats and mice to carcinogens have been documented.[2,3,51,78,91,92,112,113] Only a few examples of differences will be cited here.

Sodium saccharin causes urinary tract tumors in ACI rats but not in B6C3F1 mice.[109] Increased DNA synthesis of urinary bladder epithelium was demonstrated in rats but not mice. Since sodium saccharin is excreted largely intact, differences other than metabolism must account for this effect.[109]

In other cases, species differences in response to a chemical can be explained by different metabolic pathways. One example is the greater sensitivity of B6C3F1 mice to perchloroethylene (PE)-induced hepatocellular carcinoma compared to Sprague-Dawley rats. Following inhalation of 10 ppm, mice were found to metabolize greater than eight times more PE per kg body weight than rats.[114] Increased DNA synthesis was observed in mice but not rats after repeated oral administration of PE at dose levels which are tumorigenic in mice in lifetime studies. In this example the species difference appears to be due, at least in part, to the rate of metabolism since ten-fold higher doses in rats will cause some histological evidence of liver damage.[114]

Arylamines, a group of occupational carcinogens for humans are also carcinogenic in rats (Table 2), but the target tissue is not always the same in humans as in other species, such as the hamster and mouse.[115] In tests of eleven substituted benzenediamines (SBD) in F344 rats and B6C3F1 mice, mice more consistently had increased incidences of hepatocellular neoplasms only. The F344 rats showed a greater range of target organ susceptibility, with treatment related neoplasms being found in the urinary tract, forestomach, liver, mammary gland, thyroid gland, skin and associated glands. It was postulated that the greater range of target organ susceptibility in the rat was related to a greater capacity of the tissues to metabolize SBD.[94]

On the other hand, when F344 rats were exposed to the known human carcinogen, vinyl chloride, the rats developed a high incidence of hemangiosarcomas, thus responding in a similar fashion to humans, mouse and hamster.[71] Nickel subsulfide is also a carcinogen in humans. In experimental animals, several species have been shown to be susceptible to nickel carcinogenesis by direct inoculation at various sites. Rats are the most susceptible species with the F344 rat being intermediate. Mice, hamsters and rabbits were also variably susceptible.[111]

Weisburger[116] reviewed results of the NCI/NTP carcinogenicity tests of a number of aromatic amines in F344 rats and B6C3F1 mice. Thirty-eight of 53 had comparable results in rats and mice; 16 were negative in both species and 22 positive in both species. For those positive in both species, the organs affected were often different. An additional 15 compounds were positive in only one species: six in mice and nine in rats.

Thus, both rats and mice will respond in a similar qualitative manner to toxicants and carcinogens in some instances, but in other cases metabolic and/or other differences will mean that the response may be quite different. Without pharmacokinetic or metabolism data, one cannot predict how different species will respond.

CONCLUSIONS

Many of the qualities that led to the selection of the B6C3F1 mouse and the F344 rat for the bioassay program including ease of production, good survival to two years, relatively low tumor incidence and large historical data base, are the same factors that lead to their continued use today. The issue of using random bred *versus* inbred animals was controversial originally, and the issue has not been resolved. In 1973, the Canadian Ministry of Health and Welfare[43] and the FDA Advisory Committee[42] recommended the use of random bred animals. The Canadian Food and Drug Directorate[117] continues to suggest the use of outbred strains as do the guidelines for carcinogen testing in the United Kingdom.[118] With the thousands of animals used in toxicity and carcinogenicity testing since 1973, it is surprising that this issue has not been resolved. The limited comparisons that the NCI/NTP program has made between B6C3F1 mouse and the Swiss mouse do not suggest major qualitative differences. On the other hand, not enough direct comparison studies have been done so that this issue can be resolved. Much of the understanding of species differences may be solved by pharmacokinetic and metabolic studies.

One of the most controversial issues involving the B6C3F1 mouse is the high incidence of hepatocellular neoplasms in the males. It has been argued that the male mouse is overly sensitive to the induction of liver tumors and a positive response in the liver of this strain should not be considered relevant for other species. Almost 15 years ago the identical question of "What is the biologic behavior of mouse hepatomas?" appeared in an article on the bioassay of pesticides and industrial chemicals.[47] This same question is discussed today.

Haseman and Huff[112] evaluated the results of 265 chemicals tested by NCI and NTP for carcinogenicity; 134 (51%) were carcinogenic. Of these, 27 induced only liver tumors in B6C3F1 mice. Eighteen of these were positive in both sexes; five were positive only in males and four were positive only in females. Ward *et al.*[91] reviewed available mutagenicity data for 24 chemicals positive in the mouse liver only. Fourteen had been tested for mutagenicity, five of which were positive in bacterial mutagenicity tests. These data suggest that the male mouse liver is not unduly sensitive to cancer induction by chemicals.[51,91,92,112,114]

Some important chemicals, when tested for carcinogenicity, caused an increase in tumors in one sex in one organ system, and one species. These chemicals need to be re-examined utilizing today's better methods for evaluating chemical disposition and metabolism. Many of the short term *in vivo* assays may also provide additional insight, and it may be worthwhile to retest selected chemicals in a variety of species and strains.[92]

Finally, an increased awareness of the biological significance of a lesion or tumor for the species in which it occurs will be also helpful in extrapolating that data for other species. In humans, patient history after surgery or biopsy gives the pathologist a good understanding about biological behavior for most morphological entities. This is in contrast to rodents where little is known about the biological behavior for a number of benign lesions. Malignant lesions with invasion or distant metastases clearly indicate to the pathologist their potential behavior. Many studies now include interim sacrifices and stop studies where the compound in question is given for the first 15 months to one group which is then held until two years. Both the interim sacrifices and stop studies should provide added insight about the biological behavior of many lesions found in the B6C3F1 mouse and F344 rat.

In the foreseeable future, rodents will continue to be used to assess possible toxicity and carcinogenicity of chemicals. Such studies need to be well designed, well conducted and carefully evaluated and interpreted. The data available suggest that the B6C3F1 mouse and F344 rat are suitable strains for these studies. Additional comparisons need to be made with other strains and species, especially when a positive response is restricted to a single sex and strain. The ultimate rationale for testing in animals is to protect the public health. This must be balanced against societal needs for progress. Only through judicious use of the data available and conduct of additional studies as needed, can the public health be protected without unduly restricting progress.

Acknowledgements

The authors express appreciation to Dr. E. McConnell, Dr. J. Mennear, Dr. J. Haseman, and Dr. H. Solleveld for access to studies and data that are being prepared for publication. The authors express their thanks to Ms. Beth deBrito for typing and retyping this manuscript. Preparation of this manuscript was supported, in part, by PHS grant RR00170.

REFERENCES

1. Smithcors, J.F., *Evolution of the Veterinary Art*. Kansas City, MO: Veterinary Medicine Publishing Co. (1957)
2. Tomatis, L., The predictive value of rodent carcinogenicity tests in the evaluation of human risks. *Ann. Rev. Pharmacol. Toxicol.* 19: 511–530 (1979)
3. Tomatis, L., Agthe, C., Bartsch, H., Huff, J., Montesano, R., Seracci, R., Walker, E., and Wilbourn, J., Evaluation of the carcinogenicity of chemicals: A review of the monograph program of the International Agency for Research on Cancer (1971 to 1977). *Cancer Res.* 38: 877–885 (1978)

4. Ivankovic, S., Eisenbrand, G., and Preussmann, R., Lung carcinoma induction in BD rats after a single intratracheal installation of an arsenic-containing pesticide mixture formerly used in vineyards. *Int. J. Cancer* 24: 786-788 (1979)
5. National Toxicology Program, Carcinogenesis bioassay of benzene.(Technical Report Series) DHHS Publication No. (NIH). (draft report)
6. Briggs, G.B., and Oehme, F.W., in: *The Laboratory Rat* (H.J. Baker, J.R. Lindsey, and S.H. Weisbroth, eds.), Vol. II, pp 104-118, Academic Press, New York (1980)
7. Peckman, J.C., in: *The Laboratory Rat* (H.J. Baker, J.R. Lindsey, and S.H. Weisbroth, eds.), Vol. II, pp 119-147, Academic Press, New York (1980)
8. Sivak, A., in: *Biomedical Research* (H.L. Foster, J.D. Small, and J.G. Fox, eds.), Vol. IV, pp 341-349, Academic Press, New York (1982)
9. Altman, N.H., and Goodman, D.G., in: *The Laboratory Rat* (H.J. Baker, J.R. Lindsey, and S.H. Weisbroth, eds.), Vol. I, pp 334-378, Academic Press, New York (1979)
10. Anver, M.R., Cohen, B.J., Lattuada, C.P., and Foster, S.J., Age-associated lesions in barrier-reared male Sprague-Dawley rats: A comparison between Hap:(SD) and Crl:COBS$^{(R)}$CD$^{(E)}$(SD) stocks. *Expl. Aging Res.* 8: 3-24 (1982)
11. Coleman, G.L., Barthold, S.W., Osbaldiston, G.W., Foster, S.J., and Jonas, A.M., Pathological changes during aging in barrier-reared Fischer 344 male rats. *J. Gerontol.* 32: 258-278 (1977)
12. Davis, R.K., Stevenson, G.T., and Busch, K.A., Tumor incidence in normal Sprague-Dawley female rats. *Cancer Res.* 16: 194-197 (1956)
13. Festing, M.F.W., in: *The Laboratory Rat* (H.J. Baker, J.R. Lindsey, and S.H. Weisbroth, eds.), Vol. I, pp 55-72, Academic Press, New York (1979)
14. Goodman, D.G., Anver, M.R., Ward, J.M., Sauer, R.M., Boorman, G.A., Bates, R.R., Strandberg, J.D., Squire, R.A., Reznik, G., Parker, G.A., Jones, S.R., and Ines, G.D., *Chemically Induced and Unusual Proliferative and Neoplastic Lesions in Rats.* Washington, DC: Registry of Veterinary Pathology, AFIP (in press)
15. Goodman, D.G., Ward, J.M., Squire, R.A., Chu, K.C., and Linhart, M.S., Neoplastic and nonneoplastic lesions in aging F344 rats. *Toxicol. Appl. Pharmacol.* 48: 237-248 (1979)
16. Goodman, D.G., Ward, J.M., Squire, R.A., Paxton, M.B., Reichardt, W.D., Chu, K.C., and Linhart, M.S., Neoplastic and nonneoplastic lesions in aging Osborne-Mendel rats. *Toxicol. Appl. Pharmacol.* 55: 433-447 (1980)
17. Haseman, J., Huff, J.A., and Boorman, G.A., personal communication
18. MacKenzie, W.F., and Garner, F.M., Comparison of neoplasms in six sources of rats. *J. Natl. Cancer Inst.* 50: 1243-1257 (1973)
19. Maekawa, A., Kurokawa, Y., Takahashi, M., Kokubo, T., Ogiu, T., Onodera, H., Tanigawa, H., Ohno, Y., Furukawa, F., and Hayashi, Y., Spontaneous tumors in F-344/DuCrj rats. *Gann* 74: 365-372 (1983)
20. NIH Rodents, 1980 Catalogue, Strains and Stocks of Laboratory Rodents Provided by the NIH Genetic Resource. NIH Pub. No. 81-606, April (1981)
21. Prejean, J.D., Peckham, J.C., Casey, A.E., Griswold, D.P., Weisburger, E.K., and Weisburger, J.H., Spontaneous tumors in Sprague-Dawley rats and Swiss mice. *Cancer Res.* 33: 2768-2773 (1973)
22. Sacksteder, M.R., Brief communication: Occurrence of spontaneous tumors in the germ-free F344 rat. *J. Natl. Cancer Inst.* 57: 1371-1373 (1976)

23. Sass, B., Rabstein, R.S., Madison, R., Nims, R.M., Peters, R.L., and Kelloff, G.J., Incidence of spontaneous neoplasms in F344 rats throughout the natural life-span. *J. Natl. Cancer Inst.* 54: 1449–1456 (1975)

24. Schardein, J.L., Fitzgerald, J.E., and Kaump, D.H., Spontaneous tumors in Holtzman-source rats of various ages. *Pathol. Vet.* 5: 238–252 (1968)

25. Squire, R.A., Goodman, D.G., Valerio, M.G., Fredrickson, T.N., Strandberg, J.D., Levitt, M.H., Lingeman, C.H., Harshbarger, J.C., and Dawe, C.J., in: *Pathology of Laboratory Animals* (K. Benirschke, F.M. Garner, and T.C. Jones, eds.), Vol. II, pp 1057–1284, Springer-Verlag, New York

26. Solleveld, H.A., Haseman, J.K., and McConnell, E.E., The natural history of body weight gain, survival and neoplasia in the Fischer 344 rat. *J. Natl. Cancer Inst.* 72: 929–940 (1984)

27. Takizawa, S., and Miyamoto, M., Observations on spontaneous tumors in Wistar Furth strain rats. *Hiroshima J. Med. Sci.* 25: 59–98 (1976)

28. Thompson, S.W., Haseby, R.A., Fox, M.A., Davis, C.L. and Hunt, R.D., Spontaneous tumors in the Sprague-Dawley rat. *J. Natl. Cancer Inst.* 27: 1037–1057 (1961)

29. Ward, J.M., Sagartz, J.W., and Casey, H.W., *Pathology of the Aging F344 Rat.* Washington, DC: Registry of Veterinary Pathology, AFIP (1980)

30. Jacobs, B.B., and Huseby, R.A., Neoplasms occurring in aged Fischer rats, with special reference to testicular, uterine, and thyroid tumors. *J. Natl. Cancer Inst.* 39: 303–309 (1967)

31. Sher, S.P., Jensen, R.D., and Bokelman, D.L., Spontaneous tumors in control F344 and Charles River-CD rats and Charles River CD-1 and B6C3F1 mice. *Toxicol. Lett.* 11: 103–110 (1982)

32. Goodman, D.G., Anver, M.R., Sauer, R.M., Boorman, G.A., Ward, J.M., Strandberg, J.D., Innes, G.D., Vonderfecht, S., and Parker, G.A., *Experimentally Induced and Unusual Proliferative and Neoplastic Lesions in Mice.* Washington, DC: Registry of Veterinary Pathology, AFIP (in press)

33. Goodman, D.G., Bates, R.R., Ward, J.M., Frith, C.H., Sauer, R.M., Jones, S.R., Strandberg, J.D., Squire, R.A., Montali, R.J., and Parker, G.A., *Common Lesions in Aged B6C3F1 (C57BL/6N x C3H/HeN)F1 and BALB/cStCrlfC3H/Nctr Mice.* Washington, DC: Registry of Veterinary Pathology, AFIP (1981)

34. Lynch, C.J., The so-called Swiss mouse. *Lab. Anim. Care* 19: 214–220 (1969)

35. Madison, R.M., Rabstein, L.S., and Bryan, W.R., Mortality rate and spontaneous lesions found in 2,928 untreated BALB/cCr mice. *J. Natl. Cancer Inst.* 40: 683–685 (1968)

36. Sheldon, W.G., and Greenman, D.L., Spontaneous lesions in control BALB/c female mice. *J. Environ. Pathol. Toxicol.* 3: 155–167 (1979)

37. Staats, J., Standardized nomenclature for inbred strains of mice: Sixth listing. *Cancer Res.* 36: 4333–4377 (1976)

38. Ward, J.M., Goodman, D.G., Squire, R.A., Chu, K.C., and Linhart, M.S., Neoplastic and nonneoplastic lesions in aging (C57BL/6N x C3H/HeN)F$_1$ (B6C3F1) mice. *J. Natl. Cancer Inst.* 63: 849–854 (1979)

39. Page, N.P., in: *Environmental Cancer* (H.F. Kraybill, and M. Mehlman, eds.), Vol. 3, pp 87–171, Wiley and Sons, New York (1977)

40. Sontag, J.M., Page, N.P., and Saffiotti, U., Guidelines for carcinogen bioassay in small rodents. NCI Carcinogenesis Technical Report Series, No. 1 (1976)

41. Weisburger, J.H., Grantham, P.H., Van Horn, E.C., Steigbigel, N.M., Rall, D.P., and Weisburger, E.K., Activation and detoxification of N-2-fluorenylacetamide in man. *Cancer Res.* 24: 475–479 (1964)

42. Food and Drug Administration Advisory Committee on Protocols for Safety Evaluation, Panel on Carcinogenesis Report on Cancer Testing in the Safety of Food Additives and Pesticides. *Toxicol. Appl. Pharmacol.* 20: 419-438 (1971)

43. Canadian Ministry of Health and Welfare, The testing of chemicals for carcinogenicity, mutagenicity and teratogenicity. [Cited in: *Environ. Cancer* (H. Kraybill and M. Mehlman, eds.), Vol. 3, pp 87-171, Wiley and Sons, New York (1973)]

44. Shimkin, M.B., in: *Carcinogenesis Testing of Chemicals* (L. Goldberg, ed.), pp 15-20, CRC Press, Cleveland, OH (1974)

45. Altman, P.L., and Katz, D.D., Inbred and genetically defined strains of laboratory animals. Part 1, Mouse and Rat. *Fed. Amer. Soc. Exp. Biol.*, Bethesda, MD (1979)

46. Weisburger, E.K., History of the bioassay program of the National Cancer Institute. *Prog. Exp. Tumor Res.* 26: 187-201 (1983)

47. Innes, J.R.M., Ulland, B.M., Valerio, M.G., Petrucelli, L., Fishbein, L., Hart, E.R., Pallotta, A.J., Bates, R.R., Falk, H.L., Gart, J.J., Klein, M., Mitchell, I., and Peters, J., Bioassay of pesticides and industrial chemicals for tumorigenicity in mice: A preliminary note. *J. Natl. Cancer Inst.* 42: 1101-1114 (1969).

48. Cameron, T., and Hickman, R., personal communication

49. Homburger, F., Russfield, A.B., Weisburger, J.H., Lim, S., Chak, S.P., and Weisburger, E.K., Aging changes in CD-1HaM/ICR mice reared under standard laboratory conditions. *J. Natl. Cancer Inst.* 55: 37-45 (1975)

50. Ihle, J.N., Arthur, L.O., and Fine, D.L., Autogenous immunity to mouse mammary tumor virus in mouse strains of high and low mammary tumor incidence. *Cancer Res.* 36: 2840-2844 (1976)

51. Maronpot, R.R., and Boorman, G.A., Interpretation of rodent hepatocellular proliferative alterations and hepatocellular tumors in chemical safety assessment. *Toxicol. Pathol.* 10: 71-78 (1982)

52. Ward, J.M., Goodman, D.G., Griesemer, R.A., Hardisty, J.F., Schueler, R.L., Squire, R.A., and Strandberg, J.D., Quality assurance for pathology in rodent carcinogenesis tests. *J. Environ. Pathol. Toxicol.* 2: 371-378 (1978)

53. Becker, F.F., Morphological classification of mouse liver tumors based on biological characteristics. *Cancer Res.* 42: 3918-3923 (1982)

54. Ward, J.M., Berral, E., Buratto, G., Goodman, D.G., Strandberg, J.D., and Schueler, R., Histopathology of neoplastic and nonneoplastic hepatic lesions in mice fed diets containing tetrachlorovinphos. *J. Natl. Cancer Inst.* 63: 111-118 (1979)

55. Reuber, M.D., and Ward, J.M., Histopathology of liver carcinomas in (C57BL/6N x C3H/HeN)F₁ mice ingesting chlordane. *J. Natl. Cancer Inst.* 63: 89-92 (1979)

56. Hoover, K.L., Ward, J.M., and Stinson, S.F., Histopathologic differences between liver tumors in untreated (C57BL/6 x C3H)F₁ mice and nitrofen-fed mice. *J. Natl. Cancer Inst.* 65: 937-948 (1980)

57. Reznik, G., and Ward, J.M., Carcinogenicity of the hair dye component 2-nitro-p-phenylenediamine (2-NPPD): Induction of eosinophilic hepatocellular neoplasms in female B6C3F1 mice. *Fd. Cosmet. Toxicol.* 17: 493-500 (1979)

58. Pattingale, P.K., and Frith, C.H., Immunomorphologic classification of spontaneous lymphoid cell neoplasms occurring in female BALB/c mice. *J. Natl. Cancer Inst.* 70: 169-179 (1983)

59. Dunn, T.B., and Deringer, M.K., Reticulum cell neoplasm, type B or the "Hodgkin's-like lesion" of the mouse. *J. Natl. Cancer Inst.* 40: 771–821 (1968)

60. Dunn, T.B., Normal and pathologic anatomy of the reticular tissue in laboratory mice with a classification and discussion of neoplasms. *J. Natl. Cancer Inst.* 14: 1281–1433 (1954)

61. Brooks, R.E., Pulmonary adenoma of strain A mice: An electron microscopic study. *J. Natl. Cancer Inst.* 41: 719–742 (1968)

62. Stewart, H.L., in: *The Pathophysiology of Cancer* (F. Homburger and W.H. Fishman, eds.), pp 18–37, Hoeber-Harper, New York (1959)

63. Kauffman, S.L., Alexander, L., and Sass, L., Histologic and ultrastructural features of the Clara cell adenoma of the mouse lung. *Lab. Invest.* 40: 708–716 (1979)

64. Dunn, T.B., Normal and pathologic anatomy of the adrenal gland of the mouse, including neoplasms. *J. Natl. Cancer Inst.* 44: 1323–1389 (1970)

65. Goodman, D.G., in: *Endocrine System* (T.C. Jones, U. Mohr, and R.D. Hunt, eds.), pp 66–68, Springer-Verlag, New York (1983)

66. Frith, C.H., in: *Endocrine System* (T.C. Jones, U. Mohr, and R.D. Hunt, eds.), pp 49–56, Springer-Verlag, New York (1983)

67. McConnell, E.E., Pathology requirements for rodent two-year studies. I. A review of current procedures. *Toxicol. Pathol.* (in press)

68. Roe, F.J.C., and Tucker, M.J., Recent developments in the design of carcinogenicity tests on laboratory animals. *Proc. Europ. Soc. Study of Drug Toxicity* 15: 171–177 (1973)

69. Vlahakis, G., Possible carcinogenic effects of cedar shavings in bedding of C3H-AvyfB mice. *J. Natl. Cancer Inst.* 58: 149–150 (1977)

70. Andervont, H.B., Studies on the occurrence of spontaneous hepatomas in mice of strains C3H and CBA. *J. Natl. Cancer Inst.* 11: 581–592 (1950)

71. Drew, R.T., Boorman, G.A., Haseman, J.K., McConnell, E.E., Busey, W., and Moore, J.A., The effect of age and exposure duration on cancer induction by a known carcinogen in rats, mice and hamsters. *Toxicol. Appl. Pharmacol.* 68: 120–130 (1983)

72. National Toxicology Program, Carcinogenesis bioassay of 1,3-butadiene (*Technical Report Series*) DHHS Publication No. (NIH) (draft report)

73. National Toxicology Program, Carcinogenesis bioassay of propylene oxide (*Technical Report Series*) DHHS Publication No. (NIH) (draft report)

74. Turek, F.W., and Desjardins, C., Development of Leydig cell tumors and onset of changes in the reproductive and endocrine systems of aging F344 rats. *J. Natl. Cancer Inst.* 63: 969–975 (1979)

75. Cockrell, B.Y., and Garner, F.M., Interstitial cell tumor of the testes in rats. *Comp. Pathol. Bull.* 8: 2–4 (1976)

76. Welsch, C.W., and Nagasawa, M., Prolactin and murine mammary tumorigenesis: A review. *Cancer Res.* 37: 951–963 (1977)

77. Van Zwieten, M.J., The rat as animal model in breast cancer research. Ph.D. thesis. Martinus Nijhoff Publishers, The Netherlands (1984)

78. Griesemer, R.A., and Cueto, C., in: *Molecular and Cellular Aspects of Carcinogen Screening Tests* (R. Montesano, H. Bartsch, and L. Tomatis, eds.), pp 259–281, IARC Sci. Publications No. 27, IARC, Lyon (1980)

79. Davey, F.R., and Moloney, W.C., Postmortem observations on Fischer rats with leukemia and other disorders. *Lab. Invest.* 23: 327–334 (1970)

80. Moloney, W.C., Boschetti, A.E., and King, V.P., Spontaneous leukemia in Fischer rats. *Cancer Res.* 30: 41–43 (1970)

81. Stromberg, P.C., and Vogtsberger, L.M., Pathology of the mononuclear cell leukemia of Fischer rats. I. Morphologic studies. *Vet. Pathol.* 20: 698–708 (1983)
82. Stromberg, P.C., Vogtsberger, L.M., and Marsh, L.R., Pathology of the mononuclear cell leukemia of Fischer rats. III. Clinical chemistry. *Vet. Pathol.* 20: 718–726 (1983a)
83. Stromberg, P.C., Vogtsberger, L.M., March, L.R., and Wilson, F.D., Pathology of mononuclear cell leukemia of Fischer rats. II. Hematology. *Vet. Pathol.* 20: 709–717 (1983)
84. Ward, J.M., and Reynolds, C.W., Large granular lymphocyte leukemia. A heterogeneous lymphocytic leukemia in F344 rats. *Am. J. Pathol.* 111: 1–10 (1983)
85. Anver, M.R., and Cohen, B.J., in: *The Laboratory Rat* (H.J. Baker, J.R. Lindsey, and S.H. Weisbroth, eds.), Vol. I, pp 378–401, Academic Press, New York (1979)
86. Squire, R.A., and Levitt, M.H., Report of a workshop on classification of specific hepatocellular lesions in rats. *Cancer Res.* 35: 3214–3223 (1975)
87. Institute of Laboratory Animal Resources (ILAR), Histologic typing of liver tumors of the rat. National Research Council/National Academy of Sciences, Washington, DC. *J. Natl. Cancer Inst.* 64: 180–206 (1981)
88. Enomoto, K., and Farber, E., Kinetics of phenotypic maturation of remodeling of hyperplastic nodules during liver carcinogenesis. *Cancer Res.* 42: 2330–2335 (1982)
89. Pitot, H.C., and Sirica, A.E., The stages of initiation and promotion in hepatocarcinogenesis. *Biochim. Biophys. Acta* 605: 191–215 (1980)
90. Teebor, G.W., and Becker, F.F., Regression and persistence of hyperplastic hepatic nodules induced by N-2-fluorenylacetamide and their relationship to hepatocarcinogenesis. *Cancer Res.* 31: 1–3 (1971)
91. Ward, J.M., Griesemer, R.A., and Weisburger, E.K., The mouse liver tumor as an endpoint in carcinogenesis tests. *Toxicol. Appl. Pharmacol.* 51: 389–397 (1979)
92. Nutrition Foundation, *The Relevance of Mouse Liver Hepatoma to Human Carcinogenic Risk*, The Nutrition Foundation, Inc., Washington, DC. (1984)
93. Eastin, W., personal communication
94. Sontag, J.M., Carcinogenicity of substituted-benzenediamines (phenylenediamines) in rats and mice. *J. Natl. Cancer Inst.* 66: 591–602 (1981)
95. Masoro, E.J., Mortality and growth characteristics of rat strains commonly used in aging research. *Exp. Aging Res.* 6: 219–233 (1980)
96. Solleveld, H.A., and Boorman, G.A., personal communication
97. Maekawa, A., and Odashima, S., Spontaneous tumors in ACI/N rats. *J. Natl. Cancer Inst.* 55: 1437–1445 (1975)
98. National Toxicology Program, Carcinogenesis bioassay of trichloroethylene (*Technical Report Series*). DHHS Publication No. (NIH) (draft report)
99. National Toxicology Program, Carcinogenesis bioassay of tetrachloroethylene (*Technical Report Series*). DHHS Publication No. (NIH) (draft report)
100. Anderson, R.L., and Kanerva, R.L., Comparisons of response of Fischer 344 and Charles River rats to 1.5% nitrilotriacetic acid and 2% trisodium nitrilotriacetate monohydrate. *Fd. Cosmet. Toxicol.* 17: 137–140 (1983)
101. Dunning, W.F., Curtis, M.R., and Segaloff, A., Strain differences in response to estrone and the induction of mammary gland, adrenal, and bladder cancer in rats. *Cancer Res.* 13: 147–152 (1953)

102. Pamukcu, A.M., Wang, C.Y., Hatcher, J., and Bryan, G.T., Carcinogenicity of tannin and tannin-free extracts of bracken fern (Pteridium aquilinum) in rats. *J. Natl. Cancer Inst.* 65: 131–136 (1980)

103. Berman, J.J., Rice, J.M., Wenk, M.L., and Roller, P.P., Intestinal tumors induced by a single intraperitoneal injection of methyl (acetoxymethyl) nitrosamine in three strains of rats. *Cancer Res.* 39: 1462–1466 (1979)

104. Reuber, M.D., Varying degrees of susceptibility of inbred strains of rats to N-2-fluorenyldiacetamide hepatic carcinogenesis. *Toxicol. Appl. Pharmacol.* 37: 525–530 (1976)

105. Roebuck, B.D., and Longnecker, D.S., Species and rat strain variation in pancreatic nodule induction by azaserine. *J. Natl. Cancer Inst.* 59: 1273–1277 (1977)

106. Weisburger, E.K., Ulland, B.M., Schueler, R.L., Weisburger, J.H., and Harris, P.N., Carcinogenicity of three dose levels of 1,4-bis(4-fluorophenyl)-2-propenyl-N-cyclooctyl carbamate in male Sprague-Dawley and F344 rats. *J. Natl. Cancer Inst.* 54: 975–979 (1975)

107. Naito, M., Naito, Y., and Ito, A., Strain differences of tumorigenic effect of neonatally administered N-ethyl-N-nitrosourea in rats. *Gann* 73: 323–331 (1982)

108. Ito, N., Arai, M., Sugihara, S., Hirao, K., Makiura, S., Matayoshi, K., and Denda, A., Experimental urinary bladder tumors induced by N-butyl-N-(4-hydroxybutyl) nitrosamine. *Gann Monogr.* 17: 367–381 (1975)

109. Fukushima, S., Arai, M., Nakanowatari, J., Hibino, T., Okuda, M., and Ito, N., Differences in susceptibility to sodium saccharin among various strains of rats and other animal species. *Gann* 74: 8–20 (1983)

110. Lijinsky, W., and Taylor, H.W., Comparison of bladder carcinogenesis by nitrosomethyldodecylamine in Sprague-Dawley and Fischer rats carrying transplanted bladder tissue. *Cancer Lett.* 5: 215–218 (1978)

111. Sunderman, F.W., Jr., in: *Organ and Species Specificity in Chemical Carcinogenesis* (R. Langenbach, S. Nesnow and J.M. Rice, eds.), pp 107–127, Plenum Press, New York and London (1983)

112. Haseman, J., and Huff, J., personal communication

113. Schumann, A.M., Quast, J.F., and Watanabe, P.G., Pharmacokinetics and macromolecular interactions of perchloroethylene in mice and rats as related to oncogenicity. *Toxicol. Appl. Pharmacol.* 55: 207–219 (1980)

114. Tomatis, L., Partensky, C., and Montesano, R., The predictive value of mouse liver tumor induction in carcinogenicity testing—a literature survey. *Int. J. Cancer* 12: 1–20 (1973)

115. Weisburger, J.H., and Fiala, E.S., Mechanisms of species, strain, and dose effects in arylamine carcinogenesis. *Natl. Cancer Inst. Monogr.* 58: 41–48 (1981)

116. Weisburger, E.K., in: *Organ and Species Specificity in Chemical Carcinogenesis* (R. Langenbach, S. Nesnow and J.M. Rice, eds.), pp 23–48, Plenum Press, New York and London (1983)

117. Draft of Preclinical Toxicologic Guidelines, Bureau of Drugs, Health Protection Branch, Health and Welfare, Canada, October 1979. [Cited in: Sher, S.P., Jensen, R.D., and Bokelman, D.L., Spontaneous tumors in control F344 and Charles River CD rats and Charles River CD-1 and B6C3F1 mice. *Toxicol. Lett.* 11: 103–110 (1982)]

118. Notes for Guidelines on Carcinogenicity Testing on Medicinal Products, MAIL 24 (Medicines Act Information Letter) (June 1979)

15

Adequacy of Syrian Hamsters for Long-Term Animal Bioassays

Freddy Homburger
Richard A. Adams

Bio-Research Institute, Incorporated
Cambridge, Massachusetts

REASONS FOR SPECIES SELECTION

The historical reasons for the selection of rats and mice for bioassays for carcinogenicity were their ready availability, cheap initial cost and cost of maintenance, and brief lifespan, with correspondingly short times of latency for tumor induction.

Following Shubik's initial paper on *Chemical Carcinogenesis as a Chronic Toxicity Test*,[1] the first guidelines for bioassays for carcinogenicity were published by the Association of Food and Drug Administration Officials in 1959[2] (Table 1). At that time, mice and rats were the only rodents in wide use in the laboratory and they represented a logical choice with few, if any, alternatives. For a long time this choice seemed adequate and subsequent guidelines, as shown in Table 1, continued to deal only with rats and mice, initially Sprague-Dawley rats and CF1 mice. As the number of long-term bioassays with these strains began to increase, it became obvious that the relatively high incidence of spontaneous tumors in control animals tended to obscure the results and make their interpretation difficult. This led to the abandonment by the National Cancer Institute (NCI) and the National Toxicology Program (NTP) of Sprague-Dawley rats and CF1 mice, which were replaced by Fischer 344 rats and B6C3F1 mice.[29,30]

Besides the high incidence of spontaneous tumors, rats and mice also suffered from the disadvantages of marked susceptibility to respiratory infections, great sensitivity to the toxicity of nicotine (which precluded their use for carcinogenesis studies of tobacco smoke at doses high enough to induce cancer) and a tendency, especially in mice, to form hepatic nodules spontaneously and at the slightest provocation. The introduction of a new species into the standard bioassay protocol was officially considered for the first time in a conference on carcinogenicity testing of chemicals at the National Academy of Sciences in 1974. The Interagency Regulatory Liaison Group (IRLG) named hamsters as a third species in 1979.[22]

Table 1: The Evolution of Methodology for Carcinogenesis Bioassay: A Review of Literature

Author(s)	Subject	Reference
Shubik, P. and Sice, J.	Chemical carcinogenesis as chronic toxicity test	1
Food and Drug Administration Officers	Appraisal of safety of chemicals in foods, drugs and cosmetics	2
Food Protection Committee, Food and Nutrition Protection Board	Problems in the evaluation of carcinogenic hazards from the use of food additives	3
Weisburger, J.H. and Weisburger, E.K.	Tests for chemical carcinogenesis	4
Arcos, J.G., Arcos, M.F., and Wolf, G.	Testing procedures	5
World Health Organization	Principles for the testing and evaluation of drugs for carcinogenicity	6
International Union Against Cancer, Panel on Carcinogenicity of Cancer Research Commission	Carcinogenicity testing	7
FDA Advisory Committee on Protocols for Safety Evaluation, Panel on Carcinogenesis	Report on cancer testing in the safety evaluation of food additives and pesticides	8
Shubik, P.	The use of Syrian golden hamsters in chronic toxicity testing	9
Hayes, W.J.	Tests for detecting and measuring long-term toxicity	10
Grasso, P. and Crampton, R.F.	The value of the mouse in carcinogenicity testing	11
Health and Welfare Canada	The testing of chemicals for carcinogenicity	12
Golberg, L. (editor)	Carcinogenesis testing of chemicals	13
Grasso, P.	Review of tests for carcinogenicity and their significance for man	14
Homburger, F.	The potential usefulness of the Syrian hamster in future toxicology	15
Sontag, J.M., Page, N.P. and Saffiotti, U.	Guidelines for carcinogenesis bioassay in small rodents	16
Munro, I.C.	Considerations in chronic testing, the chemical, the dose, the design	17

(continued)

Table 1: (continued)

Author(s)	Subject	Reference
Food and Drug Administration	Good laboratory practices regulations	18
Food Safety Council, Scientific Committee	Proposed system for food safety assessment	19
Loomis, T.A.	Toxicologic testing methods	20
Environmental Protection Agency	Proposed health effects tests standards for Toxic Substances Control Act Test Rules	21
Interagency Regulatory Liaison Group	Scientific bases for identification of potential carcinogens and estimation of risk	22
Weisburger, J., and Williams, G.M.	Chemical carcinogenesis	23
Robens, J.F., Joiner, J.D., and Schueler, R.L.	Methods in testing for carcinogenicity	24
Homburger, F., Adams, R.A., Bernfeld, P., Van Dongen, C.G., and Soto, E.	A new first-generation hybrid Syrian hamster, BIO F1D Alexander for *in vivo* carcinogenesis bioassay, as a third species or to replace the mouse	25
Homburger, F., Van Dongen, C.G., Adams, R.A., and Soto, E.	Standardizing Syrian hamsters for toxicology	26
Adams, R.A. and Homburger, F.	Design and logistics of lifetime carcinogenesis bioassay using hamsters	27
Homburger, F.	Carcinogenesis, concepts, and *in vivo* testing in the study of toxicity and safety evaluation	28

Shubik had suggested the hamster for chronic toxicity testing as early as 1956. In 1968,[31] 1969[32] and 1972[33] one of the authors of this paper (F. Homburger) reviewed the literature on carcinogenesis in the Syrian hamster since its beginning in 1939, compared it with that available from studies in other species, and suggested that most inconsistencies of results obtained in hamsters could be explained by the dependence on genetic factors of the hamster's susceptibility to carcinogens. He postulated that the study of chemical carcinogens, if pursued in inbred lines of Syrian hamsters, could yield reproducible information of real pertinence to humans.[32] Shubik advocated hamsters specifically for bioassays for carcinogenicity in 1972,[9] and in 1978 a conference was held in Cambridge, Massachusetts, on the Syrian hamster in Toxicology and Carcinogenesis Research.[34]

While the paradoxical combination of high susceptibility to carcinogens and low spontaneous tumor incidence has long been recognized in the Syrian hamster,[35] this unique property of hamsters has not been used to improve bioassays for carcinogenicity because of the belief that hamsters were difficult to handle and keep alive during long-term experiments. Hyperplastic ileitis and severe amyloidosis prematurely decimated early studies that had been planned for long-term bioassay, and there was apprehension about lymphocytic chorio-meningitis virus, which could be carried by hamsters and cause human infections. Hamsters available from certain commercial sources were of ill-defined background and tended to be in poor health.

With the development of better husbandry methods[36] and health screening procedures, the quality of commercially available hamsters has greatly improved. Inbred strains available from several sources now permit the use of standardized biological material, just as is possible with mice and to some extent with rats. [37,38] The susceptibility of certain inbred strains of hamsters to carcinogens has been quantitated,[15,39] and hybrids of carcinogen-susceptible strains have been developed which constitute ideal animals for long-term bioassay. These hybrids are characterized by long survival, freedom from intercurrent diseases, reduced amyloidosis and, with the exception of modest rates of lymphoma and adrenal tumor in senescent animals (neoplasms not of the type frequently encountered in a bioassay for carcinogenicity), a greatly reduced spontaneous neoplasm profile.[25]

This is an appropriate time to review the studies which have been done in recent years in hamsters [with special emphasis on work done under the Good Laboratory Practices (GLPs) of the Food and Drug Administration (FDA) since 1978] and to analyze this body of work to determine the adequacy of hamsters for such assays.

Comparative Studies in Different Species

A relatively small number of compounds has been tested in comparative lifetime bioassays that include Syrian hamsters as one of the test species. An interesting example is a study of 2,3,7,8-tetrachloro-dibenzo-p-dioxin (TCDD), in which hamsters proved to be the most resistant species tested.[40] Toxicokinetic studies[41] have shown that hamsters metabolize dioxin faster than any other species. This has made possible the long-term administration of this highly toxic chemical, to hamsters, with the resultant demonstration, never before made in either rats or mice, that intraperitoneal or subcutaneous injections of dioxin at four week intervals resulted in perioral squamous cell cancer with pulmonary metastases.[42]

Amitrole (Aminotriazole) was also studied comparatively in rats, mice and hamsters[43] in lifetime bioassays in which 0.1 ppm, 10 ppm and 100 ppm of the chemical were administered in the diet. While there were effects upon the thyroid of the three species at the high dose, tumors of the thyroid and/or pituitary occurred only in rats.

Formaldehyde was administered to monkeys, rats and hamsters by inhalation.[44] At concentrations of 2.95 ppm, but not lower, formaldehyde produced epithelial squamous metaplasia within 26 weeks in monkeys and rats, but not in hamsters. This instance of hamster "resistance" must be accepted guardedly, however, since the test animals were random bred and marked variation in susceptibility to respiratory carcinogens, for example, tobacco smoke, is known to occur among different inbred strains of hamsters.[45]

Hamsters also proved less sensitive than guinea pigs to the acute lethal effects of polybrominated biphenyls,[46] but no data are available resulting from comparative lifetime bioassays.

An instance of a compound having greater toxicity for hamsters is that of perfluoro-n-decanoic acid. Greater numbers of fat vacuoles appear in the liver when perfluoro-n-decanoic acid is administered to hamsters than in other species.[47]

Other differences in the toxicity of various compounds have been noted but are not well studied or understood, such as the resistance of hamsters, especially that of certain inbred strains, toward nicotine,[48] or the fact that hamsters are at least as susceptible as rats, but more susceptible than mice, to the acute toxicity of intraperitoneal injection of citrinin.[49]

Long-Term Bioassays in Hamsters of Various Substances Without Simultaneous Testing in Other Species

Some aromatic amines cause bladder cancer in hamsters[50,51] whereas, though not tested simultaneously, they are known not to do so in rats and mice. In hamsters with atypical proliferative colitis, such substances also caused intestinal cancer.[52]

Coumarin, previously reported as carcinogenic in rats, was not carcinogenic when tested in hamsters.[53] Rotenone, given orally and intraperitoneally to rats and in the diet to hamsters was non-carcinogenic in hamsters.[54,55]

Quantitative differences in the rate of excretion of similar metabolites of N-butyl-N-(4-hydroxybutyl)nitrosamine[56] and Quazepam[57] in rats, mice and hamsters have been noted, with hamsters being the most rapid metabolizers.

Hein[58] noted that among inbred strains of hamsters there are marked differences in the rate of hepatic acetylation.

Mice were sensitive to tumor induction with DDT, whereas hamsters were not and in one study rats reacted marginally,[59] although others have induced liver tumors in rats with DDT.[60] Studies of the metabolites of DDT excreted by mice and hamsters showed that though similar end products were produced by both species, the hamster was not nearly as efficient as the mouse in converting DDT to the tumorigenic metabolite 1,1-dichloro-2,2-bis(p-chlorophenyl)ethane, which causes liver tumors in mice and hamsters and adrenal tumors in hamsters.[61,62]

Recently, certain food additives have been examined in hamsters. In lifetime studies in rats and hamsters, carrageenan was non-carcinogenic in both species.[63] In the rat, however, spontaneous mammary and testicular tumors occurring in untreated control animals as well as in treated animals obscured the results, whereas in hamsters spontaneous tumors of these types did not occur. The food additive AF2 [2-(2-furyl)-3-(5-nitro-2-furyl)acrylamide] was fed for 660 days to hamsters and caused forestomach and esophageal tumors.[64]

Aflatoxin B₁ in large doses induced cholangiocellular carcinomas in hamsters as well as in rats (1 mg/kg to 2 mg/kg given five times per week for six weeks). In hamsters the latent period was longer than in rats, and one-third of the hamsters developed bile duct and/or liver cancer after 78 weeks.[65]

N-δ-(N-methyl-N-nitrosocarbamoyl)-L-ornithine caused mammary and skin cancers in hamsters, but they were less susceptible than rats.[66]

Essentially negative results were obtained in hamsters given quercetin and rutin orally[67] or Praziquantel, which also did not cause cancer in rats.[68]

Hydrazine, carcinogenic in mice and rats, does not produce tumors in the hamster. The metabolic reason for this difference is not as yet fully understood and is only partially illuminated by recent studies on the methylation of liver DNA guanine in hamsters given hydrazine.

Respiratory Carcinogenesis

Inhalation of cigarette smoke by suitable Syrian hamsters results in carcinoma of the larynx in a high percentage of the animals. Lesions are never found in untreated control hamsters or hamsters placed in smoking machines but not exposed to cigarette smoke. This method of inducing laryngeal cancer with cigarette smoke, first reported by Dontenwill,[69] was refined by Bernfeld and associates,[45,70,71] who were the first to demonstrate significant differences in susceptibility to respiratory cancer by tobacco smoke among several strains of inbred Syrian hamsters. In animals exposed for more than a year to smoke from American reference cigarettes, the incidences of larynx cancer varied from nearly 20% in susceptible animals to about 4% in resistant animals.[45] In a later study,[70] nearly 50% of animals exposed to higher concentrations of smoke from British reference cigarettes developed cancer of the larynx. The same authors[71] also reported that the laryngeal epithelial hyperplasia produced by exposure to cigarette smoke for only three months was of greater severity in animals exposed to types of cigarettes that had been previously shown to produce cancer in long-term studies than in animals exposed to cigarettes previously shown to be innocuous. This suggests that subacute exposure to tobacco smoke might serve to select those smoking products likely to be less carcinogenic than others. The techniques might permit selection of smoking materials deserving more refined safety evaluation.

Hamsters are eminently suitable for safety evaluation of smoking products since the endpoint of such studies, laryngeal cancer, is a close model of the laryngeal cancer which is demonstrably associated with cigarette smoking in humans.[72] Furthermore, the epithelial cells so transformed are of the same embryonic origin as those that in humans give rise to bronchogenic carcinoma, the most common form of human lung cancer, and one which shows strong association with cigarette smoking.

The hamster's special suitability for such studies is based on the absence of spontaneous respiratory tumors, the great susceptibility of certain inbred strains to respiratory carcinogens, and the resistance of these inbred strains to the toxicity of nicotine.[48] Another important factor is the marked resistance of the hamster to pulmonary infections. This is in contrast to the great susceptibility of rats and mice to such infections which tend to reduce the value of inhalation studies performed with those species. The lesions of murine pneumonia also tend to mimic epithelial proliferation and atypia, rendering evaluation still more difficult. In dogs, a species in which lung tumor can also be induced by exposure to cigarette smoke through tracheostomies, spontaneous lung tumors are known to occur. Furthermore, large scale studies with significant numbers of dogs are difficult and expensive.

The identity of the carcinogenic agents in cigarette smoke remains elusive, although there are numerous candidates among the hundreds of known chemical components therein. One possible mechanism to explain species and strain differences might be the way in which benzo(a)pyrene and its metabolites bind to

DNA. Kaufman[73] found this to differ in laryngeal mucosa from resistant and susceptible hamster strains and Mass[74] described an 18-fold difference between rats and hamsters in activation of benzo(a)pyrene and its binding to DNA.

Nitrosamines could also be a factor in the carcinogenicity of tobacco smoke. For example, studies of up to 16 weeks' duration[75] suggest that doses of up to 24 mg of diethylnitrosamine given subcutaneously during that period affected argyrophilic cells and neuroepithelial bodies and caused hyperplasia of the epithelia of the respiratory tract in lungs of hamsters. It has not been established, however, that such changes are precursors of lung cancers.

Long-term inhalation bioassays employing hamsters have recently been carried out on several compounds of interest. Bleomycin induced pulmonary fibrosis similar to that observed in humans,[76] and inhalation of dimethylcarbamoyl chloride by Syrian hamsters caused carcinomas of the nasal tract, with a latent period considerably longer than that observed in rats.[77]

Nitrosamines and Other Nitroso Compounds as Carcinogens for the Respiratory Tract and Other Organs

In Syrian (and also European) hamsters, most nitrosamines so far tested are organotropic for the respiratory tract. For example, N-nitrosodiethanolamine, described by Pour and Wallcave[78] as an upper respiratory tract carcinogen, caused nasal and tracheal carcinomas in hamsters,[79] regardless of the site of application.

Other nitroso compounds subjected to chronic tests in hamsters and found to be carcinogenic are nitrosomorpholine, which caused dose-related tumors in the larynx, trachea, digestive tract, and liver when given in the drinking water;[80] 4-(methylnitrosoamino)-1-butanone and N'-nitrosonornicotine, shown by Hoffmann et al.[81] to be carcinogenic environmental contaminants; and nitrosopyrrolidine, which caused hepatocellular cancer even in low doses.[82] Nitrosomethyldodecanylamine caused mucoepidermoid lung cancers, bladder cancers and tumors at the injection sites in European hamsters.[83]

Certain co-carcinogenic factors were observed to intensify the carcinogenicity of nitroso compounds, namely chronic ethanol consumption which intensified the carcinogenic effects of N-nitrosopyrrolidine and N-nitrosonornicotine,[84] and formaldehyde which accentuated the carcinogenic effects of diethylnitrosamine, increasing the numbers of induced respiratory cancers per animal.[85]

Asbestos and Other Particulates as Respiratory Carcinogens

These appeared to be weakly active in several life-time exposure bioassays in hamsters. However, the exact genetic background of these hamsters was usually not known, so that it is quite possible that inappropriate (carcinogen-resistant) animals were inadvertantly used in some instances. Thus, inhaled organic fibers, asbestos and fiber glass produced few tumors, asbestos appearing to be the most fibrogenic of these substances.[86] Although the addition of benzo(a)-pyrene to intratracheally instilled foundry particulates caused small numbers of lung tumors in long-term inhalation studies, such dusts were not carcinogenic when instilled alone.[87] Intratracheal instillation of 10 mg of milled chrysotile twice monthly induced benign tumors, the incidence of which was increased by the addition of benzo(a)pyrene. Intrapleural injections of the asbestos, however, produced mesotheliomas, the incidence of which was unaffected by the addition of benzo(a)pyrene.[88] When nickel-enriched fly ash was administered to hamsters for 20 months by inhalation, non-significant numbers of rare lung tumors were observed.[89]

The carcinogenicity of asbestos was also tested by the intraperitoneal route.[90,91] In one instance,[90] only intraperitoneal fibrosis occurred, but other investigators induced mesotheliomas. The studies of Smith and his associates [92-95] demonstrated carcinogenicity for chrysotile, tremolite, and glass fibers and reduced fiber length meant reduced carcinogenicity. The same group also showed a co-carcinogenic effect of chrysotile for intratracheally instilled benzo(a)pyrene.[96] They also fed various fibers in the drinking water and found that some tumors were thereby induced with amosite (not a statistically significant incidence, however), whereas the shorter fibers of cumingtonite and taconite had no effect.[93,95]

Inhaled Radioactive Substances

Little[97] (who has intensively studied polonium as a pulmonary carcinogen) pointed out the importance of non-carcinogenic secondary factors. Intratracheal instillation of physiological saline solution,[98] for example, increased radiation-induced pulmonary carcinoma from 2% to 36%. Little's group successfully demonstrated the carcinogenic properties of inhaled polonium in hamsters, but others, upon exposing hamsters to radon daughters and uranium ore dusts found only metaplastic changes and a few squamous cancers at the highest radiation levels, and concluded that hamsters might not be suitable animals for such studies. The genetic background of the hamsters used by these investigators is unspecified; they may well have dealt with resistant animals, since no positive controls were included in their studies.[99] In contrast, Smith *et al.*[94] found that radionuclides clearly induced cancer in the respiratory tract of the hamster, whereas the rat seemed to be a poor species for assessment of pulmonary effects, including carcinogenesis, that could be extrapolated to man.

The Direct Application of N-Methyl-N-Nitrosourea to a Well Defined Segment of the Hamster Trachea

This method, a standardized testing procedure, has recently been employed to study the morphogenesis of induced tumors.[100] Topically applied, ethylnitrosourea caused benign papillomas, whereas methylnitrosourea induced frank cancers.[101]

Besides the respiratory tract of hamsters, the kidney of the male, the exocrine pancreas, the gallbladder and the skin have all been more or less extensively studied and present special opportunities for bioassay of carcinogenic activity.

Peculiar Behavior of Hamster Kidney Suggesting Suitability for Certain Bioassays for Carcinogenicity

Following the observation of Vasquez-Lopez[102] that prolonged treatment with estrogens caused renal cancer in male hamsters, and Kirkman's later observation regarding the similar effects of diethylstilbestrol (DES),[103] Burrows commented on the failure of most investigators to induce renal carcinoma and on the uniqueness of hamsters in this respect.[104] This subject has been reviewed several times.[31,32,105] If safety evaluation studies had been carried out in the 1940s with protocols such as are currently in use, and if estrogens, including diethylstilbestrol, had been tested in hamsters, the high incidence of renal carcinomas occurring in the males would definitely have led to labeling this compound as a carcinogen. Thus, it is doubtful whether diethylstilbestrol would ever have been prescribed, as it later was, to prevent threatened abortion. Such studies in hamsters might have prevented the tragedy which has in recent years struck the offspring of many women who received DES during pregnancy. While the mechanisms of sex-dependent renal carcinogenesis remain unclear, recent work employing a fluorinated analogue of DES (which in male hamsters causes clear cell kidney cancer) suggests that quinones are the probable carcinogenic metabolite of DES.[106]

Hamster Pancreas as Target Organ for Certain Nitrosamines

Pour and associates administered weekly subcutaneous injections of from 125 mg/kg body weight to 500 mg/kg body weight of 2,2'-dihydroxy-di-n-propylnitrosamine to 8 week old hamsters for life. They induced pancreatic neoplasms in all of their animals.[107] This opened a field that has been extensively explored and reviewed.[66,108-111] The nitrosamine model of pancreatic carcinogenesis in hamsters is one in which the lesions produced are histologically the equivalent of those of the human disease. Because hamsters are more susceptible than other species to this type of lesion, they are more suitable for long-term bioassay whenever the pancreas is a suspected target organ, and when test substances or their metabolites are related to nitrosamines.

The Gallbladder as a Susceptible Site for Methylcholanthrene Carcinogenesis

Bain and associates[112-114] demonstrated a high incidence of papillary adenocarcinoma in gallbladders of hamsters implanted with beeswax pellets containing methylcholanthrene. High cholesterol diets had co-carcinogenic effects. More recently, this has been confirmed by Japanese workers who found that more than half of the animals developed carcinoma within 220 days after implantation of such pellets into their gallbladders.[115,116] They also found that a lithogenic diet proved to be co-carcinogenic.[117] Because rats do not have gallbladders, and gallbladder surgery is far easier to perform in hamsters than in mice, hamsters should be the species of choice for long-term bioassays in this site. Furthermore, in hamsters the topical dose for induction of gallbladder cancer may be well defined.

Species-Specific Properties of Hamster Skin Possibly Useful in Long-Term Bioassays

The expectation has not been completely fulfilled that the innate resistance of Syrian hamsters to the toxicity of nicotine might make them useful for lifetime skin painting assays of tobacco smoke condensates:[118] Massive and long-continued application of cigarette smoke condensate, which readily induces skin cancer in various strains of mice, fails to do so in hamsters. On the other hand, certain inbred lines of hamsters exhibit dermal melanomas within a few weeks following application of single doses of small amounts of dimethylbenzanthracene (DMBA).[119] This reaction was much more rapid than development of papilloma in the most sensitive SenCar mice, following application of much larger doses of DMBA in combination with phorbol esters as promoters. Phorbol esters were ineffective as promoters of melanoma in the hamster skin.[120]

Because of the growing importance of human melanoma, which has been increasing in frequency in recent years, and because of the proven susceptibility of hamsters to melanogenesis, skin painting in DMBA-susceptible hamsters deserves to be included in the safety evaluation of products having the potential for contact with the skin.

The Hamster Cheek Pouch as a Bioassay for Carcinogenicity

The cheek pouch of hamsters has long been used both for studies on mechanisms of carcinogenesis and to a limited extent for bioassays for carcinogenicity (the subject was reviewed in 1979).[105]

This unique organ might well be standardized for testing for carcinogenicity since Solt[121] has shown that cheek pouch cells rapidly respond with induction of gamma-glutamyl transpeptidase when exposed to carcinogens. This would provide in one system a combination of an early marker for carcinogenicity and the eventual oncogenic response (squamous cell carcinoma).

DISCUSSION

In reviewing the historical background and the present performance of *in vivo* bioassays for carcinogenicity, we must conclude that the species of laboratory animals currently employed in such tests were chosen for expedience rather than for valid scientific reasons. In addition, the results of an important proportion of recently performed tests are equivocal or at least difficult to interpret[122] indicating the need for further study.

It is legitimate to ask whether the use of new species of laboratory animals could improve the outcome of bioassays, especially since we may assume that for the foreseeable future, *in vivo* bioassays will remain the most important single determinant in the evaluation of the safety of chemicals. Hence, efforts leading to the improvement of the methodology of such tests are important, but the realization of such improvements is likely to require much time.

Under the twin pressures of increasing public awareness of the carcinogenic hazards of many environmental and occupational pollutants and the enactment of legislation to meet the resulting demands for safety regulation, a set of laws and the inevitable bureaucracy to administer them and to formulate regulations have developed. Guidelines have appeared, accreditation bodies have been formed, and good laboratory practices have been prescribed. Today, the conduct of long-term bioassays intended to establish the safety of chemicals for clearance by various government regulatory agencies has become so standardized and institutionalized that any contemplated change in procedures threatens to become a major undertaking. For these reasons, the long-term bioassay *in vivo*, widely thought to be inherently unsatisfactory, continues to be used and will undoubtedly continue to be used for some time before improvements can become possible.

Many results of lifetime bioassays are equivocal because the lesions presumably induced by the test substance develop in untreated animals as well, in many instances with varying incidences from one laboratory to another, or even within the same laboratory in different studies.

This unduly great incidence of spontaneous tumors in control mice and rats is the principal deficiency of the *in vivo* bioassay method in use today by the National Toxicology Program and by the many chemical, pharmaceutical and consumer-goods manufacturers wishing to comply with existing regulations. (The other drawbacks which made the search for short-term *in vitro* bioassays so attractive are the high costs and long duration of the *in vivo* tests.)

The literature on the hamster reveals the hamster's uniquely low incidence of spontaneous tumors, especially of the type known to be induced by administered carcinogens, combined with a marked susceptibility to the carcinogenic effects of administered polycyclic hydrocarbons, aniline derivatives, nitroso compounds and other classes of chemical carcinogens.

The use of Syrian hamsters as a third species or to replace mice, could no doubt, in some instances, help to make the lifetime bioassay more sensitive and more rapid. This would certainly be the case for test substances related to compounds towards which hamsters have been shown to be highly sensitive, such as aniline derivatives, nitrosamines or other nitroso compounds and substances yielding quinones. Because in hamsters the incidence of spontaneous tumors of the type most likely to be induced by such compounds is extremely low, small numbers of induced tumors suffice to bring about statistically significant results. In the case of substances such as dioxin, both rats and mice would be long dead before a carcinogenic effect could possibly occur. The pharmacodynamics of test substances should therefore be studied in hamsters as well as in rats and mice before decisions are made as to which species should be committed to long-term bioassay.

Since the hamster offers such obvious advantages for more sensitive and rapid bioassay, the question arises, why has it not been used more frequently in bioassays for carcinogenicity? Historically, the hamster is a latecomer to the laboratory, having been introduced only in the 1940's when the use of mice and rats was already firmly entrenched. Hamsters mistakenly acquired a sullied reputation because of the very qualities which gave them an advantage for use in microbiology, their great susceptibility to viral infections and protozoan infestations. They also were misrepresented by the uninitiated as combative and hard to handle, all too often it seems, considered to be subject to the mysterious affliction of "wet-tail", or in other cases, amyloidosis. Furthermore, the sources of most commercially available hamsters were poorly identified. Only randombred animals were obtainable and it was therefore uncertain that experimental results could ever be replicated at different times.

Over the years, sustained experience in hamster husbandry has resulted in the production of predictably healthy animals. Inbred lines, bred by pedigreed brother x sister matings for more than 20 generations are available from several commercial sources. Most recently, a carcinogen-susceptible hybrid has been produced which is longer-lived than most other hamsters, has a low incidence of adrenal tumors and lymphomas but practically no other spontaneous neoplasms and, especially in the males, shows only minimal terminal amyloidosis. Such animals could be most suitable in testing for carcinogenicity and in some instances could very well replace mice.[25]

In addition to its general suitability on the basis of the advantages cited so far, the Syrian hamster has certain species-specific properties which make it especially useful for specific types of bioassay. Among these are:

(1) Great resistance to pulmonary infections coupled with susceptibility of the respiratory epithelium to known carcinogens, making the species ideal for inhalation studies.

(2) The responsiveness of hamster kidneys (especially in males) to the carcinogenic effect of estrogens, offering a unique tool for bioassays of related agents.

(3) The susceptibility of the respiratory and gallbladder epithelia to topical application of carcinogens, highly exploitable for bioassays in these areas.

(4) The proven responsiveness of the exocrine pancreas, which offers opportunities for bioassay of carcinogens with possible organotropism for the pancreas.

(5) The uniqueness of the skin as a model for dermal melanogenesis.

(6) The specific greater resistance to the toxicity of certain substances, permitting the easy demonstration of the carcinogenicity of certain substances, such as cigarette smoke and dioxin. This little studied characteristic of hamsters might be of future importance in improving the long-term bioassay.

(7) The uniqueness of the cheek pouch as a site for topical induction of cancer with opportunity for *in vivo* direct inspection.

We conclude that the Syrian hamster is not merely adequate but eminently suitable for long-term bioassays for carcinogenicity, and offers opportunities to improve the standard long-term bioassay, especially for compounds which are demonstrably metabolized by hamsters as they are by humans. The hamster could well replace the mouse as a second species and eliminate some of the confusion which results from high spontaneous tumor incidences in mice, their high susceptibility to carcinogens,[123] and from a tendency of their liver cells to be altered by various mechanisms which are perhaps unrelated to carcinogenesis.

REFERENCES

1. Shubik, P., and Sice, J., Chemical carcinogenesis as a chronic toxicity test. *Cancer Res.* 16: 728–742 (1956)
2. Food and Drug Officials of the USA, *Appraisal of Safety of Chemicals in Food, Drugs and Cosmetics.* Assoc. of Food and Drug Officials of the USA. Austin, Texas (1959)

3. Food Protection Committee, Food and Nutrition Board, Problems in the evaluation of carcinogenic hazards from the use of food additives. National Academy of Sciences, National Research Council, Pub. No. 749, *Cancer Res.* 21: 429-456 (1960)

4. Weisburger, J.H., and Weisburger, E.K., in: *Methods in Cancer Research* (H. Busch, ed.), Vol. 1, pp 307-387, Academic Press, New York (1967)

5. Arcos, J.G., Arcos, M.F., and Wolf, G., *Testing Procedures in Chemical Induction of Cancer*, New York: Vol. 1, pp 340-463, Academic Press (1968)

6. World Health Organization, Principles for the Testing and Evaluation of Drugs for Carcinogenicity. WHO Technical Reports Series No. 426 (1969)

7. International Union Against Cancer, Panel on Carcinogenicity of Cancer Research Commission. Carcinogenicity Testing, UICC Technical Report Series, Vol. 2, pp 1-43 (1969)

8. Food and Drug Administration Advisory Committee on Protocols for Safety Evaluation, Panel on Carcinogenesis, Report on Cancer Testing in the Safety Evaluation of Food Additives and Pesticides. *Toxicol. Appl. Pharmacol.* 20: 419-438 (1971)

9. Shubik, P., The use of Syrian golden hamsters in chronic toxicity testing. *Prog. Exp. Tumor Res.* 16: 176-184 (1972)

10. Hayes, W.J., in: *Essays in Toxicology* (W.J. Hayes, ed.), Vol. 3, Academic Press, New York (1972)

11. Grasso, P., and Crampton, R.F., The value of the mouse in carcinogenicity testing. *Fd. Cosmet. Toxicol.* 10: 418-426 (1972)

12. Health and Welfare Canada, The Testing of Chemicals for Carcinogenicity, Mutagenicity and Teratogenicity. Ministry of Health and Welfare, Ottawa, Canada (1973)

13. Golberg, L. (ed.), *Carcinogenesis Testing of Chemicals*. Cleveland, Ohio: CRC Press (1974)

14. Grasso, P., Review of tests for carcinogenicity and their significance to man. *Clin. Toxicol.* 9: 745-760 (1976)

15. Homburger, F., in: *Advances in Modern Toxicology* (M.A. Mehlman, ed.), pp 35-60, Hemisphere Pub. Co., Washington, DC (1976)

16. Sontag, J.M., Page, N.P., and Saffiotti, U., Guidelines for carcinogenesis bioassay in small rodents. *NCI Carcinogenesis Technical Report Series* No. 1 (1976)

17. Munro, I.C., Considerations in chronic testing, the chemical, the dose, the design. *J. Environ. Pathol. Toxicol.* 1: 183-197 (1977)

18. Food and Drug Administration, Good Laboratory Practice Regulations. *Fed. Register* 43: 59986-60025 (1978)

19. Food Safety Council, Scientific Committee, Proposed system for food safety assessment. *Fd. Cosmet. Toxicol.* (Suppl) 16: 1-136 (1978)

20. Loomis, T.A., in: *Essentials of Toxicology*, 3rd ed. (T.A. Loomis, ed.), pp 195-237, Lea & Febiger, Philadelphia (1978)

21. Environmental Protection Agency, Proposed Health Effects Tests Standards for Toxic Substances Control Act Test Rules. *Fed. Register* 44: 27334-27374 (1979)

22. Interagency Regulatory Liaison Group, Scientific Bases for Identification of Potential Carcinogens and Estimation of Risk. *Fed. Register* 44: 39858-39879 (1979)

23. Weisburger, J.H., and Williams, G.M., in: *Casarett and Doull's Toxicology*, 2nd ed., pp 84-138, Macmillan Pub. Co., Inc., New York (1980)

24. Robens, J.F., Joiner, J.D., and Schueler, R.L., in: *Principles and Methods of Toxicology* (W. Hayes, ed.), Raven Press, New York (1982)

25. Homburger, F., Van Dongen, C.G., Adams, R.A., and Soto, E., in: *Survey and Synthesis of Pathology Research* 1: 125-133 (1983)
26. Homburger, F., Van Dongen, C.G., Adams, R.A., and Soto, E., in: *Safety Evaluation and Regulation of Chemicals* (F. Homburger, ed.), pp 225-232, S. Karger Publishers, Basel/New York (1983)
27. Adams, R.A., and Homburger, F., in: *Skin Painting Techniques and in vivo Carcinogenesis Bioassays* (F. Homburger, ed.), Vol. 26, pp 202-207, *Prog. Exp. Tumor Res.*, S. Karger Publishers, Basel/New York (1983)
28. Homburger, F., Hayes, J.A., and Pelikan, E.W. (eds.), *A Guide to General Toxicology*, S. Karger Publishers, Basel/New York (1983)
29. Tarone, R.E., Chu, K.C., and Ward, J.M., Variability in the rates of some common naturally occurring tumors in Fischer 344 rats and (C57BL/6 x C3H/HeN)F1 (B6C3F1) mice. *J. Natl. Cancer Inst.* 66: 1175-1181 (1981)
30. Sher, S.P., Tumors in control hamsters, rats and mice. Literature tabulation. *CRC Crit. Rev. Toxicol.* 10: 49-79 (1982)
31. Homburger, F., in: *Prog. Exp. Tumor Res.*, (F. Homburger, ed.), Vol. 10, pp 163-237, S. Karger Publishers, Basel/New York (1968)
32. Homburger, F., Chemical carcinogenesis in the Syrian hamster, a review. *Cancer* 23: 313-338 (1969)
33. Homburger, F., in: *Pathology of the Syrian Hamster*, (F. Homburger, ed.), Vol. 16, pp 152-175, *Prog. Exp. Tumor Res.*, S. Karger Publishers, Basel/New York (1972)
34. Adams, R.A., DiPaolo, J.A., and Homburger, F., The Syrian hamster in toxicology and carcinogenesis research. *Cancer Res.* 38: 2642-2645 (1978)
35. Van Hoosier, G.L., Jr., Spjut, H.J., and Trentin, J.J., Spontaneous Tumors of the Syrian hamster: Observations in a Closed Breeding Colony and a Review of the Literature in Defining the Laboratory Animal. National Academy of Sciences. Washington, D.C. (1972)
36. Committee on Care and Use of Laboratory Animals of the Institute of Laboratory Animal Resources, National Research Council. *Guide for the Care and Use of Laboratory Animals*. USD of Health, Education and Welfare, USPHS 1978, NIH 78-23 (rev. 1978)
37. Altman, P.L., and Katz, D.D. (eds.), *Inbred and Genetically Defined Strains of Laboratory Animals. Biological Handbooks III, Part 2: Hamster, Guinea Pig, Rabbit and Chicken*. Federation of American Societies for Experimental Biology, Bethesda, Maryland (1979)
38. Festing, M.F.W., *Inbred Strains in Biomedical Research*. New York: Oxford University Press (1979)
39. Homburger, F., in: *Skin Painting Techniques and In Vivo Carcinogenesis Bioassays*, Vol. 26, pp 259-265, *Prog. Exp. Tumor Res.*, S. Karger Publishers, Basel/New York (1983)
40. Henk, J.M., New, M.A., Kociba, R.J., and Rao, K.S., 2,3,7,8-Tetrachlorodibenzo-p-dioxin: Acute oral toxicity in hamsters. *Toxicol. Appl. Pharmacol.* 59: 405-407 (1981)
41. Olson, P.R., Gasiewica, T.A., and Neal, R.A., Tissue distribution, excretion and metabolism of 2,3,7,8-tetrachlorodibenzo-p-dioxin in the golden Syrian hamster (abs) #1361, *Fed. Proc.* 39: 524, (1980); *Toxicol. Appl. Pharmacol.* 56: 78-85 (1980)
42. Rao, S., and Subbarao, V., Carcinogenicity of 2,3,7,8-tetrachlorodibenzo-p-dioxin (TCDD) in Syrian golden hamsters (abs), Hamster Soc. Ann. Mtg. (1983)

43. Steinhoff, D., Weber, H., Mohr, U., and Boehme, K., Evaluation of amitrole (aminotriazole) for potential carcinogenicity in orally dosed rats, mice and golden hamsters. *Toxicol. Appl. Pharmacol.* 69:161–169 (1983)

44. Rusch, G.M., Clary, J.J., Rinehardt, W.E., and Bolte, H.F., A 26 week inhalation toxicity study with formaldehyde in the monkey, rat and hamster. *Toxicol. Appl. Pharmacol.* 68: 329–343 (1983)

45. Bernfeld, P., Homburger, F., and Russfield, A.B., Strain differences in the response of inbred Syrian hamsters to cigarette smoke inhalation. *J. Natl. Cancer Inst.* 53: 1141–1157 (1974)

46. Collins, J.E., Sleight, S.D., and Aust, S.D., Acute pathologic effects of polybrominated biphenyls (PBB) in guinea pigs and golden hamsters (abs). *The Pharmacologist* 24: 149 (1982)

47. Van Rafelghem, M., Andersen, M., Bruner, R., and Mattie, D., Comparative toxicity of perfluoro-n-decanoic acid in rats and hamsters. *The Toxicologist* (abs) 2: 148 (1982)

48. Bernfeld, P., and Homburger, F., High nicotine tolerance of Syrian golden hamsters (abs). *Toxicol. Appl. Pharmacol.* 22: 324 (1972)

49. Jordan, W.H., Carlton, W.W., and Sausing, G.A., Critinin mycotoxicosis in the Syrian hamster. *Fd. Cosmet. Toxicol.* 16: 355–363 (1978)

50. Saffiotti, U., Cefis, F., Montesano, R., and Sellakumar, A.R., in: *Bladder Cancer, a Symposium* (W.B. Deichmann, *et al.*, eds.), Aesculapius Publishing Company, Birmingham, Alabama (1967)

51. Homburger, F., Hsueh, S.S., Soto, E., and Van Dongen, C.G., Induction of transitional cell carcinoma of the urinary bladder by feeding beta-naphthylamine to inbred Syrian hamsters. *J. Inter-American Med.* 2: 30 (1977)

52. Williams, G.M., Chandrasekawan, V., Katayam, S., and Weisburger, J.H., Carcinogenicity of 3-methyl-2-naphthylamine and 3,2'-dimethyl-4-aminobiphenyl to the bladder and gastrointestinal tract of the Syrian golden hamster with atypical proliferative enteritis. *J. Natl. Cancer Inst.* 67: 481–486 (1981)

53. Ueno, I., and Hirono, I., Non-carcinogenic response to coumarin in Syrian golden hamsters. *Fd. Cosmet. Tox.* 19: 353–355 (1981)

54. Freudenthal, R.I., Leber, A.P., Thake, D.C., and Baron, R.L., Carcinogenic potential of rotenone subchronic oral and peritoneal administration to rats and chronic dietary administration to Syrian golden hamsters. Natl. Tech. Information Service, Springfield, VA, Pub. 81–190936 (1981)

55. Leber, A.P., and Persing, R.L., Carcinogenic potential of rotenone. Phase I: Dietary administration to hamsters. U.S. Dept. of Commerce, National Technical Information Service (NTIS) PB 83–800680 (October 1982)

56. Suzuki, E., Anjo, T., Aoki, J., and Okada, M., Species variations in the metabolism of N-butyl-N-(4-hydroxy-butyl)nitrosamine and related compounds in relation to urinary bladder carcinogenesis. *Gann.* 74: 60–68 (1983)

57. Hilbert, J., Symchowicz, S., and Zanpaglione, N., The metabolic fate of ^{14}C-Quazepam in hamsters and mice (abs). *The Pharmacologist* 23: 196 (1981)

58. Hein, D.W., Ominchinski, J.G., Brewer, J.A., and Weber, W., A unique pharmacogenetic expression of the N-acetylation polymorphism in the inbred hamster. *J. Pharmacol. Exp. Therap.* 220: 8–15 (1982)

59. Gold, B., and Brunk, G., Metabolism of 1,1,1-trichloro-2,2-bis(p-chlorophenyl)ethane, (DDT), 1,1-dichloro-2,2-bis(p-chlorophenyl)ethane and 1-chloro-2,2-bis(p-chlorophenyl)ethene in the hamster. *Cancer Res.* 43: 2644–2647 (1983)

60. Cabral, J.R.P., Hall, R.K., Rossi, L., Broncyk, S., and Shubik, P., Comparative chronic toxicity of DDT in rats and hamsters (abs). Ann. Meetg. Toxicol. Soc. (1980)
61. Rossi, L., Barbieri, O., Sanguineti, M., Cabral, J.R.P., Bruzzi, P., and Santi, L., Carcinogenicity study with technical-grade dichlorophenyltrichloroethane and 1,1-dichloro-2,2-bis(p-chlorophenyl)ethylene in hamsters. *Cancer Res.* 43: 776–781 (1983)
62. Gingell, R., and Wallcave, L., Species differences in the acute toxicity and tissue distribution of DDT in mice and hamsters. *Toxicol. Appl. Pharmacol.* 28:385–394 (1974)
63. Rustia, M., Shubik, P., and Patil, K., Lifespan carcinogenicity test with native carrageenan in rats and hamsters. *Cancer Lett.* 11: 1–10 (1980)
64. Kinebuchi, M., Kawachi, T., Matsukura, N., and Sugimura, T.S., Further studies on the carcinogenicity of the food additive AF-2 in hamsters. *Fd. Cosmet. Toxicol.* 17: 339–341 (1979)
65. Moore, M.R., Pitot, H.C., Miller, E., and Miller, J.A., Cholangiocellular carcinomas induced in Syrian golden hamsters administered aflatoxin B_1 in large doses. *J. Natl. Cancer Inst.* 68: 271–277 (1982)
66. Longnecker, D.S., Carcinogenesis in the pancreas. *Arch. Pathol. Lab. Med.* 107: 54–58 (1983)
67. Morino, K., Matsukura, N., Kawachi, T., Ogaki, H., Sugimira, T., and Hirono, A., Carcinogenicity test of quercetin and rutin in golden hamsters by oral administration. *Carcinogenesis* 3: 93–97 (1982)
68. Ketkar, M., Althoff, J., and Mohr, U., A chronic study of praziquantel in Syrian golden hamsters and Sprague Dawley rats. *Toxicology* 24: 345–350 (1982)
69. Dontenwill, W., Chevalier, H.J., and Harke, H.P., Investigations on the effects of chronic cigarette smoke inhalation in Syrian golden hamsters. *J. Natl. Cancer Inst.* 51: 1781–1832 (1973)
70. Bernfeld, P., Homburger, F., Soto, E., and Pai, K.J., Cigarette smoke inhalation studies in inbred Syrian golden hamsters. *J. Natl. Cancer Inst.* 63: 675–689 (1979)
71. Bernfeld, P., Homburger, F., and Soto, E., Subchronic cigarette smoke inhalation studies in inbred Syrian golden hamsters that develop laryngeal carcinoma upon chronic exposure. *J. Natl. Cancer Inst.* 71: 619–623 (1983)
72. Homburger, F., Soto, E., Althoff, J., and Heitz, P., Animal model of human disease, carcinoma of the larynx in hamsters exposed to cigarette smoke. *Am. J. Pathol.* 95: 845–848 (1979)
73. Kaufman, D.G., Genta, V.M., and Harris, C.C., in: *Experimental Lung Cancer, Carcinogenesis and Bioassays* (E. Karbe and J.F. Park, eds.), pp 564–574, Springer Verlag, Berlin (1974)
74. Mass, M.J., Species differences in the activation of carcinogen in respiratory epithelium. A possible explanation for the unequal susceptibility of tracheal epithelium of rats and hamsters to carcinogenesis by benzo(a)pyrene (*Diss. abs. Int. B.*), 42: 547–B (1981)
75. Linnoila, R.I., Effects of diethylnitrosamine on lung neuroendocrine cells. *Exp. Lung Res.* 3: 225–236 (1982)
76. Tryka, A.F., Godleski, J.J., Skornik, W.A., and Brain, J.D., Progressive pulmonary fibrosis in hamsters (abs), 2034 *Fed. Proc.* 41: (March, 1982)
77. Sellakumar, A.R., Laskin, S., Kuschner, M., Rusch, G., Katz, G.V., Snyder, G.A., and Albert, R.E., Inhalation carcinogenesis by dimethylcarbamoyl chloride in Syrian hamsters. *J. Environ. Pathol. Toxicol.* 4: 107–115 (1980)

78. Pour, P., and Wallcave, L., The carcinogenicity of N-nitrosodiethanolamine, an environmental pollutant, in Syrian hamsters. *Cancer Lett.* 14: 23–27 (1981)

79. Hoffmann, D., Rivenson, A., Adams, J.D., Juchatz, A., Vinchkoski, N., and Hecht, S.S., Effects of route of administration and dose on the carcinogenicity of N-nitrosodiethanolamine in the Syrian golden hamster. *Cancer Res.* 43: 2521–2524 (1983)

80. Ketkar, M.B., Holste, J., Preussmann, R., and Althoff, J., Carcinogenic effect of nitrosomorpholine administration in the drinking water to Syrian golden hamsters. *Cancer Lett.* 17: 333–338 (1983)

81. Hoffmann, D., Castonguay, A., and Hecht, S.S., Comparative carcinogenicity and metabolism of 4-(methylnitrosamino)-1-(3-pyridyl)-1-butanone and N'-nitrosonornicotine in Syrian golden hamsters. *Cancer Res.* 41: 2386–2396 (1981)

82. Ketkar, M.B., Schneider, P., Preussmann, R., Plass, C., and Mohr, U., Carcinogenic effect of low doses of nitrosopyrrolidine administered in drinking water to Syrian golden hamsters. *J. Cancer Res. Clin. Oncol.* 104: 75–79 (1982)

83. Ketkar, M.B., Althoff, J., and Lijinsky, W., The carcinogenic effect of nitrosomethyldodecylamine in the European hamster. *Cancer Lett.* 13: 165–168 (1981)

84. McCoy, G.D., Hecht, S.S., Chen, C.B., Katayama, S., Rivenson, A., Hoffmann, D., and Wynder, E.D., Influence of chronic ethanol consumption on the metabolism and carcinogenicity of N-nitrosopyrrolidine and N-nitrosomethyldodecylamine in the European hamster. *Cancer Lett.* 13: 165–168 (1981)

85. Dalbey, W., and Nettesheim, P., Influence of nitrogen dioxide and formaldehyde on incidence of diethylnitrosamine-induced tumors in hamster respiratory tract (abs). *Toxicologist* 1: 138 (1981)

86. Lee, K.P., Barraras, C.E., Griffith, F.D., Waritz, R.S., and Lapin, C.A., Comparative pulmonary responses to inhaled organic fibres, asbestos and fibreglass. *Environ. Res.* 24: 167–191 (1981)

87. Niemeier, R.W., Stettler, L.E., Mulligan, L.T., and Rowland, J., Cocarcinogenicity of foundry particulates (abs), Sec. Ann. NCI/EPA/NIOSH Collaborative Workshop: Progress on Joint Environmental and Occupational Cancer Studies, Sept. 9–11, Rockville, MD, 1981 (33 pp)

88. Pyley, L.N., Pretumorous lesions and lung and pleural tumors induced by asbestos in rats, Syrian golden hamsters and Macaca Mulatta (rhesus) monkeys. *IARC Sci. Pub.* 1: 343–355 (1980)

89. Wehner, A.P., Dagle, G.E., and Millman, E.M., Chronic inhalation exposure of hamsters to nickel-enriched fly ash. *Environ. Res.* 26: 195–216 (1981)

90. Pott, F., Huth, F., and Spurny, K., Tumor induction after intraperitoneal injection of fibrous dusts. *IARC Sci. Pub.* 1: 337–342 (1980)

91. Gross, P., Kociba, R.J., Sparschu, G.L., and Norris, J.M., The biologic response to titanium phosphate. *Arch. Pathol. Lab. Med.* 101: 550–554 (1977)

92. Smith, W.E., and Hubert, D.D., in: *Experimental Lung Cancer Carcinogenesis and Bioassay* (E. Karbe and J.F. Parks, eds.), pp 93–101, Springer Verlag, Berlin (1974)

93. Smith, W.E., Hubert, D.D., and Sobel, H.J., Dimensions of fibers in relation to biological activity. *IARC Sci. Pub.* 1: 357–360 (1980)

94. Smith, D.M., Thomas, R.G., and Anderson, E.C., Respiratory tract carcinogenesis induced by radionucleides in the Syrian hamster. Proc. 19th Ann. Hanford Life Sciences Symposium, Richland, VA, Oct. 22, 1979. National Technical Information Service, Springfield, VA. LA-UR-79-3281, Conf. 791002-2. 1980. Also LA-UR-79-3378, Conf. 800304 (1980)

95. Smith, W.E., Hubert, D.H., Sobel, H.J., Teters, E.T., and Doerfler, T.E., Health of experimental animals drinking water with and without amosite asbestos and other mineral particles. *J. Environ. Pathol. Toxicol.* 3: 277-300 (1980)

96. Smith, W.E., Miller, L., and Churg, J., in: *Morphology of Experimental Respiratory Carcinogenesis. AEC Symposium Series 21* (P. Nettesheim, M.G. Hanna, and J.W. Deatherage, Jr., eds.), pp 299-316 USAEC Div. of Technical Information Extension, Oak Ridge, TN (1970)

97. Little, J.B., and Gossman, B.N., in: *Morphology of Experimental Respiratory Carcinogenesis* (P. Nettesheim, M.G. Hanna, and J.W. Deatherage, Jr., eds.), AEC Symposium Series Vol. 21, pp 383-394, (1970)

98. Little, J.B., Influence of noncarcinogenic secondary factors on radiation carcinogenesis. *Radiation Res.* 87: 240-250 (1981)

99. Cross, F.T., Palmer, F., Busch, R.H., Filipy, R.E., and Stuart, B.O., Development of lesions in Syrian golden hamsters following exposure to radon daughters and uranium ore dust. *Health Physics* 42: 135-153 (1981)

100. Stinson, F.S., and Lilga, J.C., Morphogenesis of neoplasms induced in the hamster trachea with N-methyl-N-nitrosourea. *Cancer Res.* 40: 609-613 (1980)

101. Grubbs, C.J., Becci, P.J., Thompson, H.J., and Moon, R.G., Carcinogenicity of N-methyl-N-nitrosourea when applied to a localized area of the hamster trachea. *J. Natl. Cancer Inst.* 66: 961-965 (1981)

102. Vasquez-Lopez, E., The reaction of the pituitary gland and related hypothalamic centre in the hamster to prolonged treatment with estrogen. *J. Pathol. Bact.* 56: 1-13 (1944)

103. Kirkman, H., and Bacon, R.L., Estrogen-induced tumors of the kidney, I. Incidence of renal tumors in intact and gonadectomized male golden hamsters treated with diethylstilbestrol. *J. Natl. Cancer Inst.* 13: 745-755 (1952)

104. Burrows, H., in: *Subcutaneous sarcomata, in Oestrogens and Neoplasia* (H. Burrows, and E.S. Horning, eds.), p 74, Charles C. Thomas, Springfield (1952)

105. Homburger, F., in: *Oncogenesis and Natural Immunity in Syrian Hamsters* (J.J. Trentin, ed.), Vol. 23, pp 100-179, *Prog. Exp. Tumor Res.*, S. Karger Publishers, Basel/New York (1979)

106. Liehr, J.G., Bellatore, A.M., McLachan, J.A., and Sirbasku, D.A., Mechanism of diethylstilbestrol carcinogenicity as studied with the fluorinated analogue E-3',3",5',5"-tetrafluorodiethylstilbestrol. *Cancer Res.* 43: 2678-2682 (1983)

107. Pour, P., Mohr, U., Cardesa, A., Althoff, J., and Kruger, F.W., Pancreatic neoplasms in an animal model: Morphological, biological and comparative studies. *Cancer* 36: 379-389 (1975)

108. Arai, H., Miyata, Y., Shibata, M., Kinoshita, H., Hosoda, M., and Takahashi, K., Preneoplastic changes in the pancreatic duct epithelium in the pancreas carcinogenesis in hamsters induced by N-nitroso-bis(2-oxopropyl)amine, (abs) *Proc. Mtg. Amer. Assoc. Cancer Res.* (1978)

109. Pour, P.M., and Raha, C.R., Pancreatic carcinogenic effect of nitrosobis(2-oxobutyl)amine and N-nitroso(2-oxobutyl) (2-oxopropyl)amine in Syrian hamsters. *Cancer Lett.* 12: 223–229 (1981)

110. Pour, P.M., Runge, R.G., Birt, D., Gingell, R., Lawson, T., and Nagel, D., Current knowledge of pancreatic carcinogenesis in the hamster and its relevance to human disease. *Cancer* 47 (Suppl.): 1573–1587 (1981)

111. Ruckert, K., Carcinogenesis in the pancreas. *Fortschr. Medizin* 99: 917–918 (1981)

112. Bain, G.O., Allen, P.B.R., Silberman, O., and Kowalewski, K., Induction in hamsters of biliary carcinoma by intracholecystic methylcholanthrene pellet. *Cancer Res.* 19: 93–96 (1959)

113. Bain, G.O., and Kowalewski, K., The anatomical pathology of experimental gallbladder carcinoma in hamsters. *Canad. J. Surg.* 4: 338–355 (1961)

114. Bain, G.O., Siegenberg, J., and Kowalewski, K., Further studies on methylcholanthrene-induced tumors of the gallbladder and liver in the golden hamster. *Canad. J. Surg.* 6: 367–371 (1963)

115. Akira, S., Studies on the histogenesis and mode of development of the gallbladder carcinoma induced in hamsters by insertion of methylcholanthrene-beeswax pellets, (abs) World Congress, Stockholm, Sweden, Swedish Soc. of Med. Sci. (1982)

116. Suzuki, A., Watanabe, M., and Takahashi, T., Induction of carcinoma of the gallbladder in hamsters by insertion of methylcholanthrene beeswax pellets. *Jap. J. Surg.* 12: 227–228 (1982)

117. Onizuka, T., and Nakazawa, S., Effect of gallstones on experimental induction of gallbladder cancer in Syrian golden hamsters (abs), The World Congress in Stockholm, Sweden, June 14–19, 1982. The Swedish Society of Medical Sciences (558 pp) (1982)

118. Bernfeld, P., and Homburger, F., in: *Skin Painting Techniques and In Vivo Carcinogenesis Bioassay* (F. Homburger, ed.), Vol. 26, pp 128–153, *Prog. Exp. Tumor Res.*, S. Karger Publishers, Basel/New York (1983)

119. Homburger, F. (ed.), *Skin Painting Techniques and In Vivo Carcinogenesis Bioassays.*, Vol. 26, *Prog. Exp. Tumor Res.*, S. Karger Publishers, Basel/New York (1983)

120. Sisskin, E.E., and Barrett, J.C., Hyperplasia of Syrian hamster epidermis induced by single but not multiple treatment with 12-o-tetradecanoylphorbol-13-acetate. *Cancer Res.* 41: 346–350 (1981)

121. Solt, L., and Solt, D., Rapid induction of gamma-glutamyl transpeptidase (GGT) rich foci in neonatal hamster buccal pouch epithelium exposed to N-methyl-N-benzyl-nitrosamine (abs), Hamster Soc. Ann. Meetg. (1983)

122. Hottendorf, G.H., and Pachter, I.J., An analysis of the carcinogenesis testing experience of the National Cancer Institute. *Toxicol. Pathol.* 10: 22–26 (1982)

123. Schach von Wittenau, M., and Estes, P.C., The redundancy of mouse carcinogenicity bioassays. *Fund. Appl. Toxicol.* 3: 631–639 (1983)

16

Quality Assurance in Pathology for Rodent Carcinogenicity Studies

Gary A. Boorman
Charles A. Montgomery, Jr.
Scot L. Eustis
Marilyn J. Wolfe
Ernest E. McConnell

National Institute of Environmental Health Sciences
National Institutes of Health
Research Triangle Park, North Carolina

Jerry F. Hardisty

Experimental Pathology Laboratories, Incorporated
Research Triangle Park, North Carolina

INTRODUCTION

The scientific quality of carcinogenicity studies has significantly improved in the past few years. This is due partly to standardization through genetic definition of laboratory animals, improved animal husbandry, expanded experimental protocols, implementation of standard operating procedures and advanced techniques for defining compounds administered to test animals (*i.e.*, purity, stability, dosage, etc.). During this same period, there has been increased emphasis on the accuracy and consistency of the pathology data from these studies.

Improvement in the quality of pathology data has been facilitated by quality assurance programs implemented by the National Cancer Institute's (NCI) Carcinogenesis Testing Program[1] and by the use of uniform standards through Good Laboratory Practices (GLPs) mandated by the Food and Drug Administration (FDA). In July 1981, the NCI Carcinogenesis Testing Program was transferred to the National Toxicology Program (NTP). The NTP now conducts studies under GLPs and the quality assurance (QA) program for the pathology portion of the studies has been expanded to assure their scientific validity.

QUALITY ASSURANCE THROUGH QUALITY CONTROL AND QUALITY ASSESSMENT

Quality assurance (QA) encompasses the establishment and monitoring of high technical standards for the performance of research and testing. An effective quality assurance program requires that quality control procedures be followed by testing laboratories during the conduct of a study and that systematic quality assessment techniques be utilized by study sponsors to monitor and audit pathology data. Quality control procedures are steps which must be taken during data collection and diagnosis to maximize the opportunity that the pathology data are accurate and valid. Quality assessment techniques are used to verify that the quality control procedures were followed and that the pathology data are accurate.

The purpose of this chapter is to describe steps that can be taken by a testing laboratory for quality control in pathology and the current NTP procedures for quality assessment. These procedures were originally described by Ward *et al.*[1] and have been expanded by the National Toxicology Program to monitor and audit the pathology data for ongoing toxicity and carcinogenicity studies. Some of the NTP procedures may not be applicable to studies designed and conducted by others, but the scientific principles upon which these procedures are based are essential to assure the scientific validity of pathology data resulting from any toxicology or carcinogenicity study. The reader is referred to articles dealing in general with procedures needed for quality control and quality assurance.[1-8]

LABORATORY QUALITY CONTROL

The quality of a study depends on accurate pathology diagnoses as well as many other factors including experimental design, proper animal care, control or elimination of disease, accurate clinical observations, and accurate collection of in-life data. This chapter, however, will be restricted specifically to procedures required by pathology. As mentioned earlier, quality control for pathology is the procedure instituted by the laboratory to assure the accuracy and validity of the pathology data.

Professional Personnel

The quality of pathology data will only be as good as the personnel responsible for the production of the data. A veterinary or medical pathologist, experienced in rodent pathology, should be responsible for coordinating all pathology procedures, evaluations, and reporting. If a less experienced pathologist is assigned to the study, it is the responsibility of the head of the pathology department to monitor and review a portion of the work to assure consistent and accurate data. The study pathologist is responsible for the gross and microscopic evaluation of all animals in the study. This includes tabulation of data for individual animals and appropriate summary tables, and preparation of a pathology narrative that describes the lesions, discusses the results, and states a final conclusion. The study pathologist is responsible for the overall quality of the pathology data. Quality control procedures at critical phases during the study are essential. Critical phases include the necropsy examination, tissue trimming, histologic preparation of microscopic slides and histopathologic evaluation of the tissues.

Necropsy Examination

The necropsy examination of each test animal is crucial to the conduct of a nonclinical laboratory study. All possible efforts should be made to assure that the necropsy and data handling during this examination are performed properly. Specimens must be correctly identified by information located on the specimen container or accompanying the specimen in a manner to avoid error in the recording and storage of data. To prevent mislabeling during the necropsy and collection of tissues, animal tissue specimen containers and individual records used to record gross observations should be prelabeled and assembled prior to the necropsy. The necropsy records and the containers of fixative should be labeled with the study number, animal number, and date of necropsy.

The pathologist or technician performing the necropsy must be capable of reading the identifying ear notches, toe clips or any other numbering system used to verify that the animal submitted for necropsy is accurately identified. Occasionally, animals are identified incorrectly. Unless the mistaken identity is noticed at necropsy, mislabeling occurs on fixed tissue containers, paraffin blocks, slide labels, etc. This not only causes confusion and necessitates correction of data but also creates the potential for additional errors that could invalidate the study. When the necropsy technician verifies that the animal number is correct, the clinical history of that animal must be reviewed. Clinical observations must be verified at necropsy. If the clinically observed lesions cannot be verified, then it is necessary to investigate whether the clinical signs were incorrectly stated or may have been associated with a different animal. It is much easier to resolve these discrepancies at this time than during a subsequent data audit.

The necropsy examination must be performed in a systematic manner. Complete postmortem examinations are required on each animal unless otherwise specified in the study protocol. All external and internal organs and tissues should be examined. The location and nature of any lesions should be carefully documented. Lesions should be described concisely and accurately using nonmedical terms to specify the weight, size, number, shape, color, consistency, structural outline, and location of lesions. Accurate descriptive lesions will enable the pathologist to match the gross observations with microscopic changes further assuring that lesions are not overlooked. Quality control procedures must be instituted to assure that each tissue required by the protocol is taken and placed in fixative.

If organ weights are required by the study protocol, it is essential that specific trimming instructions are followed. These should be included in the study protocol and the laboratory's standard operating procedures. In studies conducted by the NTP, organ weights are taken from all animals surviving to the end of subchronic toxicity studies. Organs weighed are the liver, thymus, right kidney, heart, brain, lungs and right testicle. These organs are weighed to the nearest 10 mg except for testicle and thymus which are weighed to the nearest 1.0 mg. Specific trimming instructions for these organs are as follows:

(1) Liver—must be free of adjacent tissues and gallbladder must be opened in mice.

(2) Thymus—must be carefully dissected from adjacent tissues.

(3) Right kidney—must be dissected from perirenal fat and adrenal gland. If one kidney is grossly affected, both should be weighed.

(4) Heart—must be removed at base and be free of pericardial sac. Gently squeeze to remove blood from chambers. If blood has clotted, chambers must be opened and clots removed.

(5) Brain—head should be removed at atlantooccipital junction. Brain must be free of olfactory lobes for weighing.

(6) Lungs—one-half of the trachea is left attached to the lung so that after weighing the lungs can be perfused with fixative.

(7) Right testicle—epididymis must be removed prior to weighing.

After tissues and/or organs have been examined *in situ*, they are dissected from the carcass, re-examined, and fixed in 10% neutral buffered formalin. Special handling of the tissues is particularly important to provide maximum fixation without introducing artifacts. Tissues are fixed at a thickness not to exceed 0.5 cm except as follows:

(1) The trachea and lungs are infused by introducing 10% buffered formalin (approximately 1 ml to 2 ml for mice and 4 ml to 8 ml for rats) into the trachea until the lungs are completely filled to normal inspiratory volume. The ideal method is to infuse at 20 mm water pressure, then submerge the trachea and lungs for forty-eight hours in 10% buffered formalin.

(2) The calvaria must be removed for examination of the brain and pituitary. The brain is removed for fixation and the pituitary left *in situ* for fixation. The nasal bones are not removed. The head is retained for decalcification.

(3) Distended urinary bladders are fixed as is. Contracted, or empty bladders are partially distended with formalin. Urinary bladders are opened and examined after fixation.

(4) Liver lobes are sliced to insure fixation. The kidneys are bisected, and the cut surfaces examined before fixation. The left kidney is bisected lengthwise and the right kidney crosswise.

(5) For chronic toxicity and carcinogenicity studies the entire mucosal surfaces of the esophagus, stomach, small and large intestines, and rectum are opened as described below:

(a) Examine oral cavity.

(b) Remove mandible to allow visualization of the tongue and posterior pharynx.

(c) Take a routine section of esophagus with thyroid, trachea and esophagus in one section. Open remaining esophagus and examine.

(d) Split the pelvis and remove the entire gastrointestinal tract including the anus.

(e) Transect stomach at pylorus and inject stomach with formalin (mouse = 2ml; rat = 5 ml). Stomach is opened and examined at trimming.

(f) The entire intestinal tract is opened and examined. Areas with lesions are individually identified and pinned flat on paper or cardboard for fixation, labeled as to location, and recorded on necropsy record. Cross sections of duodenum, jejunum, ileum, cecum, colon, and rectum are taken to include a Peyer's patch when possible.

(6) Multiple representative portions of large or variable tissue masses including surrounding unaffected tissues must be fixed. Very small masses may be fixed intact.

(7) Several thoraco-lumbar vertebrae are fixed with the spinal cord *in situ.*

(8) A section of the heart is sliced from the base through the apex so that all four chambers are visualized.

(9) Oral cavity, pharynx and larynx are carefully examined grossly. If any abnormalities including tumors are noted the tissues are examined microscopically. The larynx is routinely examined microscopically for all inhalation studies.

The quality of the necropsy examination of each test animal may be the single most important technical aspect of a study. All of the efforts extended in animal care, toxicology, experimental design, and more importantly, the actual test results are contained in the tissues of the animal at the end of the study. It cannot be overemphasized that the outcome of the study hinges upon the pathologic findings in the test animal. If a protocol-required tissue or a gross lesion is not taken during the necropsy examination, in most instances it will be lost forever. Improper or incomplete necropsy examinations can seriously influence the outcome of a toxicity or carcinogenicity experiment.

Histology Procedures

The histology laboratory is responsible for the preparation of animal tissues for microscopic examination by a pathologist. These tissues are submitted to the histology laboratory in special tissue preservatives or fixatives. Conscientious care and handling of these animal tissues are absolutely essential to assure accurate individual animal tissue identification, accountability and high quality standards throughout the various histologic processing steps. Tissues must be processed according to instructions in the study protocol and standard operating procedures for the histology laboratory. Accurate records must be kept during the course of the tissue processing. All equipment must be functioning properly and according to established standards. The reagents and chemical mixtures must be properly identified, measured and mixed, and changed or rotated according to specification. It is important that tissue specimens be identified through the various steps during the histologic processing of tissue. Important quality control steps for the histology laboratory are verification that all required tissues and gross lesions are present, tissues are trimmed in a standard manner, all blocks and slides are identified and properly labeled and the quality of the section and stain is adequate. Recuts from wet tissue and/or block recuts should be made when necessary to assure these steps. The histology laboratory should assemble the slides and records of gross findings from each animal for the pathologist to evaluate.

Tissue Trimming

The histology technician responsible for tissue trimming must have the study protocol available, as well as the gross necropsy observations. All protocol-required tissues should be trimmed for embedding in a standard uniform manner. Specific instructions for tissue trimming should be included in the histology laboratory standard operating procedures. The National Toxicology Program has developed specific guidelines for studies it sponsors to improve tissue accountability and assist in comparison of studies conducted by different testing laboratories. These guidelines are applicable to most toxicity and carcinogenicity studies which require histopathologic evaluation. Specific methods for tissue trimming required by the NTP are as follows:

(1) Multiple portions of tumors or masses are trimmed if they are large or variable in appearance. Adjacent normal tissue is included, if possible, with the tumors.

(2) Parenchymal organs (*e.g.*, liver) should be free of adjacent tissues and trimmed to allow the largest surface area possible for examination. For liver and lung, one section of each nodule (tumor) is trimmed, up to five for each organ. Section the five largest tumors if more than five lesions. Include adjacent normal tissue along with the tumor. Prepare at least two sections of normal liver including sections through left and right lobes. In mice, one section of liver should include the adjacent common bile duct or gallbladder. Longitudinal sections of each preputial or clitoral gland are prepared from rats.

(3) Each kidney is trimmed to include the entire cortex and medulla.

(4) Three cross-sections of the brain include: (a) Frontal cortex and basal ganglia; (b) parietal cortex and thalamus; and (c) cerebellum and pons. Lesions observed after sectioning must be recorded.

(5) Entire coronal (perpendicular to a sagital plane and parallel to the long axis of the body) section of both right and left lungs including mainstem bronchi is trimmed.

(6) Hollow organs are trimmed and blocked to allow a cross-section slide from mucosa to serosa.

(7) Following fixation, the trachea is opened to the level of the hilus and grossly examined. Any tumors or abnormalities in the trachea are to be examined microscopically.

(8) Following fixation, the pituitary is carefully removed and trimmed to allow a transverse section.

(9) After decalcification of the head, three separate sections of the nasal cavity are taken at (a) the level of the incisor teeth, (b) midway between incisors and first molar, and (c) middle of second molar (olfactory region). The remainder of the nasal cavity and turbinates are carefully examined for gross lesions at this time. Gross lesions observed after sectioning must be recorded.

(10) Tissues are trimmed to a maximum thickness of 0.3 cm for processing. Small (<0.3 cm) endocrine organs, lymph nodes, and tissue masses may be submitted intact. One cross section is prepared from each thyroid, adrenal, ovary, testis and the pituitary. The left testis includes the epididymis.

All gross lesions must be trimmed and cassettes used for each lesion should be identified. This is especially important for multiple lesions of the same organ. For example, record that the 1 cm mass of the left lobe of the lung is in cassette number seven while the 0.75 cm mass from the right diaphragmatic lobe of the lung is in cassette number eight. Only in this manner can the pathologist make an accurate correlation of the gross observations with microscopic lesions. The technician doing the trimming should note specificially any lesions described grossly that are not found (*i.e.*, irregular darkened area of left lateral lobe of liver not found at trimming). Also, any new lesions found at trimming must be described and recorded (*i.e.*, 1 mm white focus median surface right apical lung lobe in cassette number seven). This is crucial to assure that all lesions are available for evaluation and that no bias exists in tissue sampling between groups.

Tissue Embedding and Slide Preparation

The technician must review the trimming records to verify that all tissues and lesions are embedded into paraffin blocks. It is also important to make certain that the correct side of the tissue is embedded down so that small lesions or tissues (*i.e.*, parathyroid glands) are on the face of the block for sectioning.

During embedding, it is essential that a standard procedure be followed to increase efficiency and tissue accountability. Multiple embedding of tissues in paraffin blocks increases the efficiency of the histology technician as well as the pathologist during histopathologic examination of the slides. It is essential, however, when using multiple embedding techniques that the tissues be appropriately grouped. Tissues should be grouped according to size and consistency to enhance the quality of the sections. One possible grouping for tissues of the male mouse is:

Slide Number	Tissues
1	Brain Pituitary Adrenal Thyroid/parathyroid Trachea/esophagus
2	Heart Kidneys Liver with gallbladder Thymus Spleen
3	Lung and mainstem bronchi
4	Stomach Small intestine Pancreas Large intestine Urinary bladder Mesenteric lymph node
5	Testes/epididymis Prostate/seminal vesicle Salivary gland with mandibular lymph node Mammary gland with skin
6	Bone Bone marrow Spinal cord (if neurologic signs are present)
7	Nasal turbinates and nasal cavity
8	Tissue masses or gross lesions
9	Blood smear (if required)

During slide preparation, care must be taken to ensure that inaccuracies are not introduced into the study. Solvents used during slide preparation necessitate that slides be identified initially by pencil on the frosted end of the slide. After the slides are stained and coverslipped, permanent labels are placed over the penciled identification. During this procedure the permanent label must be compared with the block number and the penciled identification to make certain all labels are identical. When the slides from one animal are complete, these should be compared with the block identification for accuracy. The face of the block must be examined to assure that all embedded tissues are on the slide. Observations recorded during the necropsy and tissue trimming must be reviewed to make sure that all gross lesions are included.

Before the slides are presented to the pathologist, a final review by the histology laboratory should be done for slide quality. Slide quality review includes examination for legible correct identification, proper placement of labels and tissues (*i.e.*, label should not cover a portion of tissue), and cover glass placement. The slides should also be examined for the presence of excess mounting media, air bubbles, tissue floaters, chatter or knife marks, folds, holes in tissue, thickness of section and stain quality. This review must also ascertain that all gross lesions and required tissues are present. During this final slide review, some recuts may be necessary. This could happen due to poor slide quality, required tissues not included on a slide or a missing gross lesion. This may require resectioning of the paraffin block and preparation of additional slides or examination of the wet tissue to obtain missing tissues or gross lesions. Any additional steps taken must be carefully documented. Care must be taken so that multiple recuts or additional tissue samplings do not create a sampling bias between experimental groups.

Histopathologic Evaluation

Histopathologic evaluation of the microscopic slides is a crucial step. During the evaluation, the pathologist should maintain a list of diagnoses used for each organ to make certain that nomenclature is consistent and uniform throughout the study. Care must be taken to address all gross lesions. When no corresponding microscopic lesion is found, it should be stated specifically (*i.e.*, a microscopic lesion to account for the mottled liver noted grossly was not present). If the lack of corresponding microscopic lesion indicates that a gross lesion was not trimmed or sectioned properly (*i.e.*, a mass or nodule noted grossly in an organ), then the pathologist must request additional sections of the paraffin block or re-examination of the wet tissue. During the microscopic examination of the slides, the pathologist must make a diagnosis for all required tissues and gross lesions. If a gross lesion (*i.e.*, amputated tail or overgrown incisor tooth) is recorded by the necropsy technician and it is decided not to prepare a microscopic section, then the pathologist should document this during the microscopic portion of the evaluation. All tissues must be evaluated and diagnosed as normal or a specific lesion diagnosis is made so that accurate tissue counts will be available for evaluation of the data. The pathologist should determine and record whether the tissues are sampled uniformly (*i.e.*, for rodent stomachs that both glandular and nonglandular portions are included), whether required tissues are present and whether the histologic quality of slides meets current standards. With increasing emphasis on GLPs, scientific validity, and study quality, the role and responsibilities of the pathologist have expanded beyond the routine evaluation of the tissues. This is appropriate since the pathologist is in the best position to assure that all the pathology data meet the study protocol requirements. Following evaluation of the tabulated data, the pathologist must assure that the data accurately reflect the study findings and must prepare an interpretive pathology narrative that describes the lesions, summarizes the data, and makes a conclusion on the study results.

SPONSOR QUALITY ASSESSMENT

A major responsibility of a study sponsor is the verification that the results of the toxicology or carcinogenicity test are supported by the raw data and that the conduct of the study is in compliance with the study protocol, laboratory Standard Operating Procedures and Good Laboratory Practices regulations. This should be accomplished by periodic monitoring during the study and quality assessment of the raw data and report upon completion. For studies sponsored at several testing laboratories by the National Toxicology Program, a multistage quality assessment program has been developed to monitor and audit studies to determine if the quality of the pathology data is in conformance with GLPs and meets NTP standards. A multistage quality assessment program allows early detection and resolution of potential problems. The review conducted by the NTP proceeds in several stages of increasing detail. Problems or findings found during each stage are resolved before the study review proceeds to the next stage. First, in a preliminary review, the quality of the pathology data is evaluated while the slides and tissues are still in the testing laboratory. Second, an assessment of the quality of the pathology materials (*i.e.*, fixed tissues, paraffin blocks, microscopic slides) is conducted. Third, a quality assessment of morphologic diagnoses is conducted by an independent pathologist who prepares a quality assessment report documenting all discrepancies. This report and slides are reviewed by a panel of pathologists (the NTP Pathology Working Group) experienced in toxicologic pathology to examine discrepancies which exist. The discrepancies are resolved by the study pathologist prior to the production of a final pathology narrative and tables. Each of these stages is described in more detail below.

PRELIMINARY REVIEW OF PATHOLOGY DATA

During the preliminary data review the individual animal records and tabulated histopathologic diagnoses are examined for errors, inconsistencies, and deviations from established NTP standards and guidelines. The individual animal records are reviewed to assure that the data have been entered correctly to eliminate entry of erroneous data into the computerized system used to tabulate the data.[9] The records are reviewed to verify that animal number, dose group, date and age of death, and disposition and condition codes are correct. The gross observations are reviewed and matched with histologic diagnoses or descriptions to confirm that each group lesion has been considered. The morphologic diagnoses are reviewed to determine that only nomenclature acceptable to the computer software has been used and that each tissue with a microscopic lesion is recorded as examined microscopically. If satisfactory, then the data are tabulated by the computerized system for preparation of individual animal incidence tables and summary tables. If not, the individual animal records are returned to the laboratory for editing.

The tabulated data are examined by the study pathologist who makes necessary changes or corrections and prepares a draft pathology narrative which describes the lesions, summarizes the data and makes conclusions on the study results. The corrected tables and narrative summary are evaluated by the NTP prior to a review of the morphologic diagnoses from an examination of the slides. Our past experience has indicated that the quality of some aspects of the pathology data can often be ascertained by simply examining the pathology tables. If this is done while the slides and tissues are still at the laboratory, the study pathologist can more easily and quickly address questions raised during this review. The tables are examined for inconsistent nomenclature used for diagnosis. These may involve inconsistencies in either topographic or morphologic nomenclature. An example of a possible inconsistency in topography would be to have some diagnoses of *Thyroid—Follicular Cell Hyperplasia* and *Thyroid Follicle—Hyperplasia*. The study pathologist must verify that these should both appear under one topography. An example of possible morphologic inconsistencies would be *Thyroid—Adenoma; C-Cell Adenoma;* and *Follicular Cell Adenoma.* The study pathologist should review the cases where adenoma was diagnosed to properly classify the cell of origin. During this preliminary review, the pathology tables are examined for tumor incidence rates in controls that are unusually low or high when compared with historical rates and all negative and positive trends that may be treatment related. The pathologist's narrative that accompanies these tables is studied to be sure that treatment-related trends and variations in control incidence rates are discussed. Deficiencies found during the preliminary review of the data are returned to the study pathologist for resolution of the problems before an evaluation of the diagnoses is conducted from an examination of the slides.

REVIEW OF PATHOLOGY MATERIALS

The purpose of an audit of the pathology materials is to confirm the authenticity of the data given in the NTP technical report. The pathology materials (*i.e.*, individual animal records, fixed tissue, paraffin blocks, microscopic slides) are inventoried upon receipt. The slides are examined macroscopically for the quality of the histotechnique. This includes a macroscopic examination of each slide to evaluate for labeling, tissue and coverglass placement, air bubbles, and cracked coverslips or broken slides. During this evaluation, the slide identification penciled on the frosted end of the slide is compared with the printed slide label. Labels are also checked that changes are initialed and dated to meet GLP standards. A microscopic evaluation of the quality of the histotechnique is conducted by a histology technician on selected slides for such aspects as section thickness, knife marks, processing artifacts, holes, stain intensity, etc. that affect slide quality. The paraffin blocks are arranged next to the slides for each animal to confirm that slide labels match block labels, number and distribution of tissues in a particular slide match the block and that all blocks have been sectioned with corresponding sections on microscopic slides. Blocks are also examined for proper resealing to assure good preservation of tissues during storage. This slide to block match-up is done for all slides and blocks in the controls and high dose animals. If any discrepancies are found, a slide to block match-up is done for all animals in other dose groups.

After inventory of the bags containing fixed tissue, 10% of the bags selected at random from each dose group are examined to assure that the label is appropriate to confirm the animal's identity from tissues (*i.e.*, ears punched, notched or tagged or toes clipped) and to correlate the bag label identification with the individual animal identification. Wet tissues from these randomly chosen animals are reviewed by a pathologist for lesions that may not have been trimmed. Additional bags are opened when the clinical history suggests a possible mix-up in animals and in all cases where a gross lesion noted at necropsy was not described microscopically to assure that gross lesions have been trimmed for evaluation. In studies where gross lesions are found that were not trimmed or tissue identity suggests possible animal mix-ups, additional bags are opened and examined until the extent of the problem is determined. For example, the animal room records show that animal number 37 was noted as dead on May 15 and two weeks later animal number 37 was noted as moribund and submitted to necropsy with a note entered later that the May 15 death was actually animal number 39 but misidentified at that time. In this example, both bags of fixed tissue would be opened to confirm that the animal numbers are correct and both individual animal records would be checked for date of death.

PATHOLOGY DIAGNOSTIC QUALITY ASSESSMENT

The Toxicity and Carcinogenesis Testing Program managed by the NTP involves many pathologists of diverse backgrounds from several laboratories throughout the country. A quality assessment program has been established to review the accuracy of the study pathologist's diagnoses. This quality assessment program utilizes a unit of independent pathologists, with extensive experience with lesions in the strains of rodents used, to assess the histopathologic diagnoses. Disagreements in diagnosis and other inconsistencies in the data are examined by a panel of toxicologic pathologists who make recommendations for resolutions.

A quality assessment pathologist examines microscopically all tissues determined to be target organs during the preliminary data review, all neoplasms diagnosed in the study, and all tissues from 10% of the animals selected randomly from each experimental group. This microscopic review may also include all tissues with tumor incidences which are unusually low or high in the control groups. During this review, the quality assessment pathologist's diagnoses are compared with the study pathologist's diagnoses and all disagreements are noted. At the same time, a technician prepares an inventory of the tissues on the slides for each animal. The quality assessment unit prepares a report of all discrepancies in tissue counts and diagnoses and an accompanying set of slides containing all target tissues and slides with noted discrepancies to be reviewed by the NTP Pathology Working Group.

The NTP Pathology Working Group (PWG) consists of a chairperson and a group of pathologists who have knowledge of rodent pathology and are experienced in the lesions in question. The chairperson reviews the report and set of slides prepared by the quality assessment unit. Representative slides of the treatment-related lesions in target tissues and discrepancies noted in the quality assessment report are reviewed by the entire group. This review is done in a "blind" fashion in that the participants do not know the diagnoses of the study pathologist or the reviewing pathologist nor the treatment group. When there is a difference of opinion between the study pathologist and the PWG, the slide is returned to the study pathologist for reexamination. The PWG also evaluates slide quality, quality of the original pathology and quality of the quality assessment review.

After the study pathologist reviews the slides in question, a final pathology table is generated and a final pathology narrative is prepared by the study pathologist. At this point the pathology is considered complete, and the drafting of the NTP technical report proceeds. During this phase, the pathology is again subject to review by interested parties and peer review by the NTP Board of Scientific Counselors. Following this intensive pathology process the *ad hoc* peer review panel can examine the technical report with confidence that all lesions have been accounted for, accurately and consistently sampled, recorded, tabulated, interpreted, and evaluated in the final report.

SUMMARY

We have focused on quality assurance in pathology utilizing extensive quality control procedures by the testing laboratory and quality assessment techniques conducted by the National Toxicology Program. Although not discussed, the National Toxicology Program also conducts extensive audits of all aspects of the study including toxicology, chemistry, health and safety and animal care. A summary of findings of the audits are included in the final technical report.

Toxicology studies are expensive and time consuming. Further, they are often pivotal pieces of evidence used in the decision-making process that concerns the use of and human exposure to many economically important compounds and mixtures. Therefore, it is important that laboratories entrusted to conduct these studies have adequate quality control procedures to assure the scientific validity of the pathology data. Agencies that utilize these data should have quality assessment procedures to verify that the laboratory pathology quality control process is adequate and to confirm the authenticity of the data used in the decision-making process.

REFERENCES

1.   Ward, J.M., Goodman, D.G., Griesemer, R.A., Hardisty, J.F., Schueler, R.L., Squire, R.A., and Strandberg, J.D., Quality assurance of pathology in rodent carcinogenesis tests. *J. Environ. Pathol. Toxicol.* 2: 371–378 (1978)
2.   Page, N.P., Chronic toxicity and carcinogenesis guidelines, *J. Environ. Pathol. Toxicol.* 1: 161–182 (1977)
3.   Guidelines for Carcinogen Bioassay in Small Rodents. NCI Carcinogenesis Technical Report Series No. 1, Bethesda, MD, National Cancer Institute (1976)
4.   Swenberg, J.A., in: *Scientific Considerations in Monitoring and Evaluating Toxicological Research* (E.J. Gralla, ed.), pp 79–88, Hemisphere Publishing Co., New York (1981)
5.   Griesemer, R.A., and Dunkel, V.C., Laboratory tests for chemical carcinogenesis. *J. Environ. Pathol. Toxicol.* 3: 565–571 (1980)
6.   Kulwich, B.A., Hardisty, J.F., Gilmore, C.E., and Ward, J.M., Correlation between gross observations of tumors and neoplasms diagnosed microscopically in carcinogenesis bioassays in rats. *J. Environ. Pathol. Toxicol.* 3: 281–287 (1980)
7.   Frith, C.H., Highman, B., and Konvicka, A.J., Advances in automation for experimental pathology. *Lab. Animal Sci.* 26: 171–185 (1976)
8.   Huff, J.E., and Moore, J.A., in: *Proceedings of the Symposium on Information Transfer in Toxicology*, pp 81–98, National Technical Information Service (NTIS), Pub. No. PB82-220922, 5285 Port Royal Road, Springfield, Virginia 22160 (1982)
9.   Linhart, M.S., Cooper, J.A., Martin, R.L., Page, N.P., and Peters, J.A., Carcinogenesis bioassay data system, *Comp. Biomed. Res.* 7: 230–248 (1974)

17

Statistical Evaluation of Long-Term Animal Bioassays for Carcinogenicity

Colin N. Park
Richard J. Kociba

Dow Chemical U.S.A.
Midland, Michigan

INTRODUCTION

This chapter will review statistical methods commonly used to evaluate oncogenicity data generated in long-term animal bioassays. The strengths, weaknesses, operating characteristics, and interpretation of the statistical methodologies will be discussed. A general conclusion is that results of statistical tests by themselves cannot be interpreted literally but must be evaluated and placed in context with the overall biological interpretation. Of course, this is true in all areas of toxicology, but it is especially important in the evaluation of oncogenicity data for reasons discussed in the chapter.

The overriding philosophy is that it is more important to supply practical, understandable methods to aid in the interpretation of biological data than to satisfy all the rigors of statistical decision theory. From a theoretical viewpoint, it would seem possible to incorporate a complete set of statistical criteria into a protocol and use these criteria to interpret objectively the results of a study. In practice, however, the confounding effects of a large number of non-independent hypothesis tests and the possible effects of differential early mortality preclude a strict statistical interpretation of the data. For this reason, simplicity and interpretability of methods are important.

In support of this philosophy, Haseman[1] recently stated that "It should be emphasized that no rigid statistical decision rule is currently being employed by the National Toxicology Program (NTP) in the evaluation of tumor incidence data."

A typical lifetime rodent bioassay involves histopathologic examination of up to fifty tissues and organs, resulting in incidence data being generated on more than one hundred tumor categories. If the expected tumor frequency in each of the 100 categories were biologically independent and a statistical procedure with a true alpha of 0.05 were used, then the overall alpha level for the experiment would be $1-(0.95)^{100} = 0.994$. Thus, there would be a 99.4% chance of seeing at least one statistical asterisk, and almost all oncogenicity studies would be positive on the basis of statistical testing. Fortunately, however, this is not the case. First, not all statistical tests operate as described above and also biological plausibility usually prevails in the interpretation of data.

The above scenario, while not quantitatively correct, does point out a conceptual problem, namely that the false positive (type I) error rate of a collection of tests is greater than that of each individual test. This lack of control over the type I error rate has led many toxicologists to either distrust statistical methods or not to endorse them as a useful interpretive tool. It is therefore important for the statistician to have a basic comprehension of toxicology in order to foster the most appropriate utilization of statistical methods in a practical situation. Similarly, toxicologists should understand the basic concepts of statistical methods to make better use of them as an interpretive tool.

It should also be the objective of statisticians to use methods that are most appropriate for the data being analyzed. The tests should be sensitive to the most likely treatment effects and the false positive error rates should be controlled or at least understood.

Various methods of analysis will be discussed in this chapter, but first there are some general principles which, if adhered to, will result in "better" statistics in the sense of more accurately reflecting the biological results. From a statistician's point of view, methods which have lower false positive and false negative error rates are better. From the toxicologist's viewpoint this means that the statistical methods don't "lie" as often and are more useful as an aid in the decision making process. Therefore, it is an objective to use methods, statistical and toxicological, which result in fewer false positive conclusions and are sensitive to treatment effects. The following general principles which relate either directly or indirectly to statistical methods can help achieve the above goal.

(1) It is inappropriate to analyze statistically redundant variables. Redundant variables are those which are highly correlated with other more appropriate or more definitive measures. The most relevant observational categories should be defined and only these should be statistically evaluated except in special cases. For example, body weight and weight gain both measure growth and are highly correlated.

Another example is based on the fact that histopathologic observations are more definitive than the preliminary gross observations made at the time of necropsy. Following this principle, both gross and histopathologic results may be tabulated, but the histopathologic interpretations are more appropriate for statistical evaluation. Still another example of a redundant variable is the secondary or metastatic lesions of certain disease processes, as typified by Fischer 344 rat leukemia. Only the organ or site of the primary lesion should be compared across treatment groups.

A corollary to this concept is that statistical analysis should only be conducted on appropriate aggregations of histogenetically similar tumors in order to achieve reasonable sensitivity and to minimize the number of statistical evaluations.

Decisions as to which lesions to combine can only be decided on a case by case basis with the full involvement of the pathologist who examined the tissues and rendered the diagnoses. Factors impacting this decision process include consideration of histogenetic tissue similarities or differences, diagnostic terminology used to categorize toxic, preneoplastic, benign and malignant lesions and historical knowledge regarding the biologic behavior of certain lesions. McConnell[2] has recently proposed draft guidelines to aid NTP toxicologists in addressing this critical issue.

(2) Variables which are highly confounded by certain factors such as spontaneous geriatric changes should not be statistically evaluated in many cases. Some of these variables may be uninterpretable because of variation introduced by uncontrolled factors. For example, clinical chemistry, hematology and urinalysis data collected in the first year of a lifetime rodent study help identify chronic toxicity and target organs, but these observations become almost uninterpretable in geriatric animals because of the effect of diseases of old age. The leukemia that occurs at a high spontaneous rate in aging Fischer 344 rats changes hematologic values to such an extent that statistical comparisons become uninterpretable. Similarly, liver weights in species with a high spontaneous incidence of liver tumors or leukemic infiltrates are often meaningless after 18 months of age.

It is also inappropriate to analyze tumor data based on aggregation of total number of tumor-bearing animals or total number of animals with benign or malignant tumors (combining of all tumor types). While this may be useful as a descriptive statistic, it should not be tested for significance because the result is not directly interpretable, regardless of whether the result is positive or negative. It should also be noted that the correct experimental unit for statistical purposes is the animal; thus, the number of tumor-bearing animals, not the number of tumors is generally recorded and analyzed.

The general principle is that for statistical tests to be useful, they must only be employed on variables for which the results can be logically interpreted.

(3) Potential target organ(s) identified in other subchronic and chronic studies should be considered during the statistical and biologic evaluation of data from oncogenicity studies. The large number of statistical comparisons necessary in lifetime oncogenicity studies make a strict statistical interpretation of the results difficult. As will be discussed later, the experiment-wise false positive error rate cannot be defined, resulting in the need for careful biological interpretation and some healthy skepticism of equivocal results. If, however, a target organ can be identified from sub-chronic studies or from metabolic and pharmacokinetic considerations, then tumor frequencies in these organs can be more rigorously used for hypothesis *testing* rather than hypothesis *generating*.

These general principles reflect biological judgements which should be made before the study is started. Use of these recommendations will result in more meaningful biological and statistical interpretations.

Many experimental designs employ three treatment groups and a control group with an approximately equal allocation of animals to all groups. This design will be used for discussion purposes and for quantitative examples. The general results and conclusions can be generalized to other designs, but specific quantitative results were generated from these assumptions.

The remainder of this chapter will compare the weaknesses, strengths and operating characteristics (false positive and false negative error rates) of statistical tests commonly used in oncogenicity bioassays. The error rates reported here have been calculated from unpublished simulation studies conducted in our laboratories. In each simulated trial a fixed tumor rate, for example 1%, was selected and a "tumor" or "no tumor" outcome was assigned to the eighty animals in each group through the use of computer generated random numbers. The resulting tumor incidence for the simulated experiment was then tabulated, statistically tested, and repeated thousands of times to determine the proportion of significant or non-significant outcomes. In this manner the effect of spontaneous tumor frequency on false positive (type I) error rates was evaluated and the ability of different statistical methods to detect underlying differences, was determined. "Good" statistical tests have type I error rates which approximate their nominal value (*e.g.*, 0.05) across a wide variety of conditions. From a statistical point of view one test is better than another if its false negative error rate is lower and its false positive error rate is correct (near its nominal level).

PAIRWISE TESTS

Historically, Fisher's Exact Probability test has been used to compare each treatment group to the concurrent control.[3] Fisher's test is an "exact" nonparametric method which is appropriate for low incidence data, but the test has rather unique operating characteristics.

Statistical procedures such as Student's t-test use a preselected type I error rate, alpha, which is defined as the probability that the experimental results will show a treatment-related effect when none exists. Alpha is constant across all applications of the t-test as long as the assumptions of the test are met. The assumptions are a normal distribution of outcomes, equal variances across treatment groups and independent observations on the individual animals. For Fisher's test applied to oncogenicity testing, even if alpha is fixed at a nominal value, for example 0.05, the true error rate varies considerably as a function of the spontaneous tumor rate. If no tumors are observed in a control group, then at least five tumors must be found in a treatment group before the difference is significant (alpha = 0.05, equal number of animals in each group). The likelihood of observing five rare tumors, for example liver angiosarcomas, in the absence of any treatment-related effect is very remote. Thus, Fisher's test (and other methods) have a false positive error rate which is very low for rare tumors and only approaches the nominal value for tumors which have a relatively high background rate. Table 1 shows the true type I error rate as a function of the background tumor incidence and number of animals per treatment group.

The table below shows the actual false positive error rates for a nominal alpha of 0.05. All probabilities shown in Table 1 should be at or near 0.05 if the test were operating at its theoretical type I error rate. In fact, it can be seen that the true type I error rate is far lower than 0.05, particularly for tumors with a low spontaneous incidence. What this means in practice is that for tumors with a low spontaneous incidence, false positives will rarely occur whereas for tumors with a spontaneous incidence rate above 10% there will be between two and five false positives for every 100 independent comparisons that are done.

Table 1: Type I Error Rates for Fisher's Exact Probability Test,
Nominal Alpha = 0.05*

| Spontaneous Tumor Rate (%) | . . . . .Type I Error Rates . . . . . | |
	50 Animals Per Group	80 Animals Per Group
1	0.00009	<0.001
2	0.0012	0.004
5	0.0112	0.022
10	0.0244	0.028

*The results for 50 animals are reproduced from Haseman[1] with the author's permission. The results for 80 animals were found by computer simulation, rather than exact calculation.

It will be shown later that the same problem exists for other statistical tests, but to a lesser degree. From a theoretical point of view it would appear that this problem seriously compromises Fisher's test for use in oncogenicity studies. In practice, however, the repetitive use of Fisher's test results in realistic statistical decisions even though it may not be the best approach. If a statistical test with a real alpha level of 0.05 were applied to 100 different tumor incidences, the resulting experiment-wise false positive error rate would approach 100%. However, this is not the case in practice, because Fisher's test, and other procedures to some extent, have a very low false positive rate for most tumor types as a result of the low spontaneous incidence. Thus, in only a small number of cases does alpha approach its nominal value. Salsburg[4], Fears et al.,[5] and Haseman[1] have discussed this issue in some detail, but the point is that this is a case of two wrongs making a right. The false positive multiple comparison problem is overcome by using a method which has a very low type I error rate for most comparisons, resulting in a reasonable experiment-wise false positive rate. Along with a low false positive rate, Fisher's test also has poor sensitivity for rare tumors. For instance, power calculations show that a 20-fold increase in a tumor with a background incidence of 0.3% has less than a 50% chance of being detected statistically by Fisher's test. It is important, therefore, that the incidence of rare tumors be evaluated carefully on a case-by-case basis. Considerations should include dose-response patterns, historical as well as concurrent control incidence, and biological plausibility including consistency across sex, strains and studies. These factors are always important in the evaluation of toxicity studies, but are especially important in the evaluation of low incidence tumors. The occurrence of two or three tumors in a particular dose group will not be significant by Fisher's test but may represent a real treatment effect or may represent chance variation, depending upon the historical background rate. These interpretations can be formalized into statistical tests against historical controls using, for instance, a Poisson frequency test, but many biological assumptions are necessary for such tests to be valid. In these instances, interpretation based upon biological judgements is likely to be more informative and appropriate.

TREND TESTS

Trend tests evaluate (linearly) increasing frequencies with increasing dose. They have the intuitive appeal that one test is made for all doses, rather than individual pairwise tests; from a statistical viewpoint they appear to have better operating characteristics. These types of tests have been used in the past, for example in National Cancer Institute (NCI) bioassay analyses, and will probably be used more extensively in the future. Peto *et al.*,[6] in an excellent review article on statistical procedures, strongly recommend the routine use of trend tests. The particular trend statistic advocated by Peto *et al.* is similar to that used in the Cochran-Armitage trend test.[7]

It is important that some of the characteristics of this test be understood before it is used routinely. A specific issue that must be addressed is the choice of dose units to be used in the test. Alternatives include actual dose units, log units with some arbitrary value for control, *e.g.*, 0, or an ordinal scale such 0, 1, 2 and 3. This decision must be made before the data are examined and must be made on biological grounds. The question to be addressed is, if a treatment-related effect exists, will it be linear with *actual* dose, or will it be linear with respect to log dose or some other choice? In most cases the dose levels used in oncogenicity studies are on a log scale, for example in multiple units such as 3, 10 and 30 implying that effects, if they exist, are expected to be proportional to log dose rather than dose itself. In this case any linear transformation of the log doses will give the same statistical results. For this reason 1, 2, and 3 is often used as a convenient scale that makes for easy calculations. The logarithm of zero is undefined so that the control dose must be arbitrarily located with respect to 1, 2, and 3; a logical and convenient choice is at zero. The simulation results presented in this chapter use dose spacings of 0, 1, 2 and 3 as well as 0, 3, 10 and 30. Other geometrical (logarithm) dose spacings give similar results to 0, 3, 10 and 30.

Table 2 shows the false positive error rates for Peto's test using different tumor rates, dose units and for different nominal alpha levels. If the test were operating at its correct type I error rate, each of the probabilities in the table would be approximately equal to the alpha level given above the actual probabilities.

The results indicate, however, that Peto's test has too low a false positive error rate for tumors with a low spontaneous background. For instance, if the true tumor rate is 0.001, then the estimated false positive error rate for a nominal alpha of 0.05 is actually 0.003 or 0.002 for actual doses or log doses (with zero for control), respectively. Thus, the test will "almost never" (two to three per thousand tests) result in a false positive. This same characteristic was noted in Table 1 for Fisher's test. As the spontaneous tumor rate in the treated and control groups increases, Peto's test quickly approaches its correct false positive rate, in contrast to Fisher's test. For instance, when the background incidence of tumors is 1%, Fisher's test has a false positive rate of less than 0.001 while the type I error rate for Peto's test is approximately 0.049 to 0.052 for a nominal alpha of 0.05. For all spontaneous tumor rates evaluated in our simulation studies, Peto's test was more accurate than Fisher's test with respect to its false positive rate.

Table 2: False Positive Error Rates for the Peto Trend Test

	. . . . Dose Units					
	0, 3, 10, 30				0, 1, 2, 3	
	. . . . Alpha (One Sided)					
	0.05	0.01	0.005	0.05	0.01	0.005
Spontaneous Tumor Rate	. . . . Error Rates					
0.001	0.003	0.002	<0.001	0.002	<0.001	<0.001
0.002	0.009	0.008	<0.001	0.007	<0.001	<0.001
0.005	0.027	0.018	0.003	0.023	0.004	0.001
0.01	0.048	0.023	0.007	0.045	0.005	0.002
0.02	0.066	0.020	0.010	0.050	0.006	0.004
0.05	0.057	0.012	0.007	0.049	0.009	0.005
0.10	0.054	0.013	0.007	0.052	0.010	0.005

Historically, the use of trend tests has not been recommended for low tumor frequencies because the chi-square statistic employed for significance testing is a large sample approximation[7,8] but the computer simulation results shown in Table 2 indicate that the problem is not nearly as bad as was originally anticipated.

Another interesting result demonstrated in Table 2 is that the trend test, when applied to actual doses, has a higher type I error rate than the nominal value would indicate over a certain range of background incidences. This is a result of the discreteness of outcomes leading to significance. For example, the results shown in Table 3 for control, low, middle and high doses, respectively, all show significant linear trends on actual doses but not log doses.

Table 3: Tumor Rates Significant at $\alpha = 0.05$ (One Sided Trend Test) Using Actual Doses but not Log Doses

	. . . . Dose Units			
	0	3	10	30
Set	. . . . Tumor Rates			
A	2/80	0/80	2/80	4/80
B	0/80	1/80	0/80	3/80
C	1/80	0/80	1/80	3/80
D	1/80	0/80	2/80	3/80

Tables 2 and 3 demonstrate a potential problem with the routine use of trend tests for oncogenicity testing. Because they operate near their nominal alpha level, the probability of at least one false positive result in a large number of tests will be very large. This is not a problem with Fisher's test because, for the lower spontaneous tumor rates that comprise most of the data, there is far less than a 5% chance of a false positive. Haseman[1] notes that "most tumor types have a low spontaneous frequency (<2%). For these tumors it is virtually impossible for a false positive result to occur."

It is important to note that this comment is true for Fisher's test but, as indicated in Table 2, is not nearly as much of a problem for the Peto trend test. Thus, the routine use of the *trend* test for all tumor incidence data at an alpha level of 0.05 will be counterproductive to the generation of interpretable statistics. Too many false positives will occur. On the positive side, however, trend tests achieve their nominal alpha level over a wider range of background frequencies as compared to Fisher's test.

Mantel[9] has credited Tukey with suggesting a Bonferroni type of correction for the multiple comparison problem encountered in toxicological testing. Tukey's suggestion is to use $alpha = \alpha/(n)^{1/2}$ where α is the nominal alpha level (0.05) and n is the number of dependent variables being tested. Strict adherence to the Bonferroni inequality for *independent* comparisons would suggest using $alpha = \alpha/n$, but in toxicity and oncogenicity testing the various outcomes (frequencies) are not independent; thus, $\alpha/(n)^{1/2}$ is suggested as a rule of thumb. Implementing this rule of thumb for oncogenicity testing with approximately 100 potential tumor sites would suggest using the trend test with an alpha of $0.05/(100)^{1/2}$, or 0.005.

The obvious drawback to the routine use of such a small alpha level is that the test would be expected to be less sensitive. Simulation results indicate, however, that the trend test is uniformly more powerful than Fisher's test, particularly for low incidence tumors. Table 4 shows some selected examples demonstrating this point.

Table 4: Power of Fisher's Test and Peto's Trend Test, Alpha = 0.05[*]

Control Tumor Rate	Top Dose Incidence Rate	Fisher's Test	Trend Test Doses = 0, 3, 10, 30	Trend Test Doses = 0, 1, 2, 3
0.001	0.03	0.08	0.65	0.64
0.001	0.05	0.35	0.89	0.88
0.005	0.03	0.06	0.49	0.45
0.005	0.05	0.28	0.78	0.71
0.01	0.05	0.22	0.64	0.55
0.01	0.10	0.75	0.96	0.92
0.02	0.08	0.40	0.73	0.62
0.02	0.12	0.75	0.95	0.89
0.05	0.10	0.23	0.44	0.36
0.05	0.15	0.59	0.83	0.73
0.10	0.20	0.47	0.69	0.57
0.10	0.25	0.76	0.92	0.83
0.20	0.35	0.63	0.81	0.69

*The results shown above depict the case of a middle dose and a low dose spontaneous incidence equal to control. The results are similar if the middle dose and the low dose follow a linear trend.

The entries shown in the table are the probability of detecting a real treatment-related effect for Fisher's test and the trend test, for different combinations of control and high dose tumor incidence rates. It can be seen that Fisher's test is far less sensitive than Peto's test, particularly when the control tumor incidence is 1% or less. Thus, Fisher's test has both a low type I error rate and poor sensitivity (high type II error rate) when applied to oncogenicity studies. The results are similar for different sample sizes and for different dose units.

Further simulation work indicates that a trend test with an alpha level of 0.005 (one-sided) is at least as sensitive in most cases as Fisher's test with a one-sided alpha of 0.05. This result holds for all cases tested in which the control tumor incidence was less than 2% (Table 5).

Table 5: Power of Fisher's Test at Alpha = 0.05 Compared to Peto's Trend Test at Alpha = 0.005 (One Sided)

. . . . . . Tumor Rate.		Probability of . . . . Detecting a Difference.		
Control, Low and Middle Dose	High Dose	Fisher's Test (Alpha = 0.05)	Trend Test (Alpha = 0.005) . Actual*	Log*
0.001	0.05	0.35	0.71	0.52
0.01	0.10	0.75	0.85	0.70
0.02	0.12	0.75	0.80	0.64
0.05	0.20	0.87	0.88	0.72
0.10	0.25	0.76	0.72	0.52

*Dose units

For control tumor frequencies greater than 2%, the Peto trend test, using actual doses and alpha = 0.005, was generally more sensitive than a Bonferroni corrected Fisher test at an alpha of 0.016 = (0.05/3). The exceptions were for background tumor incidences greater than about 15%. It would appear, therefore, that the trend test, even at a smaller alpha level, has several distinct advantages over Fisher's pairwise test. These advantages include:

(1) Having a more uniform false positive error rate, thereby not "weighting" common tumors more heavily.

(2) The use of a single test, rather than a comparison for each of the dose levels.

(3) The ability to formulate a more sensitive method, while controlling the overall type I error rate in a more reasonable fashion.

It must be emphasized that the trend test must be interpreted with some caution, however. For instance, a significant linear trend does *not* imply that the dose-response effect persists across all dose levels. For example 0, 0, 0 and 4 tumors is significant at alpha = 0.005, but certainly does not mean a linear dose-response exists over the entire dose range. The correct interpretation of a significant trend test is that some differences may exist at some dose level(s).

In conjunction with the linear trend test, a lack-of-fit statistic should be calculated to rule out "significant" effects caused by extremely nonlinear responses. For example, 10, 1, 6 and 12 tumors occurring in control, low, middle and high dose groups, respectively, results in a significant linear trend using actual doses, but a significant lack of fit is also found. When lack of fit is indicated, Fisher's test should be used, not the trend test.

It must be kept in mind that lack-of-fit tests are non-specific and tend to have low power. As an example, 4, 1, 2, and 9 tumors out of 80 animals for control, low, middle and high dose groups, respectively does not yield a significant lack of fit, but is significant by the linear trend test. Therefore, significant linear trends for data which appear to be non-linear must be interpreted carefully.

MORTALITY ADJUSTMENTS

Mortality differences among treatment groups can have a large impact on the number of observed tumors. Those groups with early mortality have fewer animals alive later in life when tumors are usually observed. Peto *et al.*[6] recommend the routine use of tumor rates adjusted for possible differences in mortality. However, they also assume that on an animal-by-animal basis, and on a tumor-by-tumor basis within each animal, the pathologist can make a correct judgment as to whether or not each tumor was a major contributor to cause of death.

If this judgment can be made with few classification errors, then Peto's method, or similar mortality adjustment methods, may be appropriate. If it is felt that these decisions cannot logically be made for certain tumor types, then crude tumor rates must be compared based on the knowledge that groups with earlier mortality will tend to show fewer tumors. The bias of the test is known if unadjusted tumor rates are used. With mortality adjustments, misclassification of cause of death may lead to a positive or negative bias unless the pathologist can determine the direction of classification errors.

The mortality problem is best demonstrated by hypothetical examples in which the underlying tumor rates are known and the number of observed spontaneous deaths is specified. The tumor rates and death rates shown in Table 6 will be used in two examples. For each example the tumor rates are the same in the control and treatment groups but there is excess non-tumor mortality in the treatment group.

Table 6: Hypothetical Tumor Rates and Observed Mortality in a Study[*]

	13-18 Months	19-24 Months	25 Months to Terminal
Tumor Rate (treatment and control)	0.10	0.20	0.30
Number of Deaths (control group)	10/100	20/90	70/70
Number of Deaths (treatment group)	20/100	40/80	40/40

*Tumor rates are defined as the probability of any animal developing a specific tumor in each time period. The number of deaths is the total number of animals dying from all causes at each time period.

Example 1. For this example it is assumed that tumors are rapidly fatal and death from the tumor occurs soon after initiation. The spontaneous deaths will therefore include deaths from tumor as well as non-tumor causes. The assumptions shown in Table 6 would result in the following expected number of tumors for each dose group and time period:

Group	13–18 Months	19–24 Months	25 Months Terminal Kill	Total
Control	10	18	21	49/100
Treated	10	16	12	38/100

Note that fewer tumors are detected in the treated group, even though the tumor rates are the same in each time period. This is a result of the decreased number of animals at risk in the treatment group. A logical way of adjusting for differential mortality from causes other than oncogenesis is to calculate the number of tumors observed divided by the number of animals at risk (*i.e.*, alive at the beginning of the time period). The resulting calculations are:

	13–18 Months	19–24 Months	Terminal Kill
Control	10/100 = 10%	18/90 = 20%	21/70 = 30%
Treated	10/100 = 10%	16/80 = 20%	12/40 = 30%

Thus, the data can be logically "corrected" to reflect the real underlying tumor rates. This is essentially what life table tests do.[10,11]

Example 2. As in the first example, the real tumor rates (probabilities) are the same in control and treated animals but more deaths are observed in the treated group. A further assumption is that the tumors never cause death. These tumors are referred to as incidental tumors.[6] Tumors independent of the cause of death would be detected only at necropsy, which may be a variable time after tumor initiation. Thus, although 10% of the animals may have a tumor at a particular time, these tumors would not be detected until the animals are necropsied subsequent to death from other causes. For this case the arithmetic is more complex since the tumor prevalence reflects the cumulative probabilities and the competing non-tumor-related deaths. The expected number of tumors observed are as follows:

Group	13–18 Months	19–24 Months	Terminal Kill	Total
Control	1	6	35	42/100
Treated	2	11	20	33/100

Here as before, fewer total tumors are detected in the treated group; however, adjusting for differential mortality as before yields the following results:

	13–18 Months	19–24 Months	Terminal Kill
Control	1/100 = 1%	6/90 = 7%	35/70 = 50%
Treated	2/100 = 2%	11/80 = 14%	20/40 = 50%

An artifactual increase in risk of the treated over the controls has been generated during the first two time periods due to incorrect mortality adjustment.

The correct way of adjusting the latter data is to divide by the number of animals necropsied, rather than the number alive.[6,12] Note, however, that this would not work in example 1. The correct method for example 2 is based completely on the hypothetical assumption that this type of tumor is nonlethal (independent of cause of death).

The point of these examples is that to adjust correctly for mortality the determination must be made, on a case-by-case basis, as to whether the tumor contributed to death (incidental *versus* nonincidental relative to death). This determination will be very difficult, but unless it can be made, any adjustment procedure can give misleading answers and should not be used unless the assumptions can be justified.

A point of misunderstanding is that it is not necessary to *determine* cause of death of each animal; it is only necessary to determine whether a given observed tumor contributed to the cause of death.

Another problem arising in mortality adjustments is that the methods commonly used assume either that the tumor causes death or is completely independent of mortality. From a practical point of view the assumption of complete independence means that the incidences of tumors in animals dying spontaneously and in those not dying spontaneously are statistically identical. The methods do not allow for animals which are susceptible *both* to tumorigenicity and early mortality, but through different mechanisms. In theory it is possible to test for this susceptibility phenomenon[13] by comparing the tumor incidence in spontaneous deaths near the end of a study to the incidence observed at terminal kill. Except for rare instances, however, the small number of tumors will not allow for a meaningful comparison.

Peto has recommended the routine use of mortality adjustment methods regardless of whether real mortality differences exist. In our simulation studies we compared the false positive error rate and sensitivity of the unadjusted statistical tests to the mortality adjusted tests. The mortality rates of the control group for four consecutive time periods were 5%, 10%, 20% and 100% (terminal) compared to 5%, 15%, 30% and 100% for the tested groups. The conclusion was that sensitivity and false positive error rates for unadjusted incidental tumor analyses were not appreciably affected by the above minor mortality differences.

For large mortality differences the sensitivity of statistical tests subsequent to adjustment procedures will be low because only tumors observed while there is some survival in both groups have any effect on the statistical comparison. Adjustments are, therefore, unnecessary for minor mortality differences and provide minimal improvement in statistical sensitivity for large differences.

In summary, mortality adjusted analyses make additional biological assumptions on the structure of the data which require judgment on relationships between individual tumors and cause of death, and these assumptions are not necessary for minor differential mortality effects. For these reasons a recommended approach would be to test first for differential mortality. If no mortality differences exist, then adjusted analyses are not necessary. If there are differences but they occur early in the study, for instance in the first year, then a simple adjustment is to use the number of animals alive before the first observed tumor. This keeps the subsequent analyses simple without sacrificing any precision or sensitivity.

DIFFERENTIAL MORTALITY TESTS

Life table methods[14] are useful as a descriptive tool for visually displaying cumulative mortality but should not generally be used for statistically comparing mortality across groups. Life table methods tend to compare whether mortality differences exist at a given point in time, rather than comparing overall differences in mortality patterns over the entire study. The solution of comparing mortality across treatment groups each month during a study leads to a large number of correlated or redundant statistical tests with the result that the interpretation of one or two asterisks in the collection of tests must be made on a judgemental basis. A better procedure is to use a single test comparing control to treatment(s). One such test is the Gehan-Wilcoxon test.[15] This is a modification of the original Wilcoxon Rank Sum Test which combines an analysis of median survival time for the animals dying spontaneously with a comparison of the percentage of animals reaching terminal sacrifice.

"TIME TO TUMOR" ANALYSES

The hypothesis being tested in these analyses is that tumors develop earlier in the treated animals. This hypothesis is very difficult to test in those cases where incidental tumors are not grossly visible upon clinical examination. Moreover, the confounding effect of spontaneous deaths make these data difficult, if not impossible, to interpret unless sufficient information can be obtained from scheduled sacrifices.

Mantel[9] has proposed an interesting argument against the biological plausibility of decreased latency without an accompanying increased frequency. Briefly, Mantel reasons that in the absence of competing causes of death, all animals would eventually develop tumors. The majority of these tumors are never observed because death interrupts the inevitable tumorigenic process. If this tumorigenic process is accelerated, tumors will be observed earlier *and* more tumors will be found because of the acceleration phenomenon. Therefore, decreased latency should be accompanied by increased frequency.

Another way to view the occurrence of decreased latency without an accompanying increase in frequency is that this implies a crossing of the hazard functions as time progresses. In other words, the treated group would be under *less* risk than the control group toward the end of the study, which does not seem plausible for a true oncogenic agent.

For these reasons, it is recommended that time-to-tumor analyses should not be done routinely and should be considered only when there are no differences in mortality rates between treatment groups or if the specific tumors are fatal. Lagakos and Mosteller[16] have written an interesting article describing a case study on Red Dye Number 40. They describe in some detail the statistical and biological problems in attempting to test for decreased latency. They express some doubt as to the validity of attempting such analyses.

In summary, it is stressed that the large number of statistical comparisons done in the analyses of oncogenicity studies necessitate a careful biological evaluation of the statistical results. The common statistical methods used in the comparison of unadjusted tumor incidence rates have very different false positive and false negative characteristics. Trend tests may be a more appropriate statistical method but their larger, albeit more correct, type I error rates indicate that a smaller alpha level should be used.

Mortality adjustment procedures, which require additional biological and statistical assumptions, are not necessary if only minor differential mortality patterns occur. Thus, they should only be used if statistically significant differences in mortality are observed and cannot be accounted for by simple patterns of mortality occurring before the first observed tumors.

REFERENCES

1. Haseman, J., A reexamination of false-positive rates for carcinogenesis studies. *Fund. Appl. Toxicol.* 3: 334–339 (1983)
2. McConnell, E.E., *Interpretation of Tumor Data.* NIEHS/NTP Position Paper (1982)
3. Gart, J.J., Chu, K.C., and Tarone, R.E., Statistical issues in the interpretation of chronic bioassay tests for carcinogenicity. *J. Natl. Cancer Inst.* 62: 957–974 (1979)
4. Salsburg, D., Use of statistics when examining lifetime studies in rodents to detect carcinogenicity. *J. Toxicol. Environ. Health* 3: 611–628 (1977)
5. Fears, T.R., Tarone, R.E. and Chu, K.C., False-positive and false-negative rates for carcinogenicity screens. *Cancer Res.* 37: 1941–1945 (1977)
6. Peto, R., Pike, M.C., Day, N.E., Gray, P.G., Lee, P.N., Parish, S., Peto, J., Richards, S., and Wahrendorf, J., *Guidelines for Simple, Sensitive Significance Tests for Carcinogenic Effects in Long-term Animal Experiments.* IARC Monographs, Supplement 2, IARC, Lyon (1980)
7. Armitage, P., *Statistical Methods in Medical Research*, New York: Blackwell Scientific Publications (1971)
8. Siegel, S., *Non-Parametric Statistics for the Behavioral Sciences*, New York: McGraw-Hill (1956)
9. Mantel, N., Assessing laboratory evidence for neoplastic activity. *Biometrics* 36: 381–399 (1980)
10. Cox, D.R., Regression models and life tables. *J. Royal Stat. Soc., Series B,* 34: 187–226 (1972)
11. Tarone, R.E., Tests for trend in life table analysis. *Biometrics* 62: 679–682 (1975)
12. Hoel, D.G., and Walburg, H.E., Jr., Statistical analysis of survival experiments. *J. Natl. Cancer Inst.* 49: 361–372 (1972)
13. Kodell, R.L., Farmer, J.H., Gaylor, D.W., and Cameron, A.M., Influence of cause-of-death assignment on time-to-tumor analyses in animal carcinogenesis studies. *J. Natl. Cancer Inst.* 69: 659–664 (1982)
14. Sachs, R., Life table technique in the analysis of response-time data from laboratory experiments on animals. *Toxicol. Appl. Pharmacol.* 1: 203–227 (1959)
15. Elandt-Johnson, R.C., and Johnson, N.L., *Survival Models and Data Analysis*, New York and London: Wiley-Interscience (1980)
16. Lagakos, S., and Mosteller, F., A case study of statistics in the regulatory process: The FD&C Red No. 40 experiments. *J. Natl. Cancer Inst.* 66: 197–212 (1981)

18

Considerations in the Evaluation and Interpretation of Long-Term Animal Bioassays for Carcinogenicity

Robert R. Maronpot

National Institute of Environmental Health Sciences
National Institutes of Health
Research Triangle Park, North Carolina

INTRODUCTION

There are no universally agreed upon ways of analyzing long-term rodent carcinogenicity studies, although several approaches have been offered.[1-4] Since the evaluative and interpretive processes involve a series of informed judgments[5] made by scientists from different disciplines, some differences of opinion regarding the importance and meaning of specific findings can be expected. What is critical, however, is that unwarranted conclusions based on inadequate study design or inconclusive results should not be made.

Two elements usually precede the formulation of valid study conclusions. One element is *evaluation* (appraisal or assessment) of the adequacy and limitations of the study. The second element is study *interpretation* (explanation or elucidation). These elements will be discussed in detail in this chapter. Occasionally, current practices of the National Toxicology Program (NTP) will be used to illustrate specific points. However, the opinions expressed in this chapter are those solely of the author and do not necessarily reflect NTP policy.

CONSIDERATIONS IN THE EVALUATION OF LONG-TERM RODENT STUDIES FOR CARCINOGENICITY

Study Audit

Few long-term studies are flawless. Discovery of weaknesses and discrepancies in the conduct of the study may raise doubts regarding the interpretation of the findings and the conclusions reached. Consequently, the scientist responsible for a long-term rodent bioassay would be well advised to conduct an audit of the in-life portions of the study prior to expending efforts to assure the quality of the pathology and interpretation of the study. Such an audit should include an examination of records to assess adherence to protocol, animal health and identification, dose preparation, accuracy of animal dosing, stability and purity of test substance, environmental conditions, identification of fixed tissues, correspondence of necropsy observations and histologic findings, and the numerous aspects of the study which fall under the general category of Good Laboratory Practices. Any deficiencies discovered should be clearly documented and ultimately should temper study conclusions.

Peer Review Process

The peer review process is an integral part of the evaluation of long-term rodent bioassays. It is necessitated because of the judgemental processes that accrue in cascading fashion during evaluation of the study. One of these considerations relates to evaluation of pathology. Another relates to assessment of the strength of the experimental evidence provided by the study. The peer review process provides for a balanced approach to the evaluation of the bioassay and minimizes the possibility of renegade or maverick interpretation.

Pathology review process. The pathology review process can be logically divided into two distinct efforts: A quality assessment review, and a panel review of microscopic diagnoses.[9] The NTP pathology review process is detailed in Chapter 16. The quality assessment review utilizes gross and microscopic pathology records and histologic slides to provide an in-depth review of necropsy findings, tumor diagnoses, target tissues, and all slides from a 10% random selection of animals. The quality of the histopathology is assessed during this exercise. Review of the quality of the tissue blocks, slide-block match up, and condition and identity of unused fixed tissues can occur simultaneously with the quality assessment review or they can be reviewed separately during study audit. In the quality assessment review, diagnostic discrepancies between the original pathologist and the quality assessment pathologist are identified for further review during the second phase of the pathology review process.

It is recommended that four to seven pathologists be formally convened for peer review of microscopic diagnoses. Diagnostic discrepancies resulting from the quality assessment review plus representative target tissue lesions can be reviewed by this panel without knowledge of animal treatment or previous diagnoses. The panel should reach a consensus on each diagnosis before being informed of the original pathologist's diagnosis. If there is no clear consensus or majority opinion, the original diagnosis generally should be accepted. If the panel is in fundamental disagreement with the original diagnosis, the slide should be sent back to the original pathologist for reconsideration. The above pathology review process has been in practice by the NTP since 1980 and has served to increase the accuracy of diagnoses and standardization of pathology nomenclature for the Program. The latter is considered a necessary procedure for any large program which obtains pathology input from a variety of laboratories, each having its own pathologists. It is strongly recommended that some form of peer review of pathology be incorporated into the evaluation of any long-term rodent bioassay.

Peer review of findings from long-term studies. The following description of a formal peer review process is currently used by the NTP and is suitable for a large program. This peer review process covers all aspects of study evaluation and interpretation. A modified version of this process may be beneficial for smaller organizations.

The technical report for a long-term rodent study is prepared by an NTP Chemical Manager with internal peer review by staff scientists. Each draft report is then reviewed by the Technical Reports Review Subcommittee of the NTP Board of Scientific Counselors. The Subcommittee is composed of disciplinary scientists from academia, industry, and private and public interest organizations. At a public meeting the Subcommittee makes recommendations regarding the NTP interpretation of the long-term study under review, and agrees or disagrees with the interpretations and conclusions put forth in the draft technical report. The technical report peer review process provides for a consensus view regarding interpretation of the long-term rodent study. This avoids organizational or individual bias in the interpretation of the study and provides for the integration of diverse viewpoints in the final conclusion on the study.

Considerations in the Conduct of Pathology

Gross examination. The gross examination is the single most important part of the pathology protocol. It provides the framework and orientation within which to select tissues for trimming and histology and thereby maximizes the probability of being able to microscopically examine small lesions that might otherwise be missed in a purely random sampling. A thorough gross examination provides ample justification for reducing the histology burden and supports current attempts by the NTP to modify histology requirements in long-term animal tests.[10] Since gross observations in small tissues, such as endocrine organs, are difficult to make, histologic examination is mandatory for these tissues. For other tissues such as skin or skeletal muscle, the probability of discovering a microscopic lesion of significance in the absence of a gross lesion is remote.

It is unfortunate that some pathologists have delegated the conduct of the gross examination to a staff of prosectors and tissue trimmers. A competent prosector can dismantle the body and document alterations within the confines of a prescribed lexicon. Tissue trimmers provide a consistent presentation of tissue orientation which carries over to the slides that the pathologist evaluates. Also, in the process of trimming, additional lesions not seen at gross examination can be documented. These prosecting and trimming functions are clearly important. With rare exceptions, if the pathologist is not physically present in the necropsy room to supervise this phase then some fundamental observations may be lost that cannot be recaptured by the most diligent interpretation of histologic material. It is strongly recommended that an adequate amount of time be allowed for a thorough necropsy and that a pathologist observe and describe all gross lesions.

Current plans of the NTP call for a deliberate attempt to "trace gross lesions". Accordingly, a statement is required during histologic evaluation to provide correlation with each gross observation. This process will serve to focus more attention on the gross observations and will improve the quality of pathology.

Histologic evaluation. Slide evaluation should be made by a pathologist experienced with rodent tissues and lesions. The evaluation should be accomplished in an efficient manner that minimizes the likelihood of introducing bias. Knowledge of the clinical history and gross lesions, including organ weights, facilitates efficient evaluation of slides. Knowing whether the animal was from a high dose group or a control group permits the pathologist the option of carefully searching for subtle changes at high microscope magnification in the animals most likely to have such changes. Once identified, similar changes can be searched for in other treatment groups as well as in control animals.

Aside from subtle microscopic changes which might be documented when the pathologist is cognizant of the animal's treatment status, there are a number of subjective or arbitrary lesions which may be documented during the course of histologic evaluation. Examples of such lesions include altered bone marrow cellularity, splenic hemosiderosis, splenic extramedullary hematopoiesis, minimal nephropathy, etc. Initial tabulations of pathology might indicate a treatment-associated change in one or more of these lesions. When this happens the pathologist should recognize the possibility of bias and re-examine the relevant tissues in a random, coded fashion. While this necessitates updating previous diagnoses, the final pathology product is worth the effort and will avoid misleading results.

INTERPRETATION OF THE STUDY

Route of Administration of the Test Substance

In carcinogenicity testing it is generally assumed that the most relevant route of administration of the test substance is the route of known or anticipated human exposure. However, considerations such as solubility and stability of the test substance, ease of administration, and accuracy of dosing may mitigate against using the route of choice based on human exposure. Chemical disposition and metabolism data may identify scientifically acceptable alternative routes which are experimentally more convenient than the route of human exposure. If there is absorption and systemic distribution, any route of administration which demonstrates carcinogenic potential is valid for qualitatively demonstrating potential human hazard.[5,6] When tumors occur only at the site of compound administration (*i.e.*, sarcomas at the site of subcutaneous injection), the potential for human hazard would generally be considered to be lower if the route is not the same as that for human exposure and if the test compound is not equally active locally in humans. The relevance of the route of compound administration in long-term rodent studies is an important qualification in the interpretation of results and conclusions reached on those studies.

Chronic Toxicity and Other Study Results

Long-term studies with interim sacrifices allow for examination of the natural history of age-related and chemically-induced lesions. The most useful non-neoplastic chronic toxicity information is derived from animals observed prior to 18 months on study. Non-neoplastic changes in the commonly sampled 18- and 24-month sacrifice intervals are often confounded by spontaneous geriatric changes, although these intervals are meaningful time points for assessment of neoplastic changes. Clinical laboratory studies (*e.g.*, hematology, urinalysis, and clinical chemistry) after 18 months of study are of limited utility because the results may reflect a constellation of age-related changes which cannot easily be sorted out from chemically-induced alterations.

Chronic toxicity, whether observed at interim or final sacrifice, provides evidence of treatment-related effects in the study. During interpretation of a long-term rodent bioassay there is a need to know if the animals were sufficiently challenged. This is particularly important in studies which are negative for carcinogenicity. Evidence of chronic toxicity is also helpful in determining if the administered dose of the test substance was too high. Organ specific chronic toxicity may explain early mortality and may also indicate alteration of organ function which may impact on the interpretation of the observed tumor responses. For example, while hepatic enzyme induction may lead to a reduction of carcinogenicity in some cases because of metabolic deactivation, increased N-hydroxylation activity associated with liver toxicity would be expected to enhance carcinogenicity from chemicals such as 2-fluorenylacetamide.[7] Also, it has been suggested that a non-neoplastic pathologic change, such as necrosis, may be a predisposing factor in the development of neoplasia.[8]

The findings of long-term rodent studies should be interpreted in conjunction with results from preceding prechronic studies with particular emphasis on toxic effects and pathologic findings. Toxic effects include increased mortality, increased behavioral and clinical abnormalities, body and organ weight changes, decreased food consumption, and changes in clinical laboratory data (*e.g.*, hematology, urinalysis, and clinical chemistry). Route of administration, chemical disposition and metabolism, genotoxicity and related short-term test information, and fertility and reproductive toxicity must also be factored into the overall interpretation of long-term rodent studies. Consideration of all these elements allows for balanced conclusions regarding the carcinogenicity of the test substance.

Significance

In terms of study interpretation, there are three operationally useful types of significance: Statistical, toxicological, and "physiological" significance. Properly used, statistical significance can provide objectivity in expression of results. In interpreting statistical significance, the scientist must be cognizant of the axiomatic precision implied by mathematical expression. Such precision is usually not associated with the original observations (*e.g.*, clinical or behavioral abnormalities, gradations of severity of lesion, food and water consumption, etc.).

Toxicologically significant results relate to alterations in body weight gain, abnormal clinical signs, changes in organ weight and function, toxic lesions, and other perturbations in homeostasis which are judged to be adverse effects. Such changes may be reversible and are not necessarily statistically significant. Toxicologically significant results should be viewed as compromising the host, generally demonstrating a dose- and time-dependent pattern of occurrence, and should be "biologically plausible", especially in the absence of a clear dose-response. Toxicologically significant lesions may be non-neoplastic (*e.g.*, toxic, degenerative, hyperplastic) or neoplastic (*e.g.*, carcinogenic).

A "physiologically significant" or "biologically significant" response differs from a toxicologically significant effect in that it does not compromise normal homeostasis and is not considered an adverse effect. Two examples are compound-induced increase in liver weight in the absence of pathological alteration and decrease in the number of circulating lymphocytes reflecting a generic reaction to stress. Other study results (*e.g.*, slight decrease in red blood cell count which would be inappropriate to classify as anemia; decreases in serum enzymes such as transaminases, phosphatases, or dehydrogenases; decreases in spontaneous tumor incidences) may be tentatively regarded as examples of "physiologically significant" effects. At the present time, there is insufficient knowledge to understand these latter effects but, since they do not seem to impact adversely on the test animal, they should not be considered toxicologically significant. It should be apparent that many marginal effects may fall into this third category of significance. However, they can become toxicologically significant as they progress in severity.

When interpreting study results, the scientist is obligated to review all data whether they are statistically significant or not. Toxicologically significant findings should be identified and, whenever possible, correlated with other available study results. When present, "physiologically" significant results may be useful to indicate that the host was sufficiently challenged by the test substance.

Historic Controls

Historic control data for pathologic lesions provide a useful means for comparing the lesion response in concurrent controls with anticipated response. Thus, an atypical frequency of lesions in concurrent controls can be identified and considered in the evaluation and interpretation of the study. The historic incidence range for a given spontaneous lesion is less useful than the average incidence accompanied by the standard deviation. The limitation of historic range rests on the observation that as control incidence data are collected over time, the range constantly increases to account for particularly high or low incidences in individual studies. Ultimately, the range can become so wide as to preclude its usefulness. Expression of historic control data in terms of measures of central tendency overcomes this limitation. Major changes in the conduct or evaluation of studies may necessitate re-establishing the historic control data base. The recently added emphasis on precision of pathologic diagnoses prompted the NTP to redefine its historic control data base by excluding control incidence data obtained prior to November 30, 1981.[12] Routine periodic deletion of the oldest control data will keep the historic data base contemporarily relevant.

In study interpretation, the NTP recognizes three types of controls. The first is the concurrent control. It is the single most critical control for evaluating the outcome of the study. Ideally, concurrent control incidences for specific lesions should be consistent with historic control incidences.

The second control is the specific laboratory historic control. Assuming that the laboratory has a sufficient data base, comparison of results from concurrent control with those of the laboratory historic control will provide an index of confidence regarding the credibility of the results obtained with concurrent control. If the laboratory historic data base is small, the third control, the Program historic control, is used to assess the credibility of the results from concurrent controls. The NTP historic control is a mathematic amalgam of control incidences from all laboratories performing long-term studies for the Program.

Historic control data are useful in interpretation of bioassays when concurrent control incidences are atypically low or high. An atypically low concurrent control incidence for a specific lesion may cause the increased incidence of that lesion in the treated group to be statistically significant. In such situations, interpretation of the toxicological or physiological significance of that lesion should be tempered to account for departure of the concurrent control incidence from the expected value based on the historic control data base. If the incidence of the lesion in the treated animals is within the expected historic control range, the response could be considered equivocal or negative under the conditions of that particular study. An atypically high concurrent control incidence for a given neoplasm might mask a carcinogenic response in the treated group(s). In these instances, the outcome is prudently regarded as equivocal. In either situation, the study under consideration has obvious limitations and consideration should be given to repeating that study.

False Positives

Concerns about increased probability of obtaining false-positive carcinogenicity results as the spontaneous tumor incidence increases have received recent attention.[11-13] This is because one is more likely to obtain statistically significant increased incidences by chance alone in treated groups when there is a high (30% to 50%) spontaneous incidence of tumors in untreated controls. This is a statistical artifact that arises from the discrete nature of the sampling distribution (*see* references 12 and 13). Consequently, when assessing the biological or toxicological significance of the outcome, the scientist must temper his interpretation of the result to account for the increased probability of statistically significant positive findings having occurred by chance alone (*i.e.*, false positive). Stronger statistical evidence is generally required for an increased incidence of a common tumor to be regarded as toxicologically significant than is the case for a rare tumor. In practice, the interpretive process should take other considerations into account such as the historic rate of the tumor, the presence or absence of a dose-response pattern, the occurrence of a definitive tumor response for the same neoplasm in the other sex or species that was tested, and time to tumor information.

False Negatives

Confidence that an apparently negative result in a long-term carcinogenicity test does not represent a false negative is increased with increasing numbers of animals in the study, increased longevity of the test animals, and better quality of pathologic examination. Consistent findings in different species, sexes, and doses plus absence of genotoxicity provide added credibility to the negative result. Although careful statistical evaluation is necessary to support any negative result, interpretive judgements are especially important when assessing small increases in tumors for a tissue site with a low historic spontaneous tumor incidence (*e.g.*, duodenal tumors in rats). Two or three duodenal carcinomas in a group of 50 chemically-treated rats may represent sufficient evidence of carcino-genicity for the pathologist even though statistical p-values exceed 0.05. This issue has been discussed in detail by Fears *et al.*[13]

Decreased Tumor Incidences

The occurrence of statistically significant decreased incidences of commonly occurring tumors as a result of exposure to a test substance and not due to re-duced survival has recently been reviewed.[14] Decreased incidences of tumors of certain endocrine organs (notably fibroadenomas of the mammary gland in female Fischer 344 rats) are often associated with decreased body weight gain while decreased incidences of leukemia/lymphoma in male and female rats are frequently associated with increased incidences of liver tumor.[14] The mechanism for this apparent association is not known, however, the response is believed to be "physiologically" significant. It is appropriate to document these changes clearly for possible future re-evaluation when we learn more about the nature of this response and can better interpret it. When statistically and "physiologi-ically" significant decreases in tumor incidences occur in a long-term study, these changes constitute a valid part of the study conclusions.

Evidence of Carcinogenicity

Some standardized approach for describing the reasoning used to arrive at a conclusion about the carcinogenicity of a chemical is desirable conceptually and for consistent interpretation. Consequently, it is recommended that study re-sults be presented along with interpretive language describing the strength of the experimental evidence. The International Agency for Research on Cancer (IARC) categorization of "sufficient" *versus* "limited" evidence of carcino-genicity[15] may be too simplistic but seems inherently more acceptable than more elaborate schemes[16] requiring a series of judgemental steps which would be diffi-cult to reproduce universally. Increasing the number of categories in any scheme automatically establishes an increased number of gray zones for the classifier thereby making final pronouncements less categorical. A potentially useful compromise[10] recently adopted by the NTP consists of:

(1) *Clear Evidence of Carcinogenicity*—demonstrated by studies that are interpreted as showing a chemically-related increased incidence of malignant neoplasms, studies that exhibit a substantially in-creased incidence of benign neoplasms, or studies that exhibit an increased incidence of a combination of malignant and benign neoplasms where each increases with dose.

(2) *Some Evidence of Carcinogenicity*—demonstrated by studies that are interpreted as showing a chemically-related increased incidence of benign neoplasms, studies that exhibit marginal increases in neo-plasms of several organs/tissues, or studies that exhibit a slight in-crease in uncommon malignant or benign neoplasms.

(3) *Equivocal Evidence of Carcinogenicity*—demonstrated by studies that are interpreted as showing a marginal increase of neoplasms.

(4) *No Evidence of Carcinogenicity*—demonstrated by studies that are interpreted as showing no chemically-related increases in malignant or benign neoplasms.

(5) *Inadequate Study of Carcinogenicity*—demonstrated by studies that show major qualitative or quantitative limitations and cannot be interpreted as valid for showing either the presence or absence of a carcinogenic effect.

The above scheme is designed for application to each definitive study. A definitive study is a test in one sex of one species. Consequently, evidence for carcinogenicity can be established for up to four definitive studies in the standard NTP long-term animal bioassay (male rats, female rats, male mice, female mice). If one study is compromised for any reason (*e.g.*, early mortality due to toxicity), the weight of evidence for carcinogenicity in other studies can be independently classified. Defining the evidence of carcinogenicity should assist in subsequent regulatory decisions pertinent to the chemical under consideration. Some version of the system for ranking animal carcinogens recently proposed by Squire[4] could be used in conjunction with that proposed by the NTP for regulatory decision-making.

Qualified Conclusions

Conclusions regarding carcinogenicity must be qualified as occurring under conditions of the specific study in question. The limitations of the particular study should be clearly pointed out. This helps reduce the natural tendency of inappropriately interpreting by today's standards a study designed two to four years earlier. Long-term studies will inevitably be caught in this sort of time warp and the scientist responsible for interpretation must not ask more of the study than it was originally designed to provide or than the data will permit. The original National Cancer Institute's bioassay was designed as a screen for carcinogenicity in the rodent[17] and generally was not intended to be used to assess risk, carcinogenic potency, subtleties of chronic toxicity, pathogenesis of lesions, xenobiotic metabolism as a function of age, etc.

The time-worn debate regarding the appropriateness of the maximum tolerated dose (MTD) or estimated maximum tolerated dose (EMTD) has not and probably never will be resolved to everyone's satisfaction. Yet, the issue must be confronted anew each time that a long-term rodent study is interpreted. Clearly, if there is an unequivocal response in the treated animals, then the chemical is carcinogenic under the conditions of the study. If one of the limitations of the study was that the MTD was exceeded, then the study conclusion should be qualified as occurring under that circumstance. While use of high doses is a necessary feature of long-term carcinogenicity testing, ideal doses should not produce lethal toxicity unrelated to carcinogenesis.[18] In the same light, a negative tumor response in the absence of any treatment-related toxicologic or physiological effect may represent a situation in which the animals were insufficiently challenged. That negative response should then be qualified appropriately.

REFERENCES

1. Shubik, P., Baker, W.O., Burger, Jr., E.J., London, I.M., and Powers, W.E., General criteria for assessing the evidence of carcinogenicity of chemical substances: Report of the Subcommittee on Environmental Carcinogenesis, National Cancer Advisory Board. *J. Natl. Cancer Inst.* 58: 461-465 (1977)

2. Chu, K.C., Cueto, C., and Ward, J.M., Factors in the evaluation of 200 National Cancer Institute carcinogen bioassays. *J. Toxicol. Environ. Health* 8: 251-280 (1981)

3. Weisburger, J.H., and Williams, G.M., Carcinogen testing: Current problems and new approaches. *Science* 214: 401-407 (1981)

4. Squire, R.A., Ranking animal carcinogens: A proposed regulatory approach. *Science* 214: 877-880 (1981)

5. Saffiotti, U., Identification and definition of chemical carcinogens: Review of criteria and research needs. *J. Toxicol. Environ. Health* 6: 1029-1057 (1980)

6. Tomatis, L., The predictive value of rodent carcinogenicity tests in the evaluation of human risks. *Ann. Review Pharmacol. Toxicol.* 19: 511-530 (1979)

7. Miller, E.C., Miller, J.A., Brown, R.R., and McDonald, J.C., On the protective action of certain polycyclic aromatic hydrocarbons against carcinogenesis by amino azo dyes and 2-acetylaminofluorene. *Cancer Res.* 18: 469-477 (1958)

8. Grasso, P., Review of tests for carcinogenicity and their significance to man. *Clin. Toxicol.* 9: 745-760 (1976)

9. Maronpot, R.R., and Boorman, G.A., Interpretation of rodent hepatocellular proliferative alterations and hepatocellular tumors in chemical safety assessment. *Toxicol. Pathol.* 10: 7-80 (1983)

10. Huff, J.E., and Moore, J.A., Carcinogenesis studies design and experimental data interpretation/evaluation at the National Toxicology Program. *Proceedings of the International Symposium on Occupational Hazards Related to Plastics and Synthetic Elastomers*, Espoo, Finland, 22-27 November (1982)

11. Solleveld, H.A., Haseman, J.K., and McConnell, E.E., The natural history of body weight gain, survival and neoplasia in the Fischer 344 rat. *J. Natl. Cancer Inst.* 72: 929-940 (1984)

12. Haseman, J.K., A reexamination of false-positive rates for carcinogenesis studies. *Fund. Appl. Toxicol.* 3: 334-339 (1983)

13. Fears, T.R., Tarone, R.E., and Chu, K.C., False positive and false negative rates for carcinogenicity screens. *Cancer Res.* 37: 1941-1945 (1977)

14. Haseman, J.K., Patterns of tumor incidence in two-year cancer bioassay feeding studies in Fischer 344 rats. *Fund. Appl. Toxicol.* 3: 1-9 (1983)

15. International Agency for Research on Cancer, *Chemicals With Sufficient Evidence of Carcinogenicity in Experimental Animals - IARC Monographs Volumes 1-17*, Lyon (IARC Internal Technical Report No. 78/003), 20 pp.

16. Griesemer, R.A., and Cueto, C., Toward a classification scheme for degrees of experimental evidence for the carcinogenicity of chemicals for animals. *International Agency for Research on Cancer, Scientific Publication* #27: 259-281 (1980)

17. Page, N., in: *Advances in Modern Toxicology* (H. Kraybill and M. Mehlman, eds.), Vol. 3, pp 87-171, Wiley and Son, New York (1977)

18. Calkins, D.R., Dixon, R.L., Gerber, C.R., Zarin, D., and Omenn, G.S., Identification, characterization, and control of potential human carcinogens: A framework for Federal decision-making. *J. Natl. Cancer Inst.* 64: 169–176 (1980)

Part VI

Bioassays for Insoluble Materials

19

Bioassays for Asbestos and Other Solid Materials

David L. Coffin

U.S. Environmental Protection Agency
Research Triangle Park, North Carolina

Lalita D. Palekar

Northrop Services, Incorporated
Research Triangle Park, North Carolina

INTRODUCTION

The induction of neoplasms by relatively insoluble solids has become important chiefly because of the profound public health implications of exposure to asbestos. Though industrial exposure presents the greatest risk,[1] risk is also associated with residence near asbestos plants[2-4] and in dwellings of those working with asbestos.[3] Furthermore, it is suspected that risk may be associated with the emission of asbestos fibers from building materials. Much attention has been given, for instance, to the widespread use of asbestos in sprayed ceilings in school buildings.[5] There is also the possibility that ambient air may be sufficiently contaminated by mineral fibers emitted during building demolition and from the waste disposal or spoil and storage sites of asbestos mines or manufacturing plants to eventually contribute to the overall tumor burden of the population.[6]

Other particulate minerals used commercially in rather large amounts also may be hazardous. These minerals may be sufficiently fibrous to be tumorigenic, *e.g.*, attapulgite,[7] or they may be contaminated by asbestos fibers, *e.g.*, mica.[8] There is a growing body of evidence which suggests that risk may be associated with exposure to asbestos or nonasbestos mineral fibers released during quarrying and road paving[9] and agricultural activities.[10] Risk may also be associated with residence in a specific locality.[11] Silica has been shown to elicit reticulum cell sarcomas when introduced into the pleural cavity of rats;[12] it also induces the production of various lung tumors in rats when exposure is by inhalation.[13] There is no clear evidence that exposure to silica or quartz is tumorigenic in humans.[14] An endemic focus of mesotheliomas has been identified in rural Turkey. In this area, the prevalence of respiratory tract tumors in the general population is as great as that observed in insulation appliers, the most affected group of industrial workers.[15] Erionite, a nonasbestos mineral of the fibrous zeolite class, is suspected to be the agent responsible for this particular focus of mesotheliomas.[14] Erionite is extremely tumorigenic in experimental animals and is present in volcanic tuffs in many locations in North America and other continents.[16]

Because of the hazard associated with the commercial use of asbestos, there is an interest in developing asbestos substitutes. The problem to be considered here is that the properties that make asbestos a superior insulator (durability and long thin fibers) confer its tumorigenic properties.[17] Very careful biological screening will be required so that substitutes with the same health hazard as asbestos are not produced. This point is vital when the latent period for mineral fiber carcinogenesis is considered: an average of 45 years for mesotheliomas.[18]

Tumorigenesis from nonfibrous inert minerals, such as metallic or plastic objects, constitutes an applicable hazard as compared to asbestos. Sporadic tumor formation has been associated with sequestered metallic objects, such as shrapnel or rifle bullets, and with the implantation of various prosthetic devices for medical purposes.[19] However, the prevalence of these tumors is low compared to the number of such accidental or surgical insertions in humans. Interestingly, certain of these materials regularly produce tumors when implanted in animals. This phenomenon is usually termed foreign body or solid state carcinogenesis. It appears to be of greater interest in experimental cancer research than as a significant public health problem.

Experiments designed to evaluate the biological activities of "commercial asbestos" have been performed over the last four decades. However, it was not until 1962 that Wagner *et al.*[20] found that intrapleural injections of chrysotile and crocidolite in rats produced mesotheliomas comparable to human lesions. In 1964, Smith *et al.*[21] reported the development of fibrosis and mesotheliomas in hamsters injected intrapleurally with amosite.

The experimental work on the biological activities of commercial asbestos was reviewed in 1964 by the Committee on Geographical Pathology of the Union Internationale Contra Cancrum (UICC).[22] The UICC determined that continuation of animal experimentation was necessary; however, they recommended that more precise and qualitative exposure be done to provide means of investigating the etiology of asbestos tumorigenesis.

The UICC also recognized that the asbestos samples tested up to that date were not representative of the dust inhaled by workers. In addition, the mineral samples obtained from various locations possessed different characteristics; thus, comparison of the data from various investigations was not appropriate. The UICC therefore decided that specific asbestos samples from known locations would be prepared for biological studies and for characterization of their physiochemical properties and size distributions.

The standard UICC reference samples were prepared in Johannesberg,

South Africa in 1966. The following samples were characterized for their physio-chemical properties by Timbrell:[23] anthophyllite (Finland); amosite (Trans-vaal, South Africa); crocidolite (North Western Cape Province, South Africa); chrysotile (Rhodesia, now known as Zimbabwe); and chrysotile (Canada). The Canadian chrysotile sample consisted of fibers from eight different mines. Re-cently, the National Institute of Environmental Health Sciences (NIEHS) has standardized samples of chrysotile of three fiber sizes.

The animals recommended by the UICC for the biological evaluations were cesarean derived (C/D) specific pathogen free (SPF) rats maintained under barrier-controlled conditions. The committee, however, emphasized that other animal species should also be investigated. The animals used most often today are C/D SPF Fischer 344 (F344) rats. These animals have a very low incidence of spontaneous lung tumors, a relatively long life span, and are known to develop lung and mesothelial tumors after proper exposure to mineral asbestos.[24] The UICC suggested that the methods of exposure be inhalation, intrapleural inoculation, intrapleural implantation, intratracheal instillation, intra-peritoneal injection, subcutaneous injection, feeding, and gavage and that the duration of the study should be the animals' life span.

ASBESTOS AND OTHER MINERAL FIBERS

Silicates comprise over 90% of the earth's crust. Of the 30 mineral silicates that crystalize in a fibrous form, some are called asbestos.[25] Mineralogically, asbestos is divided into two classes: amphibole and serpentine.

The amphiboles constitute a large and important group of rock-forming minerals. Amphiboles consist of double chains or ribbons of linked tetrahedral groups of atoms having the unit composition $(Si_4 O_{11})_n$ along the fiber axis. These chains or ribbons are laterally bonded by planes of cations and by some hydroxyl ions. The cleavage planes are parallel to the silica chains. The three main amphibole subgroups are: 1) iron-magnesium, *e.g.*, anthophyllite and amosite (also known as grunerite); 2) calcium, *e.g.*, tremolite and actinolite; and 3) alkali, *e.g.*, crocidolite (also known as ribeckite).[26] The surface charge of most amphiboles is negative.[27]

Serpentines include a large number of common minerals such as micas, talc, pyrophyllite, and clays. Serpentine minerals consist of sheet silicate structures formed by linking three corners of each tetrahedron in the basal plane to its neighbors. In chrysotile asbestos, the silicate layer is bonded to a magnesium hy-droxide layer. The interatomic dimension in these layers is slightly different. Their bonding therefore results in the curving of the layers, with the silicate sheets on the inner side and magnesium hydroxide (brucite) layers on the out-side. This curving results in the formation of scrolls and cylinders referred to as fibrils. A large number of fibrils form fiber bundles.[26] The surface charge of chrysotile is positive.[27]

In addition to asbestos, many other naturally occurring minerals may form fibers. Examples are fibrous clays such as sepeolite and attapulgite and fibrous zeolites such as erionite. Minerals are also fabricated into fibrous materials for use in insulation and other purposes, for example, vitreous fibers such as fibrous glass and rock wool. These products together with asbestos are collectively termed mineral fibers. Mineral fibers are usually defined as inorganic material having particles with parallel sides at least three times longer than wide (aspect ratio of ⩾3). By this definition, fibers may vary from short and relatively wide (*e.g.*, 3-μm long x 1-μm wide) to very long and narrow (*e.g.*, >50-μm long x <0.25-μm wide) and include all intermediate lengths and widths. In all natural fibrous material relatively short fibers predominate.

The mineralogical properties often considered for their influence on biological systems are fiber size, chemical content, surface area, and surface charge.

INFLUENCE OF MINERALOGICAL PROPERTIES ON BIOLOGICAL ACTIVITIES

Tumorigenicity and Fiber Size

Among several mineralogical properties, fiber size appears to exert a strong effect on tumorigenicity. It has been difficult to determine the influence of size and shape of the natural mineral fibers because of the heterogeneity of the particles. However, studies with man-made materials such as fiberglass (in which such factors can be controlled) have indicated that an association exists between long thin fibers and tumorigenicity.[28] Fiberglass composed of fibers >8 μm long and <0.25 μm wide induced the highest incidence of tumors when introduced into the pleural cavity.[29] Data suggest, however, that effect diminishes as fibers become shorter and/or broader.[30] It is uncertain at this time whether the relationship between fiber size and tumorigenicity is a continuum or whether the relationship ends at a specific particle length. This point is of great toxicological importance because shorter, thicker fibers predominate in airborne dusts of any fibrous mineral. If these fibers possess even diminished activity, their effect in aggregate might be greater than that imparted by the fewer, longer, thinner fibers. It appears that at least in experiments using artificial intrapleural injection, induction of mesothelial tumors is a function of the geometric characteristic of the mineral fibers rather than of their specific chemical constituents.[30] These criteria also appear to hold true for human exposure; Timbrell[31] reported that the thicker fibers of inhaled anthophyllite elicited pleural plaques but not mesothelial tumors in humans. It is not apparent that these criteria are operant for the induction of lung tumors, although there is a report suggesting that tumorigenicity results only from fibers longer than 5 μm.[32]

Studies completed in our laboratory[33] using intratracheal modes of exposure indicated a phenomenon of "*in vivo*" splitting. Both UICC amosite and ferroactinolite fibers split longitudinally during their residence in the lung. Quantitative analysis of the lung revealed that the number of ferroactinolite fibers increased ten-fold, with a corresponding decrease in diameter. The degree of splitting of UICC amosite was much less. Since the clearance of UICC amosite was much higher than the rate of splitting, the number of fibers was actually reduced during the experimental period. It is noteworthy that although the initial fiber dose of ferroactinolite was much lower than UICC amosite, the incidence of tumors was higher following ferroactinolite treatment, with well differentiated squamous cell carcinomas and mesothelioma.

Tumorigenicity and Magnesium (Acid Leaching)

It has been recognized that the structural magnesium of chrysotile can be dissolved rapidly in acid media. The removal of magnesium (leaching) can be accomplished not only by hydrochloric acid,[34] but also by oxalic acid, one of the organic acids of the Krebs cycle.[35,36] It has also been noted that fibers recovered from human lungs were also stripped of magnesium.[37-39] The relationship between the magnesium content and tumorigenicity has been reported by Morgan *et al.*[40] and Monchaux *et al.*[41]

Monchaux *et al.* leached chrysotile fibers by percolation in 0.1 N oxalic acid or 0.1 N hydrochloric acid and confirmed the findings of Morgan *et al.* that the amount of magnesium leached can differ depending on the time of percolation in acid. It was also evident from both studies that the morphology and the total number of fibers were also changed. Specifically, the mean length of UICC chrysotile A was reduced from 3.21 μm to 1.94 μm in the oxalic acid treatment, in which 89% magnesium was leached. Chrysotile A fibers were reduced to 1.67 μm in hydrochloric acid treatment, in which 81% magnesium was removed. The fiber diameter was increased from 0.063 μm to 0.0685 μm and 0.0684 μm in oxalic acid and hydrochloric acid treatment, respectively. The mean aspect ratio was reduced from 61.54 to 34.22 and 3.20 and the number of fibers in 20 mg was reduced from 23×10^{10} to 13.9×10^{10} and 4.73×10^{10} in the oxalic acid-treated and hydrochloric acid-treated groups, respectively.

The animal studies revealed that pleural tumors and sometimes peritoneal tumors were observed in the rats treated by intrapleural injection of unleached and leached chrysotile fibers.[41] Also, the number of mesotheliomas was the same with unleached chrysotile A and with chrysotile A leached by oxalic acid to 10% magnesium. When the particles were leached further, fewer mesotheliomas were observed. Concomitantly, the survival time also increased with the proportion of magnesium leached. The authors thus concluded that although the size of the acid-leached fibers was changed and may be responsible for tumorigenicity, the magnesium content may also play an important role in such manifestations.

IN VITRO BIOASSAYS

Application of short term *in vitro* bioassays has contributed some information regarding the relationship of the mineralogical properties on the cellular basis. However, these reactions do not always correlate with *in vivo* tumorigenicity.

Influence of Surface Property

It is now well accepted that the surface charge of serpentine and amphiboles is opposite in polarity, but almost similar in magnitude.[27] This difference seems to play no role in tumorigenicity, as both are thought to be equally tumorigenic. In *in vitro* systems, however, chrysotile is found to be extremely toxic compared to other mineral fibers.[42-44] Light and Wie[45] pointed out that chrysotile was hemolytic in the sheep erythrocyte hemolysis system. In their later studies, Light and Wie[46] coated asbestos fibers with dipalmitoyl phosphatidylcholine (main component of pulmonary surfactant) and demonstrated that the surface charge of chrysotile changed from positive to negative and that it was no longer hemolytic to sheep erythrocytes. These findings are in agreement with those reported by Desai and Richards,[47] who also demonstrated that preincubation of chrysotile and crocidolite in a culture medium reduced their hemolytic activity.

Similarly, Jaurand et al.[48] showed that when asbestos fibers were incubated in phospholipids their hemolytic activity was considerably decreased. Hemolytic activity was also considerably reduced when the chrysotile fibers were subjected to acid leaching. It was interesting, however, that acid-treated amphiboles were found to be more hemolytic.[45,49] Light and Wei[45] also indicated that zeta potential of chrysotile is reduced with acid leaching, along with hemolytic activity. A decrease in cytotoxicity of acid-leached chrysotile to cultures of I-407 (human intestine) or ARL 6 (adult rat liver) cells was also reported by Reiss et al.[50]

Langer et al.[51] noted that changes in the surface properties of chrysotile by ball milling also reduced hemolytic activity. Palekar et al.[52] reported that the crystallization habit of mineral rock can also influence hemolysis. Among the four grunerite samples of various degrees of fibrous crystalline nature, the most fibrous grunerite (amosite) was most hemolytic to erythrocytes and cytotoxic to Chinese hamster ovary (CHO) cells; the degree of hemolysis increased with the increase in surface area.

Fibrogenesis is one of the well-known manifestations of asbestos exposure in humans[53] and animals.[54,55] It is speculated that the mechanism of fibrogenesis is a two-stage phenomenon. First, lung macrophages ingest the inhaled particles; these cells, in turn, liberate a factor that stimulates collagen synthesis by fibroblasts. This continuous deposition of collagen in the lung leads to scar tissue that infiltrates the interalveolar spaces and interferes with normal alveolar functions. However, this theory is not yet proven. This phenomenon could not be demonstrated when macrophages were exposed to silica.[56-58] The possibility that mineral fibers stimulate fibroblasts directly has been examined by Richards et al.[59] and Richards and Morris.[60] They found that exposure of rabbit lung fibroblasts to several types of mineral fibers caused increased collagen synthesis in the cell mat, as judged by hydroxyproline in hydrolysate. They also emphasized that synthesis and laying down of collagen is a complex process *in vitro*. It can be affected by many variables including the composition of the medium, the role of growth of the cells, the proportion of collagen synthesized that is bound in the cell mat, and the breakdown of collagen.

Asbestos is toxic to macrophages, causing them to release secondary lysosomal enzymes. Chrysotile rendered an earlier and higher degree of cytotoxicity than did amphiboles in guinea pig peritoneal macrophages.[61-65] Pernis and Castano[66] reported that chrysotile and crocidolite are readily phagocytized by guinea pig peritoneal macrophages. They demonstrated by transmission electron microscopy that the fibers accumulated in the secondary lysosomes. Allison[67] exposed mouse peritoneal macrophages to UICC standard reference fibers. In the absence of serum there was early cytotoxicity and loss of the lysosomal enzyme lactate dehydrogenase within one hour. In contrast, he found that during the same time the levels of acid phosphatase and β-glucuronidase increased. In the presence of 10% serum, early cytotoxicity was reduced and many fibers were taken up by secondary lysosomes. It was postulated that the serum coated the fibers, thus protecting the plasma membranes from damage. Also, it was emphasized that the relatively early release of lysosomal enzymes from macrophages suggests that lysosomes are involved in the cytotoxicity; however, it does not imply that lysosomes are necessarily disrupted within the cells. Similar results have been reported by Miller and Harrington.[68]

Reduction of cytotoxicity was also noted when macrophages were exposed to acid-leached chrysotile.[46,69] It was demonstrated that the cells did not release lysosomal enzymes. Treatment with acid-leached amphiboles, on the other hand, enhanced release of lysosomal enzymes.

Morphological alterations such as hyperplasia and metaplasia of hamster tracheal epithelium in organ culture after exposure to amosite and crocidolite have been demonstrated by Mossman and Craighead,[70] as well as hypertrophy and hyperplasia of mucin-secreting cells with increased secretion of mucin into the culture medium.[71]

Genetic Manifestations

The specific molecular mechanism of oncogenesis associated with asbestos and other inert substances is at this time unknown. While it is reasonable to presume that asbestos and other tumorigenic inorganic minerals exert their influence by means of alterations of the genetic mechanism, this point is by no means clear.

With respect to chemical carcinogenesis, the experimental data indicate that a modification of DNA can occur either directly or indirectly (requiring metabolic enhancement by a cellular enzyme system interaction), producing genotoxicity. Altered DNA is now strongly suspected as one of the factors involved in chemical carcinogenesis.

On the other hand, there is no evidence to date that a similar DNA alteration occurs as a result of cellular interaction with insoluble solids. In-depth studies reported by Hart et al.[72] have failed to demonstrate any unscheduled DNA synthesis or single strand or double strand breakage of DNA in mammalian cells exposed to a variety of asbestos and nonasbestos mineral fibers. Mossman et al.[73] have shown no DNA strand breaks in hamster tracheal cells exposed to UICC samples of crocidolite and chrysotile. These findings are further supported by Lechner et al.,[74] who reported no DNA strand breakage in human bronchial organ cultures exposed to UICC samples of crocidolite, chrysotile, and amosite.

Although DNA alteration has not been proven, chromosomal aberrations have resulted from exposure of mammalian cells to asbestos. Livingston et al.[75] found that CHO cells incubated with UICC samples of crocidolite and amosite showed slight but statistically significant increases in sister chromatid exchange (SCE) levels. Studies with Chinese hamster lung (V79) cells, however, showed no SCE even at high doses of UICC crocidolite or Min-U-Sil.[76] Casey[77] also detected no SCE in V79 cells treated with crocidolite, chrysotile, or fiberglass.

Chromatid and chromosomal damage in CHO cells treated with mineral fibers have been reported by several investigators. UICC crocidolite-treated and Canadian superfine chrysotile A (SFA chrysotile)-treated CHO cells revealed several chromosomal aberrations. No change in chromosomes, however, was observed in CHO cells treated with glass fibers or glass powder.[78]

Similar chromosomal aberrations were reported in V79 cells treated with crocidolite, amosite, or chrysotile.[79,80] In addition, it was demonstrated that these mineral fibers, although weak mutagens, did induce gene mutation at the hypoxanthine-guanine phosphoribosyl transferase (HGPRT) locus. Chromosomal aberrations were also reported in V79 cells treated with UICC crocidolite and Min-U-Sil.[76]

A time response study by Valerio *et al.*[81] has shown that lymphocytes from normal male and female rats exposed to UICC chrysotile A (Rhodesian) reveal chromosomal aberrations, namely numerical alterations and chromatid and chromosome breaks. After a 48-hour exposure, numerical alterations were more frequent; after 72 hours, chromatid breaks were most frequently noted. However, Sincock *et al.*[82] reported cultured human lymphoblasts or human fibroblasts did not show any chromosomal changes when treated with UICC crocidolite, SFA chrysotile, or glass fibers.

Morphologic Transformation

Information regarding the ability of mineral fibers to induce morphologic transformation in mammalian cells is limited. DiPaolo *et al.*[83] have observed a very low level of morphologic transformation in Syrian hamster embryo (SHE) cells exposed to UICC samples of crocidolite, anthophyllite, amosite, or Canadian chrysotile B. However, it has been questioned whether this change is real. Since clastogenesis can occur in mammalian cells exposed to mineral fibers, the change observed here may simply be due to the chromosomal alterations.

Morphologic transformation of SHE cells exposed to chrysotile and crocidolite has been reported by Hesterberg *et al.*[84] Chrysotile was more cytotoxic than crocidolite and the degree of transformation was proportional to the degree of cytotoxicity. These authors also noted that fiberglass and quartz transformed SHE cells; however, the required dose of fiberglass was much higher than that needed for other asbestos samples. In their later study, Hesterberg *et al.*[85] reported a dose-response relationship between the morphologic transformation of SHE cells and chrysotile treatment. Cellular transformation also depended on fiber dimension. Code 100 fiberglass (mean diameter 0.2 μm $\pm$ 0.1 μm) was ten times more potent than code 110 fiberglass (mean diameter 0.8 μm $\pm$ 0.1 μm). When code 110 fiberglass was ground to give shorter fibers of the same diameter, no morphologic transformation was observed.

In another system, Poole *et al.*[86] exposed C3H-10T½ mouse cells to several asbestos particles and to erionite; none of the asbestos samples induced morphologic transformation. A significant degree of transformation, however, was noted in cultures treated with erionite.

Bacterial Mutagenic Response

Ames tests using *Salmonella typhimurium* and WP2 assays using *E. coli* gave negative results even when asbestos was coupled with rat liver S9 microsomal fractions.[87,88] Szyba and Lang[89] demonstrated, however, that when cultures of *S. typhimurium* were exposed to asbestos fibers coated with benzo(a)pyrene [B(a)P] together with the S9 microsomal fraction, a significant increase in the number of transformed colonies appeared over those treatments in which only B(a)P and S9 fraction were added. It was speculated that asbestos fibers enhanced penetration of the B(a)P into the bacterial cells.

Asbestos as a Co-Carcinogen

Synergism between cigarette smoke and exposure to asbestos fibers in the induction of lung cancer is well recognized in humans.[1] Animal studies also indicate enhancement of lung tumors when exposure to mineral fiber is coupled with exposure to B(a)P. The mechanism of this interaction is not yet identified.

In vivo experiments employing intratracheal injection of B(a)P and asbestos indicate that there is a slight increase in tumorigenicity when these substances are administered together over that when asbestos or B(a)P is given alone.[21,90] Experiments in which inhalation of radon 222 was combined with intrapleural inoculation of chrysotile, crocidolite, amosite, glass fibers, or quartz particles suggested that interaction of asbestos with the radon 222 increased the number of pleural tumors over previous studies performed with glass fibers or asbestos alone.[91]

Interaction of asbestos with other carcinogens has also been shown *in vitro*. In bacterial mutagenicity tests using *S. typhimurium*, microcrystals of B(a)P adsorbed on chrysotile, crocidolite, or amosite produced a significant number of revertants. Neither asbestos nor microcrystals of B(a)P alone (without dimethyl sulfoxide) produced this reaction. This indicates a carrier effect of asbestos fibers.[92] Daniel et al.[93] reported that when NIEHS chrysotile was added, prior to B(a)P, to cultures of human fibroblasts, the level of B(a)P-DNA binding was increased. Similar observations were made by Eneanya et al.,[94] where enhancement of B(a)P-DNA binding was observed when SHE cells were preincubated with NIEHS "intermediate" chrysotile prior to B(a)P treatment. Enhancement of SHE cell transformation was also reported by DiPaolo et al.[83] when asbestos fibers were added after B(a)P treatment. It is of interest that simultaneous addition of NIEHS chrysotile and B(a)P to normal human fibroblasts did not increase the B(a)P-DNA binding levels[72,93] or B(a)P metabolite profiles.[93]

With the use of fluorescence spectroscopy, Lakowicz and Hylden[95] measured the rate of transport of B(a)P into phospholipid vesicles of dipalmitoyl phosphatidylcholine (DPPC). Since lung surfactant contains at least 70% DPPC, this artificial membrane provides a model to investigate the fate of particle-adsorbed B(a)P in the lungs. A special technique was used to adsorb B(a)P to asbestos and other mineral fibers. Asbestos samples showed a greater ability to adsorb B(a)P in a monomeric state than did silica. In addition, both amosite and silica enhanced the uptake of B(a)P; however, the uptake of B(a)P was higher with amosite than with silica although the surface area of silica was six times higher than that of amosite. In a later study, Lakowicz et al.[96] demonstrated that B(a)P coated on asbestos samples (anthophyllite, crocidolite, chrysotile, and amosite) was transported better to membrane vesicles than B(a)P coated on nonfibrous particles (hematite, silica, titanium dioxide, porous glass, and talc). It was evident that adsorption of B(a)P to the surface of the particles is necessary for its enhanced transport into membranes. Simple mixtures of B(a)P microcrystals and particulates do not show enhanced transport.

The rate of uptake of B(a)P into rat liver microsomes when it was coated on asbestos fibers was studied by Lakowicz and Bevan.[97] Concurrent with their other findings, they demonstrated that anthophyllite, Canadian chrysotile, iron oxide, and carbon black enhanced B(a)P uptake by liver microsomes in comparison to uptake from aqueous dispersions of B(a)P microcrystals. Moreover, B(a)P uptake was higher with asbestos fibers than with iron oxide. In an attempt to investigate whether B(a)P uptake by microsomes had any influence on their metabolic activity, Kandaswami and O'Brien[98] studied microsomal aryl hydrocarbon hydroxylase (AHH) activities and found a marked inhibition of AHH. These results were confirmed by Pawlak.[99] Despite the decrease in the metabolism of B(a)P with chrysotile asbestos, there was a six-fold increase in the association of B(a)P metabolites with DNA. Eneanya *et al.*[94] also reported a decrease in B(a)P metabolism in SHE cells when the cells were incubated with B(a)P and chrysotile. However, further analysis revealed that when asbestos was added with B(a)P, there was a six-fold increase in B(a)P association with DNA over that observed when B(a)P was added alone.

The authors thus concluded that the greatly increased association of the B(a)P metabolite(s) with DNA may be indicative of a shift of B(a)P metabolite(s) to a more carcinogenic state. This new metabolite(s) may compensate for the decrease of B(a)P metabolism and may be responsible for a higher incidence of lung tumors in asbestos workers who also smoke.

Synergistic interaction between 3-methylcholanthrene (3-MC) and asbestos as well as nonasbestos mineral fibers has been investigated by Mossman and Craighead.[100] Hamster tracheal tissues were exposed for four weeks to crocidolite, hematite, kaolin, or carbon coated with 3-MC prior to implantation into syngeneic animals. Several squamous cell carcinomas were produced in the trachea; the numbers of tumors were similar for 3-MC-coated asbestos, hematite, or kaolin. When other lesions such as sarcomas and undifferentiated malignant tumors were added to the carcinomas, the incidence of neoplasms was greater for crocidolite, hematite, kaolin, and carbon, ranked in a decreasing order. A careful evaluation of the relative amounts of 3-MC adsorbed to and released from the particles indicated that carcinogenicity did not relate to either the affinity of the particle for 3-MC or the elution of 3-MC from the dust. Carbon adsorbed more 3-MC than the other particulates, but the elution was minimal. Kaolin and asbestos eluted smaller quantities; hematite released the greatest amounts. These findings suggest that there must be another mechanism of carcinogenesis than just availability of a chemical carcinogen.

In support of this theory, Landesman and Mossman[101] demonstrated that when an amount of crocidolite and chrysotile which did not inhibit growth was added to tracheal epithelial cells there was a two-to-three-fold increase in ornithine decarboxylase (ODC) activity. Addition of hematite had no effect. It is now speculated that the induction of ODC, a rate limiting enzyme in the biosynthesis of polyamines, might be intrinsic to the promotion phase of carcinogenesis. In the mouse skin, the magnitude of induction of ODC has been correlated with the promoting capabilities of a number of phorbol and nonphorbol compounds.

The possibility that asbestos may act as a promoter in the respiratory tissue after exposure to chemical carcinogens has been demonstrated in tracheal transplants of F344 rats.[102] The transplants were first exposed to dimethylbenz-(a)anthracene (DMBA) at various doses and then to 200 µg of chrysotile. No enhancement of tumor production at 100 µg of DMBA, a dose tumorigenic by itself, was reported.[102] At lower doses of DMBA (50 µg and 25 µg) there was a 15% and 23% enhancement of tracheal carcinomas, respectively. At 12.5 µg

DMBA, however, this response was not observed. Chrysotile alone, at even a high dose of 2.0 mg, was weakly carcinogenic.[103] Unlike previous studies where the higher induction of tumors was ascribed to the carrier effect of asbestos, this study clearly demonstrated a role of asbestos as a promoter since DMBA was administered prior to the asbestos exposure.

In Vitro Interactions with Human Bronchial Cells

Effects of asbestos and glass fibers on bronchial epithelium have been reported by Haugen *et al.*[104] The bronchial epithelium was found to be much more reactive than bronchial fibroblasts. Among the mineral samples, chrysotile was more toxic than crocidolite and amosite. The glass fibers were relatively non-toxic. By means of the scanning electron microscope they were able to demonstrate various focal lesions such as hyperplasia, epidermoid metaplasia, and dysplasia in human bronchial explants exposed to asbestos.

FOREIGN BODY TUMORIGENICITY

The reports by Oppenheimer *et al.*[105,106] that the insertion of various plastic films into the subcutaneous tissue of rats and mice readily induced sarcomas stimulated interest in exploring the tumorigenic mechanisms. Tumors were elicited by a large array of materials: cellophane, dacron, nylon, polyethylene, and silk films. Purification of the polymers to eliminate plasticizers, stabilizers, residual monomers, and the like, did not reduce the tumorigenicity. According to several authors, the physical form rather than the specific chemical appeared to be the inciting factor. In order to explain this phenomenon, various modes of tumorigenicity were postulated: mechanical irritation, interference with nutrition, blocking growth-controlling substances, or electrostatic or electrokinetic disturbances near the implanted plastic.[107] The tumor induction appeared to be proportional to the size of the implants. Another view was expressed by Alexander and Horning[108] in a study of 17 polyurethanes implanted into the peritoneal cavity of male NBR rats. These authors observed a correlation between induction of fibrosarcoma and the presence of aromatic compounds or substituted amine groups in the structure of the polymer. Later, Autian *et al.*[109] reported induction of pulmonary cancer by implantation of strips of polyurethane (#Y-238), a chlorinated polyether polyurethane. On the basis of these two experiments, the authors suggest that tumorigenicity is a function of specific chemical characteristics.

Brand *et al.*[110,111] examined the origin of foreign body tumors and reported that the tumors arise from specific cell clones firmly attached to the surface of the implanted polymer. Within two weeks after the subcutaneous implantation of a plastic, granulocytes and monocytic macrophages infiltrate on the implant. The macrophages form a layer of binucleated and multinucleated cells. These may be interspersed with polymorphonuclear leukocytes, fibroblasts and cells resembling smooth muscle precursor cells. Subsequently, a thin membrane consisting of fibroblasts forms on the inner surface of the plastic and the macrophage layer adjacent to the plastic implant. This membrane thickens and there is blood vessel ingrowth and dormancy of the macrophages with fibrotic incapsulation of the implant. This is followed in 6 months to 12 months by the formation of nidi of proliferating fibroblasts. Brand et al.[110] implanted rigid films made of various plastics or glass subcutaneously in CHA/H or CBA/H-T6 mice. These two substrains are histocompatible, but are distinguishable on the basis of the T6 marker chromosome. After various time intervals, they removed the transplants and introduced them into mice of the opposite subline. Resulting tumors were grown *in vitro* for chromosomal analysis. It was noted that the first implant carrier was the animal from which the tumor cells originated.

IN VIVO BIOASSAYS

Inhalation Exposure

A number of biological procedures have been utilized to confirm human disease, compare activity of various mineral fibers, and to seek mineralogical determinants and mechanisms of fibrosis and tumorigenicity of asbestos and various surrogate mineral fibers. Experiments involving exposure of animals to asbestos by inhalation began rather early since this method most naturally replicates human exposure to dusts in industrial plants. Interest in pulmonary fibrosis (asbestosis) stimulated the earlier studies since the association of this lesion with asbestos exposure was known before the significance of the tumorigenicity. In 1941, Nordman and Sorga[112] reported that deposition of fibers in the pulmonary alveoli, alveolar ducts, and bronchi of mice was associated with lesions such as atypical hyperplasia of the bronchial epithelium, bronchiolization of the alveoli, epithelial metaplasia, and squamous cell carcinoma.

Additional studies in which inhalation or intratracheal injection were used in attempts to produce asbestosis and/or asbestos bodies in mice, guinea pigs, rats, and rabbits have been reviewed by Holt et al.[113] Different degrees of fibrosis and asbestos body formation were reported, as follows: guinea pigs–fibrosis and asbestos bodies; mice–fibrosis but no asbestos bodies; rats–slight fibrosis but no asbestos bodies; rabbits–no response.

An experiment designed to show the oncogenic potential of various asbestos minerals in animals was reported in 1963 by Wagner.[114] Guinea pigs, rabbits, and vervet monkeys were exposed to South African chrysotile, amosite, and impure crocidolite; the latter contained a high proportion of quartz. Earlier fibrotic lesions were induced by amosite than by chrysotile, while exposure to crocidolite produced more severe lesions in guinea pigs and monkeys. It was notable that the animals in the exposed groups were more susceptible to respiratory infection.

With the recognition of the association of exposure to asbestos and pulmonary cancer beginning in the 1940's and exposure to asbestos and mesotheliomas in the 1960's, experimental studies were specifically designed to reflect an interest in the development of neoplasia. Data were collected on deposition and clearance of the mineral fibers and the degree of carcinogenesis induced by the various types of asbestos and nonasbestos mineral fibers and particles. These data from inhalation exposure show that all the commercial asbestos fibers are tumorigenic. A very basic study was reported in 1974 by Wagner et al.[115] in which barrier-protected Wistar rats were exposed to UICC reference samples of amosite, anthophyllite, crocidolite, Canadian chrysotile, and Rhodesian chrysotile by inhalation exposure. The dust was administered by a specially designed aerosol generator.[116] Exposures were scheduled for 7 hours per day, 5 days per week. Samples of respirable dusts were collected and evaluated at the end of each daily exposure. Determination of the cumulative respirable dose was computed on the basis of chamber concentration x time of exposure. The retained dose was determined by the silicon content of the lungs of sacrificed animals using the method of Morris *et al.*[117] Mean respirable dose ranged from 68 mg/m^3 to 103 mg/m^3 for one day up to 33,700 mg/m^3 for 24 months with no appreciable difference between amphibole and chrysotile. However, the retention in the lung at 24 months was approximately 15 mg for the amphiboles and 0.3 mg and 0.6 mg for the Canadian and Rhodesian chrysotile samples, respectively. The authors suggested that faster clearance results in the lack of accumulation with time. Data were presented for tumor induction after exposure times of 1 day, 3 months, 6 months, 12 months and 24 months in animals permitted to live their entire life span. Lesions were categorized as asbestosis, adenoma, adenomatosis, adenocarcinoma, squamous cell carcinoma, and mesothelioma. The total tumor incidence for the combined categories varied from 26% to 41% for the asbestos-treated animals and was 6% for control animals that lived at least 300 days after the beginning of the exposure. The authors did not indicate significant differences in tumorigenicity among the various asbestos types. This study showed a strong association of pulmonary tumors with asbestosis.

Deposition and clearance of asbestos fibers have been assayed by Evans *et al.*[118] by means of inhalation exposure to radiolabelled UICC crocidolite. Immediately after the exposure, deposition of crocidolite (measured by detection of ^{59}Fe) was split about equally between the upper and lower respiratory tract, with the remainder in the esophagus, stomach, and small intestine. This was presumably the result of fast clearance and subsequent swallowing of material deposited in the upper respiratory tract during the period of exposure. After 30 days following the exposure, more than 70% of the total dose had been excreted in the feces and somewhat less than 30% remained in the lungs. Autoradiographs of lesions taken immediately after cessation of exposure showed that the most fibers were located at the bifurcation of the smaller bronchioles. Those fibers on the epithelium were frequently associated with macrophages, while fibers in lung parenchyma appeared to be deposited in the region of the alveolar ducts and entrance to the alveoli. Fibers deposited in the bronchioles were longer and thicker than those in the region of the alveoli. These observations are in accord with those of Timbrell *et al.*,[119] who reported that there was a reduction of length in comparison to that of the dust cloud as airways were descended. Additionally, Evans *et al.*[120] suggested that after 30 days, all fibers in the alveolar regions were intracellular and appeared to be relatively long compared with those seen in autoradiographs prepared from animals killed at earlier periods.

The site of the early lesions following inhalation exposure to asbestos tends to confirm the observations made concerning the preference for deposition. A number of investigators have reported that the earliest lesions are noted at the level of the terminal bronchiole, the alveolar ducts, and proximal alveoli.[112,114] Electron microscopic studies performed by Davies[120] show similar locations for the early lesions and the greatest concentration of fibers in these areas, while similar foci for the inhalation of fiberglass have been reported by Lee *et al.*[121] By means of a transmission and scanning electron microscopic study, Brody *et al.*[122,123] also noted the earliest concentration of chrysotile asbestos fibers at the bifurcation of the alveolar duct where lesions first appeared.

Pathological sequences in the early phases of exposure to asbestos have been studied by Brody *et al.*[122,123] Within five hours following exposure there was uptake of the fibers by Type I alveolar epithelial cells via development of microvillous projections and incorporation in small membrane-bound vesicles. During this phase, asbestos fibers were also incorporated within macrophages. Davis[120] has indicated that the earliest lesions are granulomatous nodules in proximity to terminal bronchioles with giant cells. These changes were followed by interstitial pneumonia and fibrosis. Wagner's light microscopic study[114] showed that the first alterations usually noted are scattered macrophages containing asbestos fibers in the alveoli adjacent to the terminal bronchioles. These changes are followed by recticulin proliferation which leads to thickening of the walls of the terminal bronchioles, later extending to the alveolar ducts and proximal alveoli. When such a section is examined three months after the beginning of exposure, this lesion can be readily seen at low magnification as a focal distributed thickening of the walls of the terminal bronchioles, alveolar ducts, and pulmonary alveoli. As time progresses, these enlarge and may become confluent, involving larger areas of the lungs with confluent compartmentalized fibrotic thickening of the alveolar walls, sometimes termed pseudo alveoli. These lesions are classified as asbestosis.

The rat would appear to be the animal of choice as a model for the detection of tumorigenicity from mineral fibers since the incidence of spontaneous lung tumors is very low for both the Wistar and F344 strains.[124,125] Furthermore, both strains of rats are obtainable as C/D barrier-protected animals in which the absence of infections ensures sufficient life span to permit the development of tumors with long induction periods, a characteristic of mineral fiber tumors. According to Wagner *et al.*,[115] there were more tumors induced in F344 rats with 12 months inhalation exposure than with six months exposure, but no essential differences occurred between 12 months and 24 months. Animals in all cases were permitted to live their natural life span.

With Wistar rats, no tumors of the lung were observed within 300 days of the start of the exposure, and only 13 rats of a total of 247 had died of any cause within the first 300 days. Lung tumors induced in rats by experimental treatment with asbestos were entirely peripheral. They were variously classified, but they were essentially derived from the prime site of the asbestos lesion (terminal bronchiole, alveolar duct and/or proximal pulmonary alveoli). The lesions observed were atypical epithelial hyperplasia, adenoma, adenomatosis, adenocarcinoma, and squamous cell carcinoma. These lesions are not unique but have been shown to occur in statistically greater numbers in groups of animals exposed to asbestos.[117,122]

Induction of mesotheliomas has been low following inhalation exposure to asbestos; Wagner *et al.*[115] reported 14 mesotheliomas from a total of 713 exposed animals compared to 247 lung tumors. On the other hand, Wagner[7] found that a nonasbestos silicate, erionite, produced 16 deaths from mesotheliomas out of a total of 28 animals surviving to one year.

Wagner[114] has reported that exposure of vervet monkeys and guinea pigs produced the most complete lesions of asbestosis, while rabbits appeared somewhat resistant. While early studies performed with random bred rats have elicited a measurable incidence of pulmonary tumors,[126] more reproducible results have been obtained with C/D barrier-protected rats in recent experiments. Wagner[125] reports a difference in tumor incidence between his early results with Wistar rats and his later experiments with F344 rats. The F344 rat appears to be the animal of choice in the most recent studies due to its availability, relatively small size, freedom from intercurrent disease, and low incidence of spontaneous pulmonary tumors. Bozelka et al.[127] exposed BALB/c mice to approximately 10.9 mg UICC chrysotile for 2 hours per day, 5 days per week for periods up to 2½ months. This regimen yielded a lung retention of an average of 39.7 μg chrysotile, as determined by X-ray diffraction after 30 exposure days. The authors report that these exposures produced early lesions or macrophage influx in the alveolar spaces surrounding the terminal and respiratory bronchioles and increased cellularity of the alveolar septae. After one year, fibrosis was evident in all animals. Ninety-two percent of the exposed mice had lung tumors 12 months to 18 months after the termination of the exposure, compared to an incidence of 10% in controls. These consisted mainly of small (3 mm to 6 mm) multiple tumors immediately beneath the visceral pleura, but occasionally they involved entire lung lobes with extension to parietal pleura and thoracic wall.

Intratracheal Instillation

Intratracheal injection of laboratory animals has been rather widely employed for evaluation of pulmonary effects of certain toxicants and carcinogens. It has been used, for instance, in evaluating the influence of organic chemicals and their interaction with various particulate materials.[128] It has the advantage of simplicity and unlike exposure by inhalation, it does not require complex exposure apparatus and monitoring equipment and gives a semblence of natural exposure of the lung. Experiments by King et al.,[129] reproduced asbestosis and demonstrated the formation of asbestos bodies; tumor induction was not mentioned. Smith et al.[130] instilled amosite or chrysotile into hamsters in a single injection of 2.5 mg or at biweekly treatments of 1.25 mg giving a total of 30 mg in the highest dose schedule. Asbestosis, but no tumors, was noted in surviving animals. Shabad et al.[90] exposed female rats beginning at one month of age, to chrysotile or chrysotile with adsorbed B(a)P. Dose schedules were: 2 mg chrysotile 3 times per month with and without adsorbed B(a)P, single injections of 2 mg asbestos with B(a)P, or 2 mg asbestos alone. They reported a few solitary precancerous lesions at the end of the experiment for chrysotile alone; with the combined chrysotile/B(a)P treatment 29% of the rats developed tumors. No tumors were induced by B(a)P alone.

Coffin et al.[131] performed intratracheal instillation studies with UICC amosite and a nonasbestos ferroactinolite in F344 rats. Treatments consisted of 12 weekly injections of 0.25 mg and 0.5 mg amosite and ferroactinolite, respectively. The total injected dose was 6.0 mg for the ferroactinolite and 3.0 mg for UICC amosite. The dose of the amosite was smaller because the longer fibers tended to block the airways and resulted in death from respiratory failure in the young rats. In these experiments, the dose was expressed both in mass units and numbers of mineral fibers of two categories, those particles of aspect ratio $\geqslant 3$ and fibers $\geqslant 8\,\mu m$ long and $\leqslant 0.25\,\mu m$ wide. After lifetime observation, 22 of 561 ferroactinolite-treated animals had lung tumors and five had pleural mesotheliomas compared to one lung tumor and two mesotheliomas in 139 amosite-treated animals. While the pulmonary tumor incidence is seemingly low, the tumor incidence from the ferroactinolite treatment was statistically significantly higher than in the UICC amosite group and in the control groups. The excess of tumors in the ferroactinolite group was related to longitudinal splitting of the ferroactinolite fibers during their residence in the lung after instillation.[33] There was a five-fold increase in the number of ferroactinolite fibers retained two years after the instillation as compared to an actual decline in the number of amosite fibers. This increase in ferroactinolite fibers was associated with a reduction in length but an increase of aspect ratio from 9 to 30 for the ferroactinolite versus 11.8 to 20.1 for the amosite.

In the same study,[131] observation of early histopathological changes showed granulomatous changes in the bronchi from both fibers in animals sacrificed after the twelfth instillation. These changes consisted of large polypoid granulomatous lesions in the smaller airways with numerous fiber-containing solitary macrophages and giant cells but with normal-appearing ciliated epithelium. This lesion was most characteristic of the amosite-treated animals. Sporadic foci of interalveolar septal thickenings adjacent to the terminal bronchiolar-alveolar ductal junctures were barely evident at the first killing period following the last of the 12 weekly intratracheal instillations, but they became more pronounced at the later killing periods. There was gradual alteration to higher epithelium; one animal showed frank atypical bronchiolo-alveolar-cell hyperplasia by one year. Squamous cell metaplasia was also evident in a few of these animals. This lesion was more common and the epithelial changes more evident for the ferroactinolite-treated group, persisting through the lifetime studies.

Later changes most commonly consisted of bronchiolo-alveolar-cell tumors and atypical bronchiolo-alveolar-cell hyperplasia. These lesions were frequently multiple and sometimes appeared to intergrade in the same lung. Squamous cell metaplasia also developed in the hyperplastic lesions. A few were carcinomatous. Other tumors noted consisted of adeno- and epidermoid carcinoma. The incidence of lung tumors in ferroactinolite-treated animals, amosite-treated animals, shams, and untreated controls was 3.9%, 0.7%, 0.6%, and 0.4%, respectively. The number of hyperplastic lesions was similar in the ferroactinolite-treated animals. There were mesotheliomas in both treatment groups.

Except for granuloma of the bronchi, the lesions resembled those reported from inhalation exposure. Long fibers, sometimes $>50\,\mu m$ in length, were observed in bronchial granulomas. Such fibers would have been trapped in the nose or upper airway if exposure was by inhalation. Among the possible causes of a lower incidence of tumors by intratracheal instillation compared to inhalation exposure might be the following: short dosing period, dosing during an inappropriate interval of the life-span, different placement of the mineral fibers in the airway, or simply a lower dose. Except for the airway granulomas, early and late lesions appeared at the same sites as those induced by inhalation, suggesting that the mineral dust followed the same depositional pattern as for inhalation.

Intrapleural Injection

The administration of mineral dusts into the pleural cavity by various means has been much used to determine the tumorigenic potential of such material since the initial report of Wagner and Berry.[132] These methods are relatively simple and yield a higher rate of pleural tumors than other methods. Tumors thus induced not only replicate the cellular pattern of those occurring in human beings[133] but they contain hyaluronic acid, another feature of the human tumors. The model has been used to study several mechanisms of tumorigenicity by various mineral fibers, *e.g.*, the association of tumorigenesis with long narrow fibers;[29] local fibrogenesis as an effect of fiber length;[134] the influence of *in vivo* leaching of chrysotile and distribution of leached products;[135,136] and the reduction of tumorigenicity by acid leaching of chrysotile.[40,41]

Three techniques for the introduction of mineral dusts into the pleural cavity have been described. Most commonly, the material suspended in saline is merely injected through the chest wall. Wagner and Berry[137] injected in the region of the right axilla at the level of the second nipple. The problem is to avoid injecting into the peritoneal cavity, the lungs, or other viscera, while penetrating to the pleural cavity. The above authors indicated that in certain of their experiments, sarcomas of the chest wall developed at the site of inoculation, indicating that the material had been injected into the chest wall rather than the pleural cavity. In subsequent experiments, they used a second method which obviated this factor. A needle was placed on a hub fitted with a two-way valve with one arm connecting to the syringe and the other connecting to a capillary manometer that showed negative pressure when the pleural cavity was pierced. The third method of pleural implants was developed by Stanton and Wrench[28] and used for the purpose of determining influence of particle shape on the induction of pleural tumors. They employed a complex method in which fiber glass disks impregnated with mineral dusts suspended in 10% gelatin were implanted against the visceral pleura of the left lung.

The tumors induced were of several cellular types, although all were believed to be derived from mesothelial tissue. They were usually classified as sarcomatous mesothelioma, tubulopapillary mesothelioma, and mixed mesothelioma. A fourth group was sometimes added, pleomorphic mesothelioma. These tumors spread throughout the pleural cavity and actively invaded the adjacent tissues. The pathological sequence has been studied by Davis.[134] The first lesions to appear following intrapleural inoculation consist of granulomas containing macrophages, giant cells, and fibroblasts which appear within one week. The cytology differs somewhat among the various laboratory animals employed. In the rat these lesions were replaced by fibrous tissue and after approximately two months persisted as rather cellular granulomas surrounded by a capsule. Electron microscopic studies showed that within a few days mesothelial cells contained asbestos fibers; some appeared to acquire a rounder appearance and seemed less attached to contiguous cells. Wagner[137] injected SPF Wistar rats with 20 mg of asbestos dust (amosite, chrysotile, crocidolite, and extracted crocidolite, and silica). They found that mesothelial hyperplasia appeared after six months; there was evidence at this time of penetration of the fibers between the mesothelial cells. Tumors appeared to originate in the submesothelial connective tissue and at first resembled primitive spindle cells, later differentiating into spinate cells or epithelial-like cells. Shabad *et al.*[90] have described the sequences of early lesions after exposure to chrysotile asbestos. Early pretumorous lesions consisted of the mesothelial cells on the visceral or parietal pleural surface. Focal growths developed within the hyperplastic areas, containing multilayered aggregations of cuboidal cells occasionally with papillomatous outgrowths containing connective tissue stroma. These areas might be associated with underlying connective tissue plaques. The authors infer that these stages comprised preneoplastic lesions.

When exposed rats are permitted to live their entire life span, death from mesothelioma begins at slightly less than 400 days; 50% of the mortality occurs during the next 300 days. Mean survival time was considerably less for animals dying with mesothelioma than for untreated controls, but this difference was much less marked for treated animals in which no mesotheliomas were found. Mean survival time was longer in all cases for SPF animals. The overall incidence of mesothelioma for the SPF rats was: amosite, 40%; chrysotile, 64%; crocidolite, 59%; and extracted crocidolite, 59%. The dose-response studies of Wagner *et al.*[138] with chrysotile and crocidolite, employed doses of 0.5, 1, 2, 4 and 8 mg and 12 rats/dose. The response was suggestive of a graded response to tumorigenicity although, as the authors mentioned, the number of animals was too small for precise results. A statistical model of Pike[139] which may have been effective for similar studies was employed.

On the other hand, Stanton and Wrench[28] reported a higher incidence of mesothelial tumors by implantation of a larger dose of asbestos fibers. Forty milligrams of amosite, chrysotile and crocidolite produced 58% to 75% mesothelial tumors. Although the technique used by Stanton and Wrench was different from the one used by Wagner, the tumors produced were similar histologically.

Intraperitoneal Injection

Intraperitoneal injections have been used less than intrapleural injections. Frederick *et al.*[140] injected mice with amosite, anthophyllite, and crocidolite. All animals were sacrificed within four months of inoculation. Granulomas that contained short, medium, and long fibers and a differential placement of short fibers only in the lymph nodes were noted. Pott *et al.*[141,142] demonstrated that intraperitoneal injections of chrysotile, glass fibers, nemalite and polygorscite produced mesotheliomas in rats. On the other hand, granular dusts such as actinolite and talcum did not produce tumors. From these results, they emphasized that the shape factor of the dust is involved in tumorigenicity. In a further study, Pott *et al.*,[141] reported that similar tumors could be produced in hamsters injected with crocidolite, but not with fiberglass. By light and electron microscopic methods Davis[143] studied the histogenesis of tumors produced by intraperitoneal injections of crocidolite and chrysotile asbestos in rats, mice, and guinea pigs. The earliest lesions consisted of numerous small pedunculated masses containing a central core of reticulin or collagen that appeared on the surface of the viscera, the diaphragm, and the body wall; lesions were covered by a single layer of cells resembling mesothelium. These lesions originated either in the areas of granulomatous reactions to mineral fibers or on unaltered mesothelial surfaces. When the tumors were more advanced, spindle cell lesion pattern was evident. These spindle cell lesions were prone to become locally invasive.

A feature of the intraperitoneal injection of animals was the tendency of the animals to develop ascites as the tumors progressed. The fluid might contain erythrocytes, but it always contained tumor cells.

Subcutaneous Injection

The induction of lesions and the migration of mineral fibers have been studied by Rowe *et al.*[144] by injecting mice subcutaneously at two sites in both flanks with 10 mg of amosite, crocidolite, or chrysotile asbestos. Local sarcomas occurred in 7 of 86 mice, 40 weeks or more after the first injection. In addition, nonmalignant mesothelial proliferation was noted. The time to death from tumor varied from 41 weeks to 109 weeks.

In these experiments, wide disbursal of the asbestos fibers was discernable by light microscopy. The authors pointed out that fibers accumulated in the visceral and parietal pleura and pericardium, with involvement of the adjacent lung. Asbestos also appeared on the serous surface of abdominal viscera and retroperitoneal surfaces. The serosal surface reacted by adhesions, thickening of fibrous capsules, and disseminated fibrotic nodules. The mesotheliomas noted were usually multifocal. Early distribution of asbestos fibers was studied by Kanazawa *et al.*[145] after subcutaneous injection of mice.

Ingestion Exposure

Human exposure to asbestos and related substances by ingestion is rather widespread and has been the subject of a recent workshop[146] that produced a summary of exposure assessment, epidemiological studies and bioassay, control, and other matters. Condie[147] reviewed various reports of laboratory experiments involving ingestion of chrysotile, crocidolite, amosite, talc, taconite tailings, cellulose fibers, contaminated tap water, and diatomaceous earth. Exposures were performed by adding the test material to the feed or drinking water in amounts that varied from 0.15% to 10% of the diet. Rats, hamsters, and in one instance baboons were used.

Mass doses in rats varied from 5 mg per week to 20 mg per day among the various studies. The reviewer concluded that despite limitation in technique and variability in the methods that "the majority of the studies were either negative or equivocal."

Long-term studies of ingestion of amosite and chrysotile using Syrian golden hamsters were also negative.[148] At the concentration of 1% in pelleted diet, no gastric tumors were observed. This study also failed to show any synergistic reactions between chrysotile and 1,2-dimethylhydrazine dihydrochloride (DMH). In another study,[149] blocky (nonfibrous) tremolite or amosite was given to the dams of F344 rats. At 21 days after birth, the pups (F1 generation) were weaned. At eight weeks of age DMH was administered by gavage to control pups and those whose dam had received tremolite or amosite. No toxicity or increase in neoplasia was observed in pups whose dam had been exposed to tremolite. Some c-cell carcinomas of the thyroid and monocytic (mononuclear cell) leukemia in male rats were observed in the pups whose dam had been exposed to amosite. No toxic or neoplastic lesions were observed in the target organs, *i.e.*, gastrointestinal tract and mesothelium. A high rate (62% to 74%) of intestinal neoplasia was observed in the animals receiving DMH alone and in those receiving DMH whose dams had received amosite. The authors failed to show either enhancement of carcinogenic response or protective effect due to DMH and amosite exposure. Thus ingestion studies have not been successful in elucidating the tumorigenic effects of mineral fibers in animals.

Bioassay for Foreign Body Tumorigenicity

The induction of foreign body tumors has been most commonly accomplished by implanting the material subcutaneously in the flank of rats or mice. Dogs are also susceptible, while guinea pigs and chickens appear resistant. Tumors thus derived are almost invariably sarcomas, with fibrosarcomas predominating.

The studies by Brand *et al.*[110,111] appear to offer the best model for determining the tumorigenic potential of such material in the shortest possible time. The plastic material (7 mm x 15 mm or 15 mm x 22 mm) with rounded corners was inserted subcutaneously in either flank of CBA/H mice, and the incision was closed with wound clips. After three months or later, the test material was removed and cultured for *in vitro* demonstration of precancerous cells from the foreign surface and the foreign body fibrous capsule. Differentiation of the precancerous cells was based on morphology and clone-specific chromosome abnormalities. Evaluation of plastic material in the induction of sarcoma has been carried out in mice by Oppenheimer *et al.*[106] and Autian *et al.*[109] Tumors induced through subcutaneous insertion have been chiefly fibrosarcoma; other tumors were induced depending on the site of insertion. Generally, the number of tumors and the shortness of the induction were proportional to the size of the implant or the total area if a number of smaller insets were employed. Roughened surfaces appeared to prolong the induction period. After insertion within the flank, a fibrous capsule surrounded the inserted material. This could be palpated within three months and any tumor mass could subsequently be detected.

EVALUATION OF BIOASSAY METHODS

In conducting a bioassay of an insoluble material, the test should be done by the most sensitive means available. In selected cases this should be followed by models designed to replicate the disease by a route comparable to that seen in humans unless it is known that the method chosen accurately predicts human carcinogenesis. The two classes of insoluble materials, inorganic mineral fibers and foreign bodies discussed herein differ in their route of exposure in humans. In the former case, it is by inhalation or possibly by the ingestion of contaminated fluids, while in the latter instance it is by accidental or intentional implantation of masses or surfaces within the tissue. In the case of mineral fibers, the most sensitive *in vivo* route appears to be by injection or by implantation within the pleural or peritoneal cavities. Since both methods are simple to conduct with high tumor yield, dose-response data can be obtained with relatively few animals at fairly low cost. There is evidence however, that these two methods may not be necessarily equal in tumor yield. For instance, Maltoni *et al.*[150]

found higher tumor yields in rats with erionite in the pleural cavity while with crocidolite the yield was highest in the peritoneal cavity. This finding is congruent with the experimental studies of Wagner who showed induction of mesothelioma following exposure by inhalation to erionite to a degree never before observed from exposure to asbestos.[7] Interestingly, in 41 malignancies noted in exposed Turkish villagers there were 27 mesothelioma *versus* 8 lung cancers.[15]

At this time, it is uncertain if injection into the pleural or peritoneal cavities adequately reflect risk from exposure to asbestos in humans. It would appear, from the limited data for erionite, that there may be a good correlation with exposure by inhalation but possibly less so for asbestos. It also seems that this system would not discriminate between such factors as differing degrees of transport from the lung into the pleura or peritoneum which might be a function of physical or chemical properties of various mineral fibers. A weakness of the data from studies by the intrapleural or intraperitoneal route is that the interaction with other carcinogenic influences which may be responsible for the major portion of the human lung cancers attributable to exposure to asbestos has not been evaluated.

The fact that the induction of lung cancer has been relatively low following exposure to asbestos by inhalation may reflect the omission of an organic carcinogen and reflect only those cancers induced by the direct influence of the asbestos fiber. It would appear likely that the most complete model for replication of exposure to tumorigenic mineral fibers in humans would be a combined exposure by inhalation to both asbestos and cigarette smoke. We can find no reports of this method in the available literature. Although the addition of B(a)P results in higher tumor yields from intratracheal instillation of asbestos fibers,[90] intratracheal instillation of asbestos alone, while replicating early lesions seen in exposed animals, has not yet been a reliable method due to low yields of pulmonary tumors.

A great deal of attention has been given to the possible role of ingestion of asbestos or other inorganic material from contaminated drinking water or beverages. Thus far no consistent epidemiologic association between amount of asbestos in water and incidence of human cancer has been observed. In some studies, contamination with asbestos has not existed long enough to account for the latent period. A complete review of the subject of exposure by ingestion is available.[146] Most experimental studies by ingestion have been negative. Additionally, non-pulmonary tumors have not seemed to be a feature of inhalation studies in animals where, according to the data, more than ½ of the inhaled dose is cleared from the respiratory tract and swallowed. Each inhalation exposure thus constitutes an ingestion experiment.

Why are the experimental results incongruent with data from humans which indicate a small but consistent increase in certain extra-pulmonary tumors in persons exposed occupationally to asbestos dust?[1] The following points might be considered: 1) The penetration through the gastrointestinal tract and transport to the target organs might be insufficient (in dose) to result in statistically significant numbers of tumor considering the relatively small number of experimental animals used; 2) the physiochemical milieu of the digestive tract might inactivate the tumorigenic properties of the mineral fibers regardless of the degree of penetration or transport. Since chrysotile is the most commonly used asbestos, it is conceivable that this mechanism might explain the low numbers of extra-respiratory tract tumors in humans due to this material. Crocidolite, on the other hand, is unaffected by such treatment; thus, acid leaching cannot explain the failure of crocidolite to induce tumors in experimental animals after exposure by ingestion. The latter view appears to fit the human situation where most such tumor incidence has been reported from occupational groups exposed by inhalation. Since acid leaching by oxalic or hydrochloric acid decreases both the tumorigenicity and cytotoxicity of chrysotile, it might be postulated that such an effect might occur in the stomach.

The demands posed by potential hazards due to evaluation of the effluents from commercial asbestos now in place in man-made environments, the problem of exposure to asbestos or non-asbestos mineral fibers in the natural environment, and the need to determine the safety of various materials to be considered as substitutes require a very large bioassay effort. This would appear to be an impossible undertaking. A number of *in vitro* tests have been utilized for a number of years to demonstrate the cytotoxicity of asbestos and related substances. These are erythrocyte lysis and toxicity testing with alveolar macrophage. When silica or quartz is assayed in the same systems, its reactivity is intermediate between chrysotile and the amphiboles.[42-44] Silica, however, is usually considered non-carcinogenic in humans. The V79 bioassay, however, appears to discriminate the silica Min-U-Sil from asbestos.[151-152] This assay may thus react to a qualitative difference between silica and asbestos. It appears certain, however, that induction of tumors by asbestos from intrapleural exposure of rats is distinctly different from that induced by Min-U-Sil. The former consistently induces mesothelioma while with the latter only reticulum cell sarcomas have been noted.

Assays for cytotoxicity using alveolar macrophages have elicited the phagocytic function of macrophages. The ability of macrophages to phagocytize a long fiber by "cooperation" with other macrophages has been demonstrated. It has been speculated that this phenomenon may cause the often observed, giant multinucleated macrophages and play a role in the production of "asbestos bodies." These assays have also been used to demonstrate the release of lysosomal enzymes as an indication of cell injury.[61-65]

Primary cells of Syrian hamster embryo (SHE) have been used to explore the phenomenon of morphologic transformation which is often used for screening chemical carcinogens. Using this method, it has been shown that transformation can occur by treatment with asbestos and that the degree of the changes is related to the number and size of the mineral fibers.[84,85]

Ames tests using *Salmonella typhimurium* and WP2 assays using *E. coli* have shown negative results after exposure with mineral fiber.[87,88] A co-carcinogenic effect, however, was observed when asbestos fibers coated with B(a)P were added in the presence of S9 microsomal fractions.[89] Experiments using artificial membranes such as dipalmitoyl phosphatidylcholine (DPPC) have demonstrated a carrier effect of asbestos.[95] A higher B(a)P transport was evident when it was coated on asbestos than on non-asbestos mineral fibers.[96] In addition to the transport, a shift of B(a)P metabolite(s) to a more carcinogenic state has also been postulated.[94]

Other methods employing *in vivo* and *in vitro* techniques have also been used for eliciting the co-carcinogenic effects of asbestos in the presence of B(a)P.

Hamster tracheal tissues which had been exposed to asbestos and 3-methyl-cholanthrene (3-MC) produced squamous cell carcinomas when the tracheal tissues were implanted into syngeneic animals.[100] Similar experiments using non-asbestos mineral fibers produced no tumors. In this study, however, it was shown that the degree of adsorption and release of the chemical carcinogens was not related to the degree of carcinogenicity. It was further demonstrated that addition of asbestos to tracheal cells induced ornithine decarboxylase (ODC), an enzyme speculated as intrinsic to promotion of carcinogenicity.[101] The role of asbestos as a promoter has also been elicited in a study using tracheal transplants of F344 rats: An enhancement of tumor production was reported when tracheal explants were exposed to 7,12-dimethylbenz(a)anthracene (DMBA) prior to exposure to asbestos.[102]

RISK ASSESSMENT

There is a need to conduct a risk assessment of the potential carcinogenic effects of inert materials with which humans may come in contact either naturally or through insertion of masses into the body. In the case of inorganic fibrillar material (asbestos and related substances) where risk is certainly greatest, there are four categories where human contact may occur. These are: (1) occupational exposure from current use; (2) non-occupational exposure to asbestos now in place; (3) exposure to asbestos or asbestos-like materials in the natural environment; and (4) exposure to man-made or man-modified asbestos substitutes.

Current Use

The evidence for severe health effects from occupational exposure to commercial asbestos is overwhelming. Asbestos workers including miners, millers, fabricators and applicators, are all at high risk.[1] A study of insulation workers by Selikoff et al.[153] has yielded the largest excess of asbestos-related deaths among any occupational groups. In this study, not only were there elevated incidences of pulmonary and mesothelial tumors, but deaths from cancer of the kidney, larynx, pharynx and buccal cavity significantly increased. Elevation of other non-thoracic tumors was evident, but did not reach statistical significance.

Risk estimates from human data have been made according to a relationship of reconstructed concentration of the dust and/or duration of exposure.[154-157] Dose-response relationships for exposure to asbestos have given different slopes but a straight-line relationship for cancer when plotted against measured cumulative dose.[158,159]

In attempting to construct cumulative dose-response relationships for mesothelioma, the factor of the latent period must be considered and separated from cumulative exposure; these two factors being concurrent. Newhouse[157] has shown that those workers exposed for two years to asbestos and having left their employment, have a much higher risk than might be expected when compared with cohorts who have remained active workers in the plant for a similar period. Thus, the factor of latency after an initial or inducing dose which may be only brief must be considered along with cumulative dose. While it is certain that direct exposure to asbestos fibers poses a high risk of pulmonary cancer, other extrathoracic cancers are also associated with exposure.

Asbestos in Place

Regardless of the possible application of control measures for new application of asbestos, measurable amounts will continue to be in the environment until it is removed from structures where it is now contained and the material disposed of in safe disposal sites. It should be noted that the very fact of its removal, as for instance by building demolition and transportation and disposal of waste, constitute a threat to the environment unless carefully controlled.

Asbestos in-place poses problems in two ways: in airborne dust within buildings and by contribution to the pollution of the ambient air. Contamination within buildings has received much attention because of the publicity given to the problem of sprayed acoustical ceilings commonly used in schools and other public buildings. Many other products are likely contributors of asbestos to indoor air.[160,161] Although asbestos fibers contaminate ambient air in urban environments, the contribution of current use sources (asbestos plants and application of new material) *versus* the contribution from asbestos in place (effluents from buildings, building demolition and disposal sites) is not well known. A recent monograph has detailed the methods and other aspects of air monitoring.[162] It is suspected that exposure to ambient air may constitute some degree of hazard in urban environments.[163] It has been stated that "there seems to be little doubt as to malignant mesothelioma caused by asbestos air pollution in the United States".[164] Fibers found in ambient air tend to be different from those associated with commercial use of asbestos. They tend to be shorter which might reduce the risk factor. Other factors might modify the potential biological effect of airborne fibers since those derived from certain asbestos products are subject to wear, or are incorporated with various binders which might alter their surface activity.

Natural Environment

Risk from asbestos or asbestos-like material in the natural environment depends on its pathogenic potential and the degree and mode of exposure of the population. Potentially, such hazard could result from non-asbestos mining, quarrying, rock crushing, dust from gravel roads and exposure to agricultural soil. Serpentine rock containing chrysotile fibers has been employed as crushed paving stone on playgrounds and gravel roads in a heavily populated area.[165] There have been frequent reports of non-tumorous pleural lesions (pleural plaques) among farm workers in situations in which the soil contained a high concentration of anthopyllite or tremolite.[166-170] Timbrell,[31] on the basis of fibrous analysis of pleura of the Finnish farmers with pleural plaques, demonstrated that the absence of mesothelioma, was a function of fiber diameter. It is interesting that fibers of large diameter penetrated to the pleura but did not cause mesotheliomas. It is conceivable that a similar situation with thinner fibers would pose a risk of mesothelioma.

Mesothelioma, however, has been reported in other places where no commercial asbestos was present.[171,172] It has also been demonstrated that a nonasbestos ferroactinolite obtained from surface rocks was at least equal to amosite in the experimental induction of tumors in rats.[131]

The high mortality from exposure to natural mineral fibers in the Turkish villages has been mentioned previously. Here, the mineral most likely to be responsible is erionite,[15] a non-asbestos fibrous silicate of the zeolite series, although one report mentioned the presence of traces of naturally occurring asbestos in the area.[165] There appears no doubt that this results from naturally occurring mineral fibers. The data from experimental animals also strongly suggest that it is the erionite which is responsible for the episode. It is evident that natural sources of asbestos or other fibrous minerals are a source of risk to a greater or lesser extent, varying from an endemic disaster in the Turkish villages to the presence of rather benign pleural plaques in the case of the Finnish farmers of Karelia. Fibrous minerals are commonly present in surface rocks or soil used for many purposes.

Asbestos Substitutes

Since the extremely hazardous nature of asbestos has become known, considerable attention has been given to the development of non-hazardous substitutes. These fall into three categories: 1) Man-made vitreous fibers such as rock or mineral wool and fibrous glass; 2) natural particulate material such as attapulgite, sepiollite, vermiculite, etc; or 3) fibrous material which has been modified by coating with other minerals. Man-made vitreous fibers made by blowing or drawing molten material[173] have been used under such names as rock or mineral wool, slagwool or fibrous glass. These have been used for insulation in building material, heat ducts and the like for many years. These fibers break transversely, but do not split longitudinally into finer diameters. They can be manufactured in various diameters.[174] The finer fibers are very expensive to manufacture and are normally used only for experimental purposes. Fibers below 1 μm readily induce mesothelioma when introduced into the pleural cavity.[7,175] In contrast, inhalation studies have been negative for induction of mesothelioma.[7] While fine fibrous glass produced mesothelioma when injected into the pleural cavity, exposure of humans by inhalation did not produce these tumors. Mesothelioma has not been produced experimentally by inhalation which contrasts strikingly with asbestos and especially erionite.[175] Data in humans were reviewed by Gross[176,177] who could see no evidence of development of lung cancer or non-malignant respiratory disease. Data from a number of authors were reviewed in a recent document and no significant pulmonary disease was reported.[178] Few of the above subjects had been exposed for a sufficient time to develop malignancies on the basis of the latent period expected for asbestos. Additional studies where longer periods of exposure existed also were reviewed. It was stated that "there is some evidence that a small excess of respiratory cancer has occurred among persons who produce (man-made mineral fibers) either fibrous glass or mineral wool." However, the report later cautions that the results are equivocal at this time.

Data in humans are available for two natural substitutes, attapulgite and talc.[178] In the case of exposure to talc, two problems exist. Talc can be contaminated with asbestos fibers or it may rarely exist as fibrous talc. Some excess of pulmonary cancer has been reported for workers exposed to talc contaminated by asbestos fibers, whereas only non-malignant disease, such as alteration in respiratory function or pulmonary fibrosis, has been reported in talc workers where the talc was not contaminated. These latter biological effects appear related to the silica content of the talc. Bilateral pleural thickening from both types of talc has been reported.

Studies in animals carried out with various substitutes indicate that man-made vitreous fibers of many types elicit mesothelioma when introduced into the pleural cavity providing they are below the width necessary to induce this reaction (<1.5 μm). Wagner[7] has tested several man-made substitutes by intrapleural inoculation. He produced mesotheliomas varying from 1% to 6% incidence with a number of vitreous materials compared to 6% for UICC chrysotile. Diameter for the positive material varied from 1.30 μm to 0.46 μm for the man-made fibers and 0.19 μm for the chrysotile. In inhalation experiments with the same material, total lung tumors were: glass microfibers, 2%; rockwool, 4%; glass wool with resin, 2%; chrysotile, 25%; and controls, 0%. The authors suggest that these data are not significantly different. The same authors studied fibrous clays by intrapleural inoculation. They found in two groups of 48 animals exposed to two samples of US attapulgite 10 and 5 developed mesothelioma, respectively *versus* 9 mesotheliomas in those animals exposed to chrysotile B. The animals exposed to sepeolite, halloysite and controls had no tumors.

Data from studies in animals appear to indicate that the man-made and natural substitutes which are sufficiently fibrous readily induce mesothelioma after intrapleural inoculation. Studies by inhalation reported to date, however, show equivocal indications of pulmonary cancer and no mesothelioma. The following points might be considered for risk by substitutes: (1) Exposure of humans appears to be low; (2) data thus far are somewhat suggestive of slight excess of pulmonary cancer in persons who have been exposed long enough for the development of pulmonary tumors, but probably insufficient time for the development of mesothelioma.

Studies in animals, while readily demonstrating mesothelioma from intrapleural inoculation, have failed to induce such tumors by inhalation. In view of the probable low exposure of humans to fibers from substitutes, naturally occurring fibrous material or effluents from asbestos in place, it would appear most likely that the risk would be manifest principally in the occurrence of mesothelioma with a long latent period[1] rather than an appreciable excess of pulmonary cancer. Another factor which might be considered, at least in the case of school room exposure of younger children, is that no concomitant exposure to tobacco smoke would be likely. This fact poses problems for epidemiological studies since many of the potential hazards have not existed for a sufficient time to equal the median latent period for mesothelioma induction by low doses of mineral fibers. Another factor to be considered is what mechanisms induce penetration of the lung and the induction of mesothelioma. Timbrell has shown that anthophyllite fibers penetrate from the lung to the pleural cavity, but are too thick to induce mesothelioma. On the other hand, natural fibers differ in the rate of induction of mesothelioma. Wagner[7] has shown vastly augmented induction of mesothelial tumors in rats by erionite as contrasted to standard UICC asbestos fibers. Studies by Coffin *et al.*[131] suggested that their sample of ferroactinolite might have an intermediate effect. It would seem clear that there must be a better understanding of the factors which lead to induction of mesothelioma on the basis of mineralogical and biological studies before adequate risk assessment of natural and artificial fibers can be made.

A large volume of materials is either being added, artificially to the environment as in the case of substitutes, or introduced by human activity in the case of natural mineral fibers. These will require a large volume of biological testing since no reliance can be placed on data where the contamination is newly introduced or where the population potentially at risk is too small for accurate epidemiological study. It would seem most prudent to carry out integrated *in vivo* and *in vitro* testing employing UICC asbestos and other materials of differing tumorigenicity in order to develop better testing procedures.

REFERENCES

1. Selikoff, I.J., and Lee, D.H.K., *Asbestos and Disease*, New York: Academic Press (1978)
2. Wagner, J.C., Sleggs, C.A., and Marchand, P., Diffuse pleural mesothelioma and asbestos exposure in North Western Cape Province. *Br. J. Ind. Med.* 17: 260-271 (1960)
3. Newhouse, M.L., and Thompson, H., Mesothelioma of the pleura and peritoneum following exposure to asbestos in the London Area. *Br. J. Ind. Med.* 22: 261-269 (1965)
4. Bohlig, H., and Hain, E., in: *Biological Effects of Asbestos*, IARC Publication No. 8, Proceedings of a Working Conference, Lyon, France 2-6, October, 1972. (P. Bogovski, J.C. Gilson, V. Timbrell, and J.C. Wagner, eds.) (1973)
5. Nicholson, W.J., Sevoszowski, Jr., E.J., Porohl, A.N., Todaro, J.D., and Adams, A., Asbestos contamination in the U.S. state schools from use of asbestos surfacing material. *Ann. N. Y. Acad. Sci.* 330: 587-596 (1979)
6. Nicholson, W.J., and Pundsack, F.L., in: *Biological Effects of Asbestos*, pp 126-130, IARC publication No. 8. Proceedings of a Working Conference, Lyon, France 2-6, October, 1972. (P. Bogovski, J.C. Gilson, V. Tembrell, and J.C. Wagner, eds.) (1973)
7. Wagner, J.C., in: *Proceedings World Symposium on Asbestos*. Montreal, Quebec, Canada. May 25-27, 1982
8. Kleinfeld, M., Messite, J., and Zaki, M.E., Mortality experiences among talc workers: A follow-up study. *J. Occup. Med.* 16: 345 (1974)
9. Rohl, A.N., Langer, A., and Selikoff, I.J., Environmental asbestos pollution related to use of quarried serpentine rock. *Science* 196: 1319-1322 (1977)
10. Kiviluoto, R., Pleural plaque and asbestos: Further observation on endemic and other non-occupational asbestos. *Ann. N.Y. Acad. Sci.* 132: 235-239 (1965)
11. Baris, Y.I., Sahin, A.A., Ozesmi, M., *et al.*, An outbreak of pleural mesothelioma and chronic fibrosis pleurisy in the Village of Karin/Urgup in Anatolia. *Thorax.* 33: 181-192 (1978)
12. Wagner, M.M.F., Pathogenesis of malignant histiocytic lymphoma induced by silica in a colony of specific-pathogen-free Wistar rats. *J. Natl. Cancer Inst.* 57: 509-517 (1976)
13. Holland, L.M., Gonzales, M., Wilson, J.S., and Tillery, M.I., in: *Health Issues Related to Metal and Non-Metallic Mining* (W.L. Wagner, W.N. Rom, and J.A. Marchant, eds.), pp 485-596, Butterworth, Boston (1983)

14. Ziskind, M., Jones, R.N., and Weil, H., Silicosis. *Am. Rev. Respiratory Disease.* 113: 643–665 (1976)
15. Artvenli and Baris, B.I., Environmental fiber-induced pleuro-pulmonary diseases in an Anatolian village: An epidemiologic study. *Arch. Environ. Health* 37: 177–181 (1982)
16. Rohl, A.N., Langer, A.M., Moncure, G., Selikoff, I.J., and Fischbein, A., Endemic pleural disease associated with exposure to mixed fibrous dust in Turkey. *Science* 216: 518–520 (1982)
17. WHO-Euro 1983, A report of the proceedings of the biological effects of man-made mineral fibers. WHO-Euro, Copenhagen, 20–22, April (1983)
18. Wagner, J.C., Epidemiology of diffuse mesothelial tumors: Evidence of an association from studies in South Africa and the United Kingdom. *Ann. N.Y. Acad. Sci.* 132: 575–578 (1965)
19. Brand, G.K., in: *Cancer, A comprehensive treatis.* (Frederick F. Becker, ed.), Vol. 2, pp 661–692, Plenum Publishing Company, New York and London (1982)
20. Wagner, J.C., Experimental production of mesothelial tumors of the pleura by implementation of dusts in laboratory animals. *Nature* 196: 180–182 (1962)
21. Smith, W.E., Miller, L., and Churg, J., Respiratory tract tumors in hamsters after intratracheal benzo(a)pyrene with and without asbestos. *Proc. Am. Assoc. Cancer Res.* 9: 65 (1968)
22. Report and recommendations of the working group on asbestos and cancer. *Br. J. Ind. Med.* 22: 165–171 (1974)
23. Timbrell, V., in: *Pneumoconiosis* (H.A. Shapiro, ed.), pp 28–36, Oxford University Press, London and New York (1970)
24. Wagner, J.C., and Berry, G., in: *Biological Effects of Asbestos* (P. Bogovski, J.C. Gilson, V. Timbrell, J.C. Wagner, and W. Davis, eds.), IARC Scientific Publications No. 8, Proceedings of a working conference held at the International Agency for Research on Cancer, Lyon, France, 2–6 October 1972, pp 85–88, International Agency for Research on Cancer, Lyon (1973)
25. Bragg, W.L., and Claringbull, G.F., *Crystal Structure of Minerals*, London: pp 314–320, Bell (1965)
26. Harington, J.S., Allison, A.C., and Badami, D.V., in: *Advances in Pharmacology and Chemotherapy* (S. Garattini, F. Hawking, A. Goldin, I.J. Kopin, and R.J. Schnitzer, eds.), Vol. 12, pp 291–402, Academic Press, New York (1975)
27. Mossmann, B.T., *In vitro* approaches for determining mechanisms of toxicity and carcinogenicity by asbestos in the gastrointestinal respiratory tracts. *Environ Health Perspect.* 53: 155–161 (1983)
28. Stanton, M.F., and Wrench, C., Mechanisms of mesothelioma induction with asbestos and fibrous glass. *J. Natl. Cancer Inst.* 48: 797–816 (1972)
29. Stanton, M.F., Layard, M., Tegeris, A., Miller, E., May, M., and Kent, E., Carcinogenicity of fibrous glass: Pleural response in the rat in relation to fiber dimension. *J. Natl. Cancer Inst.* 58: 587–603 (1977)
30. Stanton, M.F., Layard, M., Tegeris, M., Miller, E., May, M., Morgan, E., and Smith, A., Relation of particle dimension to carcinogenicity in amphibole asbestoses and other fibrous minerals. *J. Natl. Cancer Inst.* 67: 965–975 (1981)
31. Timbrell, V., Deposition and retention of fibres in the human lung. *Ann. Occup. Hyg.* 26: 347–369 (1982)

32. Gross, P., Is short-fibered asbestos dust a biological hazard? *Arch. Environ. Health* 29: 115-117 (1974)

33. Cook, P.M., Palekar, L.D., and Coffin. D.L., Interpretation of the carcinogenicity of amosite asbestos and ferroactinolite on the basis of retained fiber dose and characteristics *in vivo. Toxicol. Lett.* 13: 151-158 (1982)

34. Morgan, A., Holmes, A., and Gold, C., Studies of the solubility of constituents of chrysotile asbestos *in vivo* using radioactive tracer techniques. *Environ. Res.* 4: 558-570 (1971)

35. Thomassin, J.H., Goni, J., Baillif, P., and Touray, J.C., An XPS study of the dissolution kinetics of chrysotile in 0.1 N oxalic acid at different temperatures. *Phys. Chem. Miner.* 1: 385-398 (1976)

36. Goni, J., Thomassin, J.H., Jaurand, M.C., and Touray, J.C., in: Origin and Distribution of the Elements (L.H. Ahrens, ed.), pp 807-817, Pergamon Press, Oxford (1979)

37. Langer, A.M., Rubin, I.B., and Selikoff, I.J., Chemical characterization of asbestos lody cores by electron microprobe analysis. *J. Histochem. Cytochem.* 20: 723-734 (1972)

38. Langer, A.M., Rubin, I.B., Selikoff, I.J., and Pooley, F.D., Chemical characterization of uncoated asbestos fibers from the lungs of asbestos workers by electron microprobe analysis. *J. Histochem. Cytochem.* 20: 734-740 (1972)

39. Juarand, M.C., Sebastien, P., Bignon, J., and Goni, J., Leaching of chrysotile asbestos in human lungs. Correlation with *in vitro* studies using rabbit alveolar macrophages. *Environ. Res.* 14: 245-254 (1977)

40. Morgan, A., Davies, P., Wagner, J.C., Berry, G., and Holmes, A., The biological effects of magnesium-leached chrysotile asbestos. *Br. J. Exp. Pathol.* 58: 465-473 (1977)

41. Monchaux, G., Bignon, J., Juarand, M.C., Lafuma, J., Sebastien, P., Masse, R., Hirsch, A., and Goni, G., Mesotheliomas in rats following inoculation with acid-leached chrysotile asbestos and other mineral fibers. *Carcinogenesis* 2: 229-236 (1981)

42. Schnitzer, R.J., and Pundsack, F.L., Asbestos hemolysis. *Environ. Res.* 3: 1-13 (1970)

43. Harington, J.S., Miller, K., and Macnab, G., Hemolysis by asbestos. *Environ. Res.* 4: 95-117 (1971)

44. Rahman, Q., Narang, S., Kaw, J.L., and Zaidi, S.H., Asbestos induced haemolysis in relation to its silica solubility. *Environ. Physiol. Biochem.* 4: 284-288 (1974)

45. Light, W.G., and Wei, E.T., Surface charge and asbestos toxicity. *Nature* 265: 537-539 (1977)

46. Light, W.G., and Wei, E.T., Surface charge and hemolytic activity of asbestos. *Environ. Res.* 13: 135-145 (1977)

47. Desai, R., and Richards, R.J., The adsorption of biological macromolecules by mineral dusts. *Environ. Res.* 16: 449-464 (1978)

48. Juarand, M.C., Thomassin, J.H., Baillif, P., Magne, L., Touray, J.C., and Bignon, J., Chemical and photoelectron spectrometry analysis of the adsorption of phospholipid model membranes and red blood cell membranes to chrysotile fibers. *Br. J. Ind. Med.* 37: 169-174 (1980)

49. Juarand, M.C., Magne, L., Boulmier, J.L., and Bignon, J., *In vitro* activity of alveolar macrophages and red blood cells with asbestos fibres treated with oxalic acid, sulfur dioxide and benzo-3,4-pyrene. *Toxicology* 21: 323-342 (1981)

50. Reiss, B., Solomon, S., Weisburger, J.H., and Williams, G.M., Comparative toxicities of different forms of asbestos in a cell culture assay. *Environ. Res.* 22: 109–129 (1983)

51. Langer, A.M., Wolff, M.S., Rohl, A.N., and Selikoff, I.J., Variation of properties of chrysotile asbestos subjected to milling. *J. Toxicol. Environ. Health* 4: 173–188 (1978)

52. Palekar, L.D., Spooner, C.M., and Coffin, D.L., in: *Health Hazards of Asbestos Exposure* (I.J. Selikoff and E.C. Hammond, eds.), Ann. N.Y. Acad. Sci. 330: 673–704 (1979)

53. Dement, J.M., Marschant, J.A., and Green, F.H.Y., in: *Occupational Respiratory Disease* (J.A. Marschant, B.A. Boelecke, and G. Taylor, eds.), National Institute for Occupational Safety and Health (in press)

54. Gross, P., and deTreville, R.T.P., Experimental asbestosis. *Arch. Environ. Health* 15: 638–649 (1967)

55. Davis, J.M.G., Long term fibrogenic effects of chrysotile and crocidolite asbestos dust injected into the pleural cavity of experimental animals. *Br. J. Exp. Pathol.* 51: 617–627 (1970)

56. Heppleston, A.G., and Styles, J.S., Activity of a macrophage factor in collagen formation by silica. *Nature* (London) 214: 521–522 (1967)

57. Heppleston, A.G., Fibrogenic action of silica. *Brit. Med. Bull.* 25: 282–287 (1969)

58. Heppleston, A.G., in: *Pneumoconiosis* (H.A. Shapiro, ed.), pp 496–498, Oxford University Press, London and New York (1970)

59. Richards, R.J., Wusteman, F.S., and Dodgson, K.S., The direct effects of dusts on lung fibroblasts grown *in vitro*. *Life Sci.* 10: 1149–1159 (1971)

60. Richards, R.J., and Morris, T.G., Collagen and mucopolysaccharide production in growing lung fibroblasts exposed to chrysotile asbestos. *Life Sci.* 12: 441–451 (1973)

61. Parazzi, E., Pernis, B., Secchi, G.C., and Vigiliani, E.C., Studies on "*in vitro*" cytotoxicity of asbestos dust. *Med. Lavoro* 59: 561–576 (1968)

62. Parazzi, E., Secchi, G.C., Pernis, B., and Vigliani, E.C., Studies on the cytotoxic action of silica dusts on macrophages *in vitro*. *Arch. Environ. Health* 17: 850–859 (1968)

63. Davies, P., Allison, A.C., Ackerman, J., Butterfield, A., and Williams, S., Asbestos induces selective release of lysosomal enzymes from mononuclear phagocytes. *Nature* 251: 423–425 (1974)

64. Juarand, M.C., Magne, L., and Bignon, J., in: *The In Vitro Effects of Mineral Dusts* (R.C. Brown, M. Chamberlain, R. Davies, and I.P. Gormley, eds.), pp 83–87, Academic Press, London, New York, Toronto, Sydney, San Francisco (1980)

65. Juarand, M.C., Magne, L., Boulmier, J.L., and Bignon, J., *In vitro* activity of alveolar macrophages and red blood cells with asbestos fibers treated with oxalic acid, sulfur dioxide and benzo-3,4-pyrene. *Toxicology* 21: 323–342 (1981)

66. Pernis, B., and Castano, P., Effecto del asbesto sulle cellule *in vitro*. *Med. Lavoro* 62: 120–129 (1971)

67. Allison, A.C., in: *Biological Effects of Asbestos* (P. Bogovski, J.C. Gilson, V. Timbrell, J.C. Wagner, and W. Davis, eds.), IARC Scientific Publications No. 8, Proceedings of a working conference held at the International Agency for Research on Cancer, Lyon, France, 2–6 October 1972, pp 89–93, International Agency for Research on Cancer, Lyon (1973)

68. Miller, K., and Harrington, J.S., Some biochemical effects of asbestos on macrophages. *Br. J. Exp. Pathol.* 53: 397–405 (1972)

69. Beck, E.G., Holt, P.F., and Nasrallah, E.T., Effects of chrysotile and acid-treated chrysotile on macrophage cultures. *Br. J. Ind. Med.* 28: 179–185 (1971)
70. Mossman, B.T., and Craighead, G.E., Use of hamster tracheal organ culture for assessing carcinogenic effect of inorganic particulates on the respiratory epithelium. *Prog. Exp. Tumor Res.* 24: 37–45 (1979)
71. Mossman, B.T., Adler, K.B., Jean, L., and Craighead, J.E., Mechanisms of hypersecretion in rodent tracheal explants after exposure to chrysotile asbestos. *Chest* 81: 235–245 (1982)
72. Hart, R.W., Fertel, R., Newman, H.A.I., Daniel, F.B., and Blakeslee, J.R., *Effects of Selected Asbestos Fibers on Cellular and Molecular Parameters,* EPA Report #600/1-79-021, Health Effects Research Laboratory, Office of Research and Development, U.S. Environmental Protection Agency, Cincinnati (1979)
73. Mossman, B.T., Eastman, A., Landesman, M.J., and Bresnick, E., Effects of crocidolite and chrysotile asbestos on cellular uptake and metabolism of benzo(a)pyrene in hamster tracheal epithelial cells. *Environ. Health Perspect.* 51: 331–336 (1983)
74. Lechner, J.F., Haugen, A., Tokiwa, T., Trump, B.F., and Harris, C.C., in: *Human Carcinogenesis* (C.C. Harris and H. Autrup, eds.), Academic Press, New York (in press)
75. Livingston, G.C., Rom, W.N., and Morris, M.V., Asbestos-induced sister chromatid exchanges in cultured Chinese hamster ovarian fibroblast cells. *J. Environ. Pathol. Toxicol.* 4: 373–382 (1980)
76. Price-Jones, M.J., Gubbings, G., and Chamberlain, M., The genetic effects of crocidolite asbestos; comparison of chromosome abnormalities and sister chromatid exchanges. *Mutation Res.* 79: 331–336 (1980)
77. Casey, G., Sister-chromatid exchange and cell kinetics in CHO-K1 cells, human fibroblasts and lymphoblastoid cells exposed *in vitro* to asbestos and glass fibre. *Mutation Res.* 116: 369–377 (1983)
78. Sincock, A., and Seabright, M., Induction of chromosome changes in Chinese hamster cells by exposure to asbestos fibers. *Nature* (London) 257: 56–58 (1975)
79. Huang, S.L., Saggioro, D., Michelmann, H., and Malling, H.V., Genetic effects of crocidolite asbestos in Chinese hamster lung cells. *Mutation Res.* 57: 225–232 (1978)
80. Huang, S.L., Amosite, chrysotile and crocidolite asbestos are mutagenic in Chinese hamster lung cells. *Mutation Res.* 68: 265–275 (1979)
81. Valerio, F., deFerrari, M., Otagio, L., Reptto, E., and Santi, L., in: *IARC Scientific Publication No. 30,* pp 485–489, International Agency for Research on Cancer, Lyon, France (1980)
82. Sincock, A.M., Delhanty, J.D.A., and Casey, G., A comparison of the cytogenetic response to asbestos and glass fibre in Chinese hamster and human cell lines. *Mutation Res.* 101: 257–268 (1982)
83. DiPaolo, J.A., DeMarinis, A.J., and Doniger, J., Asbestos and benzo(a)pyrene synergism in the transformation of Syrian hamster embryo cells. *J. Environ. Pathol. Toxicol.* 5: 535–543 (1982)
84. Hesterberg, T.W., Cummings, T., Brody, A.R., Barrett, J.C., Asbestos induces morphological transformation in Syrian hamster embryo cells in culture. *J. Cell Biol.* 95: 449 (1982)
85. Hesterberg, T.W., Tsutsui, T., and Barrett, J.C., Neoplastic transformation of Syrian hamster embryo (SHE) cells by asbestos and fiberglass: The importance of fiber dimension. *Proc. Am. Assoc. Cancer Res.* (in press)

86. Poole, A., Brown, R.C., Turver, C.J., Skidmore, J.W., and Griffiths, D.M., *In vitro* genotoxic activities of fibrous erionite. *Br. J. Cancer* 47: 697–705 (1983)
87. Chamberlain, M., and Tarmy, E.M., Asbestos and glass fibers in bacterial mutation tests. *Mutation Res.* 43: 159–164 (1977)
88. Light, W.G., and Wei, E.T., in: *The In Vitro Effects of Mineral Dusts* (R.C. Brown, I.P. Gormley, M. Chamberlain and R. Davies, eds.), pp 139–145, Academic Press, New York (1980)
89. Szyba, K., and Lange, A., A carrier function of asbestos fibres in benzo(a)-pyrene mutagenicity. *Arch. Immunol. Ther. Exp.* 30: 257–260 (1982)
90. Shabad, L.M., Pylev, L.N., Krivosheeva, L.V., Kulagina, T.F., and Nemenko, B.A., Experimental studies on asbestos carcinogenicity. *J. Natl. Cancer Inst.* 52: 1175–1187 (1974)
91. Bignon, J., and Juarand, M.C., Biological *in vitro* and *in vivo* responses of chrysotile versus amphiboles. *Environ. Health Perspect.* 51: 73–80 (1983)
92. Szyba, K., and Lange, A., Presentation of benzo(a)pyrene to microsomal enzymes by asbestos fibers in the *Salmonella*/mammalian microsome mutagenicity test. *Environ. Health Perspect.* 51: 337–341 (1983)
93. Daniel, F.B., *In vitro* assessment of asbestos genotoxicity. *Environ. Health Perspect.* 53: 163–167 (1983)
94. Eneanya, D.T., Daniel, F.B., and Hart, R.W., Effect of asbestos (chrysotile intermediate) on the metabolism of benzo(a)pyrene in Syrian hamster embryo cells. *Fed. Proc.* 38: 542 (1979)
95. Lakowicz, J.R., and Hylden, J.L., Asbestos-mediated membrane uptake of benzo(a)pyrene observed by fluorescence spectroscopy. *Nature* 275: 446–448 (1978)
96. Lakowicz, J.R., Bevan, D.R., and Riemer, S.C., Transport of a carcinogen, benzo(a)pyrene, from particulates to lipid bilayers. *Biochem. Biophys. Acta* 629: 243–258 (1980)
97. Lakowicz, J.R., and Bevan, D.R., Effects of asbestos, iron oxide, silica, and carbon black on the microsomal availability of benzo(a)pyrene. *Biochemistry* 18: 5170–5176 (1979)
98. Kandaswami, C., and O'Brien, P.J., Effects of asbestos on membrane transport and metabolism of benzo(a)pyrene. *Biochem. Biophys. Res. Commun.* 97: 794–801 (1980)
99. Pawlak, A.L., Factors affecting benzo(a)pyrene activation in mammalian cells. *Arch. Immunol. Ther. Exp.* 30: 247–255 (1982)
100. Mossman, B.T., and Craighead, J.F., in: *Inhaled Particles. Annals. Occupational Hygiene*, Vol. 26, pp 572–585, Pergamon Press, London (1982)
101. Landesman, J.M., and Mossman, B.T., Induction of ornithine decarboxylase in hamster tracheal epithelial cells exposed to asbestos and 12-0-tetradecanoyl phorbol acetate. *Cancer Res.* 42: 3669–3675 (1982)
102. Topping, D.C., and Nettesheim, P., Two-stage carcinogenesis studies with asbestos in Fischer 344 rats. *J. Natl. Cancer Inst.* 65: 627–630 (1980)
103. Topping, D.C., Nettesheim, P. and Martin, D.H., Toxic and tumorigenic effects of asbestos on tracheal mucosa. *J. Environ. Pathol. Toxicol.* 3: 261–275 (1980)
104. Haugen, A., Schafer, P.W., Lechner, J.F., Stoner, G.D., Trump, B.F., and Harris, C.C., Cellular ingestion, toxic effects, and lesions observed in human bronchial epithelial tissue and cells cultured with asbestos and glass fibers. *Int. J. Cancer* 30: 265–272 (1982)
105. Oppenheimer, B.S., Oppenheimer, E.T., and Stout, A.P., Sarcomas induced in rodents by embedding various plastic films. *Proc. Soc. Exp. Biol. Med.* 79: 366–369 (1952)

106. Oppenheimer, B.S., Oppenheimer, E.T., Danishefsky, I., Stout, A.P., and Eirich, R., Further studies of polymers as carcinogenic agents in animals. *Cancer Res.* 15: 333–340 (1955)

107. Kordon, H.A., Localized interfacial forces resulting from implanted plastics as possible physical factors involved in tumor formation. *J. Theor. Biol.* 17: 1–11 (1967)

108. Alexander, P., and Horning, E.S., in: *Ciba Foundation Symposium on Carcinogenesis: Mechanisms of Action* (G.E.W. Wolstenholme, and N. O'Connor, eds.), pp 12–25, Little, Brown, & Co., Boston (1959)

109. Autian, J., Singh, A.R., Turner, J.E., Hung, G.W.C., Nunez, L.J., and Lawrence, W.H., Carcinogenesis from polyurethane. *Cancer Res.* 35: 1591–1596 (1975)

110. Brand, K.G., Buoen, L.C., and Brand, I., Foreign-body tumorigenesis in mice: most probable number of originator cells. *J. Natl. Cancer Inst.* 51: 1071–1074 (1973)

111. Brand, K.G., Buoen, L.C., and Brand, I., Multiphasic incidence of foreign-body-induced sarcomas. *Cancer Res.* 36: 3681–3683 (1976)

112. Nordmann, M., and Sorge, A., Lungenkrebs durch Asbestastaub in Tierversuch (Pulmonary cancer produced by asbestos dust in animal experiments) *Z. Krebsforsch.* 51: 168–182 (1941)

113. Holt, P.F., Mills, J., and Young, D.K., The early effects of chrysotile asbestos dust on the rat lung. *J. Pathol. Bacteriol.* 87: 15–23 (1964)

114. Wagner, J.C., Asbestosis in experimental animals. *Br. J. Ind. Med.* 20: 1–12 (1963)

115. Wagner, J.C., Berry, G., Skidmore, J.W., and Timbrell, V., The effects of the inhalation of asbestos in rats. *Br. J. Cancer* 29: 252–268 (1974)

116. Timbrell, V., Skidmore, J.W., Hyett, A.W., and Wagner, J.C., Exposure chambers for inhalation experiments with standard reference samples of asbestos of the International Union Against Cancer (UICC). *Aerosol Sci.* 1: 215–223 (1970)

117. Morris, T.G., Roberts, W.H., Silverton, R.E., Skidmore, J.W., Wagner, J.C., and Cook, G.W., in: *Inhaled Particles and Vapours* II (C.N. Davies, ed.), pp 205, Pergamon Press, Oxford (1967)

118. Evans, J.C., Evans, R.J., Holmes, A., Hounam, R.F., Jones, D.M., Morgan, A. and Walsh, M., Studies on the deposition of inhaled fibrous material in the respiratory tract of the rat and its subsequent clearance using radioactive tracer techniques. 1. UICC Crocidolite asbestos. *Environ. Res.* 6: 180–201 (1973)

119. Timbrell, V., Pooley, F., and Wagner, J.C., in: *Pneumoconiosis: Proceedings of the International Conference Johannesberg* (1969) (H.A. Shapiro, ed.), pp 120–125, Oxford University Press, Capetown (1970)

120. Davis, J.M.G., The ultrastructural changes that occur during the transformation of lung macrophages to giant cells and fibroblasts in experimental asbestosis. *Br. J. Exp. Pathol.* 44: 568–575 (1963)

121. Lee, K.P., Barras, C.E., Griffith, F.D., and Waritz, R.S., Pulmonary response to glass fiber by inhalation exposure. *Lab. Invest.* 40: 123–133 (1979)

122. Brody, A.R., Hill, L.H., Adkins, B., Jr., and O'Connor, R.W., Chrysotile asbestos inhalation in rats: deposition pattern and reaction of alveolar epithelium and pulmonary macrophages. *Am. Rev. Respir. Dis.* 123: 670–679 (1981)

123. Brody, A.R., and Hill, L.H., Interstitial accumulation of inhaled chrysotile asbestos fibers and consequent formation of microcalcifications. *Am. J. Pathol.* 109: 107–114 (1982)

124. Coleman, G.L., Barthold, S.W., Osbaldiston, G.W., Foster, S.J., and Jonas, A.M., Pathological changes during aging in barrier-reared Fischer 344 male rats. *J. Gerontology* 32: 258–278 (1977)
125. Wagner, J.C., Experimental studies and the pathology of asbestos-induced lung diseases. *Archivum Immunol. Ther. Exp.* 30: 221–228 (1982)
126. Gross, P., de Treville, R.T.P., and Cralley, L.J., in: *Pneumoconiosis: Proceedings Intl. Conf., Johannesburg, 1969* (H.A. Shapiro, ed.), pp 220–224, Oxford University Press, Capetown (1970)
127. Bozelka, B.E., Sestini, P., Gaumer, H.R., Hammad, Y., Heather, C.J., and Salvaggio, J.E., A murine model of asbestosis. *Am. J. Pathol.* 112: 326–337 (1983)
128. Saffiotti, V., Montesano, R., Sellakumar, A.R., and Kaufman, D.G., Respiratory tract carcinogenesis in hamsters induced by different numbers of administration of benzo(a)pyrene and ferric oxide. *Cancer Res.* 32: 1073–1078 (1972)
129. King, E.J., Mohanty, G.P., Harrison, C.V., and Nagelschmidt, G., The actions of different forms of pure silica on the lungs of rats. *Br. J. Ind. Med.* 10: 9–17 (1953)
130. Smith, W.E., Miller, L., Elasser, R.E., and Hubert, D.D., Tests for carcinogenicity of asbestos. *N.Y. Acad. Sci.* 132: 456–487 (1967)
131. Coffin, D.L., Palekar, L.D., and Cook, P.M., Tumorigenesis by a ferroactinolite mineral. *Toxicol. Lett.* 13: 143–150 (1982)
132. Wagner, J.C., and Berry, G., Mesotheliomas in rats following inoculation with asbestos. *Br. J. Cancer* 23: 567–581 (1969)
133. Wagner, J.C., Tumors in experimental animals following exposure to asbestos dust. *Ann. d'Anatomie Pathologique* 21: 211–214 (1976)
134. Davis, J.M.G., The fibrogenic effects of mineral dusts injected into the pleural cavity of mice. *Br. J. Exp. Pathol.* 53: 190–201 (1972)
135. Morgan, A., Holmes, A., and Gold, C., Studies of the solubility of constituents of chrysotile asbestos *in vivo* using radioactive tracer techniques. *Environ. Res.* 4: 558–570 (1971)
136. LaFuma, J., Morin, M., Poncy, J.L., Masse, R., Hirch, A., Bignon, J., and Morchaux, G., in: *IARC Scientific Publication Vol. 30, Biological Effects of Mineral Fibers*, Vol. 1, pp 311–320, International Agency for Research on Cancer, Lyon (1980)
137. Wagner, J.C., Berry, G., and Timbrell, V., Mesothelioma in rats following inoculation with asbestos. *Br. J. Cancer.* 23: 567–581 (1969)
138. Wagner, J.C., Berry, G., and Timbrell, V., Mesothelioma in rats after inoculation with asbestos and other material. *Br. J. Cancer* 28: 173–185 (1973)
139. Pike, M.C., A method of analysis of a certain class of experiments in carcinogenesis. *Bionetics* 22: 142–161 (1966)
140. Friedrichs, K.H. *et al.*, Study of tissue reaction and fiber distribution in abdominal granulomas and lymph nodes of the rat following intraperitoneal administration of various amphiboles. *Int. Arch. Arbeitsmed.* 28: 341–354 (1972)
141. Pott, F., Huth, F., and Friedrichs, K.H., Tumorigenic effects of fibrous dust in experimental animals. *Environ. Health Perspect.* 9: 313–315 (1974)
142. Pott, F., Huth, F., Spurny, K., in: IARC Scientific Publications No. 30, *Biological Effects of Mineral Fibers*, Vol. 1 (J.C. Wagner, ed.), pp 337–342, International Agency for Research on Cancer, Lyon (1980)
143. Davis, J.M.G., Histogenesis and fine structure of peritoneal tumors produced in animals by injections of asbestos. *J. Natl. Cancer Inst.* 52: 1823–1837 (1974)

144. Roe, F.J.C., Carter, R.L., Walters, M.A., and Harington, J.S., The pathological effects of subcutaneous injections of asbestos fibres in mice: Migration of fibres to submesothelial tissues and induction of mesotheliomata. *Int. J. Cancer* 2: 628-638 (1967)

145. Kanazawa, K., Birbeck, M.S.C., Carter, R.L., and Roe, F.J.C., Migration of asbestos fibres from subcutaneous injection sites in mice. *Br. J. Cancer* 24: 96-106 (1970)

146. Lucier, G.W., and Hook, G.E.R. (eds.), Summary Workshop on Ingested Asbestos, October 13-14, 1982, Cincinnati, Ohio, *Environ. Health Perspect.,* Vol. 53, U.S. Dept. of Health and Human Services, Public Health Service—National Institute of Health, National Institute of Environmental Health Sciences (1983)

147. Condie, L.W., Review of published studies of orally administered asbestos. *Environ. Health Perspect.* 53: 3-9 (1983)

148. McConnell, E.E., Shefner, A.M., Rust, J.H., and Moore, J.A., Chronic effects of dietary exposure to amosite and chrysotile asbestos in Syrian golden hamsters. *Environ. Health Perspect.* 53: 11-25 (1983)

149. McConnell, E.E., Rutter, H.A., Ulland, B.m., and Moore, J.A., Chronic effects of dietary exposure to amosite asbestos and tremolite in F344 rats. *Environ. Health Perspect.* 53: 27-44 (1983)

150. Maltoni, C., Minardi, F., and Morisi, L., Pleural mesotheliomas in Sprague-Dawley rats by erionite: First experimental evidence. *Environ. Res.* 29: 238-244 (1982)

151. Palekar, L.D., Brown, B.G., and Coffin, D.L., Correlation of *in vivo* tumorigenesis and V79 cytotoxicity. EPA Symposium on short-term bioassays for complex environmental mixtures (In press)

152. Chamberlain, M., and Brown, R.C., The cytotoxic effects of asbestos and other mineral dust in tissue culture cell lines. *Br. J. Exp. Pathol.* 59: 183-189 (1978)

153. Selikoff, I.J., Hammond, E.C., and Seidman, H., Mortality experiences of insulation workers in the United States and Canada. (1943-1969) *Ann. N.Y. Acad. Sci.* 330: 91-116 (1979)

154. Peto, J.H., in: *Biological Effects of Mineral Fibers* (J.C. Wagner, ed.), Vol. II, pp 829-836, IARC, Lyon (1980)

155. Peto, J., Seidman, H., and Selikoff, I.J., Mesothelioma mortality in asbestos workers. Implication for models of carcinogenesis and risk assessment. *Br. J. Cancer* 45: 124-135 (1982)

156. Nicholson, W.J., Selikoff, I.J., Seidman, H., Lilis, R., and Formby, P., Long term mortality experience. *Ann. N.Y. Acad. Sci.* 330: 11-21 (1979)

157. Newhouse, M.L., and Berry, G., Patterns of mortality in asbestos factory workers in London. *Ann. N.Y. Acad. Sci.* 330: 53-60 (1979)

158. Dement, J.M., Harris, R.L., Symons, M.J., and Shy, C., Estimates of dose-response for respiratory cancer among chrysotile asbestos textile workers. *Ann. Occup. Hyg.* 26: 869-887 (1979)

159. Henderson, V., and Enterline, P.E., Asbestos exposure: Factors associated with excess cancer and respiratory disease mortality. *Ann. N.Y. Acad. Sci.* 330: 117-126 (1979)

160. Nicholson, W.J., Rohl, A.N., Sawyer, E.J., Swoszowski, J.D., Control of sprayed asbestos surfaces in school buildings: A feasibility study. Report to the National Institute of Environmental Health Sciences, June 15, (1978)

161. Sawyer, R.N., Indoor asbestos pollution. Application of hazard criterion. *Ann. N.Y. Acad. Sci.* 330: 129-132 (1979)

162. Chatfield, E.J., Measurement of asbestos fibre concentrations in ambient atmospheres. A study prepared for the Royal Commission on Matters of Health and Safety Arising from the Use of Asbestos in Ontario. pp 1-115 (1983)
163. Bohlig, H., and Haine, E., in: *Biological Effects of Asbestos.* IARC Scientific Publication No. 8, (P. Bogovski, J.C. Gilson, V. Timbrell, and J.C. Wagner, eds.), Proceedings of a Working Conference held at the International Agency for Research on Cancer, Lyon, France, 2-6 October (1972)
164. Enterline, P.E., and Marsh, G.M., The health of workers in the man-made mineral fiber industry. Presented at the biological effects of man-made mineral fibers, Occupational Health Conference, WHO-EURO, Copenhagen, April 20, (1982)
165. Rohl, A.N., Langer, A.M., Moncure, G., Selikoff, I.J., and Fischbein, A., Endemic pleural disease associated with exposure to mixed fibrous dust in Turkey. *Science* 216: 518-520 (1982)
166. Kiviluoto, R., Pleural calcification as a roentgenological sign of non-occupational endemic anthophyllite-asbestosis. *Acta Radiol. Suppl.* 194: 1-67 (1960)
167. Kiviluoto, R., Pleural plaques and asbestos: Further observations on endemic and non-occupational asbestosis. *Ann. N.Y. Acad. Sci.* 132: 235-239 (1965)
168. Burilkov, T., and Michailova, L., Asbestos content of the soil and endemic pleural asbestosis. *Environ. Res.* 3: 443-451 (1970)
169. Navratil, M., and Trippe, F., Prevalence of pleural calcification in persons exposed to asbestos dust, and in the general population in the same district. *Environ. Res.* 5: 210-216 (1972)
170. Becklake, M.R., Asbestos-related diseases of the lungs and pleura. Editorial. *Am. Rev. Resp. Dis.* 126: 187-194 (1982)
171. Das, P.B., *et al.*, Mesothelioma in a community in India. A clinico-pathological study. *Aust. N.Z. J. Med.* 6: 218-225 (1976)
172. Milne, J.E.H., Thirty-two cases of mesothelioma in Victoria, Australia: A retrospective survey related to occupational asbestos exposure. *Br. J. Ind. Med.* 33: 115-121 (1976)
173. Klingholz, R., Technology and production of man-made mineral fibres. *Ann. Occup. Hyg.* 20: 153-159 (1977)
174. Cameron, J.D., Man-made mineral fibres: Medical Research—CIRFS/Eurima Initiative, *Ann. Occup. Hyg.* 20: 149-152 (1977)
175. Pigott, G.H., and Ishmael, J., A strategy for the design and evaluation of a 'safe' inorganic fibre. *Ann. Occup. Hyg.* 26: 371-380 (1982)
176. Gross, P., Theodos, P.A., Murphy, R.L.H., Cooper, W.C., and Morgan, W.K.C., The pulmonary response to fiberglass dust: *Chest* 69: 216-219 (1976)
177. Gross, P., Man-made vitreous fibers: Present status of research on health effects. *Int. Arch. Occup. Environ. Health.* 50: 103-112 (1982)
178. Nonoccupational health risks of asbestiform fibers, Report of committee on nonoccupational health risks of asbestiform fibers, National Academy Press. Washington, D.C., pp 1-334 (1984)

Part VII

Assays with Potential Utility

20

In Vitro Assay to Detect Inhibitors of Intercellular Communication

James E. Trosko
Cy Jone
Charles Aylsworth
Chia-cheng Chang

Michigan State University
East Lansing, Michigan

INTERCELLULAR COMMUNICATION: AN IMPORTANT BIOLOGICAL PROCESS

Intercellular communication within and between cells of various tissues is a fundamental biological process in multicellular organisms which is required to orchestrate complex mechanisms regulating cell proliferation and differentiation.[1-5] The regulation of proliferation and differentiation in various stem cells and their terminally differentiated daughter cells is accomplished by various forms of cell to cell communication mechanisms[6] (Figure 1). One form of intercellular communication is mediated by the transfer of molecules over a distance from the "signaling" cell to the "target" cell. The production of a growth factor or hormone by one cell type and the transversing of the molecule to a distal cell with a receptor is an example of this form of communication. Another form of communication is mediated by the transfer of small molecular weight molecules or ions through gap junctions.[7]

In effect, cellular and physiological homeostasis is maintained by these forms of intercellular communication, as they provide the means for feedback and cybernetic control of a multicellular organism. Normal disruption of either of these forms of intercellular communication appears to lead to adaptive responses of cells to proliferate or to perform specific differentiated functions. Inhibition of intercellular communication can be, in principle, brought about by physical removal of cells, cell death, physical blockage or isolation of cells from other cells, and by endogenous or exogenous chemicals.[8]

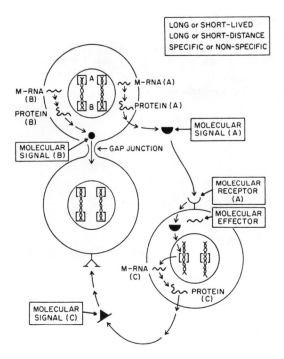

Figure 1: This heuristic diagram illustrates two general forms of inter-cellular communication. One involves the production and transmission of "signal" molecules over a distance through extracellular space to a target tissue. The other involves the transfer of "signal" molecules via permeable intercellular junctions between coupled cells.

Under certain circumstances, inhibition of intercellular communication can, in theory, be non-adaptive or harmful to the organism. During early organo-genesis, intercellular communication could lead to irreversible developmental consequences, leading either to embryo lethality or to teratogenesis.[9] With the demonstration that some teratogens can inhibit intercellular communication, and that some are cytotoxins (which can indirectly inhibit intercellular communi-cation),[10,11] it has been speculated that chemicals which can interfere with normal intercellular communication processes can be teratogens.[12]

In the developed organism, many specialized processes; *i.e.*, spermato-genesis, depend on delicate intercellular communication mechanisms to affect the proper maturation of sperm cells from the spermatogonia. The observation that this maturation is dependent on gap junction-mediated communication be-tween the Sertoli-Leydig cells and the maturing sperm-forming cells[13] implies that disruption of this form of intercellular communication would lead to a-spermia. It has been speculated that many reproductive toxicants might act by inhibiting this form of intercellular communication.[14]

Of the many significant observations which relate to carcinogenesis is the fact that cancer cells do not seem to respond to normal body signals (*i.e.*, they appear to be a "disease of homeostatic dysfunction";[15] a "disease of differentiation"[16]), nor do they contact inhibit properly.[17,18] With the demonstration of the multi-stage nature of carcinogenesis,[19-21] being conceptualized as the result of the conversion of a normal cell to a premalignant cell (initiation phase) and the clonal amplification of the premalignant cell to a "critical" mass (promotion phase) where a premalignant cell is transformed to a malignant cell,[8] it has been possible to demonstrate that the mechanisms of initiation and promotion are quite distinct.[22,24]

The recent observation that many tumor promoters,[25-46] but not tumor initiators,[36,45] can inhibit a form of intercellular communication *in vitro*, led Yotti *et al.*[25] and Murray and Fitzgerald[26] to speculate that chemicals which block intercellular communication have the potential of being tumor promoters.

Therefore, based on the aforementioned evidence, it seems that a technique to detect, *in vitro*, chemicals having the ability to inhibit intercellular communication, has the potential of detecting potential teratogens, tumor promoters and reproductive toxicants (as well as other disease states which might be the result of dysfunctional intercellular communication).

METABOLIC COOPERATION: *IN VITRO* MEANS TO MEASURE INTERCELLULAR COMMUNICATION

Based on the assumption that disruption of intercellular communication can lead to potentially harmful biological consequences, it has been postulated that by using various means *in vitro*, one could measure intercellular communication.[39] We will limit both the review and discussion to gap junction-mediated intercellular communication (not that the non-gap junction-mediated form is unimportant).

There have been several approaches to measure gap junction-mediated intercellular communication. One is to label donor cells with either radioactive or fluorescent molecules which can be transferred via gap junctions after co-cultivation with unlabeled recipient cells. Another is to co-cultivate cells with and without functional hypoxanthine guanine-phosphoribosyltransferase (HG-PRT). The phenomenon of "metabolic cooperation" was observed to occur when HG-PRT$^+$ cells (those cells having HG-PRT) were co-cultivated with HG-PRT$^-$ cells (mutant cells lacking HG-PRT) in the presence of the drug 8-azaguanine or 6-thioguanine (*i.e.*, the "kiss of death").[47,48] In this situation, if the HG-PRT$^+$ (6-thioguanine-sensitive) cell is coupled by gap junctions to the HG-PRT$^-$ (6-thioguanine-resistant) cell, the 6-thioguanine-sensitive cell (6TG^s can metabolize the 6-thioguanine (6TG) to a lethal substrate which, if transferred to the 6-thioguanine-resistant cell (6TG^r) by functional gap junctions, will kill not only itself, but the heretofore 6TG^r cell. We and others[25-46] have shown that many known tumor promoters have the ability to inhibit metabolic cooperation and intercellular communication.

EXPERIMENTAL PROTOCOL TO MEASURE METABOLIC COOPERATION

Rationale

The phenomenon of metabolic cooperation is a form of intercellular communication in which a mutant phenotype of enzyme-deficient cells is corrected by normal cells or by different mutant cells. Two types of metabolic cooperation are known: one which requires cell to cell contact; the other does not. The specific kind of metabolic cooperation to be used to detect chemicals capable of interfering with intercellular communication is the hypoxanthine-guanine phosphoribosyltransferase (HG-PRT) system described by Subak-Sharpe *et al.*[47]

Cells, lacking HG-PRT activity (designated HG-PRT⁻), are resistant to the drug, 6-thioguanine (6TG) and will form colonies under conditions in which wild-type cells, HG-PRT⁺, are killed. If a mixture of HG-PRT⁺ and HG-PRT⁻ cells is co-cultivated in medium containing 6TG such that physical contact is made between the two types of cells, metabolic cooperation can take place between HG-PRT⁺ and HG-PRT⁻ cells by which the phosphorylated 6TG is transferred from HG-PRT⁺ cells to the HG-PRT⁻ cells. Under these circumstances, the HG-PRT⁻ cells are killed even though they lack a functional HG-PRT gene.

Using this system, Yotti *et al.*[25] observed that tumor promoting phorbol esters could rescue HG-PRT⁻ Chinese hamster V79 cells at non-cytotoxic doses in a stoichiometric manner after a "no-effect" level of the chemicals is used. The interpretation of this phorbol ester-induced rescue of HG-PRT⁻ cells was that these tumor promoters blocked the transfer of the metabolized and phosphorylated 6TG from the HG-PRT⁺ cells to the HG-PRT⁻ cells. Since the phosphorylated 6TG could only be transferred via gap junctions from one cell to the other,[49] it was inferred that these phorbol esters somehow interfered with gap junction-mediated intercellular communication. Yancey *et al.*[50] and Enomoto *et al.*,[36,40] using freeze fracture and electrocoupling techniques, respectively, showed that the phorbol esters did reduce gap junction structures/function.

Using a wide variety of techniques to measure intercellular communication in a number of cell systems *in vitro*, several investigators independently[27] or subsequently have verified these observations.[27,30,31,35,36,38,40,42,45] Based on the assumption that all tumor promoters, which act at non-cytotoxic levels (see later discussion concerning cytotoxicity as an "indirect promoter"), might act by inhibiting intercellular communication, a number of chemicals, either known or subsequently shown to be tumor promoters, have been shown to inhibit metabolic cooperation. Discrepancies, either false-positives or false-negatives, will be discussed later when we examine the limitations of the system.[39]

Cytotoxicity and Range-Finding Studies

The basic principle of this assay is the ability of a chemical to inhibit metabolic cooperation without killing cells. Consequently, prior to testing a chemical in the metabolic cooperation assay, one must determine the cytotoxicity of the chemical. Clearly, if one uses a cytotoxic level, one will reduce the density of the co-cultivated cells, thereby not only affecting the possibility of an HG-PRT⁺ and HG-PRT⁻ cell from contacting each other, but also by potentially preventing some (or all) of the HG-PRT⁻ cells from growing into colonies.

The standard and original protocol for determining cytotoxicity was to check various concentrations of the test chemicals on the colony-forming ability of 100 to 500 6TG^r cells after they had been placed in nine cm plates for four hours. The original medium was Eagle's minimal essential medium with Earle's salts, supplemented with a 100% increase of all non-essential amino acids, 50% increase of all vitamins and essential amino acids except glutamine, 1.0 mM pyruvate and 5% fetal bovine serum. The bicarbonate concentration was 1.0 g/liter.

Since the original publications on this assay,[51] we have modified it to accommodate newer findings. First, since the normal density of cells to test cytotoxicity is much less than that needed to test for metabolic cooperation (*i.e.*, 100 cells/plate compared to $4x10^5$ cells/plate), the effective concentration/cell in the two assays is not the same. For some chemicals, the concentration to kill 100 cells will be less than that needed to inhibit intercellular communication between $4x10^5$ cells.

There are two ways to bypass this potential problem. One is to use a dose of the chemical which allows approximately 60% recovery in the cytotoxicity plates for the highest dose in the metabolic cooperation cells. Just by observing the number and size of the colonies in the metabolic cooperation plates, as well as the dose response curve, one could determine if the chemical might be a non-cytotoxic inhibitor of metabolic cooperation. The other way is to co-cultivate 100 6TG^r, metabolic cooperation-deficient (MC$^-$) mutants[52] with $4x10^5$ 6TG^s Chinese hamster V79 cells in 6 cm petri dishes in the presence of 6TG and the test chemical. Under these conditions, assessment of cytotoxicity is more accurate since the cell densities will be identical to the metabolic cooperation assay. It should be noted that even with MC$^-$ cells, the survival curves for some chemicals were essentially the same as those obtained for the studies using one hundred 6TG resistant cells. The two methods should complement each other.

The protocol for conducting the cytotoxicity assays consists of three subsequent steps. The first is an approximate determination of the dose range (over several logs), wherein 100 to 500 6TG^r cells are inoculated into a few 6 cm plates, allowed to attach for four hours, and exposed to either the solvent or the solvent-chemical to be tested. Visual inspection is made after three to four days for cell division or the physical appearance of the cells.

After this preliminary experiment is performed, a second more elaborate test is done, using the aforementioned approach, but with four 60 mm plates. The test sample is added using a suitable solvent, along with 10 μg/ml of 6TG and the cells are incubated for three days. After this period, medium is removed, and fresh medium containing 10 μg/ml of 6TG is added. After two days of incubation, selective medium is replaced with additional selective medium. Following another two to three days of incubation, medium is decanted, and cells are fixed and stained with Giemsa or another suitable stain (*i.e.*, crystal violet). Surviving colonies are counted and recorded. A final cytotoxicity determination is done to "fine tune" the dose range to determine a series of non-cytotoxic concentrations and one cytotoxic (approximately 60% survival) concentration, which can be used in the metabolic cooperation assay.

The stock 6TG^s cultures should periodically be placed in HAT (hypoxanthine-aminopterin-thymidine) containing medium to remove spontaneously mutated 6TG^r cells. Later, after a few generations in HAT medium, the 6TG^S cells should be placed back into normal medium to re-adapt before being used in the assay.

Assay for Inhibition of Metabolic Cooperation

After a determination of the maximum non-cytotoxic concentration of the drug which can be used (plus one concentration giving 60% survival), a series of plates with 100 HG-PRT$^-$ (6TG^r) and 4×10^5 HG-PRT$^+$ (6TG^S) cells are plated into 6 cm cell culture dishes. Ten to twenty dishes are prepared for each test sample concentration and for the negative and positive controls. It is best to use as little solvent as possible (less than 0.5% under ideal conditions). In addition, the same amount of solvent should be used for each concentration of chemical to be tested. After four hours of incubation to allow for cell attachment, the test chemical in a suitable solvent (see later discussion on limitations of assay) is added along with 6TG at 10 μg/ml.

Following three days of incubation, the medium is removed, cells are washed and medium containing only 6TG is added. After two days, medium is replaced with additional medium containing 6TG. After an additional two to three days of incubation, surviving colonies are fixed and stained with Giemsa. Table 1 outlines the details of the assay and the use of the proper controls. Figure 2 is a photographic representation of a completed assay for inhibition of metabolic cooperation in Chinese hamster V79 cells by the test chemical, phenobarbital. The plating efficiency plates (bottom row) demonstrate that phenobarbital had no appreciable cytotoxicity to these cells over this concentration range. Positive, negative and plating efficiency controls for this assay are shown in the top row of the picture.

Table 1: Details of Assay for Inhibition of Metabolic Cooperation

Compound Added	Concentration	HGPRT$^+$ Cells (4×10^5)	HGPRT$^-$ Cells (100)	Expected No. of 6-TG^r Colonies per Dish (Theoretical)
Solvent (negative control)	highest used	+	+	0–20
Solvent (plating efficiency control)	highest used	−	+	100
Test chemical (experiment)	1	+	+	not known
	2	+	+	not known
	3	+	+	not known
	4	+	+	not known
	5	+	+	not known
Test chemical (plating efficiency)	1	−	+	90–100
	2	−	+	90–100
	3	−	+	90–100
	4	−	+	90–100
	5	−	+	90–100
TPA (positive control)	0.010 μg/ml	+	+	100

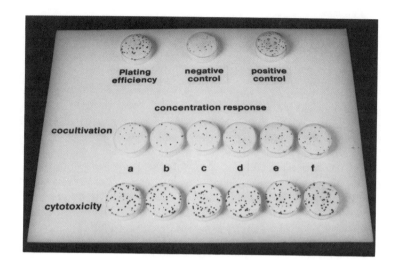

Figure 2: Photograph of sample plates of each treatment in the metabolic cooperation assay using Chinese hamster V79 cells. Negative control plates tested the effect of the solvent carrier, whereas the positive control plates tested the phorbol ester, 12-tetradecanoylphorbol-13-acetate. The test chemical was phenobarbital.

INTERPRETATION OF RESULTS: POTENTIAL AND LIMITATIONS OF THE ASSAY

In order to understand the significance of the results, there are several major concepts of which one must be aware: (a) *In vitro* assays can never be a perfect predictor of *in vivo* phenomena, since *in vivo* systems include physiological, immunological and other higher order phenomena not found in *in vitro* systems; (b) chemicals which inhibit intercellular communication might do so in the original or metabolized form; (c) *ergo*, species differences in drug metabolism and distribution *in vivo* might not be detected by a given cell line or strain *in vitro*; (d) chemicals which can inhibit intercellular communication in epithelial cells might not inhibit intercellular communication in fibroblast cells; (e) inhibition of intercellular communication, *in vivo*, can be the result of cell removal or cell death, as well as non-cytotoxic modulation of gap junctions; therefore, the *in vitro* assay to measure non-cytotoxic inhibitors of metabolic cooperation will not detect cytotoxic inhibitors; (f) modulators of gap junction-mediated intercellular communication can be useful and adaptive chemicals, as well as harmful agents, since it would depend on circumstances such as time of modulation and duration; (g) promotion appears to be a membrane-triggered process, therefore, solvents used to dissolve the test chemicals should be carefully controlled; and (h) not all chemicals which inhibit intercellular communication act the same way.

To elaborate on these points, we first must recall that it has been shown that there is species and strain specificity to the response of tumor promoters.[53-57] The basis of that specificity is not known, however, drug disposition and metabolism, as well as basic differences in cellular responses or receptors to various chemicals must be considered as likely candidates. As a result, the use of Chinese hamster V79 cells to detect all potential non-cytotoxic promoters of all cell types in all organs in all species seems highly unlikely. However, to date, most of the non-cytotoxic inhibitors of metabolic cooperation in the Chinese hamster V79 cells seem to be tumor promoters, teratogens or reproductive toxicants of various organ systems in many rodent systems [*i.e.*, 12-0-tetradecanoyl phorbol-13-acetate (TPA) as a mouse skin tumor promoter; dichlorodiphenyltrichloroethane (DDT), polybrominated biphenyls (PBB), polychlorinated biphenyls (PCB), phenobarbital as rat liver promoters and rat reproductive toxicants; oleic and linoleic acids as rat breast tumor promoters; butylated hydroxytoluene (BHT) as a rat lung tumor promoter; bile acids as rat colon tumor promoters; and saccharin as a rat bladder tumor promoter].

Tumor promoters have been shown in several model systems *in vivo* to act only if they are given at a high enough concentration to the initiated tissue, in a regular fashion and for chronic periods of time.[58]

Several *in vivo* experiments have now implicated at least three classes of chemicals which could be tumor promoters. TPA[58] and phenobarbital[59] have to be given above a threshold level, regularly and for chronic periods of time, since they are metabolized and excreted. To be physiologically effective as promoters, the organ must be constantly exposed to the effective level, or else, the organ and tissue behave as though they were never exposed to the chemical, since these kinds of tumor promoters appear to act reversibly (at least in the early stages).

Saccharin represents another class of promoters, in that it does not seem to be metabolized appreciably. However, it is rapidly excreted. Therefore, for it to be effective, it must be present at effective levels, regularly and for an extended length of time. Certain congeners of polybrominated biphenyls (PBB's) on the other hand, which are not appreciably metabolized or excreted, do not have to be given chronically or regularly if a single exposure is high enough.[60] In this case, once ingested, the PBB's are deposited in the body fat and constantly "flush" the body as it sets up an equilibrium with the blood stream and the body fat. The *in vitro* metabolic cooperation assay is based on a very short (acute) phenomenon; namely the non-inhibition or inhibition of transfer of a lethal metabolite via gap junctions.

It is now clear that tumor promoters such as TPA can induce opposite effects, such as cell proliferation or differentiation, in different cell types[61,62] (*see* reference 63). In addition, it is clear from the literature that the TPA-like promoters can induce one kind of response in epithelial cells and either no response or an opposite response in fibroblast cells.[42,64,65] Conceptually, epithelial-derived tumors might have different types of promoters from fibroblast-derived tumors. Therefore, it is imperative that a battery of *in vitro* tests be derived, using both epithelial and fibroblast cells, to detect promoters of carcinomas and sarcomas. On the basis of the results of the Chinese hamster V79 cell system, it appears it is a good predictor of epithelial-derived tumors of rodents.

In vivo experiments defining the process of tumor promotion in various organ systems[24] suggest that the process involves, at the very least, selective or clonal amplification of the initiated cell.[8,66] In some tissues, sustained hyperplasia, caused by a variety of means (*see* reference 14 for review), appears sufficient to cause promotion. On the other hand, some hyperplasia-inducing chemicals do not seem to cause promotion in the animal models tested.[67]

Physical removal of cells, such as surgery or abrasion,[68] has been shown to act as tumor-promoters. Cell death, caused either by genotoxic or non-genotoxic chemicals (*i.e.*, chloroform, viruses, carbon tetrachloride, ethanol) could cause surviving initiated cells to regenerate the dead tissue (*i.e.*, compensatory hyperplasia).[69]

An example which illustrates the two distinct potential mechanisms of tumor promotion (namely, non-cytotoxic and cytotoxic inhibition of intercelllular communication) has been reported.[70] Two congeners of polybrominated biphenyls have been shown to have dramatically different cytotoxicities *in vitro* [2,4,5,2',4',5'-hexabromobiphenyl (HBB) is less toxic than 3,4,5,2',4',5'-HBB[32]]. At non-cytotoxic doses, 2,4,5,2',4',5'-HBB is a powerful liver tumor promoter,[71] whereas 3,4,5,3',4',5'-HBB is not.[70] However, at cytotoxic doses, the 3,4,5,3'4',5'-HBB has been shown to be a promoter of liver tumors.[70] This implies that if an agent or chemical can induce cell killing, then it has the potential of inducing compensatory hyperplasia and of being a tumor promoter. For this reason, caution must be exercised in stating that just because a given chemical does not inhibit intercellular communication at non-cytotoxic doses, that it could not be a tumor promoter or teratogen at cytotoxic levels.

In the case of TPA-like promoters, the general induction of hyperplasia of both the initiated and non-initiated tissue (*see* reference 72 for operational definitions) appears to be accompanied by the inability of the initiated cells to terminally differentiate, causing a selective accumulation of the abnormal initiated cells. On the other hand, phenobarbital-type promoters of the liver seem to affect promotion differently. Phenobarbital does not cause a general hyperplasia of the total liver (non-initiated cells), but only the initiated cells.[73] There is even evidence that TPA-induced promotion of initiated cells is dependent on the stage of promotion, in that receptors might be present for discreet periods of time during the promotion phase.[42,56]

It has been previously mentioned that disruption of intercellular communication is basically an adaptive mechanism by which cells can homeostatically respond to environmental changes. For that reason, one must recognize that this *in vitro* assay can be utilized not only to detect potentially harmful chemicals but also potentially useful chemicals. It appears that the very mechanism by which a chemical can be potentially harmful is the reason it can be useful; namely, as an acute perturber of intercellular communication, a chemical might be pharmacologically beneficial (*i.e.*, anticonvulsant, pain-killer, tranquilizer, pesticide, etc.). However, given at a "critical period" of development or chronically in a regular fashion at high enough levels, these same chemicals can be either teratogens,[12] tumor promoters[25] or reproductive toxicants.[14] In other words, chemicals which are judged useful are those which effect a specific biological function we desire. If they are used out of context, they can have the aforementioned negative side effects.

Since the gap junctional-mediated metabolic cooperation assay is based on a membrane-dependent process, care must be exercised when using solvents to dissolve test chemicals. Dimethyl sulfoxide (DMSO) is considered a very good solvent for chemicals, many of which have been shown to be tumor promoters. DMSO (which to our knowledge has not been rigorously tested as a potential tumor promoter[74]) does inhibit metabolic cooperation at a certain dose level (Trosko, unpublished observations), as do ethanol and most other solvents which we tested. In many *in vitro* test systems, DMSO has been shown to alter patterns of differentiation[75] and is a known teratogen.[76] In addition, it seems to act as an "anti-tumor" promoter inhibiting the promoting action of phorbol esters in two-stage mouse skin carcinogenesis experiments.[77] Ethanol is suspected of being a tumor promoter from epidemiological and experimental studies,[78] as well as being a teratogen.[79] Ethanol is suspected of being a general cytotoxin at high concentrations, possibly by its membrane-disrupting potential.[80,81] Neither ethanol nor DMSO are classic gene mutagens or genotoxins.[82] Consequently, the assay, having detected the metabolic cooperation inhibitory effects of these chemicals, is doing what it is designed to do, detect potentially harmful chemicals.

The fact that some chemicals have been shown to inhibit metabolic cooperation *in vitro* using Chinese hamster cells (*i.e.*, Valium®, DMSO), but not shown to act as tumor promoters *in vivo* in a given animal system,[83] can be interpreted as a "false positive", due to the inadequacy of various *in vivo* test systems or not being tested properly. Clearly, DDT, 2,3,7,8-tetrachlorodibenzo-p-dioxin (TCDD), and phenobarbital, which are tumor promoters in rat liver, are not promoters of certain mouse skin systems, but of others (*i.e.*, references 84 and 85). There is no way, at present, to predict, *a priori*, from the Chinese hamster (or any other cell system), where a positive chemical will act as a tumor promoter. Only knowledge of *in vivo* metabolism, disposition, concentration and receptors, will allow one to make better educated guesses. In the case of DMSO and Valium®, if one knew where these two chemicals might most effectively induce either hyperplasia or selective growth of cells, one might be able to test if they could act as tumor promoters by initiating those tissues.

Quantitative studies of various chemicals such as TPA and toxaphene have indicated significant differences in the manner in which they inhibit intercellular communication. TPA has been shown to be mediated by membrane receptors,[86] whereas, to our knowledge, chemicals such as toxaphene do not have such specific plasma membrane receptors. "Down regulation" is a phenomenon associated with many membrane receptors.[87,88] Down regulation of TPA effects on the biochemical level has been observed.[89] We have also observed a "biological down regulation" of the TPA-inhibited metabolic cooperation in intercellular communication but not of other non-receptor inhibition of intercellular communication. In general, the doses needed to inhibit metabolic cooperation seem to be related to whether or not the chemicals are receptor-dependent (*i.e.*, TPA, teleocidin at ng levels) and the mechanisms by which they inhibit gap-junction function (*i.e.*, pesticides, etc. at μg levels; saccharin at mg levels).

Acknowledgements

Research on which this manuscript is based was supported by grants from the U.S. Environmental Protection Agency (R811269) and the National Cancer Institute (CA21104). Although the information described in this article has been funded wholly or in part by the United States Environmental Protection Agency under assistance agreement (R811269) to James E. Trosko, it has not been subjected to the Agency's required peer and administrative review and therefore does not necessarily reflect the views of the Agency and no official endorsement should be inferred.

REFERENCES

1. Loewenstein, W.R., Junctional intercellular communication and the control of growth. *Biochim. Biophys. Acta* 560: 1–65 (1979)
2. Evans, W.H., Communication between cells. *Nature* 283: 521–522 (1980)
3. Goodenough, D.A., in: *Membrane-Membrane Interactions* (N.B. Gilula, ed.), pp 167–178, Raven Press, New York (1980)
4. Revel, J.-P., Yancey, S.B., Meyer, D.J., and Nicholson, B., Cell junctions and intercellular communication. *In Vitro* 16: 1010–1017 (1980)
5. Mazet, F. and Ehrhart, J.-C., Importance physiologique des jonctions communicantes. *J. de Physiologie* 76: 529–549 (1980)
6. Potter, V.R., Initiation and promotion in cancer formation: The importance of studies on intercellular communication. *Yale J. Biol. Med.* 53: 367–384 (1980)
7. Loewenstein, W.R., Junctional intercellular communication: The cell-to-cell membrane channel. *Physiol. Res.* 61: 829–913 (1981)
8. Trosko, J.E. and Chang, C.C., An integrative hypothesis linking cancer, diabetes and atherosclerosis: The role of mutations and epigenetic changes. *Med. Hypoth.* 6: 455–468 (1980)
9. Trosko, J.E., and Chang, C.C., in: *Tumor Promotion and Cocarcinogenesis In Vitro* (T.S. Slaga, ed.), CRC Press, Boca Raton, Florida (in press)
10. Wilson, J.G., in: *Handbook of Teratology* (J.G. Wilson and F.C. Fruser, eds.), pp 47–74, Plenum Press, New York (1977)
11. Freese, E., Use of cultured cells in the identification of potential teratogens. *Teratogenesis, Carcinogenesis, and Mutagenesis* 2: 355–360 (1982)
12. Trosko, J.E., Chang, C.C., and Netzloff, M., The role of inhibited cell-cell communication in teratogenesis. *Teratogenesis, Carcinogenesis, and Mutagenesis* 2: 31–45 (1982)
13. Sharpe, R.M., Fraser, H.M., Cooper, I., and Rommerts, F.F.G., Sertoli-Leydig cell communication via an LHRH-like factor. *Nature* 290: 785–787 (1981)
14. Trosko, J.E., Chang, C., and Medcalf, A., Mechanism of tumor promotion: Potential role of intercellular communication. *Cancer Invest.* 1: 511–526 (1983)
15. Iversen, O.H., in: *Progress in Biocybernetics* (N. Weiner and J.P. Schade, eds.), Vol. 2, pp 76–110, Elsevier Publ. Comp., Amsterdam (1965)
16. Pierce, G.B., Neoplasms, differentiation and mutations. *Am. J. Pathol.* 77: 103–118 (1974)

17. Borek, C., and Sachs, L., The difference in contact inhibition of cell replication between normal cells and cells transformed by different carcinogens. *Proc. Natl. Acad. Sci. U.S.A.* 56: 1705–1711 (1966)
18. Corsaro, C.M., and Migeon, B.R., Comparison of contact-mediated communication in normal and transformed human cells in culture. *Proc. Natl. Acad. Sci. U.S.A.* 74: 4476–4480 (1977)
19. Foulds, L., The experimental study of tumor progression: A review. *Cancer Res.* 14: 327–339 (1954)
20. Fialkow, P.J., Clonal origin of human tumors. *Biochim. Biophys. Acta* 458: 384–421 (1976)
21. Cairns, J., Mutation, selection and the natural history of cancer. *Nature* 225: 197–200 (1975)
22. Berenblum, I., and Shubik, P., A new, quantitative approach to the study of the stages of chemical carcinogenesis in the mouse's skin. *Br. J. Cancer* 1: 383–391 (1947)
23. Boutwell, R.K., The function and mechanism of promoters of carcinogenesis. CRC *Crit. Rev. Toxicol.* 2: 419–443 (1974)
24. Pitot, H.C., Goldsworthy, T., and Moram, S., The natural history of carcinogenesis: Implications of experimental carcinogenesis in the genesis of human cancer. *J. Supramol. Struct. Cellul. Biochem.* 17: 133–146 (1981)
25. Yotti, L.P., Chang, C.C., and Trosko, J.E., Elimination of metabolic cooperation in Chinese hamster cells by a tumor promoter. *Science* 206: 1089–1091 (1979)
26. Murray, A.W., and Fitzgerald, D.J., Tumor promoters inhibit metabolic cooperation in cocultures of epidermal and 3T3 cells. *Biochem. Biophys. Res. Commun.* 91: 395–401 (1979)
27. Umeda, M., Noda, K., and Ono, T., Inhibition of metabolic cooperation in Chinese hamster cells by various chemicals including tumor promoters. *Gann* 71: 614–620 (1980)
28. Trosko, J.E., Dawson, B., Yotti, L.P., and Chang, C.C., Saccharin may act as a tumor promoter by inhibiting metabolic cooperation between cells. *Nature* 284: 109–110 (1980)
29. Trosko, J.E., Dawson, B., and Chang, C.C., PBB inhibits metabolic cooperation in Chinese hamster cells *in vitro*: Its potential as a tumor promoter. *Environ. Health Perspect.* 37: 179–182 (1981)
30. Newbold, R.F., and Amos, J., Inhibition of metabolic cooperation between cells in culture by tumor promoters. *Carcinogenesis* 2: 243–249 (1981)
31. Kinsella, A.R., Investigation of the effects of the phorbol ester TPA on carcinogen-induced forward mutagenesis to 6-thioguanine-resistance in V79 Chinese hamster cells. *Carcinogenesis* 2: 43–48 (1981)
32. Tsushimoto, G., Trosko, J.E., Chang, C.C., and Aust, S.D., Inhibition of metabolic cooperation in Chinese hamster V79 cells in culture by various polybrominated biphenyl (PBB) congeners. *Carcinogenesis* 3: 181–185 (1982)
33. Trosko, J.E., Yotti, L.P., Warren, G., Tsushimoto, G., and Chang, C.C., in: *Carcinogenesis* (E. Hecker, N.E. Fusening, W. Kunz, F. Marks, and H.W. Thielmann, eds.), Vol. 7, pp 565–585, Raven Press, New York (1982)
34. Warren, S.T., Doolittle, D.J., Chang, C.C., Goodman, J.I., and Trosko, J.E., Evaluation of the carcinogenic potential of 2,4-dinitrofluoro-benzene and its implications regarding mutagenicity testing. *Carcinogenesis* 3: 139–145 (1982)
35. Williams, G.M., Telang, S., and Tong, C., Inhibition of intercellular communication between liver cells by the liver tumor promoter 1,1,1-trichloro-2,2-bis(p-chlorophenyl) ethane. *Cancer Lett.* 11: 339–344 (1981)

36. Enomoto, T., Sasaki, Y., Kanno, Y., and Yamasaki, H., Tumor promoters cause a rapid and reversible inhibition of the formation and maintenance of electrical cell coupling in culture. *Proc. Natl. Acad. Sci. U.S.A.* 78: 5628–5632 (1981)

37. Slaga, T.J., Klein-Szanto, A.S.P. Triplett, L.C., Yotti, L.P., and Trosko, J.E., Skin tumor promoting activity of benzoyl peroxide: a widely used free radical generating compound. *Science* 213: 1023–1025 (1981)

38. Noda, K., Umeda, M., and Ono, T., Effects of various chemicals including bile acids and chemical carcinogens on the inhibition of metabolic cooperation. *Gann* 72: 772–776 (1981)

39. Trosko, J., Jone, C., Aylsworth, C., and Tsushimoto, G., Elimination of metabolic cooperation is associated with the tumor promoters, oleic acid and anthralin. *Carcinogenesis* 3: 1101–1103 (1982)

40. Enomoto, T., Sasaki, Y., Shiba, Y., Kanno, Y., and Yamasaki, H., Inhibition of the formation of electrical cell coupling of FL cells by tumor promoters. *Gann* 72: 631–634 (1982)

41. Tsushimoto, G., Trosko, J.E., Chang, C.C., and Matsumura, F., Inhibition of intercellular communication by chlordecone (Kepone) and Mirex in Chinese hamster V79 cells *in vitro. Toxicol. Appl. Pharmacol.* 64: 550–556 (1982)

42. Friedman, E.A., and Steinberg, M., Disrupted communication between late-stage premalignant human colon epithelial cells by 12-0-tetradecanoyl phorbol-13-acetate. *Cancer Res.* 42: 5096–5105 (1982)

43. Jone, C.M., Trosko, J.E., Chang, C.C., Fujiki, H., and Sugimura, T., Inhibition of intercellular communication in Chinese hamster V79 cells by teleocidin. *Gann* 73: 874–878 (1982)

44. Tsushimoto, G., Asano, S., Trosko, J.E., and Chang, C.C., in: *PCB's: Human and Environmental Hazards* (F. Ditri and M. Kamrin, eds.), pp 241–252, Ann Arbor Science Publ., Ann Arbor, Michigan (1983)

45. Telang, S., Tong, C., and Williams, G.M., Epigenetic membrane effects of a possible tumor promoting type on cultured liver cells by the non-genotoxic organochlorine pesticides, chlordane and heptachlor. *Carcinogenesis* 3: 1175–1178 (1982)

46. Tsushimoto, G., Chang, C.C., Trosko, J.E., and Matsumura, F., Cytotoxic, mutagenic, and tumor-promoting properties of DDT, lindane and chlordane on Chinese hamster cells *in vitro. Arch. Environ. Contam. Toxicol.* 12: 721–730 (1983)

47. Subak-Sharpe, J.H., Burk, R.R., and Pitts, J.D., Metabolic cooperation between biochemically marked mammalian cells in tissue culture. *Cell Sci.* 4: 353–367 (1969)

48. Hooper, M.L., Metabolic cooperation between mammalian cells in culture. *Biochim. Biophys. Acta* 651: 85–103 (1982)

49. Cox, R.P., Krauss, M.R., Balis, M.E., and Dancis, J., Evidence for transfer of enzyme product as the basis of metabolic cooperation between tissue culture fibroblast of Lesch-Nyhan disease and normal cells. *Proc. Natl. Acad. Sci. U.S.A.* 67: 1573–1579 (1970)

50. Yancey, S.B., Edens, J.E., Trosko, J.E., Chang, C.C., and Revel, J.-P, Decreased incidence of gap junctions between Chinese hamster V79 cells upon exposure to the tumor promoter 12-0-tetradecanoyl phorbol-13-acetate. *Exp. Cell Res.* 139: 329–340 (1982)

51. Trosko, J.E., Yotti, L.P., Dawson, B., and Chang, C.C., in: *Short-Term Tests for Chemical Carcinogens* (H. Stich and R.H.C. San, eds.), pp 420–427, Springer-Verlag, New York (1981)

52. Aylsworth, C.F., Jone, C., Trosko, J.E., Meites, J., and Welsch, C.W., Promotion of dimethylbenz(a)anthracene-induced mammary tumorigenesis by high dietary fat in the rat; possible role of intercellular communication. *J. Natl. Cancer Inst.* 72: 637–645 (1984)

53. Sisskin, E.E., Gray, T., and Barrett, J.C., Correlation between sensitivity to tumor promotion and sustained epidermal hyperplasia of mice and rats treated with 12-0-tetradecanoylphorbol-13-acetate. *Carcinogenesis* 3: 403–407 (1982)

54. Ashman, L.K., Murray, A.W., Cook, M.G., and Kotlarski, I., Two-stage skin carcinogenesis in sensitive and resistant mouse strains. *Carcinogenesis* 3: 99–102 (1982)

55. Yuspa, S.H., Spangler, E.F., Donahoe, R., Geusz, S., Ferguson, E., Wenk, M., and Hennings, H., Sensitivity to two-stage carcinogenesis of SENCAR mouse skin grafted to nude mice. *Cancer Res.* 42: 437–439 (1982)

56. Shoyab, M., Warren, T.C., and Todaro, G.J., Tissue and species distribution and developmental variation of specific receptors for biologically active phorbol and ingenol esters. *Carcinogenesis* 2: 1273–1276 (1981)

57. Warren, S.T., Yotti, L.P., Moskal, J.R., Chang, C.C., and Trosko, J.E., Metabolic cooperation in CHO and V79 cells following treatment with a tumor promoter. *Exp. Cell Res.* 131: 427–430 (1981)

58. Verma, A.K., and Boutwell, R.K., Effects of dose and duration of treatment with the tumor-promoting agent, 12-0-tetradecanoylphorbol-13-acetate on mouse skin carcinogenesis. *Carcinogenesis* 1: 271–276 (1980)

59. Peraino, C., Staffeldt, E.F., Haugen, D.A., Lombard, L.S., Stevens, F.J., and Fry, R.F.M., Effects of varying the dietary concentration of phenobarbital on its enhancement of 2-acetylaminofluorene-induced hepatic tumorigenesis. *Cancer Res.* 40: 3268–3273 (1980)

60. Jensen, R., Sleight, S.D., and Aust, S., Effect of varying the length of exposure to polybrominated biphenyls on the development of γ-glutamyl transpeptidase enzyme-altered foci. *Carcinogenesis* 5: 63–66 (1984)

61. Miao, R.M., Fieldsteel, A.H., and Fodge, D.W., Opposing effects of tumor promoters on erythroid differentiation. *Nature* 274: 271–272 (1978)

62. Yuspa, S.H., Ben, T., Hennings, H., and Lichti, U., Divergent responses in epidermal basal cells exposed to the tumor promoter 12-0-tetradecanoylphorbol-13-acetate. *Cancer Res.* 42: 2344–2349 (1982)

63. Trosko, J.E., and Chang, C.C., in: *Mechanisms of Tumor Promotion* (T.J. Slaga, ed.), Vol. 4, pp 119–145, CRC Press, Boca Raton, Florida (1984)

64. Lechner, J.F., and Kaighn, M.E., EGF growth promoting activity is neutralized by phorbol esters. *Cell Biol. Intern. Rep.* 4: 23–28 (1980)

65. Mosser, D.D., and Bols, N.C., The effect of phorbols on metabolic cooperation between human fibroblasts. *Carcinogenesis* 3: 1207–1212 (1982)

66. Potter, V.R., A new protocol and its rationale for the study of initiation and promotion of carcinogenesis in rat liver. *Carcinogenesis* 2: 1375–1379 (1981)

67. Mufson, R.A., Fischer, S.M., Verma, A.K., Gleason, G.L., Slaga, T.J., and Boutwell, R.K., Effects of 12-0-tetradecanoylphorbol-13-acetate and mezerein on epidermal ornithine decarboxylase activity, isoproterenol-stimulated levels of cyclic adenosine 3':5'-monophosphate, and induction of mouse skin tumors *in vivo*. *Cancer Res.* 38: 4791–4795 (1979)

68. Frei, J.V., Some mechanisms operative in carcinogenesis: A review. *Chem. Biol. Interactions* 12: 1–25 (1976)

69. Argyris, T.S., and Slaga, T.J., Promotion of carcinogenesis by repeated abrasion in initiated skin of mice. *Cancer Res.* 41: 5193–5195 (1981)

70. Jensen, R.K., Sleight, S.D., Aust, S.D., Goodman, J.I., and Trosko, J.E. Hepatic tumor promotion by 3,3',4,4'5,5'-hexabromobiphenyl: The interrelationship between toxicity, induction of microsomal drug metabolizing enzymes and tumor promotion. *Toxicol. Appl. Pharmacol.* 71: 163-176 (1983)

71. Jensen, R.K., Sleight, S.D., Goodman, J.I., Aust, S.D., and Trosko, J.E., Polybrominated biphenyls as promoters in experimental hepatocarcinogenesis in rats. *Carcinogenesis* 3: 1183-1186 (1982)

72. Trosko, J.E., Jone, C., and Chang, C.C., The role of tumor promoters on phenotypic alterations affecting intercellular communication and tumorigenesis. *Ann. New York Acad. Sci.,* 407: 316-327 (1983)

73. Schulte-Hermann, R., Ohde, G., Schuppler, J., and Timmermann-Trosiener, I., Enhanced proliferation of putative preneoplastic cells in rat liver following treatment with the tumor promoters phenobarbital, hexachlorocyclohexane, steroid compounds and nafenopin. *Cancer Res.* 41: 2556-2562 (1981)

74. Stenback, F., and Garcia, H., Studies on the modifying effect of dimethyl sulfoxide and other chemicals on experimental skin tumor induction. *Ann. New York Acad. Sci.* 243: 209-227 (1975)

75. Collins, S.J., Ruscetti, F.W., Gallagher, R.E. and Gallo, R.C., Terminal differentiation of human promyelocytic leukemia cells induced by dimethyl sulfoxide and other polar compounds. *Proc. Natl. Acad. Sci. U.S.A.* 75: 2458-2462 (1978)

76. Ferm, V.H., Congenital malformations induced by dimethyl sulfoxide in the golden hamster. *J. Embryol. Exp. Morphol.* 16: 49-54 (1966)

77. Iversen, O.H., Thorud, E., and Volden, G., Inhibition of methylcholanthrene-induced skin carcinogenesis in hairless mice by dimethyl sulfoxide. *Carcinogenesis* 2: 1129-1133 (1981)

78. Rothman, K.J., in: *Persons at High Risk of Cancer* (J.F. Fraumeni, Jr., ed.), pp 139-150, Academic Press, New York (1975)

79. Sulik, K.K., Johnston, M.C., and Webb, M.A., Fetal alcohol syndrome: Embryogenesis in a mouse model. *Science* 214: 936-938 (1981)

80. Goldstein, D.B., and Chin, J.H., Interaction of ethanol with biological membranes. *Fed. Proc.* 40: 2073-2076 (1981)

81. Schanne, F.A.X., Zucker, A.H., Farber, J.L., and Rubin, E., Alcohol-dependent liver cell necrosis *in vitro:* A new model. *Science* 212: 338-340 (1981)

82. Halkka, O., and Eriksson, K., in: *Genetic Damage in Man Caused by Environmental Agents* (K. Berg, ed.) pp 327-334, Academic Press, New York (1979)

83. Hino, O., and Kitagawa, T., Effect of diazepam on hepatocarcinogenesis in the rat. *Toxicol. Lett.* 11: 155-157 (1982)

84. Berry, D.L., Slaga, T.J., DiGiovanni, J., and Juchau, M.R., Studies with chlorinated dibenzo-p-dioxins, polybrominated biphenyls, and polychlorinated biphenyls in a two stage system of mouse skin tumorigenesis: Potent anticarcinogenic effects. *Ann. New York Acad. Sci.* 320: 405-414 (1979)

85. Poland, A., Palen, D., and Glover, E., Tumor promotion by TCDD in skin of HRS/J hairless mice. *Nature* 300: 271-273 (1982)

86. Blumberg, P.M., *In vitro* studies on the mode of action of the phorbol esters, potent tumor promoters. Part 2. *CRC Critical Rev. Toxicol.* 9: 199-234 (1981)

87. Fox, C.F., and Das, M., Internalization and processing of the EGF receptor in the induction of DNA synthesis in cultured fibroblasts: The endocytic activation hypothesis. *J. Supramol. Struct.* 10: 199–214 (1979)
88. Caro, J.F., and Amatruda, J.M., Insulin receptors in hepatocytes: Postreceptor events mediate down regulation. *Science* 210: 1029–1031 (1980)
89. Yamasaki, H., Drevon, C., and Martel, N., Specific binding of phorbol esters to friend erythroleukemia cells—general properties, down regulation and relationship to cell differentiation. *Carcinogenesis* 3: 905–910 (1982)

21

Alpha-Fetoprotein: A Marker for Exposure to Chemical Hepatocarcinogens in Rats

Harold A. Dunsford
Stewart Sell

University of Texas Medical School
Houston, Texas

INTRODUCTION

Alphafetoprotein (AFP), a glycoprotein that is the predominant serum protein during fetal life, has been shown to be a marker for exposure to hepatocarcinogens in adult rats. AFP is found in very low levels in normal adult serum, but becomes elevated in individuals with liver or yolk sack cancer.[1] It is made predominantly in the yolk sac and fetal liver, and to a lesser extent in the gastrointestinal tract.[2] In humans, serum levels peak at 3,000 μg/ml at the 35th week of gestation and decline to 30 μg/ml at birth.[3] In rats, elevation of AFP also occurs in animals with hepatocellular cancer. Elevations of AFP are seen after exposure to chemical carcinogens but prior to development of an obvious malignancy.

CHEMISTRY

AFP is an alpha 1 globulin with a molecular weight between 65,000 daltons and 74,000 daltons and an electrophoretic mobility between alpha 1 globulin and beta globulin. In most species AFP is heterogeneous with a slow and fast electrophoretic band, has slight variations in molecular weight, and differs in degree of glycosylation.[4] Glycosylation of AFP by liver cells increases with age due to maturation of glycosylating enzymes. The affinity of AFP for the lectin concanavalin-A (con-A) is related to the structure of the oligosaccharide units. Con-A reactive-AFP contains a terminal mannose residue. In con-A non-reactive-AFP, the mannose residue is linked to additional sugars, galactose and sialic acid, which prevent binding of AFP to con-A.[4] Thus, con-A non-reactive-AFP represents production by "more mature" tisssue.

Rat AFP can be divided by con-A binding and electrophoretic migration into four fractions, slow and fast con-A reactive and slow and fast con-A non-reactive. Each type is produced in slightly varying concentrations during fetal life and during chemical carcinogenesis. All are immunologically identical.[4] In the human, the affinity of AFP to con-A appears to separate yolk sac derived AFP from liver derived AFP. Yolk sac AFP is con-A non-reactive and is the major fraction appearing early in gestation. Liver derived AFP rises during gestation until the time of delivery when it makes up nearly 100% of amniotic fluid AFP.[5] The degree of glycosylation of AFP made by the liver increases with gestational age.

FUNCTION

The biological function of AFP is not known. It appears to serve as a substitute for albumin as the main serum protein in fetal life. Although some investigators feel that AFP may be immunosuppressive and thereby protect the fetus from the mother's immune system, other investigators have been unable to confirm that AFP is immunosuppressive.[6] Rat and mouse AFP have the ability to bind estrogens, and it has been suggested that AFP protects the fetus from maternal estrogens; however, human AFP does not have strong estrogen binding.[7-9] There is some recent evidence that AFP may have weak enzyme activity, but the significance of this is not clear.

REGULATION OF PRODUCTION

The production of AFP appears to be directly proportional to the tissue content of AFP mRNA.[10] In the fetal rat liver there is an inverse relationship between albumin and production of AFP, with production of albumin increasing as production of AFP decreases with age. In the newborn rat, serum AFP remains elevated ($>$1,000 μg/ml) for four weeks after parturition and then drops to normal ($>$0.06 μg/ml). During this period AFP mRNA decreases as albumin mRNA increases.[11] Studies using recombinant DNA techniques have demonstrated sufficient homology between albumin and AFP gene products to suggest that albumin and AFP come from a common precursor gene family, although they are under different controls.[12,13] Mouse AFP may be under the control of two genes.[14]

An example of the complexity of control of production of AFP is seen in chemical carcinogenesis. While a reciprocal relationship in the production of AFP and albumin exists in newborn rat liver, this does not appear to be the case during hepatocarcinogenesis. During chemical carcinogenesis, as the production of AFP increases with increased AFP mRNA, there is no simultaneous decrease in the production of albumin or levels of albumin mRNA.[11]

The explanation for this is not clear. The elevation of AFP which is seen (usually rising to 1 to 10 μg/ml) represents only a minuscule amount compared to the serum concentration of albumin (40 mg/ml). An increase of 500-fold in the serum concentration of AFP represents less than 0.1% of the serum concentration of albumin. Thus, a massive prolonged inhibition of albumin synthesis would be required to affect the serum levels of AFP.

In addition, production of AFP is localized to a new cell population, so called oval cells, not hepatocytes, during chemical hepatocarcinogenesis. Not only is the albumin made by the hepatic parenchymal cell, but it is also produced by oval cells. Thus, analysis of the relative production of AFP and albumin during carcinogenesis is subject to complex interpretations.

PURIFICATION OF AFP

Amniotic fluid or serum from rats with AFP producing primary hepatocellular carcinoma (PHC) provide a good source of AFP. The content of protein (in mg/ml) of the original fluid should be recorded. This can be done by measuring the optical density (O.D.) at 280 nm, or by the Lowry method with bovine serum albumin as the standard.[15]

AFP has a pI of 4.9 and a molecular weight of 70,000 daltons, therefore is difficult to separate from albumin which has a molecular weight of 60,000 daltons and a pI of 5.6. Two successive fractionations by isoelectric focusing (IEF) will produce reasonably pure AFP.[16, 17] Other methods include electrophoresis,[17] the use of a Concanavalin A column which binds AFP but not albumin,[18] or affinity chromatography with purified anti-rat AFP.[19]

We use affinity chromatography in our laboratory. Goat antiserum against rat AFP is cut with ammonium sulfate to yield a semi-pure anti-AFP IgG preparation. This preparation is then coupled to an agarose gel (Affi-Gel 10) column, and the agarose gel washed with phosphate buffered saline (PBS) to pH 7.4 to remove the unbound IgG.

Serum from rats bearing Morris hepatoma 7777, containing high concentrations of AFP, is passed over the agarose gel column coupled with goat anti-rat AFP. The flow-through is discarded and the gel is washed with PBS until the O.D. at 280 nm is zero.

The "affinity pure" AFP is then eluted with 4.5 M magnesium chloride in PBS, pH 7.4. The eluate is monitored at 280 nm and fractions containing protein absorbing at 280 nm are dialyzed against PBS. The fractions are tested by immunodiffusion. Those fractions demonstrating strong precipitation lines against goat anti-rat AFP are pooled and concentrated.

PREPARATION OF ANTI-RAT AFP

Once purified AFP has been obtained it can be used to raise specific antisera. Our assay is based on goat anti-rat AFP. The animals are immunized by intramuscular injections of 50 µg of purified AFP in complete Freunds adjuvant, divided into four one ml doses in four sites. They are boosted at six weeks with 50 µg of AFP in incomplete Freunds adjuvant in four divided doses, intramuscularly. A test bleed is drawn ten days later. Initial tests are done by immunodiffusion. Boosting and test bleeding are continued at four week intervals until there is a strong line of precipitation against the AFP source. There should be no reaction with normal adult serum. An antibody dilution curve (see below) should give 50% binding with a 1:8,000 or higher dilution, before the antibody will be suitable for the assay. Successive bleeds and tests can be done until sufficient antisera are collected. Five hundred ml will provide several years of assays if stored at $-20°$C.

RADIOLABELING OF AFP

AFP can be labeled with ^{125} I by protein iodination with lactoperoxidase.[20] Fifty μl of stock AFP (1 mg/ml PBS) is added to 40 μl PBS and 10 μl lactate peroxidase 4 B (Worthington). In a hood, five μl Na ^{125} I (0.5mCi) and 10 μl 10^{-4} M H_2O_2 are mixed and incubated for 30 minutes at 25°C with occasional mixing. The reaction is terminated with 5 μl of 10% sodium azide in PBS. The bound AFP is separated from the unbound AFP on a Sephadex G-50 column. One ml fractions are collected. Five μl aliquots are counted on a gamma counter and usually yield between 40,000 cpm and 100,000 cpm.

The most active one to two tubes are saved. The labeled AFP is stabilized by a 1:1 dilution with 1% human serum albumin (HSA) in PBS, and stored frozen in an appropriate container. The preparation can be used for about six weeks.

ANTIBODY DILUTION CURVE

Each time a new batch of labeled AFP is made an antibody dilution curve is carried out to determine the appropriate antibody dilution to use in the assay. Serial dilutions of goat anti-rat AFP are made with 1% HSA in PBS as the diluent. Each dilution is run in duplicate. To each tube is added 0.1 ml of 1:20 dilution of normal goat serum (NGS) and 0.1 ml labeled AFP (diluted with 1% HSA in PBS so that 0.1 ml has 10,000 cpm). Total counts are measured and recorded. The non-specific binding tube contains 0.9 ml 1/20 of NGS and 0.1 ml of labeled AFP. This tube is precipitated with 10% trichloroacetic acid.

Twenty-four hours later the tubes are precipitated with 1.5 ml 30% sodium sulfate in borate buffer pH 8.0, incubated for 15 minutes at 25°C, then centrifuged at 3,000 R.P.M. (International PR centrifuge rotor 276) at 25°C for 1 hour. The supernate is aspirated and the pellet washed in 0.5 ml 18% Na_2SO_4 in borate buffer pH 8.0, spun as above, but for 30 minutes. The supernate is aspirated and the precipitates counted for one minute in a gamma counter.

The percent binding is plotted on semilog paper. The antibody dilution is chosen which caused 50% binding. This is usually 1/8,000 to 1/10,000. Generally, the more dilute the antibody, the more sensitive is the assay.

RADIOIMMUNOASSAY

The radioimmunoassay (RIA) used in our laboratory is capable of measuring 6 ng/ml AFP, and therefore, is able to measure the levels of AFP in normal adult rats.[21,22] The sensitivity is achieved by pre-incubating the samples and standards with the anti-rat AFP for 24 hours before the addition of ^{125}I labeled AFP. The standards can be prepared from known quantities of purified AFP, or dilutions of serum containing high levels of AFP standardized against purified AFP. We use dilutions of such a serum standardized to 0.004 μg/ml to 1.280 μg/ml.

One tenth of one ml of standard or sample is added to 0.8 ml of diluted antibody. After 24 hours incubation at 25°C, 0.1 ml of ^{125}I labeled AFP containing 10,000 cpm is added. After another 24 hours incubation at 25°C the tubes are precipitated with Na_2SO_4 and the precipitates counted as described under "Antibody Dilution Curve". All samples and standards are run in duplicate. The standard curve is plotted on semilog paper. Generally, the curve is linear from 0.008 to 0.128 μg/ml.

The AFP of the normal adult rat is 0.025 to 0.065 μg/ml with our assay. Levels above 0.100 μg/ml would be considered abnormal. The levels of AFP during administration of several chemical carcinogens will be detailed in the remainder of the chapter. In following animals in long-term bioassays whose levels of AFP have returned to near normal and in which an elevation would indicate the presence of PHC, a level above 0.2 μg/ml is used to select animals for sacrifice.

Since the range of the assay is small, dilutions of the serum must be run if the inhibition value does not come out in the linear portion of the curve. In situations when the sample is limited and when the 0.2 μg/ml point is being determined, then it is satisfactory to screen with a 5 x dilution.

Enzyme linked assays (ELISA) have also been developed which had a similar sensitivity and a linear curve from 0.008 to 0.50 μg/ml. However, the ELISA assay was markedly affected by even mild hemolysis of the serum and so could not be used. The RIA is unaffected by hemolysis.

There are several recent reports of assays for AFP based on monoclonal antibodies (MoAb) to AFP.[23-26] Because AFP has several antigenic determinants, two or more MoAb must be used, each one recognizing only one determinant. MoAb have less affinity and therefore some of the assays are less sensitive.[25] Some assays can give false negative results in the presence of high levels of AFP due to binding of all available free labeled antibody by the AFP, and preventing binding of AFP to the immobilized antibody.[26] For the purposes of RIA and for immunohistochemical studies, the polyclonal antibody appears to be superior to monoclonal antibodies.

APPLICATION OF AFP IN EXPERIMENTAL CARCINOGENESIS

AFP has been found to be a useful marker of exposure to chemical hepatocarcinogens and development of chemically-induced hepatocellular carcinoma. The study of chemical carcinogenesis by standard morphology is complicated by the long time interval between the initial exposure to the carcinogen and the occurrence of tumors, often many months, or even years later.

Most chemical hepatocarcinogens cause an early prolonged rise in production of AFP during the feeding of the carcinogen, which falls to near normal levels during the latent period, and rises again with the appearance of primary hepatocellular carcinoma.[27] Transient elevations of AFP in serum occur after a stimulus to hepatocellular proliferation such as partial hepatectomy (PH), or toxic injury with regeneration such as with carbon tetrachloride.[28] The following paragraphs will review serum AFP and some of the morphologic events which occur with liver injury and several different chemical carcinogens.

Hepatocellular Proliferation

The rise in serum AFP associated with hepatocellular proliferation is slight (0.2 μg/ml) and falls off promptly within one or two weeks.[29-31] Cellular localization of production of AFP by immunofluorescence following PH or injury by galactosamine, has demonstrated that AFP is produced in a few large hepatocytes.[27] These cells closely resemble the AFP producing hepatocytes seen in fetal livers, and suggest that the production of AFP represents derepression of control of the AFP genes in the proliferating cells.

N-2-Acetylaminofluorene (AAF)

AAF is a potent carcinogen which elicits PHC in rats after prolonged exposure.[32-34] Generally, the carcinogen is given mixed in the diet for four three week cycles with one week rest periods in order to ensure survival.[32] Male Sprague-Dawley (SD) and ACI rats demonstrate similar results.[35] Female rats are less affected because they lack arylsulfotransferase needed to convert AAF to its active metabolite.[36] Fischer 344 rats are more susceptible and have to be fed the diet in two week cycles.[37] Levels of AFP rise to $>$10 μg/ml in the Fischer 344, which is higher than in the ACI rats ($>$1μg/ml) (Figure 1). The rise is dose related (Figure 2). In both SD and ACI rats, serum AFP falls before the end of administration of the carcinogen, whereas in Fischer 344 rats, the levels of AFP remain elevated for the full 14 weeks of AAF feeding (Figure 3).[37-38]

Before describing the cellular localization of production of AFP, it is important to review the histology of the AAF carcinogenesis model.[34, 39, 40] The earliest changes visible in the liver include a proliferation of bile duct-like cells which appear in the portal areas, and infiltrate out into the parenchyma. These cells are present throughout the feeding of the carcinogen and then persist in decreased numbers until the appearance of PHC. In most descriptions of AAF carcinogenesis these cells have been ignored, or felt to be part of cholangiofibrosis, caused by the carcinogen, but unrelated to PHC.[34, 41]

The earliest changes visible in the hepatocytes are areas or foci of pale staining hepatocytes. Although there are many histochemical differences among these altered hepatocytes and normal cells, the most studied cells are those positive for gamma glutamyltranspeptidase (GGT)[42] and those that exclude iron after an iron loading.[43] Many of these foci persist throughout the experiment, others disappear or change back to normal, and others are believed to change into atypical foci with more basophilic cytoplasm. By the second or third cycle large hyperplastic nodules of normal appearing hepatocytes appear, which compress the surrounding parenchyma. Some of the nodules are GGT positive and exlude iron.[42, 43] They will disappear if the full carcinogenic dose of AAF is not given, but after five cycles, some will persist. Since some of these nodules are quite large, and they cytologically resemble some well differentiated hepatomas, many investigators have concluded that PHC arise from these nodules. This conclusion

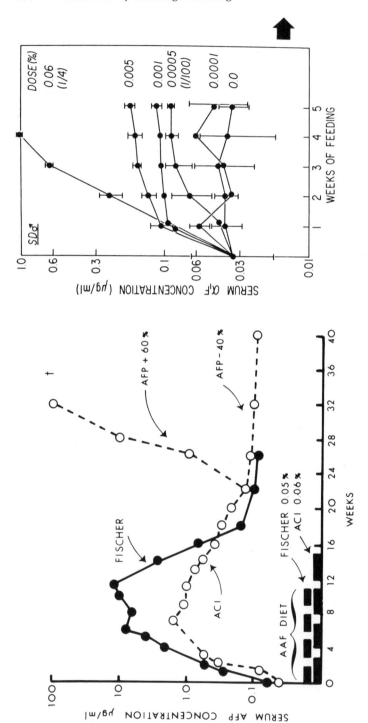

Figure 2: Serum AAF concentrations in Sprague-Dawley male rats fed different doses of AAF. At the 0.06% level the rats have received ¼ of a carcinogenic dose; at 0.0005% they have received 1/100 of a carcinogenic dose.

Figure 1: Comparison of serum AFP concentrations of Fischer 344 and Sprague-Dawley male rats fed four cycles of AAF.

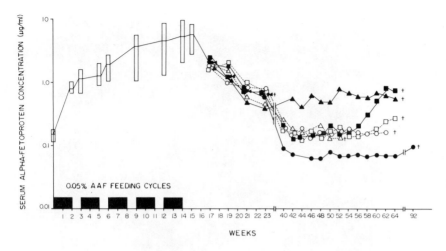

Figure 3: Serum AFP concentrations of a group of Fischer 344 male rats fed five cycles of AAF and allowed to develop hepatocellular carcinomas.

has been supported by the occasional finding of carcinoma within nodules. Serial sections of these tumors within nodules have not been performed to exclude the possibility that they represent tumor growing into the nodules from the outside.[44] Other investigators feel that the nodule is a form of benign hyperplasia and that PHC arise from the basophilic atypical foci.[45] Studies using the cellular localization of AFP as well as other markers have suggested another hypothesis.[44] Production of AFP has been identified in the oval cells, some of the atypical ductular structures, and in some atypical foci (Figure 4).[37] Significantly, the hyperplastic nodule does not produce AFP. Serum AFP falls prior to the appearance of nodules (Figure 5). Oval cells are also positive for albumin, and are surrounded by increased fibronectin and laminin (Figure 6).[37] PHC stains positively for AFP and albumin, and has increased fibronectin and laminin. Nodules and normal liver cells stain positively for albumin but not for AFP, and are not surrounded by less intensely stained zones of fibronectin or laminin. These findings are summarized in Table 1. Using these markers, the oval cell appears to have more in common with PHC than do hyperplastic nodules.[44]

Further studies of oval cells were performed in Fischer 344 rats fed AAF in a choline-deficient (CD) diet.[46] This diet alone provides a stimulus to hepatocellular proliferation which causes a mild transient elevation of AFP after two weeks of feeding. Combined with AAF, it causes a rapid rise in AFP levels two logs higher than AAF alone, (Figure 7), and a massive proliferation of oval cells. Autoradiography has demonstrated proliferation of primitive appearing cells adjacent to the bile duct, within two or three days of CD-AAF diet. Proliferation of bile duct cells can be demonstrated a few days later with extension of duct-like cells filling out the portal area and infiltrating out into the parenchyma (Figure 8).[47] By the third week the liver is filled with a new population of cells,

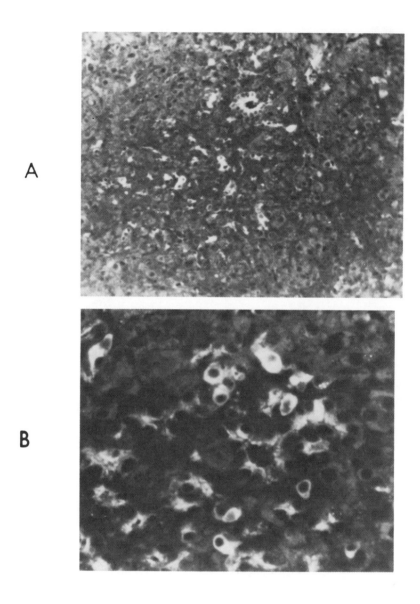

A) CD-AAF 21 days (x 160)
B) CD-AAF 21 days (x 400)

Figure 4: Localization of AFP in livers of Fischer 344 male rats by immunofluorescence.

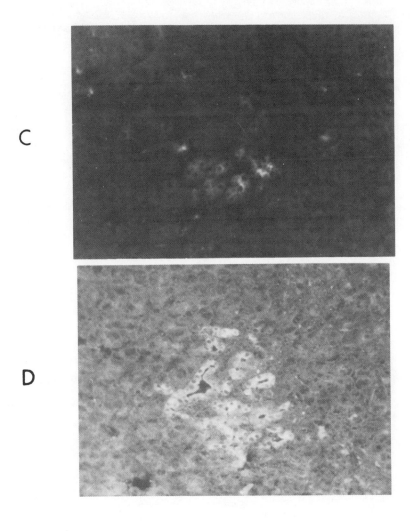

C) AAF-4 cycles (x 160)
D) AAF-3 cycles (x 160)

Figure 4: (continued).

most of which resemble bile duct cells, with microvilli and basement membranes, but which still are producing AFP and albumin (Figure 9).[48] Most of these cells disappear in time, leaving a normal appearing liver, with a few nests of these cells out in the parenchyma. These studies have suggested that the oval cell or its precursor may be the progenitor of PHC.

Table 1: Comparative Properties of Oval Cells, Neoplastic Nodules
and Hepatocellular Carcinomas

Property	Oval Cells	Nodules	Hepatomas
Appear on exposure to carcinogen	Yes, early	Yes, later	Yes, even later
Proliferation	Rapid	Rapid	Variable
Involution	Yes	Yes	No
AFP	Yes	No	Yes and no
Aldolase C	Yes	No	Yes and no
GGT	Yes	Yes	Yes
Albumin	Yes	Yes	Yes and no
Invasive	Yes	No	Yes
Fibronectin	High	Low	Variable
Transplantation	Limited growth	Limited growth	Progressive growth
In vitro	Limited growth	Survival	Progressive growth

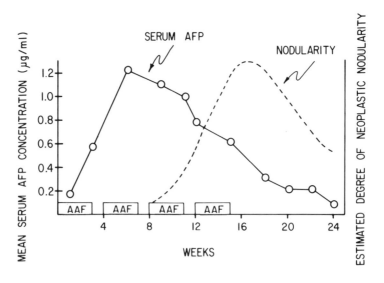

Figure 5: Lack of correlation of serum AFP concentration and of nodule formation in male ACI rats fed four cycles of AAF.

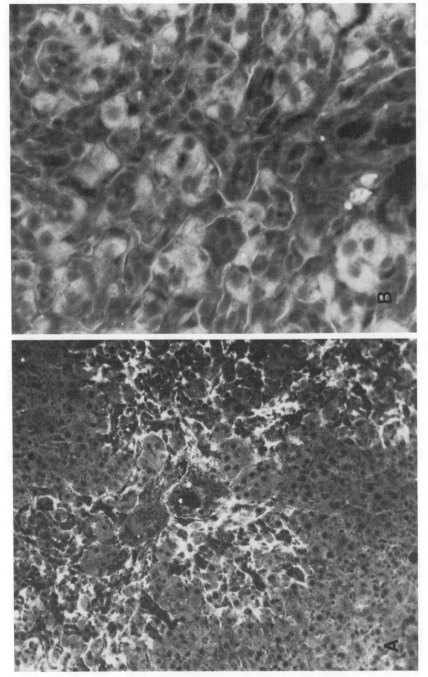

Figure 6: Fibronectin (A) (x 160) and laminin (B) (x 400) in areas of oval cell proliferation 16 days after feeding Fischer 344 male rats CD-AAF.

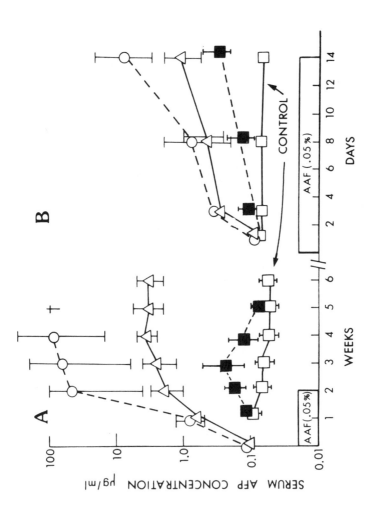

Figure 7: Serum AFP concentrations in male Fischer 344 rats fed AAF in choline devoid diets: A) Experiment 1; B) Experiment 2. The serum AFP concentrations are plotted as a function of time after feeding in a two week cycle of AAF in different diets. □—□, choline supplemented (CS); ■—■, choline devoid (CD); △—△, AAF in choline supplemented diet (CS-AAF); ○—○, AAF in choline deficient diet. The cross (+) indicates time of death of the animals fed CD-AAF. [Reproduced from reference (47).]

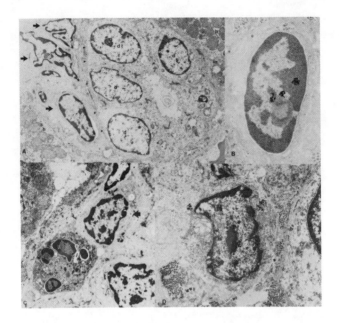

Figure 8: Electron microscopic autoradiographs of periductular cells after feeding CD-AAF for 1 or 2 days to Fischer 344 male rats: A) Day 1, B) Day 2, C) Day 1, D) Day 2.

Ethionine

Ethionine fed to rats in their diet produces an effect similar to that of AAF.[49] The serum levels of AFP (>0.3 µg/ml) (Figure 10) and cellular events are also enhanced by a choline-deficient diet.[50]

3'-Methyl-4-Dimethylaminoazobenzene (3'MDAB)

3'MDAB causes a rise in AFP which is dose dependent and has different kinetics from that which follows exposure to AAF (Figure 11).

Figure 12 shows the comparison of serum levels of AFP in rats exposed to 3'MDAB (>3µg/ml) and to its non-carcinogenic analogues 2-methyl-4-dimethyl-aminoazobenzene (2MDAB) and p-aminoazobenzene (PAAB), given following 2/3 partial hepatectomy.[51] The partial hepatectomy stimulated a transient elevation of serum AFP, as expected. Neither exposure to 2MDAB nor to PAAB caused an elevation of serum AFP, whereas 3'MDAB produced a rapid elevation.

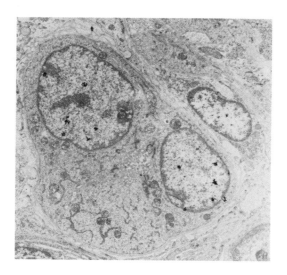

Figure 9: Electron microscopic autoradiography of midlobular duct-like structure in liver of rat fed CD-AAF for 14 days. Such structures morphologically resemble ducts but have other properties more like hepatocytes.

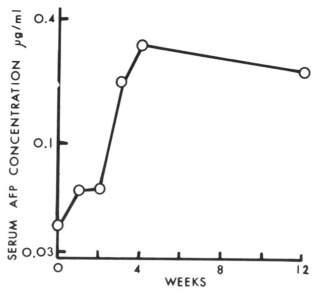

Figure 10: Serum AFP concentrations in male Sprague-Dawley rats fed 0.05% ethionine.

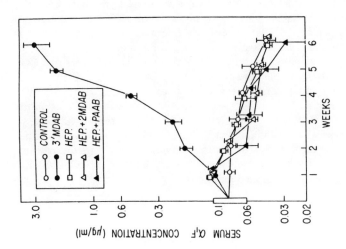

Figure 12: Serum AFP concentrations in male Sprague-Dawley rats fed 0.06% 3'MDAB, and PAAB in a riboflavin free diet. Rats fed 2MDAB and PAAB were 2/3 hepatectomized on day 0.

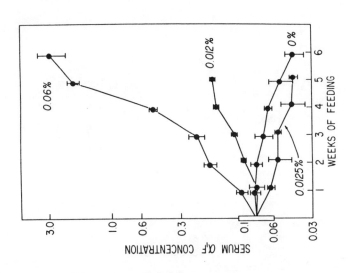

Figure 11: Serum AFP concentrations in male Sprague-Dawley rats fed different concentrations of 3'MDAB.

Diethylnitrosamine (DEN)

In contrast to other chemical carcinogens, DEN produces no early rise in serum AFP unless high doses are given (Figure 13).[38, 52] Continuous administration of a low dose of DEN in the drinking water leads to a late rise in serum AFP ($>1\mu g/ml$) which is associated with the appearance of PHC.[38] The phase of normal serum AFP is associated with micronodule formation, with essentially no proliferation of oval cells. At the earliest time of elevation of AFP, AFP may be localized in focal adenomatous hyperplastic or glandular areas similar to those seen after exposure to AAF (Sell and Becker, unpublished data). DEN injected weekly into rats on a choline-deficient diet produces a rapid elevation of serum AFP ($>10\mu g/ml$) (Figure 14) and is associated with a massive proliferation of oval cells.[52] This is in contrast to the absence of elevation of serum AFP or proliferation of oval cells when lower doses of DEN are administered in the drinking water of ACI rats. Recent studies demonstrate moderate proliferation of oval cells when higher doses of DEN (100 ppm) are administered in the drinking water (Dunsford and Sell, unpublished data).

Wy-14,643

The hypolipidemic agent Wy-14,643 produces an early temporary elevation of serum AFP ($>0.5\mu g/ml$) (Figure 15) which is associated with hepatocyte proliferation.[54] After two weeks the serum AFP falls to normal and remains low for the long latent period of 60 or more weeks before the appearance of non-AFP producing tumors.

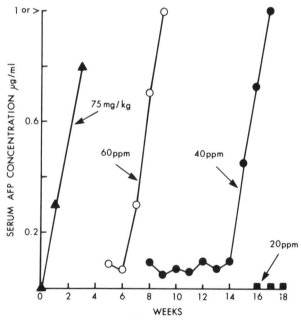

Figure 13: Serum AFP concentrations of male Sprague-Dawley rats injected intraperitoneally with 75 mg/kg DEN on Day 0 and in male ACI rats given different doses of DEN in their drinking water.

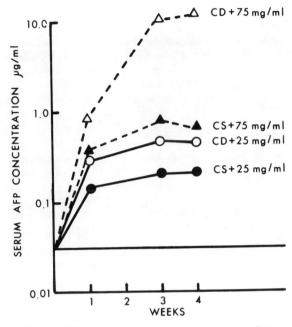

Figure 14: Serum AFP concentrations in male Sprague-Dawley rats fed a choline-deficient (CD) or choline-supplemented (CS) diet and injected with 25 mg/kg or 75 mg/kg DEN.

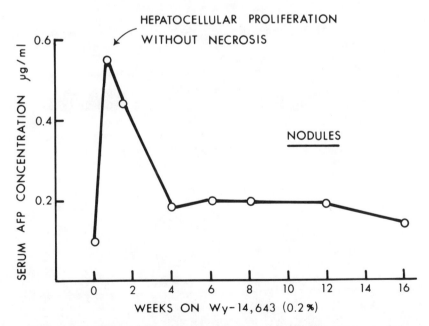

Figure 15: Serum AFP concentrations in male Fischer 344 rats fed 0.2% Wy-14,643 for 16 weeks. [Reproduced from reference (53).]

Diaminodiphenylmethane (DDPM)

Because earlier experiments indicated that oval cells were derived from duct cells,[34, 53, 55] the effect of DDPM, an agent which stimulates bile duct proliferation, was tested.[56] The marked bile duct proliferation induced is not associated with production of serum AFP or proliferation of oval cells.[56] Table 2 gives a comparison of the properties of duct-like structures appearing after CD-AAF induced proliferation of oval cells, bile ducts stimulated by DDPM, and normal bile ducts. The duct-like structures associated with proliferation of oval cells clearly demonstrate different properties and probably represent the differentiation of oval cells into bile-duct-like cells rather than the origin of cells from normal bile ducts.

Table 2: Comparison of Duct Structures Appearing After
CD-AAF or DDPM Exposure

	CD-AAF	DDPM	Normal Ducts
AFP	++	0	0
Albumin	++	0	0
GGT	++	++	+
Laminin	+	+++	+++
Fibronectin	+++	+	+
Location	Mid-lobular	Portal	Portal

CHEMICAL CARCINOGENS IN MICE

Serum AFP and histologic changes in mice following exposure to chemical hepatocarcinogens or in strains with a high incidence of spontaneous hepatocellular carcinomas are summarized in Table 3.[57-61] Although there are some differences, perhaps due to different strains or to the use of different chemicals, it may be concluded that elevations of serum AFP do not consistently occur early in mice after exposure to chemical carcinogens, but rapid elevations are essentially always associated with the development of hepatocellular carcinomas. Also, proliferation of oval cells is not a common feature during chemical hepatocarcinogenesis in the mouse and rapid elevations are essentially always associated with the development of hepatocellular carcinomas. Thus, proliferation of oval cells is not as obvious a feature during chemical carcinogenesis in the mouse as compared to the rat but the production of AFP by PHC is more consistent in the mouse.

DISCUSSION

Figure 16 summarizes the levels of serum AFP after exposure of rats to different carcinogens. The associated morphologic changes are summarized in Table 4. The different morphologic changes and levels of serum AFP appear to indicate that different hepatocarcinogens produce hepatocellular carcinomas by different mechanisms. One should keep an open mind as to the nature of the

Table 3: Summary of Serum AFP and Liver Cancer in Mice

Becker, Stillman & Sell
Cancer Res. 37:870 (1977)[57]

No early elevations in C3H-Avy fB mice, elevations above 100 ng/ml always predictive of "spontaneous" hepatocellular cancer.

Jalanko *et al.*
Int. J. Cancer 21:453 (1978)[58]

C3H/A/BOM male and female mice with a high spontaneous incidence of liver cell cancer. Demonstrated elevated serum AFP in association with preneoplastic lesions and hepatomas.

Becker & Sell
Cancer Res. 39:3491 (1979)[59]

No early elevations in C57BL/6 N mice after exposure to AAF or chlordane although nodular lesions present. Elevation of AFP > 100 ng/ml predictive of cancer.

Jalanko & Ruoslahti
Cancer Res. 39:3494 (1979)[60]

Early low elevation reported with C3H/A/BOM mice exposed to o-aminoazotoluene, later higher elevation associated with cancer. In C3HeB/FeJ mice, spontaneous hepatomas preceeded by slight increase in AFP; high elevations when PHC present. GGT elevations after carcinogen; not with spontaneous hepatocellular cancers.

Princler *et al.*
Eur. J. Cancer 17:1241 (1981)[61]

C3H-Avy fB mice have elevations of AFP associated with spontaneous PHC. Transient earlier AFP elevation is not associated with later development of PHC. Some mice with high AFP have later decline with evidence of tumor regression.

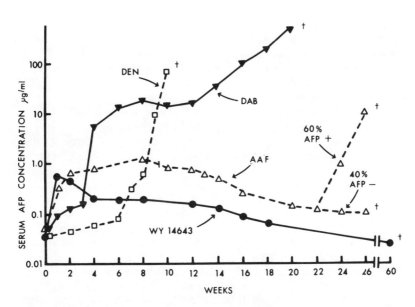

Figure 16: Composite graph showing serum AFP concentrations of rats fed different carcinogens.

DAB = 3'-Methyl-4-dimethylaminoazobenzene
AAF = N-2-Acetylaminofluorene
DEN = Diethylnitrosamine

Table 4: AFP Production and Morphologic Changes After Exposure of Rats to Chemical Hepatocarcinogens

| Carcinogen | . . . . Liver Morphology . . . . | | . . . AFP Production . . . . | | |
	Early	Late	Early (1–4 wk)	Late (10–18 wk)	Hepatomas
AAF	Foci, oval cells (OC)	Nodules, OC, ADH	++	+	+++ to 0
Ethionine	Foci, OC	Nodules, OC, ADH	++	+	+++ to 0
DEN	Foci	Nodules, ADH, ?OC	0	++	+++
3'MDAB	Necrosis, Prolif. OC	Nodules, OC, ADH	++	+++	+++
Wy-14,643	Hepatocyte Prolif.	Nodules	+	0	0
Choline-Def. (CD)	Hepatocyte Prolif.	0	+	0	0
CD + carcinogen (AAF, ETH, DEN)	Massive Oval Cell Prolif.	Nodules, OC	+++	++	+++

pre-neoplastic cells. Oval cells, more differentiated cell types derived from the oval cells, foci, and nodules, as well as normal appearing hepatocytes, must all be considered as possible precursors of PHC.

Regardless of the controversy over the nature of pre-neoplastic lesions, serum AFP appears to be a reliable marker of exposure to chemical hepato-carcinogens in rats. Every carcinogen so far tested that produces hepatomas causes an elevation in AFP at some time during the exposure. However, the interpretations of the kinetics of elevations of serum AFP are not simple. Carcinogens, such as AAF, 3'MDAB, or ethionine produce early prolonged elevations prior to development of cancers. DEN, however, causes no rise during the latent period with low dose exposure, and a rapid rise when tumors appear. Azaserine[62] and Wy-14,643 cause a small rise in AFP which cannot be differentiated from the effects of hepatocyte proliferation, when fed in a commercial diet. However, like DEN, both azaserine and Wy-14,643 cause a larger early rise in serum AFP when fed in a choline-deficient diet.[62] The choline-deficient diet appears to alter the effect of azaserine so that it becomes carcinogenic.[62] It is possible that the combination of high doses of a carcinogen combined with a choline-deficient diet may bring out some early effects of weak hepatocarcinogens. Serum AFP levels are elevated when high doses (1,000 ppm) of the carcinogen benzo(a)pyrene are administered in a purified diet to rats, suggesting that chemical carcinogens that do not act primarily on the liver may also be detected by this means.[63]

Studies of the molecular mechanisms of production of AFP in conjunction with the morphologic changes during carcinogenesis strongly suggest that expression of the AFP gene is the result of a transcriptional control in a new cell population.[10, 64-66] Levels of AFP mRNA are increased in livers containing pre-neoplastic cell populations including oval cells.[67] Studies in normal cells or hepatocellular carcinomas producing AFP have provided no evidence for gene duplication or rearrangement,[66] or for changes in mRNA processing.[68] AFP and albumin gene fragments obtained from PHC and normal livers of the same rat strain have the same restrictive endonucleic patterns.[69] However, there are differences in the restriction endonuclease patterns obtained from liver DNA of different rat strains.[66, 70]

SUMMARY

The ability to use sensitive radioimmunoassays has permitted detection of elevation of AFP during chemical hepatocarcinogenesis in rats and mice. For practical purposes, early prolonged elevations of serum AFP or sudden rapid elevations above 1 μg/ml are conclusive evidence of carcinogenic activity in rats. Weak carcinogens may not produce such patterns unless given in high doses or in combination with a potentiating system such as a choline-deficient diet. Short term determination of serum AFP may be used as a definitive marker for carcinogenic doses of AAF, ethionine, 3'MDAB, and perhaps benzo(a)pyrene. For carcinogens such as DEN, either very high initial doses must be used, or levels of AFP in the serum must be followed for the lifetime of the animal. For carcinogens such as Wy-14,643 or azaserine it may be necessary to administer high doses along with a potentiating diet to stimulate production of AFP.

Acknowledgements

Figures have been reproduced, with permission, from *Application of Biological Markers to Carcinogen Testing* (H.A. Milman and S. Sell, eds.), Plenum Publishing Corp., New York and London (1983).

REFERENCES

1. Abelev, G.I., Perova, S.D., and Khramkova, N.I., Production of embryonal α globulin by transplantable mouse hepatomas. *Transplantation* 1: 174-180 (1963)
2. Gitlin, D., and Boseman, M., Sites of serum α-fetoprotein synthesis in the human and in the rat. *J. Clin. Invest.* 46: 1010 (1967)
3. Gitlin, D., Perricelli, A., and Gitlin, G.M., Synthesis of α-fetoprotein by liver, yolk sac, and gastrointestinal tract of the human conceptus. *Cancer Res.* 32: 979-982 (1972)
4. Smith, C.J.P., and Kelleher, P.C., Alpha-fetoprotein molecular heterogeneity. Physiologic correlations with normal growth, carcinogenesis, and tumor growth. *Biochim. Biophys. Acta* 605: 1-32 (1980)
5. Ishiguro, T., Sakaguchi, H., and Sugitachi, I., Developmental changes of amniotic fluid alpha-fetoprotein subfractions in early gestation. *Amer. J. Repro. Immunol.* 3: 61-64 (1983)
6. Sell, S., Sheppard, H.W., and Poler, M., Effects of α-fetoprotein on murine immune responses. II. Studies of rats. *J. Immunol.* 119: 98 (1977)
7. Mizejewski, G.J., Vonnegut, M., and Jacobson, H.I., Estradiol-activated alpha-fetoprotein suppresses the uterotropic response to estrogens. *Proc. Natl. Acad. Sci., USA* 80:2733-2737 (1983)
8. Castelli, D., Aussel, C., Lafaurie, M., Ayraud, N., and Stora, C., Immunolocalization of alpha-fetoprotein in the ovary and hypophysis of immature female rats. *Histochem. J.* 14: 879-887 (1982)
9. Uriel, J., De Nechaud B., and Dupiers, M., Estrogen binding properties of rat, mouse and man fetospecific serum proteins. Demonstration by immunoautoradiographic methods. *Biochim. Biophys. Res. Commun.* 46: 1175-1180 (1972)

10. Sell, S., Sala-Trepat, J.M., Sargent, T., Thomas, K., Nahon, J.L., Goodman, T., and Bonner, J., Molecular mechanisms of control of albumin and alpha-fetoprotein production: A system to study the early effects of chemical hepatocarcinogens. *Cell Biology Intl. Reports* 4: 235-254 (1980)

11. Selten, G.C., Princen, H.M., Selten-Versteegen, A.M., Mol-Backy, G.P., and Yap, S.H., Sequence content of alpha-fetoprotein, albumin and fibrinogen polypeptide mRNAs in different organs, developing tissues and in liver during carcinogenesis in rats. *Biochim. Biophys. Acta* 699: 131-137 (1982)

12. Beattie, W.G., and Dugaiczyk, A., Structure and evolution of human alpha-fetoprotein deduced from partial sequence of cloned cDNA. *Gene* 20: 415-422 (1982)

13. Jagodzinski, L.L., Sargent, T.D., Yang, M., Glackin, C., and Bonner J., Sequence homology between RNAs encoding rat alpha-fetoprotein and rat serum albumin. *Proc. Natl. Acad. Sci. USA* 78: 3521-3525 (1981)

14. Belayew, A., and Tilghman, S.M., Genetic analysis of alpha-fetoprotein synthesis in mice. *Mol. Cell. Biol.* 2: 1427-1435 (1982)

15. Lowry, O.H., Rosebrough, N.J., Farr, A.L., and Randall, R.J., Protein measurement with the folin phenol reagent. *J. Biol. Chem.* 193: 265-275 (1951)

16. Haglund, H., Isoelectric focusing in natural pH gradients—A technique of growing importance for fractionation and characterization of proteins. *Sci. Tools* 14: 1-7 (1967)

17. Sell, S., Jalowayski, I., Bellone, C., and Wepsic, H.T., Isolation and characterization of rat α-fetoprotein. *Cancer Res.* 32: 1184-1189 (1972)

18. Smith, C.J., and Kelleher, P.C., α-Fetoprotein: Separation of two molecular variants by affinity chromatography with concanavalin A-agarose. *Biochim. Biophys. Acta* 317: 231-235 (1973)

19. Hudig, D., and Sell, S., Isolation, characterization and radioimmunoassay of rat alpha-macrofetoprotein (acute phase A_2 macroglobulin). *Mol. Immunol.* 16: 547-554 (1979)

20. David, G.S., and Reisfeld, R.A., Protein iodination with solid state lactoperoxidase. *Biochemistry* 13: 1014-1021 (1974)

21. Sell, S., Radioimmunoassay of rat α_1-fetoprotein. *Cancer Res.* 33: 1010-1015 (1973)

22. Sell, S., and Gord, D., Rat α-fetoprotein III. Refinement of radioimmunoassay for detection of 1 ng rat α_1 F. *Immunochem.* 10: 439-442 (1973)

23. Brock, D.J., Barron., L., and van Heyningen, V., Enzyme-linked immunospecific assays for human alphafetoprotein using monoclonal antibodies. *Clin. Chim. Acta* 122: 353-358 (1982)

24. Nomura, M., Imai, M., Takahashi, K., Kumakura, T., Tachibana, K., Aoyagi, S., Usuda, S., Nakamura, T., Miyakawa, Y., and Mayumi, M., Three-site sandwich radioimmunoassay with monoclonal antibodies for a sensitive determination of human alpha-fetoprotein. *J. Immunol. Methods* 58: 293-300 (1983)

25. van Heyningen, V., Barron, L., Brock, D.J., Crichton, D., and Lawrie, S., Monoclonal antibodies to human alpha-fetoprotein: Analysis of the behavior of three different antibodies. *J. Immunol. Methods* 50: 123–131 (1982)

26. Nomura, M., Imai, M., Usuda, S., Nakamura, T., Miyakawa, Y., and Mayumi, M., A pitfall in two-site sandwich 'one-step' immunoassay with monoclonal antibodies for the detection of human alpha-fetoproteins. *J. Immunol. Methods* 56: 13-17 (1983)

27. Sell, S., Becker, F.F., Lombardi, B., Shinozuka, H., and Reddy, J., in: *Carcino-Embryonic Proteins* (F.-G. Lehmann, ed.), Vol. 1, pp 129-136, Elsevier/North Holland Press, Amsterdam (1979)

28. Sell, S., Heterogeneity of alphafetoprotein and albumin containing cells in normal and pathological permissive states for AFP production: AFP containing cells in carcinogen fed rats recapitulate the appearance of AFP containing hepatocytes in fetal rats. *Oncodevelop. Biol. Med.* 1: 93-105 (1980)

29. Matray, F., Saufer, F., Borde, J., Mitrofanoff, P., Grosley, M., Laumonier, R., and Hemet, J., Presence of alpha-fetoprotein during liver regeneration following left hepatectomy for hepatoma in an infant. *Pathol. Biol.* (Paris) 20: 253-356 (1972)

30. Watanabe, A., Miyazaki, M., and Taketa, K., Increased α-fetoprotein production in rat liver injuries induced by various hepatotoxins. *Gann* 67: 279-287 (1975)

31. Sell, S., Stillman, D., and Gochman, N., Serum alpha fetoprotein: A diagnostic and prognostic indicator of liver cell necrosis and regeneration following experimental injury by galactosamine in rats. *Am. J. Clin. Pathol.* 66: 847-853 (1976)

32. Teebor, G.W., and Becker, F.F., Regression and persistence of hyperplastic hepatic nodules induced by N-2-fluorenylacetamide and their relationship to hepatocarcinogenesis. *Cancer Res.* 31: 1-3 (1971)

33. Reuber, M.D., Development of preneoplastic and neoplastic lesions of the liver in male rats given 0.025 percent N-2-fluorenyldiacetamide. *J. Natl. Cancer Inst.* 34: 697-724 (1965)

34. Farber, E., Similarities in the sequence of early histological changes included in the liver of the rat by ethionine, 2-acetylaminofluorene, and 3'-methyl-4-dimethylaminobenzene. *Cancer Res.* 16: 142-148 (1956)

35. Becker, F.F., and Sell, S., Early elevation of alphafetoprotein in N-2-fluorenylacetamide hepatocarcinogenesis. *Cancer Res.* 34: 2489-2494 (1974)

36. Weisburger, J.H., Yamamoto, R.S., Williams, G.M., Grantham, P.H., Matsushima, T., and Weisburger, E.K., On the sulfate ester of N-hydroxy-N-2-fluorenylacetamide as a key ultimate hepatocarcinogen in the rat. *Cancer Res.* 32: 491-500 (1972)

37. Sell, S., Distribution of α-fetoprotein- and albumin-containing cells in the livers of Fischer rats fed four cycles of N-2-fluorenylacetamide. *Cancer Res.* 38: 3107-3113 (1978)

38. Becker, F.F., and Sell, S., Differences in serum α-fetoprotein concentrations during the carcinogenic sequences resulting from exposure to diethylnitrosamine or acetylaminofluorene. *Cancer Res.* 39: 1437-1442 (1979)

39. Farber, E., and Cameron, R., The sequential analysis of cancer development. *Advances Cancer Res.* 31: 125-226 (1980)

40. Reuber, M.D., and Firminger, H.I., Morphologic and biologic correlation of lesions obtained in hepatic carcinogenesis in A X C rats given 0.025 percent N-2-fluorenyldiacetamide. *J. Natl. Cancer Inst.* 31: 1407-1429 (1963)

41. Squire, R.A., and Levitt, M.H., Report of a workshop on classification of specific hepatocellular lesions in rats. *Cancer Res.* 35: 3214-3223 (1975)

42. Farber, E., The sequential analysis of liver cancer induction. *Biochim. Biophys. Acta* 605: 149-166 (1980)

43. Williams, G.M., and Yamamoto, R.S., Absence of stainable iron from preneoplastic and neoplastic lesions in rat liver with 8-hydroxyquinoline-induced siderosis. *J. Natl. Cancer Inst.* 49: 685-692 (1972)

44. Sell, S., and Leffert, H.L., An evaluation of cellular lineages in the pathogenesis of experimental hepatocellular carcinoma. *Hepatology* 2: 77-86 (1982)

45. Williams, G.M., The pathogenesis of rat liver cancer caused by chemical carcinogens. *Biochim. Biophys. Acta* 605: 167-189 (1980)

46. Sell, S., Leffert, H.L., Shinozuka, H., Lombardi, B., and Gochman, N., Rapid development of large numbers of α-fetoprotein-containing "oval" cells in the liver of rats fed N-2-fluorenylacetamide in a choline-devoid diet. *Gann* 72: 479-487 (1981)

47. Sell., S., Osborn, K., and Leffert, H.L., Autoradiography of "oval cells" appearing rapidly in the livers of rats fed N-2-fluorenylacetamide in a choline devoid diet. *Carcinogenesis* 2: 7-14 (1981)

48. Sell, S., and Salman, J., Light and electron microscopic autoradiographic analysis of proliferating cells during the early stages of chemical hepato-carcinogenesis in the rat induced by feeding N-2-fluorenylacetamide in a choline deficient diet. *Am. J. Pathol.* 44: 287-300 (1984)

49. Shinozuka, H., Lombardi, B., Sell, S., and Iammarino, R.M., Modification of ethionine liver carcinogenesis by choline deficiency: Early histological and functional alterations. *Cancer Res.* 38: 1092-1098 (1978)

50. Shinozuka, H., Lombardi, B., Sell, S., and Iammarino, R.M., Enhancement of DL-ethionine-induced liver carcinogenesis in rats fed a choline devoid diet. *J. Natl. Cancer Inst.* 61: 813-818 (1978)

51. Becker, F.F., Horland, A.A., Shurgin, A., and Sell, S., A study of α_1-feto-protein levels during exposure to 3'-methyl-4-dimethylaminoazobenzene and its analogs. *Cancer Res.* 35: 1510-1513 (1975)

52. Shinozuka, H., Sells, M.A., Katyal, S.L., Sell, S., and Lombardi, B., Effects of a choline-devoid diet on the emergence of γ-glutamyltranspeptidase positive foci in the liver of carcinogen treated rats. *Cancer Res.* 39: 2515-2521 (1979)

53. Schaffner, F., and Popper, H., Electron microscopic studies of normal and proliferated bile ductules. *Amer. J. Pathol.* 38: 393-410 (1961)

54. Reddy, J.K., Sambasiva Rao, M., Azarnoff, D.L., and Sell, S., Mitogenic and carcinogenic effects of a hypolipidemic peroxisome proliferator, [4-chloro-6-(2,3-xylidino)-2-pyrimidinylthio] acetic acid (Wy-14,643), in rat and mouse liver. *Cancer Res.* 39: 152-161 (1979)

55. Grisham, J.W., and Hartroft, W.S., Morphologic identification by electron microscopy of "oval" cells in experimental hepatic degeneration. *Lab. Invest.* 10: 317-332 (1961)

56. Sell, S., A comparison of oval cells induced by feeding N-2-fluorenyl-acetamide in a choline devoid diet and bile duct cells induced by feeding 4,4'-diaminodiphenylmethane: Evidence that oval cells are not of bile duct origin. *Cancer Res.* 43: 1761-1767 (1983)

57. Becker, F.F., Stillman, D., and Sell, S., Serum α-fetoprotein in mouse strain (C3H-Avy fB) with spontaneous hepatocellular carcinomas. *Cancer Res.* 37: 870-872 (1977)

58. Jalanko, H., Virtanen, I., Engvail, E., and Ruoslahti, E., Early increases of serum alpha-fetoprotein in spontaneous hepatocarcinogenesis in mice. *Int. J. Cancer* 21: 453-459 (1978)

59. Becker, F.F., and Sell, S., Alphafetoprotein levels and hepatic alterations during chemical carcinogenesis in C57BL mice. *Cancer Res.* 39: 3491-3494 (1979)

60. Jalanko, H., and Ruoslahti, E., Differential expression of α-fetoprotein and γ-glutamyltranspeptidase in chemical and spontaneous hepatocarcino-genesis. *Cancer Res.* 39: 3495-3501 (1979)

61. Princler, G.L., Vlahakis, G., Kortright, K.H., Okada, S., and McIntire, K.R., Dynamics of serum alpha-fetoprotein during spontaneous hepatocellular carcinoma development in mice. *Eur. J. Cancer Clin. Oncol.* 17: 1241-1248 (1981)

62. Shinozuka, H., Katyal, S.L., and Lombardi, B., Azaserine carcinogenesis: Organ susceptibility change in rats fed a diet devoid of choline. *Int. J. Cancer* 22: 36-39 (1978)

63. Boyd, J.N., Misslbeck, N., Babish, J.G., Campbell, T.C., and Stoewsand, G.S., Plasma α-fetoprotein elevation and mutagenicity of urine as early predictors of carcinogenicity in benzo(a)pyrene fed rats. *Drug Chem. Toxicol.* 4: 197-205 (1981)

64. Sala-Trepat, J.M., Sargent, T.D., Sell, S., and Bonner, J., α-Fetoprotein and albumin genes of rats: No evidence for amplification-deletion or rearrangement in rat liver carcinogenesis. *Proc. Natl. Acad. Sci. USA* 76: 695-699 (1979)

65. Sell, S., Thomas, K., Michalson, M., Sala-Trepat, J., and Bonner, J., Control of albumin and α-fetoprotein expression in rat liver and in some transplantable hepatocellular carcinomas. *Biochim. Biophys. Acta* 564: 173-178 (1979)

66. Sala-Trepat, J.M., Dever, J., Sargent, T.D., Thomas, K., Sell, S., and Bonner, J., Changes in expression of albumin and α-fetoprotein genes during rat liver development and neoplasia. *Biochemistry* 18: 2167-2178 (1979)

67. Atryzek, V., Tamaoki, T., and Fausto, N., Changes in polysomal polyadenylated RNA and α-fetoprotein messenger RNA during hepatocarcinogenesis. *Cancer Res.* 40: 3713-3718 (1980)

68. Nahon, J.L., Gal, A., Frain, M., Sell, S., and Sala-Trepat, J.M., No evidence for post-transcriptional control of albumin and α-fetoprotein gene expression in developing rat liver and neoplasia. *Nucleic Acids Res.* 10: 1895-1911 (1982)

69. Boutler, J., and Sell, S., Abstract, AACR Meeting, 1982. Unpublished Data.

70. Lucotte, G., Gal, A., Nahon, J.L., and Sala-Trepat, J.M., EcoRI restriction-site polymorphism of the albumin gene in different inbred strains of rat. *Biochem. Genetics* 20: 1105-1115 (1982)

22

Ornithine Decarboxylase as a Marker of Carcinogenesis

Diane H. Russell

University of Arizona
Tucson, Arizona

INTRODUCTION

Ornithine decarboxylase (ODC, EC 4.1.1.17) serves as a unique, early marker of the action of complete chemical carcinogens or tumor promoters. Usually, peak ODC activity is expressed within four to six hours after exposure to the carcinogen or promoter,[1,2] and the extent of the increase in the enzyme activity exhibits a dose-dependent relationship to the chemical carcinogen or promoter. Boutwell et al.[3] and Slaga et al.[4] have reported not only a close correlation between tumor-promoting potency of a compound and the induction of ODC activity but also between the inhibitory action of retinoids on both ODC and tumor promotion and expression.[5] These correlations are likely a result of a fundamental requirement for expression of ODC and/or biosynthesis of polyamines to affect changes in nucleic acid synthesis, proliferation and differentiation—all parameters altered by carcinogens.

Ornithine decarboxylase, the initial and rate-limiting enzyme in the polyamine biosynthetic pathway, appears to be a key regulatory enzyme in growth and differentiation.[6-10] Its activity is regulated by all known classes of hormones acting on their specific target organ(s).[10-12] Hormones with dramatically different mechanisms of action work on their target tissues to effect the rapid enhancement of certain common pathways such as the coupled induction of ODC and increased RNA polymerase I activity.[10] These enhancements lead to marked, early sequential increases in putrescine, spermidine and ribosomal RNA biosynthesis and accumulation.[13-19] In cell culture, the induction of ODC and the accumulation of putrescine are initiated in the G_1 phase of the cell cycle and appear to be required for the progression of cells into S phase (DNA synthesis) and for later cell division.[20-23]

The product of ODC catalysis, putrescine, is the precursor of the poly-amines, spermidine and spermine.[24] Polyamines are the organic cations of the cell, are probably integral to the regulation of cellular pH, and have a variety of well-documented physiological and biochemical effects.[7] Putrescine long has been known to be both a procaryotic and eucaryotic growth factor,[25-29] is accumulated in tissues in response to a growth stimulus,[20,30] is conjugated to discrete nuclear proteins intracellularly,[31,32] and is excreted by cells undergoing mitosis.[10,33] The major urinary form is monoacetylputrescine.[34,35] Spermidine accumulates in a parallel fashion to ribosomal RNA,[14,15] is acetylated and excreted as monoacetylspermidine derivatives,[34-36] has been shown to increase the rate of chain elongation of DNA, RNA and protein synthesis, and is a specific translational factor for fidelity of protein synthesis.[37-41] Increased extracellular concentrations of spermidine appear related to cell toxicity and cell death processes with the major urinary conjugates being N^1-acetylspermidine and N^8-acetylspermidine.[35,36] Spermine, on the other hand, is highest in differentiated cells and increases the efficiency of the acylation of transfer RNA, a process required for optimal protein synthesis.[42,43] Spermine has the capacity to be reconverted to putrescine and spermidine.[44,45] So far, acetylated spermine has not been detected in urine, and in most abnormal growth processes such as non-differentiated malignancies; the excretion of spermine is low relative to putrescine and spermidine.[10]

Determination of ODC activity alone does not always reflect the changes in the patterns and concentrations of polyamines. Therefore, induction of ODC may be an essential component of complete carcinogenesis, but elevations in putrescine and spermidine also are required and can occur from the back conversion of spermidine and spermine as well as possibly by altered turnover of putrescine.[44-46] The ability to rapidly inhibit ODC activity by cations,[47] including the polyamines themselves,[48] by protein-protein interactions,[49,50] or by post-translational modification of the molecule[50-53] underlines the importance of careful experimentation in order to fully characterize the involvement of ODC in carcinogenesis. Nevertheless, in most instances, it serves as an accurate biochemical marker of carcinogen action.

THE ROLE OF ORNITHINE DECARBOXYLASE IN CARCINOGENESIS

Ornithine decarboxylase is rapidly and markedly elevated in target organs and cells in culture by tumor-producing concentrations of chemical carcinogens,[2] by agents which result in tumors such as dose-dependent exposure of mouse skin to ultraviolet B light,[54,55] after oncogenic viral transformation,[23,56-58] and in response to promoters of carcinogenicity.[3]

Classic studies of alterations in ODC activity and levels of polyamines in chick embryo fibroblasts after viral transformation were reported by Bachrach and coworkers in 1975.[56,57] Transformation with an oncogenic virus, Rous sarcoma virus (RSV), resulted in a 2- to 3-fold elevation of cellular putrescine and spermidine but did not alter the levels of spermine. Such elevations in polyamines are characteristic of tumor cell lines such as mouse L1210 leukemia cells[30] and rat hepatomas.[9,59] Of interest, normal and transformed cells had a similar proliferation rate but differed in the content of polyamines and in ODC activity.[56] In human patients with renal carcinomas, the concentrations of polyamines were measured in tumor nodules and in samples from the same kidney that were judged free of tumor by histological examination.[60] As in the case of cells after oncogenic viral transformation, an elevated concentration of spermidine was detected in the carcinomas compared to normal renal tissue.[60]

In a cell line transformed by a temperature-sensitive mutant of RSV, increased ODC activity and transformation occurred only at the permissive temperature.[56] Later studies of ODC in normal and virus-transformed rat fibroblasts corroborated the ability to detect a rapid alteration in ODC activity in response to virus transformation and demonstrated distinct differences in induction requirements after transformation.[23] The ODC activity was induced to a much greater extent during progression of G_1 phase and was maintained at a higher level during the transition of G_1 to S phase in transformed cells. Further, induction of ODC was dependent on serum-medium addition in Rat-1 cells, whereas after transformation, medium alone resulted in a substantial elevation of enzyme activity. Lastly, induction of ODC was less sensitive to repression of putrescine in the RSV-transformed cells. These alterations in characteristics of the expression of ODC were found to be a consequence of the transforming function of RSV in the Rat-1 fibroblast since a cell line transformed by a thermosensitive mutant, LA24/RSV, exhibited altered expression of ODC only at the permissive temperature. Transformation of chick embryo fibroblasts by a temperature-sensitive mutant of RSV has been shown also to more than double the half-life of ODC at the permissive temperature.[58] The relatively short half-life of ODC, 10 to 20 minutes, first reported in regenerating rat liver,[61] also was more than doubled after refeeding normal, starved chick embryo fibroblasts.[58]

In an extensive study of effects of antitumor agents on tumor development in L1210 leukemic mice, it was shown that the increase in survival time of the mice inoculated with L1210 leukemia tumor cells was proportional to a decrease in the content of polyamine of tumor cells.[30,62,63] Russell and Levy[30] were the first to demonstrate that the inhibition of the accumulation of putrescine and spermidine paralleled the attenuation of the growth rate of the tumor, a fact whose implications only recently have begun to be explored in terms of the development of drugs which block the enzymes in the polyamine biosynthetic pathway as possible antitumor agents. Agents such as α-difluoromethylornithine (DFMO) and methylglyoxal-bis(guanylhydrazone) (MGBG) are specific inhibitors of polyamine biosynthesis being tested as antitumor agents. Further evidence that rapid proliferation of cancers is reflected in elevated concentrations of putrescine and spermidine and elevated spermidine-to-spermine ratios is represented in a recent review[64] which also summarizes the data substantiating the utility of measuring urinary excretion of polyamine to assess tumor growth fraction and cell loss fraction and response to therapy in human cancer patients.

Increased ODC activity can be demonstrated in target organs within hours of the administration of organ-specific carcinogens (Table 1). For certain carcinogens, such as diethylnitrosamine, the elevation of liver ODC activity was dose-dependent.[1] Daily treatment with noncarcinogenic doses of diethylnitrosamine for four or seven days resulted in elevated ODC activity measured 24 hours after the last injection. Further, the serial injection of diethylnitrosamine for seven days produced a greater increase in the induction of ODC than did four days of treatment. Interestingly, a single injection of a carcinogenic dose of diethylnitrosamine (200 mg/kg) resulted in 8- to 14-fold elevation of liver ODC activity for seven days.[1] These studies which report elevated concentrations of putrescine and spermidine after viral transformation and in carcinomas suggest that carcinogenesis requires elevated polyamine biosynthesis.

Table 1: Carcinogen-Induced Increase in Ornithine Decarboxylase Activity

System	Reference
DMBA-induced breast carcinoma	Andersson *et al.*, 1976[65]
Dimethylhydrazine-treated colon, AAF-treated liver	Salser *et al.*, 1976[66]
4-Dimethylaminoazobenzene-treated rat liver	Scalabrino *et al.*, 1978[67]
Diethylnitrosamine-induced liver carcinogenesis and tumor foci formation	Olson & Russell, 1979[1] Olson & Russell, 1980[2]
Carcinogen-treated mouse bladder	Matsushima & Bryan, 1980[68]
DMBA-induced pancreatic tumor	Black & Chang, 1981[69]
Addition of carcinogens, diethylnitrosamine, benzo[a]pyrene, methylmethanesulfonate and ethylmethanesulfonate to monolayers of adult rat liver cells	van Wijk *et al.*, 1981[70]
Asbestos-treatment hamster tracheal epithelial cells—synergism with TPA	Landesman & Mossman, 1982[71]

ORNITHINE DECARBOXYLASE AS A MARKER OF PROMOTION OF CARCINOGENESIS

Since the 1940's chemical carcinogenesis has been known to occur as a two-stage process of initiation and promotion.[72,73] It was demonstrated that the application of promoting agents subsequent to the exposure of mouse skin to sub-carcinogenic doses of polycyclic aromatic hydrocarbons (initiating agents) was more effective in eliciting tumorigenic responses than hydrocarbons alone. The promoting agent used in these early experiments was croton oil, which was obtained from the seeds of the plant *Croton tiglium*, indigenous to India and Ceylon. The active tumor promoting components of croton oil were isolated by Hecker and partially characterized as phorbol esters.[74] The most potent phorbol ester characterized to date remains 12-O-tetradecanoylphorbol-13-acetate (TPA).

Induction of ODC has been shown also to be a consistent event in response to tumor promoters such as TPA, a diterpene compound (Table 2). Boutwell and co-workers[76] first linked TPA-stimulated ODC activity in mouse skin to tumor promotion; application of TPA directly to the mouse skin resulted in a 230-fold elevation of ODC within four hours.[75] The induction was dependent on protein synthesis but not RNA synthesis since it was blocked by pretreatment with cycloheximide but not affected by pretreatment with actinomycin D. The half-life of ODC in skin after induction with TPA was 17 minutes, similar to that first reported by Russell and Snyder[61] for ODC in regenerating rat liver. Cordycepin

Table 2: Ornithine Decarboxylase (ODC) Induction by Promoters of Carcinogenicity

Organ or Cell Line	Extent of ODC Elevation	Reference
TPA application to mouse skin	200–400-fold	O'Brien et al., 1975[75]
		O'Brien et al., 1975[76]
		O'Brien, 1976[77]
		Mufson et al., 1977[78]
TPA addition to mouse epidermal cells	10-fold	Yuspa et al., 1976[79]
Hexa-analog	10-fold	Yuspa et al., 1976[79]
Phorbol dibenzoate	10-fold	Yuspa et al., 1976[79]
Phorbol dibutyrate	3-fold	Yuspa et al., 1976[79]
TPA addition to hamster embryo cells, 3T3 mouse cells, and HE68BP cells	7–10-fold	O'Brien et al., 1979[80]
		O'Brien et al., 1980[81]
Mouse skin after HHPA (12-O-hexadecanoyl-16-hydroxy-phorbol-13-acetate) and 4-deoxy-HHPA application	60–110-fold	Fujiki et al., 1980[82]
TPA application to rat skin	4-fold	Lesiewicz et al., 1980[83]
TPA administration on rat brain, liver and lung, and mouse liver	8–250-fold	Weiner & Byus, 1980[84]
		Byus & Weiner, 1982[85]
Rat liver after i.p. injection of TPA	5-fold	Bisschop et al., 1981[86]
Teleocidin B application to mouse skin	300-fold	Fujiki et al., 1981[87]
TPA addition to bladder cancer cell cultures	39-fold	Izumi et al., 1981[88]
Rat liver after topical TPA	30-fold	Kishore & Boutwell, 1981[89]
TPA on proliferating basal cells of mouse epidermis	10–25-fold	Lichti et al., 1981[90]
Mouse skin explants in culture in response to TPA	40-fold	Verma & Boutwell, 1981[91]
TPA addition to Reuber H35 hepatoma cells	10–33-fold	Wu et al., 1981[92]
TPA addition to Chinese hamster ovary cells	13-fold	Lichti & Gottesman, 1982[93]
TPA administration to mouse embryo fibroblasts	2-fold	Lillehaug & Djurhuus, 1982[94]
Swiss 3T3 cells after TPA administration	7-fold	Lockyer & Magun, 1983[95]
Mouse liver after TPA administration	9–30-fold	Raunio & Pelkonen, 1983[96]
Multiple applications of TPA to mouse skin	600-fold*	Takigawa et al., 1983[97]

*After 5th application

(3'-deoxyadenosine), a compound that partially blocks the synthesis of mRNA, partially blocked the elevation in ODC activity. The increase was not dependent on elevations of either cyclic AMP or cyclic GMP.[78] Both phospholipase and lipoxygenase activities have been implicated as intermediates in the ability of TPA to induce ODC in mouse skin.[98-101] Pretreatment with colchicine or other microtubule-disrupting agents[102] also inhibited the ability of TPA to induce ODC in mouse epidermis, suggesting that an intact microtubular structure is required for the TPA-stimulated induction of ODC. In explants of mouse skin maintained in serum-free Eagle's HeLa cell medium, chelation of extracellular calcium by EGTA prevented the induction of ODC by TPA.[91] Addition of calcium to the medium, but not magnesium, restored the induction. Trifluoperazine, a calmodulin inhibitor, also was able to inhibit induction of ODC in the presence of TPA.

Further evidence that induction of ODC was relevant to the promotion phase of carcinogenesis was suggested by studies of a series of phorbol esters with different abilities to promote tumor formation. Their relative promoting capacity was directly related to the magnitude of the induction of ODC.[3] Other weaker promoters, such as Tween 60, anthralin, and iodoacetic acid, also induced ODC activity but at doses 100- to 1000-fold greater than TPA.

Multiple applications of TPA to mouse skin resulted in induction of ODC after each application with similar kinetic parameters. However, after eight applications, the induction reached a level 600-fold above controls.[3] Boutwell *et al.*[3] hypothesized that induction of ODC was specifically associated with tumor promotion. They maintained that the demonstrated induction of ODC activity by carcinogens, such as application of 7,12-dimethylbenz(a)anthracene (DMBA) to mouse skin, was related not to their initiation properties but to their promoter capacity. Promoters stimulate growth-related events such as protein, RNA and DNA synthesis, and decrease terminal cell differentiation events. A long-term study of dietary phenobarbital as a promoter of diethylnitrosamine-induced hepatic carcinogenesis did not demonstrate elevated ODC activity monitored at one, 11 and 20 weeks after 500 ppm phenobarbital in the diet.[103] However, evidence that dietary phenobarbital significantly increased the number of neoplastic nodules or hepatic cellular carcinomas was not presented either. It is possible that the timing of monitoring of ODC activity related to tumor-like phenotypic expression was premature. Olson and Russell[2] found that dietary 2-acetylaminofluorene (2-AAF) after the initiation of liver carcinogenesis with diethylnitrosamine also did not result in an early elevation of ODC activity. Other studies which do not support the correlation of induction of ODC to tumor promotion are difficult to interpret.[104,105]

The correlation between the potency of phorbol esters to promote tumor formation and their ability to induce ODC and to stimulate DNA synthesis has been shown to be dependent upon the dose of phorbol ester.[79] For instance, the addition of 0.1 μg/ml TPA to epidermal cells resulted in the same extent of induction of ODC as a 10-fold higher amount of TPA, 1.0 μg/ml. At the lower concentration of TPA, there was a consistent relationship between the induction of ODC and subsequent DNA synthesis and tumor promotion. However, at high concentrations, the relationship was less clear and certain phorbol esters and hyperplastic agents without promoting ability resulted in small increases of ODC activity. Boutwell[106,107] suggested that tumor promotion itself might consist of more than one stage. Since that time, Slaga and co-workers[108-111] have provided evidence that tumor promotion can be divided into at least two stages, designated stage I and II. They suggested that promotion is reversible in stage I but later becomes irreversible. Limiting applications of TPA act as stage I promoters, whereas mezerein, an analog of TPA, is a weak stage I promoter but an effective stage II agent when given after stage I promotion. The characteristic, apparently common to the stage I promoters, is the ability to stimulate altered function and proliferation of keratinocytes.[112-114] This selective ability to stimulate a particular type of cell may be characteristic of stage I promotion whereas stage II promotion now appears related to the accumulation of polyamines, particularly that of putrescine, since stage II promoters such as mezerein can be blocked by the administration of a suicide inhibitor of ODC, α-difluoromethylornithine (DFMO), resulting in the inhibition of ODC activity, decreased accumulation of putrescine, marked reduction in papilloma size and number, followed by a dramatic reduction in tumor incidence. It is important to note that the concentration of putrescine returned to normal within 24 hours after a single application of TPA, and that putrescine significantly enhanced tumor yield when given with TPA whereas putrescine alone did not affect epidermal ODC or result in formation of papilloma. Therefore, ODC activity marks both stage I and stage II promoter events. Blocking of stage I-specific ODC activity blocks tumor promotion and limits tumor expression whereas blocked ODC in stage II selectively can be overcome by the addition of putrescine. Further, the tumor promoter potency of TPA can be markedly enhanced by the simultaneous administration of putrescine. That both expression of ODC and the capacity for marked accumulation of putrescine may be characteristic of the expression of tumor phenotype now has been carefully demonstrated both in response to oncogenic viral transformation and after tumor development in response to sequential initiation and promotion events.

There is no doubt that tumor promoters, particularly TPA, are powerful inducers of ODC. Although carcinogens elevate ODC, this elevation has been attributed to their capacity as promoters and not to their initiating properties. The ability to block induction by ODC of initiated mouse skin in response to tumor promoters such as TPA is highly correlated with the inhibition of tumor formation. This will be discussed in more detail later in relation to the effect of analogs of vitamin A on ODC activity. Retinoid analogs have been widely studied as blockers of the induction by TPA of ODC activity as well as for their growth inhibitory properties.

ORNITHINE DECARBOXYLASE ACTIVITY AS A MARKER OF THE CARCINOGENIC AND PROMOTING PROPERTIES OF ULTRAVIOLET LIGHT

ODC activity may serve as a biochemical marker of the carcinogenic and promoting effects of ultraviolet B (UVB) light.[54,115-117] A marked induction of ODC occurs in mouse skin after exposure to UVB radiation. Maximal increases in ODC activity (250- to 400-fold above basal level) are comparable to those after application of TPA to mouse skin.[54] Again, epidermal induction of ODC was related to the dose of radiation from 0.02 joule/cm^2 to 0.18 joule/cm^2 and could be blocked by treatment with cycloheximide.

ODC activity and concentrations of polyamines were monitored in mouse skin after exposure to an amount of UVB known to be carcinogenic in hairless mice.[115] Epidermal ODC was induced within six hours and peaked at 24 hours after a single irradiation with UVB.[116] However, after 20 irradiations, ODC activity peaked at six hours and had returned to control level within 24 hours. Peak accumulation of putrescine paralleled the fluctuation in ODC activity, and the level of putrescine continued to increase with increasing numbers of irradiations. Levels of spermidine also were elevated and spermine decreased, a pattern reminiscent of rapid growth processes, viral transformation and of known tumor cell lines, as previously discussed. A spermidine/spermine ratio of 5.7 compared to 1.8 in nonirradiated controls was detected 48 hours after a single irradiation with UVB.[116] Seiler and Knödgen[118] have shown that UV light actually increased the turnover rate of spermidine and spermine in the epidermis of hairless mice.

Elevated activity of ODC and elevated concentrations of putrescine, spermidine and spermine also occur in hyperplastic skin disorders such as human psoriasis.[119-122] Therefore, elevated ODC activity and altered patterns of accumulation of polyamine mark both normal and carcinogenic growth processes, and these alterations underscore the difficulty in evaluating ODC as a specific tumor-promoting event. Careful studies, however, still point to increased ODC activity as a necessity for the activity of tumor-promoting agents.[97] Further, the requirement for expression of ODC is compatible with the effect of tumor promoters to enhance the biosynthesis and proliferation of polyamine in certain cell types.

EFFECTS OF ANALOGS OF VITAMIN A ON ORNITHINE DECARBOXYLASE ACTIVITY

Because of the implications of analogs of vitamin A as anticarcinogenic agents, a discussion of their effects on ODC and carcinogenesis is in order. Vitamin A and several of its analogs were shown to inhibit induction of ODC in the G_1 phase of the cell cycle of synchronous cultures of Chinese hamster ovary cells.[123,124] Inhibition of ODC by retinol appeared not to be a result of the general inhibition of protein synthesis, since protein synthesis was inhibited by only 20%. After the addition of retinol, not only was ODC inhibited but also DNA synthesis and cell proliferation. Therefore, the inhibition of ODC by retinoids may be related to known prophylactic and therapeutic effects on the induction and growth of benign and malignant tumors in whole animals by chemicals.[125-127] In general, there is a direct inverse relationship between the level of retinoid in the diet and the incidence of neoplasms after a chemical carcinogen.[128] Carcinogenesis is a prolonged multistage process, as previously discussed, and retinoids apparently act to inhibit the promotion phase and do not affect initiation. Table 3 demonstrates various cell types and tissues in which retinoids have been shown to inhibit ODC activity. In general, the extent of inhibition of ODC activ-

Table 3: Retinoids Inhibit Ornithine Decarboxylase (ODC) Activity

System	Analog (dose)	Reference
TPA-induced ODC in bovine lymphocytes	Retinoic acid (100 μM) Juvenile hormone (100 μM)	Kensler et al., 1978[129] Kensler et al., 1978[129]
TPA-induced ODC in mouse epidermis	7 retinoic acids, retinal, and cyclopentenyl analogs	Verma et al., 1978[130]
ODC in Chinese hamster ovary cell cycle	Retinol (10^{-5} M)	Haddox & Russell, 1979[123]
ODC in neuroblastoma and glioma cell cultures (5- to 10-fold less sensitive)	Retinoic acid (50–250 μM) Retinol (50–250 μM) Retinal (5–50 μM)	Haddox et al., 1979[124] Russell & Haddox, 1981[131] Chapman, 1980[132]
TPA-stimulated ODC in mouse skin	Retinoic acid (0.17 nmol) (topically)	Verma et al., 1980[99]
PTH-stimulated ODC in chondrocytes (pretreatment for 3–4 days)	Retinyl acetate (0.2–1 μM)	Takigawa et al., 1980[133]
Parathyroid hormone-induced ODC in rabbit costal chondrocytes	Retinyl acetate (0.2–1 μM) Retinoic acid (0.2 μM)	Takigawa et al., 1980[133] Takigawa et al., 1980[133]
Carcinogen-induced ODC in urinary bladder	13-cis-retinoic acid (0.28–28 μM)	Matsushima & Bryan, 1980[68]
TPA-induced liver ODC	Retinyl acetate (0.2–2 μg/kg)	Bisschop et al., 1981[86]
TPA- and UV-stimulated ODC in primary mouse epidermal cell cultures	Retinoic acid (0.1–1 μM)	Lichti et al., 1981[134]
MSH-stimulated ODC in mouse melanoma cells	Retinoic acid (0.1–1 μM) Retinoic acid (86 M)	Scott et al., 1982[135] Scott et al., 1983[136]
UVB-induced ODC in mouse epidermis	Retinoic acid (1.7–3.4 nmol) (topically)	Breeding & Lowe, 1982[137]
TPA-induced ODC in Swiss mouse 3T3 fibroblasts	Retinoic acid (10^{-8} to 10^{-6} M)	Bolmer & Wolf, 1982[138]

ity in response to the retinoid analog corresponds to the subsequent extent of inhibition of DNA synthesis and cell proliferation. Inhibition of ODC by retinoic acid in initiated and promoted mouse skin also positively correlates with inhibition of DNA synthesis and of tumor formation.[3,54]

The role of both induction of ODC and accumulation of putrescine in stage I and stage II tumor promotion as well as the point(s) in the promotion of inhibition of these processes by vitamin A and of inhibition of tumor formation are still difficult to fit into one cohesive theory. A further complexity seems to be the requirement (or generality) of a defined rapid increase in ODC activity in initiated tissues in response to a carcinogenic dose of a carcinogen. In synchronized CHO cells, the G_1 phase block of cell cycle progression in response to retinol administration could not be reversed by the addition of putrescine suggesting that the excursion of ODC itself, as well as accumulation of putrescine, was required for normal cell cycle progression.[131] Byus and co-workers[139] have noted and discussed the evidence in TPA-stimulated Reuber H35 cells, as a function of days in culture, which demonstrated a negative correlation between the level of induction of ODC and intracellular concentrations of putrescine. Therefore, any meaningful interpretation of the requirement of induction of ODC following treatment with TPA in the process of DNA synthesis and tumor promotion must assess the ability of the cell to accumulate putrescine, spermidine and spermine.

Nevertheless, in a physiological response system such as mouse skin, induction of ODC in response to treatment with TPA appears required for stage I promotion of an initiating agent. For stage II promotion, putrescine can be added to substitute for the increase in ODC and subsequent synthesis of putrescine.[111] The suicide substrate inhibitor of ODC, DFMO, which prevents both TPA-induced ODC activity and the accumulation of putrescine, blocks tumor formation after initiation with DMBA and treatment with TPA.[140] Also, in the skin model of tumorigenesis, retinoids appear to block stage II promotion, and the block can be reversed by the addition of putrescine.[110]

In summary, ODC can serve as a useful marker of carcinogen and promoter activity. Its key position in the early cascade regulating ribosomal RNA and ultimate new protein synthesis, coupled with its rapid response are suggestive of its importance and underline its predictability as a biochemical marker. Because ODC may be a multi-functional protein that can be modified to serve other purposes, and because metabolism of polyamines is complex, its activity may not always correlate with alterations in the polyamine pools. Monitoring both ODC activity and concentrations of polyamines assists in defining the actions of carcinogens and promoters and may in time provide us with new leads to assist in an understanding of the process of carcinogenesis.

REFERENCES

1. Olson, J.W., and Russell, D.H., Prolonged induction of hepatic ornithine decarboxylase and its relation to cyclic adenosine $3':5'$-monophosphate-dependent protein kinase activation after a single administration of diethylnitrosamine. *Cancer Res.* 39: 3074–3079 (1979)

2. Olson, J.W., and Russell, D.H., Prolonged ornithine decarboxylase induction in regenerating carcinogen-treated liver. *Cancer Res.* 40: 4373-4380 (1980)

3. Boutwell, R.K., O'Brien, T.G., Verma, A.K., Weekes, R.G., DeYoung, L.M., Ashendel, C.L., and Astrup, E.G., in: *Naturally Occurring Carcinogens-Mutagens and Modulators of Carcinogenesis* (E.C. Miller, J.A. Miller, I. Hirono, T. Sugimura, and S. Takayama, eds.), pp 287-300, Japan Sci. Soc. Press, Tokyo/Univ. Park Press, Baltimore (1979)

4. Yuspa, S.H., Lichti, U., Hennings, H., Ben, T., Patterson, E., and Slaga, T.J., in: *Carcinogenesis* (T.J. Slaga, A. Sivak, and R.K. Boutwell, eds.), Vol. 2, pp 245-255, Raven Press, New York (1978)

5. Verma, A.K., Shapas, B.G., Rice, H.M., and Boutwell R.K., Correlation of the inhibition by retinoids of tumor promoter-induced mouse epidermal ornithine decarboxylase activity and of skin tumor promotion. *Cancer Res.* 39: 419-425 (1979)

6. Russell, D., and Snyder, S.H., Amine synthesis in rapidly growing tissues: Ornithine decarboxylase activity in regenerating rat liver, chick embryo, and various tumors. *Proc. Natl. Acad. Sci. USA* 60: 1420-1427 (1968)

7. Cohen, S.S., *Introduction to the Polyamines*, New Jersey: Prentice-Hall, Inc. (1971)

8. Bachrach, U., *Function of Naturally Occurring Polyamines*, New York: Academic Press (1973)

9. Russell, D.H., in: *Polyamines in Normal and Neoplastic Growth* (D.H. Russell, ed.), pp 1-13, Raven Press, New York (1973)

10. Russell, D.H., and Durie, B.G.M., *Polyamines as Markers of Normal and Malignant Growth*, New York: Raven Press (1978)

11. Haddox, M.K., and Russell, D.H., in: *Cold Spring Harbor Conferences on Cell Proliferation—Protein Phosphorylation*, Book B (O.M. Rosen, and E.G. Krebs, eds.), Vol. 8, pp 1013-1035, Cold Spring Harbor Laboratory, New York (1981)

12. Russell, D.H., in: *Polyamines in Biology and Medicine* (D.R. Morris, and L.J. Marton, eds.), pp 109-125, Marcel Dekker, Inc., New York (1981)

13. Cohen, S.S., Hoffner, N., Jansen, M., Moore, M., and Raina, A., Polyamines, RNA synthesis, and streptomycin lethality in a relaxed mutant of *E. coli* strain 15 TAU. *Proc. Natl. Acad. Sci. USA* 57: 721-728 (1967)

14. Cohen, S.S., and Raina, A., in: *Organizational Biosynthesis* (H.J. Vogel, J.O. Lampen, and V. Bryson, eds.), pp 157-182, Academic Press, New York (1967)

15. Dion, A.S., and Herbst, E.J., The localization of spermidine in salivary gland cells of *Drosophila melanogaster* and its effect on H^3-uridine incorporation. *Proc. Natl. Acad. Sci. USA* 57: 2367-2371 (1967)

16. Tsang, B.K., and Singhal, R.L., Polyamine and cAMP metabolism in rat ventral prostate (VP) following administration of cyproterone acetate (CA). *The Pharmacologist* 18: 164 (1976)

17. Seiler, N., and Schroeder, M., Relations between polyamines and nucleic acids. II. Biochemical and fine structural studies on peripheral nerve during wallerian degeneration. *Brain Res.* 22: 81-103 (1970)

18. Russell, D.H., Putrescine and spermidine biosynthesis in the development of normal and anucleolate mutants of *Xenopus laevis*. *Proc. Natl. Acad. Sci. USA* 68: 523-527 (1971)

19. Russell, D.H., and McVicker, T.A., Polyamines in the developing rat and in supportive tissues. *Biochim. Biophys. Acta* 259: 247-250 (1972)

20. Russell, D.H., and Stambrook, P.J., Cell cycle specific fluctuations in adenosine 3':5'-cyclic monophosphate and polyamines of Chinese hamster cells. *Proc. Natl. Acad. Sci. USA* 72: 1482–1486 (1975)
21. Fuller, D.J.M., Gerner, E.W., and Russell, D.H., Polyamine biosynthesis and accumulation during the G_1 to S phase transition. *J. Cell. Physiol.* 93: 81–88 (1977)
22. Chapman, S.K., Martin, M., Hoover, M.S., and Chiou, C.Y., Ornithine decarboxylase activity and the growth of neuroblastoma cells. The effects of bromoacetylcholine, bromoacetate, and 1,3-diaminopropane. *Biochem. Pharmacol.* 27: 717–721 (1978)
23. Haddox, M.K., Magun, B.E., and Russell, D.H., Ornithine decarboxylase induction during G_1 progression of normal and RSV-transformed cells. *Cancer Res.* 40: 604–608 (1980)
24. Tabor, H., and Tabor, C.W., Spermidine, spermine and related amines. *Pharmacol. Rev.* 16: 245–300 (1964)
25. Herbst, E.W., and Snell, E.E., Putrescine as a growth factor for *Hemophilus parainfluenzae. J. Biol. Chem.* 176: 989–990 (1948)
26. Sneath, P.H.A., Putrescine as an essential growth factor for a mutant of *Aspergillus nidulans. Nature* 175: 818 (1955)
27. Ham, R.G., Putrescine and related amines as growth factors for a mammalian cell line. *Biochem. Biophys. Res. Commun.* 14: 34–38 (1964)
28. Ham, R.G., Clonal growth of mammalian cells in a chemically defined synthetic medium. *Proc. Natl. Acad. Sci. USA* 53: 288–293 (1965)
29. Pohjanpelto, P., and Raina, A., Identification of a growth factor produced by human fibroblasts *in vitro* as putrescine. *Nature New Biol.* 235: 247–249 (1972)
30. Russell, D.H., and Levy, C.C., Polyamine accumulation and biosynthesis in a mouse L1210 leukemia. *Cancer Res.* 31: 248–251 (1971)
31. Haddox, M.K., and Russell, D.H., Differential conjugation of polyamines to calf nuclear and nucleolar proteins. *J. Cell. Physiol.* 109: 447–452 (1981)
32. Haddox, M.K., and Russell, D.H., Increased nuclear conjugated polyamines and transglutaminase during liver regeneration. *Proc. Natl. Acad. Sci. USA* 78: 1712–1716 (1981)
33. Manen, C.A., and Russell, D.H., Early cyclical changes in polyamine synthesis during sea urchin development. *J. Embryol. Exp. Morph.* 30: 243–256 (1973)
34. Seiler, N., and Knödgen, B., Determination of the naturally occurring monoacetyl derivatives of di- and polyamines. *J. Chromatogr.* 164: 155–168 (1979)
35. Russell, D.H., Ellingson, J.D., and Davis, T.P., Analysis of polyamines and acetyl derivatives by a single automated amino acid analyzer technique. *J. Chromatogr.* 273: 263–274 (1983)
36. Abdel-Monem, M.M., and Ohno, K., Polyamine metabolism III: Urinary acetyl polyamines in human cancer. *J. Pharm. Sci.* 67: 1671–1673 (1978)
37. Abraham, A.K., Studies on DNA-dependent RNA polymerase from *Escherichia coli.* I. The mechanism of polyamine induced stimulation of enzyme activity. *Eur. J. Biochem.* 5: 143–146 (1968)
38. So, A.G., Davie, E.W., Epstein, R., and Tissieres, A., Effects of cations on DNA-dependent RNA polymerase. *Proc. Natl. Acad. Sci. USA* 58: 1739–1746 (1967)
39. Igarashi, K., Hikami, K., Sugawara, K., and Hirose, S., Effect of polyamines on polypeptide synthesis in rat liver cell-free system. *Biochim. Biophys. Acta* 299: 325–330 (1973)

40. Fillingame, R.H., Jorstad, C.M., and Morris, D.R., Increased cellular levels of spermidine or spermine are required for optimal DNA synthesis in lymphocytes activated by concanavalin A. *Proc. Natl. Acad. Sci. USA* 72: 4042-4045 (1975)

41. Goldemberg, S.H., and Algranati, I.D., Polyamines and antibiotic effects on translation. *Med. Biol.* 59: 360-367 (1981)

42. Cohen, S.S., Morgan, S., and Streibel, E., The polyamine content of the tRNA of *E. coli. Proc. Natl. Acad. Sci. USA* 64: 669-676 (1969)

43. Lövgren, T.N.E., Petersson, A., and Loftfield, R.B., The mechanism of aminoacylation of transfer ribonucleic acid. The role of magnesium and spermine in the synthesis of isoleucyl-tRNA. *J. Biol. Chem.* 253: 6702-6710 (1978)

44. Siimes, M., Studies on the metabolism of 1,4-^{14}C-spermidine and 1,4-^{14}C-spermine in the rat. *Acta Physiol. Scand. supp.* 298: 1-66 (1967)

45. Seiler, N., Bolkenius, F.N., and Rennert, O.M., Interconversion, catabolism and elimination of the polyamines. *Med. Biol.* 59: 334-346 (1981)

46. Russell, D.H., Medina, V.J., and Snyder, S.H., The dynamics of synthesis and degradation of polyamines in normal and regenerating rat liver and brain. *J. Biol. Chem.* 245: 6732-6738 (1970)

47. Canellakis, E.S., Kyriakidis, D.A., Heller, J.S., and Pawlak, J.W., The complexity of regulation of ornithine decarboxylase. *Med. Biol.* 59: 279-285 (1981)

48. Heller, J.S., Chen, K.Y., Kyriakidis, D.A., Fong, W.F., and Canellakis, E.S., The modulation of the induction of ornithine decarboxylase by spermine, spermidine and diamines. *J. Cell. Physiol.* 96: 225-234 (1978)

49. Heller, J.S., and Canellakis, E.S., Cellular control of ornithine decarboxylase activity by its antizyme. *J. Cell. Physiol.* 107: 209-217 (1981)

50. Kuehn, G.D., and Atmar, V.J., in: *Advances in Polyamine Research* (U. Bachrach, A. Kaye, and R. Chayen, eds.), Vol. 3, pp 615-629, Raven Press, New York (1983)

51. Russell, D.H., Posttranslational modification of ornithine decarboxylase by its product putrescine. *Biochem. Biophys. Res. Commun.* 99: 1167-1172 (1981)

52. Russell, D.H., Ornithine decarboxylase: A key regulatory protein. *Med. Biol.* 59: 286-295 (1981)

53. Russell, D.H., in: *Advances in Enzyme Regulation*, (G. Weber, ed.), Vol. 21, pp 201-222, Pergamon Press, Oxford-New York (1983)

54. Boutwell, R.K., O'Brien, T.G., Verma, A.K., Weekes, R.G., DeYoung, L.M., Ashendel, C.L., and Astrup, E.G., in: *Advances in Enzyme Regulation* (G. Weber, ed.), Vol. 17, pp 89-112, Pergamon Press, Oxford-New York (1979)

55. Lowe, N.J., Epidermal ornithine decarboxylase, polyamines, cell proliferation, and tumor promotion. *Arch. Dermatol.* 116: 822-825 (1980)

56. Don, S., and Bachrach, U., Polyamine metabolism in normal and in virus-transformed chick embryo fibroblasts. *Cancer Res.* 35: 3618-3622 (1975)

57. Don, S., Weiner, H., and Bachrach, U., Specific increase in polyamine levels in chick embryo cells transformed by Rous sarcoma virus. *Cancer Res.* 35: 194-198 (1975)

58. Bachrach, U., Polyamines and neoplastic growth: Stabilization of ornithine decarboxylase during transformation. *Biochem. Biophys. Res. Commun.* 72: 1008-1013 (1976)

59. Williams-Ashman, H.G., and Canellankis, Z.N., Polyamines in mammalian biology and medicine. *Perspect. Biol. Med.* 22: 421-453 (1979)

60. Dunzendorfer, U., and Russell, D.H., Altered polyamine profiles in prostatic hyperplasia and in kidney tumors. *Cancer Res.* 38: 2321–2324 (1978)

61. Russell, D.H., and Snyder, S.H., Amine synthesis in regenerating rat liver: Extremely rapid turnover of ornithine decarboxylase. *Mol. Pharmacol.* 5: 253–262 (1969)

62. Heby, O., and Russell, D.H., Depression of polyamine synthesis in L1210 leukemic mice during treatment with a potent antileukemic agent, 5-azacytidine. *Cancer Res.* 33: 159–165 (1973)

63. Heby, O., and Russell, D.H., in: *Polyamines in Normal and Neoplastic Growth* (D.H. Russell, ed.), pp 221–237, Raven Press, New York (1973)

64. Russell, D.H., Clinical relevance of polyamines. *CRC Crit. Rev. Clin. Lab. Sci.* 18: 261–311 (1983)

65. Andersson, A.C., Henningsson, S., Lundell, L., Rosengren, E., and Sundler, F., Diamines and polyamines in DMBA-induced breast carcinoma containing mast cells resistant to compound 48/80. *Agents & Actions* 6/5: 577–583 (1976)

66. Salser, J.S., Ball, W.J., Jr., and Balis, M.E., Biochemical changes in premalignant intestines. *Cancer Res.* 36: 3495–3498 (1976)

67. Scalabrino, G., Pösö, H., Hölttä, E., Hannonen, P., Kallio, A., and Jänne, J., Synthesis and accumulation of polyamines in rat liver during chemical carcinogenesis. *Int. J. Cancer* 21: 239–245 (1978)

68. Matsushima, M., and Bryan, G.T., Early induction of mouse urinary bladder ornithine decarboxylase activity by rodent vesical carcinogens. *Cancer Res.* 40: 1897–1901 (1980)

69. Black, O., Jr., and Chang, B., Ornithine decarboxylase and its role in pancreatic cancer. *Med. Ped. Oncol.* 9: 93 (1981)

70. van Wijk, R., Louwers, H.A.P.M., and Bisschop, A., The induction of ornithine decarboxylase and DNA synthesis in rat hepatocytes after a single administration of diethylnitrosamine. *Carcinogenesis* 2: 27–31 (1981)

71. Landesman, J.M., and Mossman, B.T., Induction of ornithine decarboxylase in hamster tracheal epithelial cells exposed to asbestos and 12-O-tetradecanoylphorbol-13-acetate. *Cancer Res.* 42: 3669–3675 (1982)

72. Mottram, J.C., A developing factor in experimental blastogenesis., *J. Pathol. Bacteriol.* 56: 181–187 (1944)

73. Berenblum, I., The cocarcinogenic action of croton resin. *Cancer Res.* 1: 44–48 (1941)

74. Paul, D., and Hecker, E., On the biochemical mechanism of tumorigenesis in mouse skin. II. Early effects on the biosynthesis of nucleic acids induced by initiating doses of DMBA and by promoting doses of phorbol-12,13-diester TPA. *Z. Krebsforsch.* 73: 149–163 (1969)

75. O'Brien, T.G., Simsiman, R.C., and Boutwell, R.K., Induction of the polyamine-biosynthetic enzymes in mouse epidermis by tumor-promoting agents. *Cancer Res.* 35: 1662–1670 (1975)

76. O'Brien, T.G., Simsiman, R.C., and Boutwell, R.K., Induction of the polyamine-biosynthetic enzymes in mouse epidermis and their specificity for tumor promotion. *Cancer Res.* 35: 2426–2433 (1975)

77. O'Brien, T.G., The induction of ornithine decarboxylase as an early, possibly obligatory, event in mouse skin carcinogenesis. *Cancer Res.* 36: 2644–2653 (1976).

78. Mufson, R.A., Astrup, E.G., Simsiman, R.C., and Boutwell, R.K., Dissociation of increases in levels of $3':5'$-cyclic AMP and $3':5'$-cyclic GMP from induction of ornithine decarboxylase by the tumor promoter 12-O-tetrade-

canoyl phorbol-13-acetate in mouse epidermis *in vivo. Proc. Natl. Acad. Sci. USA* 74: 657–661 (1977)

79. Yuspa, S.H., Lichti, U., Ben, T., Patterson, E., Hennings, H., Slaga, T.J., Colburn, N., and Kelsey, W., Phorbol esters stimulate DNA synthesis and ornithine decarboxylase activity in mouse epidermal cell cultures. *Nature* 262: 402–404 (1976)

80. O'Brien, T.G., Lewis, M.A., and Diamond, L., Ornithine decarboxylase activity and DNA synthesis after treatment of cells in culture with 12-O-tetradecanoylphorbol-13-acetate. *Cancer Res.* 39: 4477–4480 (1979)

81. O'Brien, T.G., Saladik, D., and Diamond, L., Regulation of polyamine biosynthesis in normal and transformed hamster cells in culture. *Biochim. Biophys. Acta* 632: 270–283 (1980)

82. Fujiki, H., Mori, M., Sugimura, T., Hirota, M., Ohigashi, H., and Koshimizu, K., Relationship between ornithine decarboxylase-inducing activity and configuration at C-4 in phorbol ester derivatives. *J. Cancer Res. Clin. Oncol.* 98: 9–13 (1980)

83. Lesiewicz, J., Morrison, D.M., and Goldsmith, L.A., Ornithine decarboxylase in rat skin: 2. Differential response to hair plucking and a tumor promoter. *J. Invest. Dermatol.* 75: 411–416 (1980)

84. Weiner, R.A., and Byus, C.V., Induction of ornithine decarboxylase by 12-O-tetradecanoylphorbol-13-acetate in rat tissues. *Biochem. Biophys. Res. Commun.* 97: 1575–1581 (1980)

85. Byus, C.V., and Weiner, R.A., Tumor promoting phorbol-ester derivatives increase ornithine decarboxylase activity and polyamine biosynthesis in the liver of the rat and mouse. *Carcinogenesis* 3: 751–755 (1982)

86. Bisschop, A., van Rooijen, L.A.A., Derks, H.J.G.M., and van Wijk, R., Induction of rat hepatic ornithine decarboxylase by the tumor promoters 12-O-tetradecanoylphorbol-13-acetate and phenobarbital *in vivo*; effect of retinyl acetate. *Carcinogenesis* 2: 1283–1287 (1981)

87. Fujiki, H., Mori, M., Nakayasu, M., Terada, M., Sugimura, T., and Moore, R.E., Indole alkaloids: Dihydroteleocidin B, teleocidin, and lyngbyatoxin A as members of a new class of tumor promoters. *Proc. Natl. Acad. Sci. USA* 78: 3872–3876 (1981)

88. Izumi, K., Hirao, Y., Hopp, L., and Oyasu, R., *In vitro* induction of ornithine decarboxylase in urinary bladder carcinoma cells. *Cancer Res.* 41: 405–409 (1981)

89. Kishore, G.S., and Boutwell, R.K., Induction of mouse hepatic ornithine decarboxylase by skin application of 12-O-tetradecanoylphorbol-13-acetate. *Experientia* 37: 179–180 (1981)

90. Lichti, U., Patterson, E., Hennings, H., and Yuspa, S.H., The tumor promoter 12-O-tetradecanoylphorbol-13-acetate induces ornithine decarboxylase in proliferating basal cells but not in differentiating cells from mouse epidermis. *J. Cell. Physiol.* 107: 261–270 (1981)

91. Verma, A.K., and Boutwell, R.K., Intracellular calcium and skin tumor promotion: Cancer regulation of the induction of epidermal ornithine decarboxylase activity by the tumor promoter 12-O-tetradecanoylphorbol-13-acetate. *Biochem. Biophys. Res. Commun.* 101: 375–383 (1981)

92. Wu, K., Wang, D., and Feinman, R.D., Inhibition of proteases by α_2-macroglobulin. The role of lysyl amino groups of trypsin in covalent complex formation. *J. Biol. Chem.* 20: 10409–10414 (1981)

93. Lichti, U., and Gottesman, M.M., Genetic evidence that a phorbol ester tumor promoter stimulates ornithine decarboxylase activity by a pathway that is independent of cyclic AMP-dependent protein kinases in CHO cells. *J. Cell. Physiol.* 113: 433–439 (1982)

94. Lillehaug, J.R., and Djurhuus, R., Effect of diethylstilbestrol on the transformable mouse embryo fibroblast C3H/10T1/2C18 cells. Tumor promotion, cell growth, DNA synthesis and ornithine decarboxylase. *Carcinogenesis* 3: 797–799 (1982)

95. Lockyer, J.M., and Magun, B.E., The effect of serum and phorbol ester tumor promoter on ornithine decarboxylase activity in Swiss 3T3 cells. *Cancer Lett.* 18: 215–220 (1983)

96. Raunio, H., and Pelkonen, O., Effect of polycyclic aromatic compounds and phorbol esters on ornithine decarboxylase and aryl hydrocarbon hydroxylase activities in mouse liver. *Cancer Res.* 43: 782–786 (1983)

97. Takigawa, M., Simsiman, R.C., and Boutwell, R.K., The difference between the effects of single and double applications of 12-O-tetradecanoylphorbol-13-acetate, a potent tumor promoter, on polyamine metabolism and nucleic acid synthesis in mouse epidermis. *Carcinogenesis* 4: 5–7 (1983)

98. Verma, A.K., Rice, H.M., and Boutwell, R.K., Prostaglandins and skin tumor promotion: inhibition of tumor promoter-induced ornithine decarboxylase activity in epidermis by inhibitors of prostaglandin synthesis. *Biochem. Biophys. Res. Commun.* 79: 1160–1166 (1977)

99 Verma, A.K., Ashendel, C.L., and Boutwell, R.K., Inhibition by prostaglandin synthesis inhibitors of the induction of epidermal ornithine decarboxylase activity, the accumulation of prostaglandins, and tumor promotion caused by 12-O-tetradecanoylphorbol-13-acetate. *Cancer Res.* 40: 308–315 (1980)

100. Yuspa, S.H., Lichti, U., and Ben, T., Local anesthetics inhibit induction of ornithine decarboxylase by the tumor promoter 12-O-tetradecanoylphorbol-13-acetate. *Proc. Natl. Acad. Sci. USA* 77: 5312–5316 (1980)

101. Nakadate, T., Yamamoto, S., Ishii, M., and Kato, R., Inhibition of 12-O-tetradecanoylphorbol-13-acetate-induced epidermal ornithine decarboxylase activity by phospholipase A_2 inhibitors and lipoxygenase inhibitor. *Cancer Res.* 42: 2841–2845 (1982)

102. O'Brien, T.G., Simsiman, R.C., and Boutwell, R.K., The effect of colchicine on the induction of ornithine decarboxylases by 12-O-tetradecanoyl-phorbol-13-acetate. *Cancer Res.* 36: 3766–3770 (1976)

103. Farwell, D.C., Nolan, C.E., and Herbst, E.J., Liver ornithine decarboxylase during phenobarbital promotion of nitrosamine carcinogenesis. *Cancer Lett.* 5: 139–144 (1978)

104. Marks, F., Bertsch, S., and Fürstenberger, G., Ornithine decarboxylase activity, cell proliferation, and tumor promotion in mouse epidermis *in vivo*. *Cancer Res.* 39: 4183–4188 (1979)

105. Savage, R.E., Jr., Westrich, C., Guion, C., and Pereira, M.A., Chloroform induction of ornithine decarboxylase activity in rats. *Environ. Health Perspect.* 46: 157–162 (1982)

106. Boutwell, R.K., Some biological aspects of skin carcinogenesis. *Prog. Exp. Tumor Res.* 4: 207–250 (1950)

107. Boutwell, R.K., The function and mechanism of promoters of carcinogenesis. *CRC Crit. Rev. Toxicol.* 2: 419–443 (1974)

108. Klein-Szanto, A.J.P., Major, S.K., and Slaga, T.J., Induction of dark keratinocytes by 12-O-tetradecanoylphorbol-13-acetate and mezerein as an indicator of tumor-promoting efficiency. *Carcinogenesis* 1: 399–406 (1980)

109. Slaga, T.J., Fischer, S.M., Nelson, K., and Gleason, G.L., Studies on the mechanism of skin tumor promotion: Evidence for several stages in promotion. *Proc. Natl. Acad. Sci. USA* 77: 3659–3663 (1980)

110. Slaga, T.J., Klein-Szanto, A.J.P., Fischer, S.M., Weeks, C.E., Nelson, K., and Major, S., Studies on mechanism of action of anti-tumor-promoting agents: Their specificity in two-stage promotion. *Proc. Natl. Acad. Sci. USA* 77: 2251–2254 (1980)

111. Weeks, C.E., Herrmann, A.L., Nelson, F.R., and Slaga, T.J., α-Difluoromethylornithine, an irreversible inhibitor of ornithine decarboxylase, inhibits tumor promoter-induced polyamine accumulation and carcinogenesis in mouse skin. *Proc. Natl. Acad. Sci. USA* 79: 6028–6032 (1982)

112. Raick, A.N., Ultrastructural, histological, and biochemical alterations produced by 12-O-tetradecanoyl-phorbol-13-acetate on mouse epidermis and their relevance to skin tumor promotion. *Cancer Res.* 33: 269–286 (1973)

113. Raick, A.N., Cell proliferation and promoting action in skin carcinogenesis. *Cancer Res.* 34: 920–926 (1974)

114. Raick, A.N., Cell differentiation and tumor-promoting action in skin carcinogenesis. *Cancer Res.* 34: 2915–2925 (1974)

115. Lowe, N.J., Connor, M., and Breeding, J., Inhibition of ultraviolet light induced epidermal ornithine decarboxylase and carcinogenesis by retinoic acid and antiinflammatory drugs. *Clin. Res.* 30: 158A (1982)

116. Lowe, N.J., Connor, M.J., Breeding, J.H., and Russell, D.H., Epidermal polyamine profiles after multiple exposures to ultra-violet irradiation. *Carcinogenesis* 4: 671–674 (1983)

117. Verma, A.K., Lowe, N.J., and Boutwell, R.K., Induction of mouse epidermal ornithine decarboxylase activity and DNA synthesis by ultraviolet light. *Cancer Res.* 39: 1035–1040 (1979)

118. Seiler, N., and Knödgen, B., Effects of ultraviolet light on epidermal polyamine metabolism. *Biochem. Med.* 21: 168–181 (1979)

119. Böhlen, P., Grove, J., Beya, M.F., Koch-Weser, J., Henry, M.H., and Grosshans, E., Skin polyamine levels in psoriasis: the effect of dithranol therapy. *Eur. J. Clin. Invest.* 8: 215–218 (1978)

120. Russell, D.H., Combest, W.L., Duell, E.A., Stawiski, M.A., Anderson, T.F., and Voorhees, J.J., Glucocorticoid inhibits elevated polyamine biosynthesis in psoriasis. *J. Invest. Dermatol.* 71: 177–181 (1978)

121. Voorhees, J.J., Polyamines and psoriasis. *Arch. Dermatol.* 115: 943–944 (1979)

122. Lowe, N.J., Breeding, J., and Russell, D., Cutaneous polyamines in psoriasis. *Br. J. Dermatol.* 107: 21–26 (1982)

123. Haddox, M.K., and Russell, D.H., Cell cycle-specific locus of vitamin A inhibition of growth. *Cancer Res.* 39: 2476–2480 (1979)

124. Haddox, M.K., Scott, K.F.F., and Russell, D.H., Retinol inhibition of ornithine decarboxylase induction and G_1 progression in Chinese hamster ovary cells. *Cancer Res.* 39: 4930–4938 (1979)

125. Bollag, W., Therapy of chemically induced skin tumours of mice with vitamin A palmitate and vitamin A acid. *Experientia* 27: 90–92 (1971)

126. Bollag, W., Prophylaxis of chemically induced benign and malignant epithelial tumours by vitamin A acid (retinoic acid). *Eur. J. Cancer* 8: 689–693 (1972)

127. Sporn, M.B., Dunlop, N.M., Newton, D.L., and Smith, J.M., Prevention of chemical carcinogenesis by vitamin A and its synthetic analogs (retinoids). *Fed. Proc.* 35: 1332–1338 (1976)

128. Sporn, M.B., Retinoids and carcinogenesis. *Nutr. Rev.* 35: 65–69 (1977)

129. Kensler, T.W., Verma, A.K., Boutwell, R.K., and Mueller, G.C., Effects of retinoic acid and juvenile hormone on the induction of ornithine decarboxylase activity by 12-O-tetradecanoylphorbol-13-acetate. *Cancer Res.* 38: 2896–2899 (1978)

130. Verma, A.K., Rice, H.M., Shapas, B.G., and Boutwell, R.K., Inhibition of 12-O-tetradecanoylphorbol-13-acetate-induced ornithine decarboxylase activity in mouse epidermis by vitamin A analogs (retinoids). *Cancer Res.* 38: 793–801 (1978)

131. Russell, D.H., and Haddox, M.K., Antiproliferative effects of retinoids related to the cell cycle specific inhibition of ornithine decarboxylase. *Ann. N.Y. Acad. Sci.* 359: 281–297 (1981)

132. Chapman, S.K., Antitumor effects of vitamin A and inhibitors of ornithine decarboxylase in cultured neuroblastoma and glioma cells. *Life Sci.* 26: 1359–1366 (1980)

133. Takigawa, M., Ishida, H., Takano, T., and Suzuki, F., Polyamine and differentiation: Induction of ornithine decarboxylase by parathyroid hormone is a good marker of differentiated chondrocytes. *Proc. Natl. Acad. Sci. USA* 77: 1481–1485 (1980)

134. Lichti, U., Patterson, E., Hennings, H., and Yuspa, S.H., Differential retinoic acid inhibition of ornithine decarboxylase induction by 12-O-tetradecanoylphorbol-13-acetate and by germicidal ultraviolet light. *Cancer Res.* 41: 49–54 (1981)

135. Scott, K.F.F., Meyskens, F.L., Jr., and Russell, D.H., Retinoids increase transglutaminase activity and inhibit ornithine decarboxylase activity in Chinese hamster ovary cells and in melanoma cells stimulated to differentiate. *Proc. Natl. Acad. Sci. USA* 79: 4093–4097 (1982)

136. Scott, K.F.F., Meyskens, F.L., Jr., and Russell, D.H., Calcium and retinoic acid modulation of α-melanocyte-stimulating hormone effects to increase G_1-specific transglutaminase and ornithine decarboxylase activities in mouse melanoma cells. *J. Nutr. Growth Cancer* 1: 47–55 (1983)

137. Breeding, J., and Lowe, N., Vitamin A acid differentially modulates ultraviolet light induced epidermal ornithine decarboxylase. *J. Invest. Dermatol.* 78: 121(1982)

138. Bolmer, S.D., and Wolf, G., Retinoids and phorbol esters alter release of fibronectin from enucleated cells. *Proc. Natl. Acad. Sci. USA* 79: 6541–6545 (1982)

139. Wu, V.S., Donato, N.J., and Byus, C.V., Growth state-dependent alterations in the ability of 12-O-tetradecanoylphorbol-13-acetate to increase ornithine decarboxylase activity in Reuber H35 hepatoma cells. *Cancer Res.* 41: 3384–3391 (1981)

140. Takigawa, M., Verma, A.K., Simsiman, R.C., and Boutwell, R.K., Polyamine biosynthesis and skin tumor promotion: Inhibition of 12-O-tetradecanoylphorbol-13-acetate-promoted mouse skin tumor formation by the irreversible inhibitor of ornithine decarboxylase α-difluoromethylornithine. *Biochem. Biophys. Res. Commun.* 105: 969–976 (1982)

23

Assay for Hepatic Peroxisome Proliferation to Select a Novel Class of Non-Mutagenic Hepatocarcinogens

Janardan K. Reddy
Narendra D. Lalwani

Northwestern University Medical School
Chicago, Illinois

INTRODUCTION

The majority of chemical carcinogens, which are capable of generating electrophilic reactants,[1-3] exhibit mutagenic activity, including the ability to induce DNA damage and chromosomal alterations.[4-6] Several chemicals, which do not yield positive results in the presently available short-term *in vitro* tests, are nevertheless carcinogenic in long-term animal bioassays.[7-8] These are designated as non-mutagenic or epigenetic carcinogens.[8] Short-term mutagenicity assays do not distinguish between a non-mutagenic carcinogen and a non-carcinogen. It becomes imperative, therefore, to recognize specific chemical, physical or biological properties of known non-mutagenic chemical carcinogens which may serve as potentially useful predictors of carcinogenicity. One such predictor appears to be the induction of proliferation of the cytoplasmic organelle peroxisome in the hepatic parenchymal cells of rodents.[9]

PEROXISOMES AND PEROXISOME PROLIFERATION

The peroxisome (microbody), a cytoplasmic organelle characterized morphologically by a single limiting membrane and a finely granular or homogeneous matrix (Figure 1) is a ubiquitous structure in animal and plant cells.[10-12] Peroxisomes in hepatic parenchymal cells of many species measure approximately 0.3 μm to 1 μm and contain within the matrix a crystalloid core or nu-

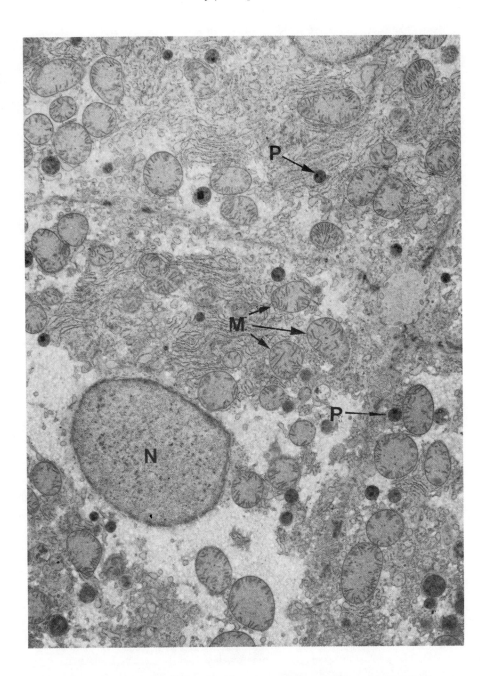

Figure 1: Electron micrograph of liver cell cytoplasm of a normal male rat. Peroxisomes (P) are few in number. (N) Nucleus, and (M) mito-chondria. (Uranyl acetate and lead citrate; magnification X 8,000).

cleoid (Figure 1). This core signifies the presence in the peroxisome of urate oxidase.[13] The crystalloid core is absent in the hepatic peroxisomes of some species, including humans, that lack the enzyme urate oxidase.[10-12] Peroxisomes can be identified positively in tissue sections by the cytochemical localization of a peroxisomal marker enzyme, catalase.[14-16] Peroxisomes, in addition to catalase, contain several other enzymes.[17-22] Of particular importance are the five hydrogen peroxide generating oxidases in rodent liver peroxisomes (Figure 2). Detailed descriptions of biological and biochemical properties of peroxisomes are available in recent reviews.[22-23]

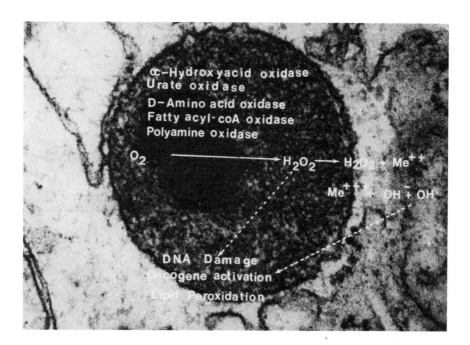

Figure 2: Model of peroxisome-mediated hepatocarcinogenesis. Peroxisome proliferators induce proliferation of peroxisomes in hepatic parenchymal cells possibly by a cytosolic receptor mechanism. Peroxisome proliferation leads to 30- to 70-fold excess generation of hydrogen peroxide in the liver as a by-product of the FAD-dependent oxidation of fatty acyl-CoA by fatty acyl-CoA oxidase, the first step in the chain reaction of peroxisomal fatty acid oxidation. The other peroxisomal oxidases may also lead to additional increases in hydrogen peroxide generation. Hydrogen peroxide generated in peroxisomes can escape degradation by catalase, since catalase is not effective in destroying hydrogen peroxide present at low concentrations.[56] Higher intracellular concentrations of hydrogen peroxide or its reduction products (OH·, etc.) resulting from interaction with metal ions may lead to DNA damage, lipid peroxidation or oncogene activation.

In normal liver cells, peroxisomes are few in number and appear somewhat insignificant in the overall cytoplasmic organization (Figure 1). The ratio of peroxisomes to mitochondria is approximately 1:5 or 1:6, but this ratio is markedly altered in hepatocytes of rats and mice fed several structurally dissimilar hypolipidemic drugs and certain phthalate ester plasticizers.[24-30] These chemicals, which serve as simple and reproducible means of increasing the number of peroxisomes (Figures 3 and 4) and of synthesis of peroxisomal enzymes in the livers of rodents and several other species, have provided considerable insight into the structure and function of peroxisomes.[26-31] The term "peroxisome proliferator" is used to designate a drug or xenobiotic which induces the proliferation of peroxisomes in liver cells.[27] The recent review by Reddy and Lalwani[23] provides a detailed account of the morphological and biochemical alterations induced by the peroxisome proliferators.

THE HYPOTHESIS

Studies from our laboratory demonstrated the hepatocarcinogenicity in rats and/or mice of six hypolipidemic compounds with hepatic peroxisome proliferative properties.[9,32] The lack of mutagenicity of these agents,[32-34] combined with the consistent coupling of proliferation of hydrogen peroxide-generating peroxisomes and formation of hepatocellular tumors led to the hypothesis that potent hepatic peroxisome proliferators as a class are carcinogenic.[9] It was further proposed that persistent proliferation of peroxisomes serves as an endogenous initiator of neoplastic transformation by increasing the intracellular production of hydrogen peroxide by the peroxisomal oxidases (Figure 2). Since the formulation of these concepts several peroxisome proliferators, including the widely used phthalate ester plasticizer di-(2-ethylhexyl)phthalate, have been found to induce hepatocellular neoplasms.[35-37] The chemical structures of carcinogenic peroxisome proliferators identified to date are illustrated in Figures 5 and 6. Accordingly, as suggested elsewhere,[9,23] the morphological finding of hepatic peroxisome proliferation seems a potentially useful indication for selecting a non-mutagenic chemical for long-term carcinogenicity testing.

EXPERIMENTAL APPROACH

General

Peroxisome proliferators identified to date are non-mutagenic, *i.e.*, they do not induce mutagenicity, DNA damage or chromosomal alterations.[33-34] Therefore, for new compounds, it is pertinent to establish that the test compound lacks activity in short-term assays for mutagenicity, and then to determine whether this compound possesses peroxisome proliferative and hepatomegalic properties.

Choice of Species and Route of Administration

Male and female F344 rats or Swiss-Webster mice, four to six weeks old, can be used for the peroxisome proliferation assay. The compound can be administered by mixing it with the powdered chow, at concentrations ranging from

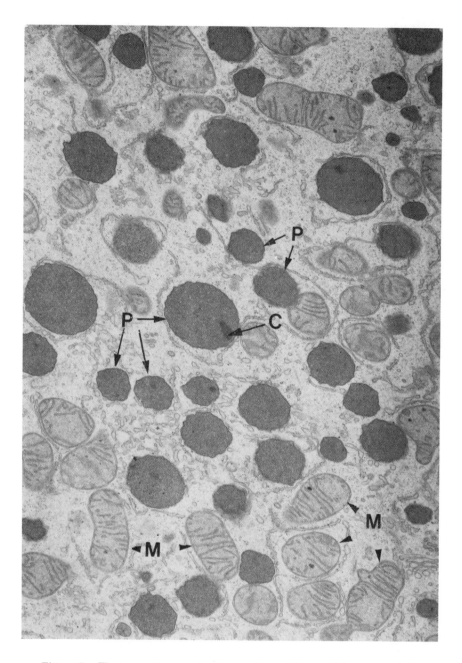

Figure 3: Electron micrograph of a portion of liver cell from a rat fed a peroxisome proliferator at 0.05% level in the diet for six weeks. Peroxisomes (P); uricase-containing crystalloid (C); mitochondria (M). (Uranyl acetate and lead citrate; magnification X 15,000).

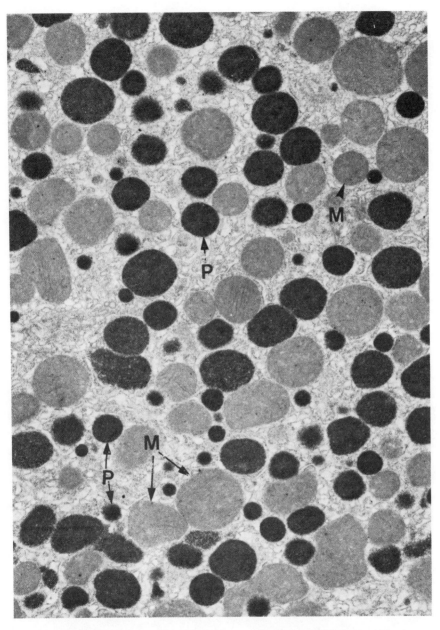

Figure 4: Liver of a rat fed a peroxisome proliferator at level of 0.05%
in powdered chow for six weeks. All proliferated peroxisomes (P)
whether they possess a nucleoid or not, stain positively for catalase,
the marker enzyme of peroxisomes. The glutaraldehyde-fixed tissue was
incubated in alkaline 3,3'-diaminobenzidine medium and post-fixed
with osmium tetroxide. Peroxisomes (P) with typical cytochemical reaction product. (Lead citrate; magnification X 15,500).

Compound No.	Name	Structure
1.	CLOFIBRATE	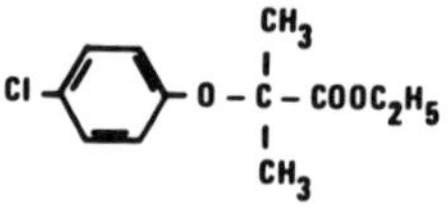
2.	NAFENOPIN	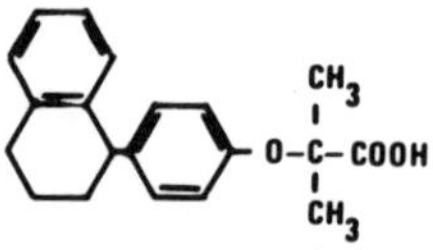
3.	METHYL CLOFENAPATE	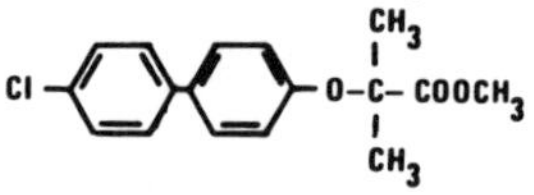
4.	WY–14,643	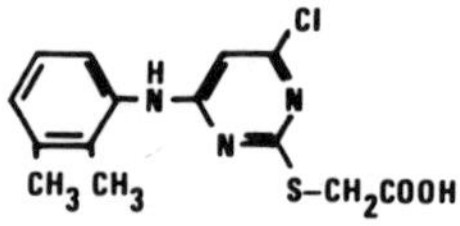
5.	BR–931	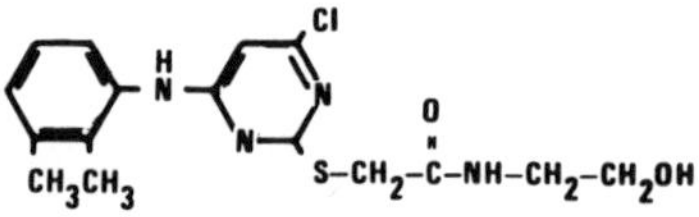
6.	TIBRIC ACID	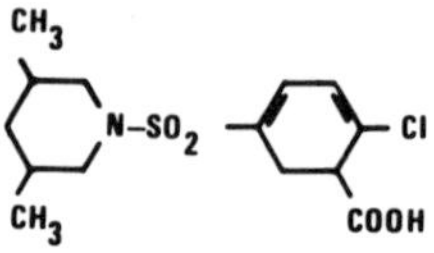
7.	FENOFIBRATE	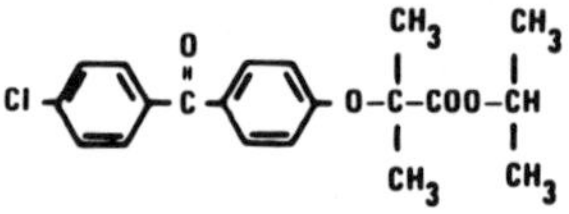
8.	GEMFIBROZIL	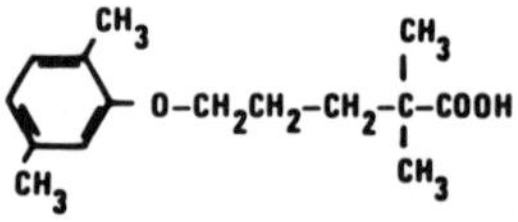
9.	BEZAFIBRATE	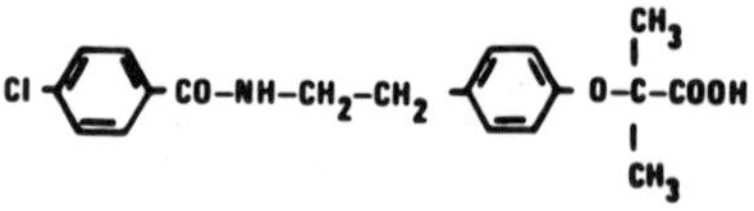
10.	CIPROFIBRATE	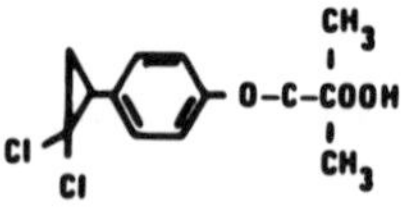

Figure 5: Chemical structures of hypolipidemic compounds which have been shown to be carcinogenic in rodent species.

Compound No.	Name	Structure
1.	DEHA	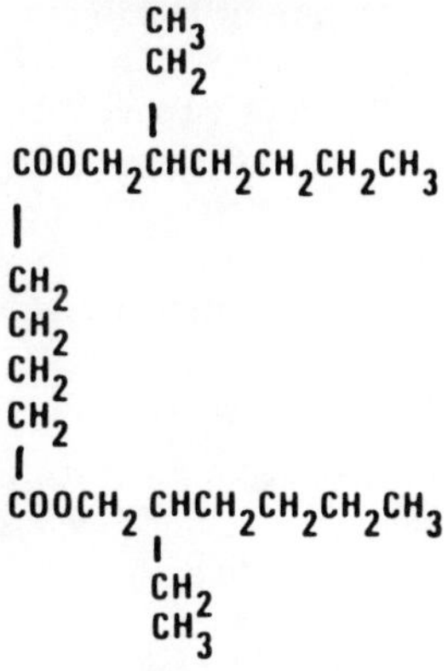
2.	DEHP	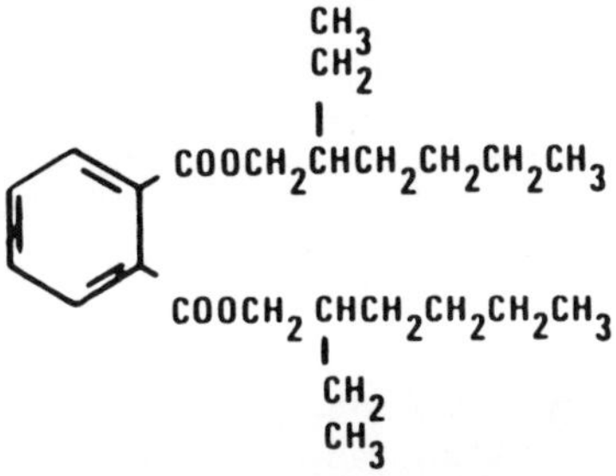

Figure 6: Chemical structures of phthalate-ester plasticizers: (1) DEHA, di(2-ethylhexyl)adipate; and (2) DEHP, di(2-ethylhexyl)phthalate. These compounds are relatively weak hepatic peroxisome proliferators. These compounds have been shown to induce a relatively low incidence of liver tumors in rats and/or mice.

0.005% to 2% (w/w) or higher, depending upon the tolerance. Available evidence indicates that at the maximum tolerated dose (MTD), the majority of peroxisome proliferators induce a maximal steady state level of hepatomegaly and peroxisome proliferation within ten days to 21 days.[38] Thus, a four to six weeks exposure period is optimal to determine whether a given chemical is capable of inducing hepatic peroxisome proliferation. These studies can be performed with two- or three-dose levels (MTD, ½ MTD and ⅓ MTD) and five animals of each species and sex per dose level. Appropriate untreated controls are necessary. Animals should be weighed at the beginning and at weekly intervals thereafter. Food consumption should be monitored. If sequential morphological and biochemical studies are planned, five males and five females of each species can be sacrificed at 1, 2, 3 and 4 or 6 week intervals. Appropriate dose for sequential studies may be selected after the initial 4 or 6 week study. At the time of sacrifice, body and liver weights should be obtained to calculate relative liver weights which range between 3.5% and 4.2% in untreated control rats and increase to 5% to 9% of the body weight when peroxisome proliferation is induced. The hepatomegaly is attributed to primary liver cell hyperplasia and cytoplasmic hypertrophy of hepatocytes due to increases in peroxisome and smooth endoplasmic reticulum volume densities.[39,40] Blood should also be collected for determination of serum cholesterol and triglycerides because peroxisome proliferation is consistently associated with hypotriglyceridemia.[23,38]

MORPHOLOGICAL ALTERATIONS IN LIVER PARENCHYMAL CELLS

Light and Electron Microscopy

For light microscopic examination, small pieces of liver from control and treated rats should be fixed in neutral buffered formalin. Large, polyhedral hypertrophic hepatocytes with granular eosinophilic cytoplasm, in 3–4 μm thick Hematoxylin and Eosin (H&E) stained paraffin-embedded tissue sections may be suggestive of peroxisome proliferation. Several liver cell mitoses may also be encountered during the first two weeks of dosing if the chemical is capable of inducing peroxisome proliferation.[41,42] Electron microscopic examination of the liver is mandatory for unequivocally establishing the peroxisome proliferative property of a chemical. For this purpose, small pieces of liver from at least three control and three treated rats (four or six weeks duration) should be fixed immediately in 2% ice-cold osmium tetroxide buffered to pH 7.4 with S-collidine buffer. After one to two hours of fixation, the tissues should be dehydrated in graded series of ethanol, and embedded in LX-112 resin (Ladd Research Industries) or any other suitable medium. Alternately, the liver pieces can be fixed in 2.5% glutaraldehyde in 0.05 M sodium cacodylate buffer, pH 7.4 for 30 minutes and then post-fixed in 2% osmium tetroxide and processed as above. Thin sections of epon-embedded tissue, following uranyl acetate and lead citrate staining, should be examined in an electron microscope and photographed randomly at selected magnifications.

Cytochemical Localization of Peroxisomal Catalase

Peroxisomes can be easily distinguished from other single-membrane limited cytoplasmic organelles in routine transmission electron micrographs. For those who are not familiar with subtle variations in the morphologic appearance of these organelles, it may be preferable to process, in parallel, tissues for cytochemical demonstration of peroxisomal marker enzyme, catalase. For this purpose, small pieces of liver (three animals per group) should be fixed in 2.5% glutaraldehyde buffered with 0.05 M sodium cacodylate, pH 7.4 for four hours at 4°C and then rinsed overnight in 0.05 M sodium cacodylate buffer containing 0.2 M sucrose. Non-frozen sections, 40 μm to 60 μm thick, should be cut using a vibratome (alternately, the tissue can be finely chopped with a razor blade) and incubated at 37°C for 45 minutes to 60 minutes in the alkaline 3,3'-diaminobenzidine oxidation medium of Novikoff and Goldfischer[43] modified from Graham and Karnovsky.[14] The composition of the medium is as follows: Ten mg to 20 mg of 3,3'-diaminobenzidine tetrahydrochloride in 10 ml of 0.05 M 2-amino-2-methyl-1,3-propanediol buffer, pH 9.4 and 0.2 ml of 1% hydrogen peroxide. Control incubation should consist of preincubation for 15 minutes in propanediol buffer containing 0.02 M 3-amino-1,2,4-triazole followed by incubation in standard 3,3'-diaminobenzidine medium also containing 0.02 M aminotriazole. Additional controls with 0.01 M potassium cyanide or 0.1 M sodium azide can be used, if necessary. After incubation, the tissue sections should be rinsed with 0.05 M sodium cacodylate buffer and postfixed for one hour in 2% osmium tetroxide, dehydrated, and embedded in Epon. Sections, 0.5 μm to 1 μm thick, can be examined with or without counterstain using a light microscope. In these sections, peroxisomes appear as yellow-brown granules. Thin sections can be examined in an electron microscope following counterstaining with lead citrate or uranyl acetate. The cytochemical reaction product is localized somewhat exclusively in peroxisomes (Figures 4 and 7).

Morphometry

Quantitative assessment of changes in the numerical and volume densities of peroxisomes requires morphometric analysis. Complete details of stereological principles for morphometry in electron microscopic cytology have been outlined by Weibel.[44] For the purpose of peroxisome proliferation assay, a simplified approach can be used. Briefly, 30 randomly photographed electron micrographs of cytoplasm of liver cells from each experimental group (ten electron micrographs from one or two blocks/animal; three animals/group) should be obtained. Micrographs should be photographed at an initial magnification of 4,000X or 8,000X and enlarged two and one-half times at printing to a final magnification of 10,000X or 20,000X. Points of intersection overlying cytoplasm, mitochondria and peroxisomes should be determined, using a 5 mm spaced lattice grid as described by Weibel.[44] The volume densities of mitochondria and peroxisomes are then determined in relation to cytoplasmic volume. Table 1 shows the representative changes in the volume density of peroxisomes and mitochondria in the livers of rats fed ciprofibrate, a hypolipidemic drug or di-(2-ethylhexyl)phthalate, an industrial plasticizer, two structurally unrelated peroxisome proliferators, with varying potency to induce hepatic peroxisome proliferation. The numerical density of peroxisomes can be determined by counting the number of peroxisome profiles and expressed as number of peroxisomes per μm^2 of cytoplasm.

BIOCHEMICAL ALTERATIONS IN LIVER

Liver enlargement resulting from the administration of peroxisome proliferators is usually associated with significant changes in the activities of mitochondrial, microsomal and peroxisomal enzymes. To assess the extent of peroxisome proliferation in liver, it would be preferable to determine the activities of catalase, carnitine acetyltransferase[30] and the peroxisomal fatty acid β-oxidation system.[21,22] Under steady-state conditions of maximum increase in peroxisome volume density (eight- to ten-fold), the catalase activity is elevated only about two-fold, whereas the activities of carnitine acetyltransferase and the peroxisomal fatty acid β-oxidation system are increased many-fold when compared to untreated controls. Increases in the activities of these three enzymes correlate positively with the increase in peroxisome population in liver cells.[30]

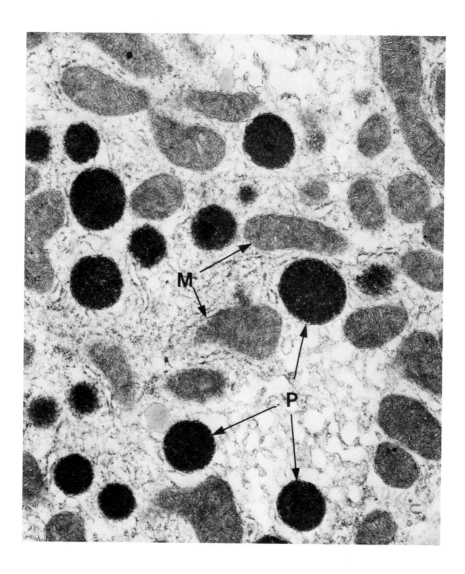

Figure 7: Cytochemical localization of catalase, by the alkaline 3,3'-diaminobenzidine medium. The reaction product is localized within the peroxisomes (P). Mitochondria (M). (Counterstained with lead citrate X 16,000).

Table 1: Morphometric Analysis of the Changes in Mitochondrial and
Peroxisome Population in the Liver Cells of Rats Fed a
Peroxisome Proliferator*

| Group | . . . . . .Volume Density** . . . . . | |
	Mitochondria	Peroxisomes
Control	18.0 ± 3.88	1.8 ± 0.62
Ciprofibrate	22.9 ± 1.57	18.8 ± 2.80
Di-(2-ethylhexyl)phthalate	17.4 ± 1.56	10.4 ± 0.39

*Male F344 rats were fed a diet containing either ciprofibrate (0.05% w/w)
or di-(2-ethylhexyl)phthalate (2% w/w) for 4 weeks.
**Points overlying cytoplasm, mitochondria and peroxisomes were deter-
mined to obtain the volume density of mitochondria and peroxisomes.
The values (mean ± standard deviation) are expressed as percent of cytoplasmic volume.

Catalase

The activity of this enzyme can be estimated spectrophotometrically by
monitoring the decomposition of hydrogen peroxide.[45] Catalase catalyzes the
reaction:

$$2H_2O_2 \xrightarrow{\text{catalase}} 2H_2O + O_2$$

The absorption maximum for hydrogen peroxide is between 230 nm and 250
nm; when hydrogen peroxide reacts with catalase, the absorption decreases with
time. The activity of catalase is calculated from the half-life of the first order
reaction.[46]

Procedure. After taking a small piece of tissue for morphology, it may be
preferable to perfuse the liver with ice-cold normal saline *via* the portal vein.
Liver homogenates (5% w/v in cold distilled water using 0.5 g to 1 g liver) are
prepared, to which 10% sodium deoxycholate (DOC) is added to give a final
DOC concentration of 0.5%. This mixture is incubated at room temperature
($20°C$ to $22°C$) for 30 minutes to extract catalase and then centrifuged at 105,000 g
for 60 minutes using Type 50 Ti rotor in a Beckman L5-65 ultracentrifuge at
$4°C$. After centrifugation, the lipid-containing layer at the top is carefully removed and the supernatant is used for determining catalase activity at $22°C$ to
$25°C$ by the spectrophotometric method described by Lück.[45] Briefly, 3 ml of
hydrogen peroxide solution (0.16 ml of 30% hydrogen peroxide in 100 ml of
0.15 M phosphate buffer, pH 7.0) is used as substrate. The optical density of
this solution is 0.500 at 240 mμ and with a 1 cm light path.[45] The reference
cuvette contains 3 ml of 0.15 M phosphate buffer without hydrogen peroxide.
To both reference and sample cuvettes, an aliquot (20 μl) of appropriately diluted liver supernatant (usually five-fold dilution for normal liver and ten-fold
dilution for treated liver) is added and the time (t) required to decrease the optical density from 0.450 to 0.400 is measured at 240 nm. One unit of catalase
is defined as the amount of enzyme which liberates half the peroxide oxygen
from a hydrogen peroxide solution at any concentration in 100 seconds at $25°C$.

Units of catalase per gram liver = 17/t multiplied by the dilution factor

The specific activity of catalase is expressed as units of catalase per mg protein in the liver supernatants. In normal Fischer 344 rat liver the catalase activity ranges between 35 units/mg protein to 42 units/mg protein.[26,30]

Carnitine Acetyltransferase

This enzyme catalyzes the readily reversible reaction:[20,48]

$$\text{Acetylcarnitine} + \text{CoA} \rightleftharpoons \text{Acetyl-CoA} + \text{carnitine}$$

Although carnitine acetyltransferase activity is found in mitochondrial, peroxisomal and microsomal fractions of normal rat liver,[46] evidence indicates that a marked increase in the activity of this enzyme occurs only in livers with peroxisome proliferation.[28,30] The activity of this short-chain carnitine acyltransferase, which is at the barely measurable level in the liver of normal rats, mice and hamsters, increases 20- to 160-fold after administration of peroxisome proliferators such as clofibrate or di(2-ethylhexyl)phthalate.[28]

Procedure. Prepare 20% liver homogenate (1 g sample of liver) in 0.25 M sucrose containing 116 mM Tris-HCl (pH 8.0) and 2.5 mM EDTA. Sonicate the homogenate, using a sonicator cell disruptor, for 2 minutes with intermittent pulse at 4°C; dilute the sonicate 1:1 (v/v) with 0.01 M sodium pyrophosphate buffer, pH 8.1, and extract the enzyme by storing this mixture at 4°C overnight. This is then centrifuged at 105,000 g for 60 minutes and the supernatant used for enzyme assay.

The enzyme activity is estimated spectrophotometrically by measuring the release of CoA-SH, both in the presence and absence of carnitine, with the general thiol reagent DTNB [5,5'-dithio-bis(2-nitrobenzoate)] at 412 nm.[47] The reaction mixture consists of 1 ml aliquot of a premixed solution containing 116 mM Tris HCl, pH 8.0; 2.5 mM EDTA; 0.5 mM DTNB; 0.2 mM acetyl-CoA and 5 mM L-carnitine to which 1 ml of doubly distilled water is added and equilibrated at 25°C. The reaction is initiated by the addition of 20 μl of liver supernatant prepared as above, and the rate of release of CoA-SH recorded on the chart (Figure 8). The difference between the rates with and without carnitine is considered as a measure of carnitine-dependent acetyltransferase activity.

The carnitine acetyltransferase activity unit is expressed as nmoles of CoA-SH released/minute using the extinction coefficient for DTNB of $E_{412m\mu} = 13,600 M^{-1} cm^{-1}$.[48]

Peroxisomal-β-Oxidation of Fatty Acids

Peroxisomal fatty acid β-oxidation system, which is different from that of mitochondria, has been identified in mammalian liver and kidney.[49,50] Like carnitine acetyl- and octanoyl-transferase, the activities of the four enzymes responsible for the overall peroxisomal fatty acid β-oxidation reaction are increased several-fold over control values. Accordingly, elevation of cyanide insensitive peroxisomal fatty acid β-oxidation system reflects an increase in peroxisome number in liver cells and also serves as a measure of hydrogen peroxide generating capacity.[21-23]

Procedure. Two methods for the measurement of peroxisomal β-oxidation of fatty acids are outlined in detail by Lazarow.[51] Briefly, the first method in-

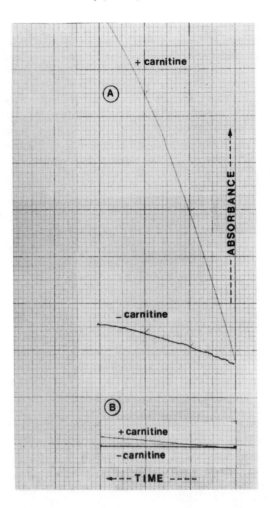

Figure 8: Spectrophotometric record at 412 nm. Typical assay for carnitine acetyltransferase of liver extracts prepared from (A) rat fed hypolipidemic drug (Wy-14,643, 0.1% in the diet for four weeks), and (B)
control rat. The assay was performed in the presence (+) or absence (-)
of carnitine, using 20 μl of liver extract. For details see the section on
carnitine acetyltransferase assay procedure.

volves the conversion of $1\text{-}^{14}C$-palmitoyl-CoA to acid soluble ^{14}C-acetyl-CoA and
the second method involves spectrophotometric measurement of enzyme-medi-
ated reduction of NAD to NADH in the presence of substrate palmitoyl-CoA.
The liver homogenates (10%, w/v) are prepared in 0.25 M sucrose using a Potter-
Elvehjem homogenizer. The homogenates are suitably diluted (to 0.5% for normal liver; or 0.1% if the enzyme activity is increased) in 0.25 M sucrose or 50
mM Tris-HCl, pH 8.0.

For the ^{14}C-palmitoyl-CoA oxidation assay, 20 μl of diluted homogenate is added to 480 μl of reaction mixture (50 mM Tris-HCl, pH 8.0, 457 μl; 20 mM NAD, 5 μl; 0.33 mM dithiothreitol, 1.5 μl; 1.5% bovine serum albumin, 2.5 μl; 2% Triton x-100, 2.5 μl; 10 mM coenzyme-A, 5 μl; 1 mM FAD, 5 μl; 5 mM s-palmitoyl-CoA, 1 μl; and 20 μCi/ml 1-^{14}C-palmitoyl-CoA, 0.5 μl) and incubated at 37°C for 10 minutes. The reaction is terminated by adding 250 μl of ice-cold perchloric acid (6%), vortexed and allowed to precipitate on ice for one hour. The precipitates are removed by centrifugation for 10 minutes at 2,000 g and the radioactivity in the supernatant is measured by liquid scintillation spectrometry.[51]

For the NAD reduction assay, 5 μl of diluted liver homogenate is added to 993 μl of reaction mixture (50 mM Tris-HCl, pH 8.0, 940 μl; 20 mM NAD, 10 μl; 0.33 mM dithiothreitol, 3 μl; 1.5% albumin, 5 μl; 2% Triton x-100, 5 μl; 10 mM CoA, 10 μl; 1 mM FAD, 10 μl; 100 mM potassium cyanide, 10 μl) maintained at 37°C in a cuvette. The reduction of NAD is monitored with and without substrate at 340 nm using a single-beam or double-beam spectrophotometer. The concentration of NAD reduced is calculated from the plot of absorbance *versus* time.

Other

Increase in peroxisome population in liver parenchymal cells can also be assessed by analyzing SDS-polyacrylamide gel electrophoretic patterns of postnuclear, light mitochondrial or microsomal fractions.[52] In the livers with peroxisome proliferation, there is a marked increase in the amount of polypeptide with an apparent molecular weight of 80,000 daltons.[52] This peroxisome proliferation-specific protein appears to be the bifunctional protein of the peroxisomal fatty acid β-oxidation system.[53] Subcellular fractionation procedures have been outlined elsewhere.[54] Fractions from three or four livers from control and experimental animals should be subjected to SDS-polyacryamide gel electrophoresis as described by Laemmli[55] using 7.5% or 10% polyacrylamide.

CARCINOGENICITY STUDIES

The ultimate proof that a chemical capable of inducing hepatic peroxisome proliferation is carcinogenic depends upon the unequivocal demonstration that it is capable of inducing hepatocellular carcinomas in rats or mice. In view of the evidence that peroxisome proliferators induce a nearly 100% incidence of liver tumors in rats and mice, a limited protocol for carcinogenicity testing can be employed if a compound is found to be a potent peroxisome proliferator. The compound can be administered by mixing in the powdered chow to groups of 15 to 20 male and female F344 rats weighing 60 g to 80 g. This limited bioassay can be performed with either one dose level (maximally tolerated dose on a chemical which may have environmental impact) or two dose levels (maximally tolerated dose and a pharmacologically active dose for a pharmaceutical agent). A potent peroxisome proliferator at the maximally tolerated dose level should induce liver tumors within 12 months to 24 months.

SUMMARY

We have outlined an approach to the testing of potential hepatic peroxisome proliferators. In view of the emerging evidence that peroxisome proliferators form a distinct class of chemical carcinogens, it would be preferable to test non-mutagenic chemicals for peroxisome proliferative property. Peroxisome proliferator carcinogens may induce cancer by mechanism(s) other than the formation of electrophiles which are capable of interacting with DNA and inducing a genetic change. Our hypothesis that peroxisome proliferators induce the development of hepatocellular carcinomas indirectly by increasing the number of hydrogen peroxide-generating peroxisomes requires further testing. Additional studies are required to determine how the excess production of hydrogen peroxide by peroxisomal oxidases leads to the initiation of neoplastic change in liver.

REFERENCES

1. Miller, E.C., Some current perspectives on chemical carcinogenesis in human and experimental animals: Presidential address. *Cancer Res.* 38: 1479-1496 (1978)
2. Weisburger, J.H., and Williams, G.M., Carcinogen testing: Current problems and new approaches. *Science* 214: 401-407 (1981)
3. Farber, E., Chemical carcinogenesis. *New Engl. J. Med.* 305: 1379-1389 (1981)
4. Pitot, H.C., The natural history of neoplastic development: The relation of experimental models to human cancer. *Cancer* 49: 1206-1211 (1982)
5. Yamasaki, H., Wilbourn, J.D., and Haroun, L., in: *Mutagens in Our Environment* (M. Sorsa and H. Vainio, eds.), pp 169-180, Alan R. Liss, Inc., New York (1982)
6. Ames, B.N., McCann, J., and Yamasaki, E., Methods for detecting carcinogens and mutagens with the *Salmonella*/mammalian-microsome mutagenicity test. *Mutation Res.* 31: 347-364 (1975)
7. Hollstein, M., McCann, J., Angelosanto, F.A., and Nichols, W.W., Short-term tests for carcinogens and mutagens. *Mutation Res.* 65: 133-226 (1979)
8. Von Borstel, R.S., and Mehta, R.D., in: *Mutagens in Our Environment* (M. Sorsa and H. Vainia, eds.), pp 47-57, Alan R. Liss, Inc., New York (1982)
9. Reddy, J.K., Azarnoff, D.L., and Hignite, C.E., Hypolipidemic peroxisome proliferators form a novel class of chemical carcinogens. *Nature* 283: 397-398 (1980)
10. Hruban, Z., and Rechcigl, M., Jr., in: *International Review in Cytology Supplement 1*, Academic Press, New York (1969)
11. DeDuve, C., and Baudhuin, P., Microbodies (Peroxisomes) and related particles. *Physiol. Rev.* 46: 323-357 (1966)
12. Shnitka, T.K., Comparative ultrastructure of hepatic microbodies in some mammals and birds in relation to species difference in uricase activity. *J. Ultrastructure Res.* 16: 598-625 (1966)
13. Hruban, Z., and Swift, H., Uricase localization in hepatic microbodies. *Science* 146: 1316-1317 (1964)
14. Graham, R.C., Jr., and Karnovsky, M.J., The histochemical demonstration of uricase activity. *J. Histochem. Cytochem.* 13: 448-453 (1965)

15. Hruban, Z., Vigil, E., Slesers, A., and Hopkins, E., Microbodies. Constituent organelles of animal cells. *Lab. Invest.* 27: 184-191 (1972)

16. Novikoff, A.B., Novikoff, P.M., Davis, C., and Quintana, J., Studies on microperoxisomes, V. Are microperoxisomes ubiquitous in mammalian cells? *J. Histochem. Cyctochem.* 21: 737-755 (1973)

17. Sies, H., Biochemistry of the peroxisome in the liver cell. *Angew. Chem. Int.* 13: 706-718 (1974)

18. Tolbert, N.E., Metabolic pathways in peroxisomes and glyoxysomes. *Ann. Rev. Biochem.* 50: 133-157 (1981)

19. Hajra, A.K., and Bishop, J.E., Glycolipid biosynthesis in peroxisomes via the acyl dihydroxyacetone phosphate pathway. *Ann. N.Y. Acad. Sci.* 386: 170-182 (1982)

20. Markwell, M.A.K., McGroaty, E.J., Bieber, L.L., and Tolbert, N.E., The subcellular distribution of carnitine acetyltransferases in mammalian liver and kidney. A new peroxisomal enzyme. *J. Biol. Chem.* 248: 3426-3432 (1973)

21. Lazarow, P.B., and DeDuve, C., A fatty acyl-CoA oxidizing system in rat liver peroxisomes; enhancement by clofibrate, a hypolipidemic drug. *Proc. Natl. Acad. Sci. USA* 73: 2043-2046 (1976)

22. Hashimoto, T., Individual peroxisomal β-oxidation enzymes. *Ann. N.Y. Acad. Sci.* 386: 5-12 (1982)

23. Reddy, J.K., and Lalwani, N.D., Carcinogenesis by hepatic peroxisome proliferators: Evaluation of the risk of hypolipidemic drugs and industrial plasticizers to humans. *CRC Crit. Rev. Toxicol.* 12: 1-58 (1983)

24. Hess, R., Stäubli, W., and Reiss, W., Nature of the hepatomegalic effect produced by ethyl-chlorophenoxyisobutyrate in the rat. *Nature* 208: 856-858 (1965)

25. Svoboda, D.J., and Azarnoff, D., Response of hepatic microbodies to a hypolipidemic agent, ethyl-chlorophenoxybutyrate (CPIB). *J. Cell Biol.* 30: 442-450 (1966)

26. Reddy, J.K., and Krishnakantha, T.P., Hepatic peroxisome proliferation: Induction by two novel compounds structurally unrelated to clofibrate. *Science* 190: 787-789 (1975)

27. Reddy, J.K., Krishnakantha, T.P., Azarnoff, D.L., and Moody, D.E., 1-Methyl-4-piperidyl-bis(p-chlorophenoxy)acetate. A new hypolipidemic peroxisome proliferator. *Res. Commun. Chem. Pathol. Pharmacol.* 10: 589-592 (1975)

28. Reddy, J.K., Moody, D.E., Azarnoff, D.L., and Rao, M.S., Di-(2-ethylhexyl) phthalate: An industrial plasticizer induces hypolipidemia and enhances hepatic catalase and carnitine acetyltransferase activities in rats and mice. *Life Science* 18: 941-945 (1976)

29. Moody, D.E., and Reddy, J.K., The hepatic effects of hypolipidemic drugs (clofibrate, nafenopin, tibric acid, and Wy-14,643) on hepatic peroxisomes and peroxisome-associated enzymes. *Am. J. Pathol.* 90: 435-446 (1978)

30. Lalwani, N.D., Reddy, M.K., Qureshi, S.A., Sirtori, C.R., Abiko, Y., and Reddy, J.K., Evaluation of selected hypolipidemic agents for the induction of peroxisomal enzymes and peroxisomal proliferation in the rat liver. *Human Toxicol.* 2: 27-48 (1983)

31. Reddy, J.K., Warren, J.R., Reddy, M.K., and Lalwani, N.D., Hepatic and renal effects of peroxisome proliferators: Biological implications. *Ann. N.Y. Acad. Sci.* 386: 81-110 (1982)

32. Reddy, J.K., Lalwani, N.D., Reddy, M.K., and Qureshi, S.A., Excessive accumulation of autofluorescent lipofuscin in the liver during hepatocarcino-

genesis by methyl clofenapate and other hypolipidemic peroxisome proliferators. *Cancer Res.* 42: 259–266 (1982)

33. Warren, J.R., Simmon, V.F., and Reddy, J.K., Properties of hypolipidemic peroxisome proliferators in the lymphocyte [^{3}H]thymidine and *Salmonella* mutagenesis assays. *Cancer Res.* 40: 36–41 (1980)

34. Warren, J.R., Lalwani, N.D., and Reddy, J.K., Phthalate esters as peroxisome proliferator carcinogens. *Environ. Health Perspect.* 45: 35–40 (1982)

35. Kluwe, W.M., McConnell, E.E., Huff, J.E., Haseman, J.K., Douglas, J.F. and Hartwell, W.V., Carcinogenicity testing of phthalate esters and related compounds by the National Toxicology Program and the National Cancer Institute. *Environ. Health Perspect.* 45: 129–133 (1982)

36. National Cancer Institute. Bioassay of di(2-ethylhexyl)adipate for possible carcinogenicity. Carcinogenesis testing program, U.S. Dept. of Health and Human Services. DHHS Publ. No. (NIH) 81–1773 (1981)

37. National Cancer Institute. Bioassay of di(2-ethylhexyl)phthalate. Carcinogenesis testing program, U.S. Dept. of Health and Human Services. DHHS Publ. No. (NIH) 81–1773 (1981)

38. Cohen, A.J., and Grasso, P., Review of hepatic response to hypolipidemic drugs in rodents and assessment of its toxicological significance to man. *Fd. Cosmet. Toxicol.* 19: 585–605 (1981)

39. Schulte-Hermann, R., Induction of liver growth by xenobiotic compounds and other stimuli. *CRC Crit. Rev. Toxicol.* 33: 97–158 (1974)

40. Golberg, L., Liver enlargement produced by drugs, its significance. *Proc. Eur. Soc. Study Drugs Toxicol.* 7: 171–177 (1966)

41. Moody, D.E., Rao, M.S., and Reddy, J.K., Mitogenic effect in mouse liver induced by a hypolipidemic drug, nafenopin. *Virch. Arch. B. Cell Pathol.* 23: 291–296 (1977)

42. Reddy, J.K., Rao, M.S., Azarnoff, D.L., and Sell, S., Mitogenic and carcinogenic effects of a hypolipidemic peroxisome proliferator [4-chloro-6-(2,3-xylidino)-2-pyrimidinylthio]acetic acid (Wy-14,643) in rat and mouse liver. *Cancer Res.* 39: 152–161 (1979)

43. Novikoff, A.B., and Goldfischer, S., Visualization of peroxisomes (microbodies) and mitochondria with diaminobenzidine. *J. Histochem. Cytochem.* 17: 675–680 (1969)

44. Weibel, E.R., Stereological principles for morphometry in electron microscopic cytology. *Int. Rev. Cytol.* 26: 235–302 (1969)

45. Lück, H., in: *Methods of Enzymatic Analysis* (H.U. Bergmeyer, ed.), pp 885–888, Academic Press, New York (1965)

46. Mittal, B., and Kurup, C.K.R., Induction of carnitine acetyltransferase by clofibrate in rat liver. *Biochem. J.* 194: 249–255 (1981)

47. Fritz, I.B., Schultz, S.K., and Spere, P.A., Properties of partially purified carnitine acetyltransferase. *J. Biol. Chem.* 238: 2509–2517 (1963)

48. Ellman, G.L., Tissue sulfhydryl groups. *Arch. Biochem. Biophys.* 82: 70–75 (1953)

49. Lalwani, N.D., Reddy, M.K., Mark, M.M., and Reddy, J.K., Induction, immunochemical identity and immunofluorescence localization of peroxisome proliferation associated polypeptide (PPA-80) and peroxisomal enoyl-CoA hydratase of mouse liver and renal cortex. *Biochem. J.* 198: 177–186 (1981)

50. Lazarow, P.B., Rat liver peroxisomes catalyze the β-oxidation of fatty acids. *J. Biol. Chem.* 253: 1522–1528 (1978)

51. Lazarow, P.B., Assay of peroxisomal β-oxidation. *Methods Enzymol.* 72: 315–319 (1981)

52. Reddy, J.K., and Kumar, N.S., The peroxisome proliferation associated polypeptide in rat liver. *Biochem. Biophys. Res. Commun.* 77: 824–829 (1979)

53. Osumi, T., and Hashimoto, T., Peroxisomal β-oxidation system of rat liver. Co-purification of enoyl-CoA hydratase and 3-hydroxyacyl CoA dehydrogenase. *Biochem. Biophys. Res. Commun.* 89: 580–584 (1979)

54. Baudhuin, P., Beaufay, H., Rahman-Li,Y., Sellinger, O.Z., Wattiaux, R., Jacques, P., and deDuve, C., Tissue fractionation studies. 17. Intracellular distribution of monoamine oxidase, asparate aminotransferase, alanine aminotransferase, d-amino acid oxidase, and catalase in rat-liver tissues. *Biochem. J.* 92: 179–184 (1964)

55. Laemmli, U.K., Cleavage of structural proteins during the assembly of the head of bacteriophage T_4. *Nature* 227: 680–685 (1970)

56. Chance, B., Sies, H., and Boveris, A., Hydrogen peroxide metabolism in mammalian organs. *Physiol. Rev.* 59: 527–605 (1979)

Part VIII

Risk Estimation

24

Examination of Risk Estimation Models

Abe Silvers

Electric Power Research Institute
Palo Alto, California

Kenny S. Crump

K.S. Crump and Company, Incorporated
Ruston, Louisiana

INTRODUCTION

It is becoming increasingly evident that many of the chemicals used by modern society are potentially hazardous to human health. This evidence comes chiefly from results from laboratory animals exposed to high doses of individual chemicals. Health effects observed in these animal studies include mutagenicity, carcinogenicity, teratogenicity, and general toxicity. Humans are constantly exposed to chemicals with the potential to cause these effects—in the workplace, in food, in water, and in air. While exposures to noxious chemicals need to be controlled, it is not feasible or even necessarily desirable to totally prevent some small levels of human exposures. For example, every gasoline or diesel-powered automobile emits benzo(a)pyrene and other substances known to cause cancer. It is safe to say that every person in the United States is exposed at some level to these exhaust constituents. To eliminate these exposures would require banning of gasoline- and diesel-powered vehicles. This is but one of many examples of exposures to toxic chemicals associated with products or services which are vital to modern society.

An acceptable level of exposure to a potentially harmful chemical is not a purely scientific question and is an appropriate subject for public debate. However, in order to have a rational basis for debating and deciding these issues, it is helpful to have some ideas of what levels of risk truly exist. In the past few years the process of risk assessment has been increasingly applied to these problems. Risk assessment involves combining scientific data on health effects and human exposures to present a picture of what the risks might be in a given situation. Regulatory agencies increasingly are using risk assessment methods to help guide their decisions. Industrial and environmental groups are also using these methods.

Risk assessment methods have been applied particularly to carcinogens. Most chemicals which are considered carcinogenic are so classified by virtue of results from lifetime animal bioassays. The human data necessary for such a determination are not available for most chemicals. Also, data from short term bioassays or from *in vitro* assays generally are not considered to be definitive. Chemicals which are found to be carcinogenic in animals from lifetime bioassays are generally considered to be putative carcinogens in humans as well.

Quantitative estimates of human risk are also made from animal bioassay data. Such estimates require two difficult steps: the extrapolation of risks from high dosages used in animal experiments to much lower doses experienced by humans; and the extrapolation of risks from animals to humans. The latter step is discussed elsewhere in this volume, and so this chapter will be confined to consideration of low dose extrapolation. This procedure is accomplished by fitting a mathematical dose-response model to animal bioassay data using statistical model fitting and confidence limit procedures. The choice of a model is critical because different models can produce vastly different results.

In this chapter, we discuss low dose extrapolation in detail. The experimental setting is described and an example of the data necessary for low dose extrapolation is given. Dose-response curves are classified with respect to their low dose properties and the critical importance of the low dose behavior of these curves in risk assessment is illustrated. Several specific dose-response models are reviewed and their biological rationale described. Various statistical procedures that are needed when fitting models to data and computing confidence limits are reviewed and evaluated. These methods are illustrated by applying them to data from a specific experiment.

These methods entail many limitations, which are described in the chapter. It seems to us that one of the potentially fruitful ways for improving these methods is through the incorporation of pharmacokinetic approaches. The last part of the chapter discusses some of the work that has been done in this area and suggests further research.

EXPERIMENTAL DESIGN

In a common laboratory study, a number of experimental groups of animals are continuously exposed to different fixed levels of a chemical. The effect of exposure may result in a response. The time to response may be observable, such as, for example, the case of the clinical appearance of a skin tumor, or the response is not directly observable, as with the appearance of a lung tumor. In the latter case, only dichotomous data, the presence or absence of the response in a given time period, is considered. Since time to response is not generally observable, we will concentrate only on studies with dichotomous data.

In this kind of study, there are N experimental subjects and n experimental groups. In each group i there are n_i subjects such that

(1)
$$\sum_{i=1}^{n} n_i = N.$$

For each group i, the dose level is d_i, i = 1, . . . n, which is different for each group. In an experimental period of length t, let U_{ij} be the dichotomous response (U_{ij} = 1 if a response occurs and U_{ij} = 0 if no response) for subject j, exposed to dose d_i, then the number of subjects that respond in group i is

(2)
$$x_i = \sum_{j=1}^{n_i} U_{ij}.$$

The National Cancer Institute's bioassay of chloroform[1] is typical of many bioassays for carcinogenicity. The reader should keep in mind that it is only the tumor incidences and doses which are of interest to us and not, for example, the fact that exposures were by gavage and might be considered of questionable import to human carcinogenesis.

This experiment's basic design consisted of administering chloroform at two dose levels, d_1 and d_2, to groups of 50 animals of each sex and species. Thus, 400 tested animals divided into eight groups were used. In addition, 20 animals per group were used as controls for each species and sex combination. Treatment was by oral gavage, five times per week for 78 weeks with sacrifice of surviving rats at 111 weeks from start of study and mice at 92 to 93 weeks. Rats were started on treatment at 52 days and mice at 35 days of age. The dose levels for male rats were d_1 = 180 mg/kg and d_2 = 90 mg/kg throughout the chronic study. For female rats, it was necessary to lower the doses from starting levels of 250 mg/kg and 125 mg/kg to d_1 = 180 mg/kg and d_2 = 90 mg/kg after 22 weeks. The initial dose levels for mice were d_1 = 200 mg/kg and d_2 = 100 mg/kg for males and d_1 = 400 mg/kg and d_2 = 200 mg/kg for females since it was considered that the animals could tolerate a higher dose. All of these factors, including the changing dose patterns, would need to be taken into account in a quantitative risk assessment for this study.

There are also additional factors to be considered. The experimental animals may be composed of different species and differing sex within species. Therefore, d_i and t may be specific for a species and sex within a species. The normal life spans of species are usually different. Most mouse bioassays for carcinogenicity currently last for at least 18 months and rat bioassays for at least 24 months. These durations are commensurate with the normal life span of these animals.

Such studies are often used to estimate a safe dose. To do so, some function P(d) relating d_i to $p_i = X_i/n_i$ is assumed, where P(d) is the probability that a subject on dose d will respond in time t.

Given a fixed low dose d, we wish to estimate the extrapolated low dose response rate P(d). Alternatively, given a fixed low response rate P*, say $0 < p < 10^{-3}$, we may wish to estimate the "safe" dose d* which produces a lifetime risk of P*. In symbols,

(3)
$$P(d^*) = P^*.$$

To do this, a parametric model $P(d) \equiv P(d,\theta)$ is assumed. The response data X_i which have a binominal distribution with parameters $P(d_i)$, N_i are used to estimate the parameter vector θ. The type of models used and the statistical estimation procedure for the inference determine the properties of the estimates. In the subsequent section we will review various models and their biological justification.

MODELS

Experimental data are used to examine and to determine the mathematical relationship between exposure effects and the test doses. This function is described by a parametric model since the estimate of safe dose typically is drawn outside of the experimental range. Models for dichotomous response data are dichotomous response models, *i.e.*, given a deterministic dose d, the model states that $P(d)$ = Probability that a subject exposed to a dose d will respond in the experimental time period. For simplicity we will initially consider models with no background response $[P(0) = 0]$ and discuss later the incorporation of background. There are two classes of dichotomous response models.

Tolerance Distribution Models

These models are based on the premise that each animal in the population has its own tolerance to the test compound. The tolerance level T is the boundary dose level. Below this level, a subject will not respond to the stimulus and above this level the subject will respond. Let $H(t)$ be the cumulative distribution of tolerance in the population. An individual who is selected at random will respond with probability $P(d)$ at dose d, where

$$(4) \qquad P(d) = Pr(\text{tolerance} < d) = H(d).$$

Except for the unknown location and scale parameters, $\ln T$ is assumed to have a known distribution F. A model can therefore be designated as

$$(5) \qquad P(d) = F(\alpha + \beta \ln d)$$

where α, β are parameters which can be estimated from data.[2] Various models of this form have been suggested. Among them is the probit, where

$$(6) \qquad F(x) = (2\pi)^{-1/2} \int_{\infty}^{x} e^{-u^2/2} \, du,$$

and where the distribution of tolerances is lognormal.[3] The logistic $F(x) = (1 + e^{-x})^{-1}$ (Reference 4) and the extreme value $F(x) = 1 - \exp[-\exp(-x)]$ (Reference 5) are others. The extreme value, with $a = e^{\alpha}$ and $b = \beta$, leads to the Weilbull

$$(7) \qquad P(d) = 1 - e^{-(ad^b)}.$$

The probit and logistic models have traditionally been applied to bioassay data but this does not alone constitute sufficient justification for their use in extrapolation to low dose.

Stochastic Models

Stochastic models are deduced from hypotheses on carcinogenic processes. For each animal, a positive response results from the random occurrence of one or more biological events. The k-hit model supposes that a target cell has to receive k "hits" of the biologically effective agent to start an irreversible change leading to the response. If it is assumed that the hits follow a homogenous Poisson process, then for k = 1 the probability P(d) that a response will occur at dose d is given by

(8) $P(d) = Pr(\text{at least one hit}) = 1-e^{-\lambda d}$

where λd is the rate at which hits occur. If $k > 1$, the probability of a response at dose d is

$$P(d) = 1 - \sum_{j=0}^{k-1} e^{-\lambda d} (\lambda d)^j / j!$$

(9)

$$= \int_0^d [\Gamma(k)]^{-1} \lambda^k t^{k-t} e^{-\lambda t} dt$$

where $\Gamma(k)$ denotes the Gamma function.[6]

If the very plausible assumption is to be made that the multihit assumptions apply to cancer in a single cell and that different cell lines compete independently to produce the first cancer, then this model reduces to the Weibull model.[7] Consequently, the Weibull model may be more plausible than the multihit model.

The multistage model is based upon the assumption that carcinogenesis is an irreversible self-replicating k-stage process originating in a single cell, with some stages dependent on the dose of the given carcinogen and the other having only spontaneous occurrences. The version of this model used for low dose extrapolation[8,9] is

(10) $P(d) = 1 - \exp(-\sum_{i=1}^{k} q_i d^i)$

where k is the number of states and q_i are parameters.

The Guess and Crump[10] model generalizes this model by allowing the number of stages to be free.

The validity of these hypotheses have not been established because current information on the mechanisms of carcinogenic processes needs further elucidation.

TYPES OF DOSE-RESPONSE FUNCTIONS

The estimation of safe doses at low doses implies that the shape of the dose-response curve is very significant. Figure 1 denotes dose-response functions P(d) with respect to their low dose shape. The characteristics of the curves discussed are threshold, low dose linear, low dose sublinear, low dose supralinear, convex and concave.

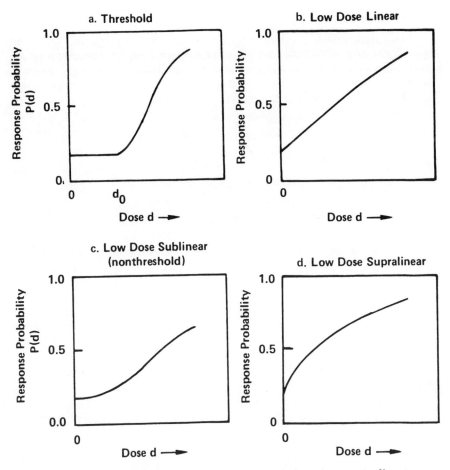

Figure 1: Characterization of dose-response functions according to their low dose properties. Source: Ricci *et al.*[7]

Threshold (Figure 1a)

A threshold dose-response function is defined when there is no increase in risk below a dose d_0 over that which exists in the absence of the dose, *i.e.*,

$$(11) \qquad P(d) = P(0) \qquad \text{for } d < d_0.$$

Low Dose Linear (Figure 1b)

A dose-response function $P(d)$ is called low dose linear if it is approximately linear at low doses and specifically, has a positive slope at $d = 0$. A mathematical description is given by:

$$(12) \qquad P(d) = P(0) + Bd + o(d)$$

where $B > 0$ and $o(d)$ satisfies $o(d)/d \to 0$ as $d \to 0$.

Low Dose Sublinear (Figure 1c)

Low dose sublinear curves satisfy $P(d) > P(0)$ for all $d > 0$, and flatten out near $d = 0$ so that the tangent line to the curve at $d = 0$ has a slope of zero. An example is given by the equation for dose-response $P(d)$,

$$(13) \qquad P(d) = 1 - \exp(-\alpha - \beta d^2), \qquad \beta > 0.$$

Note that, $P(0) = 1-\exp(-\alpha)$, $P'(0) = 0$ and $P''(0) = 2 \exp(-\alpha) > 0$, so that $P(d)$ behaves like a quadratic function of dose near $d = 0$.

Low Dose Supralinear (Figure 1d)

This type of dose-response curve $P(d)$ has an infinite slope at $d = 0$, such that

$$(14) \qquad \frac{P(d) - P(0)}{d} \to \infty \qquad \text{as } d \to 0.$$

Additional risk levels $P(d) - P(0)$ near $d = 0$ predict corresponding greater increases than dose-response predictions from the other three classes. This classification is not considered to be desirable from biologic mechanisms.

The low dose linear class is further classified as those which are convex near $d = 0$ (Figure 2a) and those which are concave near zero dose (Figure 2b). The convex subclass is defined by functions $P(d)$ for which $P''(d) > 0$ for doses sufficiently close to zero. The concave sub-class contains other low dose linear dose response functions. If responses at lower doses are linearly estimated, the response probabilities at lower doses will be underestimated if the curve is concave and overestimated if the curve is convex.

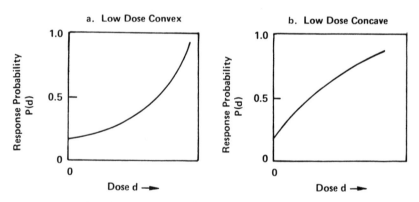

Figure 2: Classification of low dose linear response functions. Source: Ricci et al.[7]

DOSE-RESPONSE FUNCTION TAIL BEHAVIOR AT LOW DOSES

Risks predicted at low doses from described dose-response curves by the different classes can differ widely, yet, these risks are practically indistinguishable in the risk range 0.01 to 0.99. Five dose-response functions describing the data in Table 1 from a benzo[a]pyrene skin painting experiment with mice illustrate this important concept.[11] In this example, the responses are infiltrating carcinomas in mice which are exposed for 69 weeks to μg units of dose of benzo[a]pyrene. The five dose response functions based on the data in Table 1 are:

$$(15) \quad P_1(d) = \begin{cases} 1 - \exp\{-2.3 \times 10^{-4}(d-6)^2 - 4.10 \times 10^{-7}(d-6)^3\} & \text{for } d > 6 \\ 0 & \text{for } d < 6 \end{cases}$$

—a multistage model[10] modified to include a threshold;

Low dose sublinear

$$(16) \qquad P_2(d) = \phi \ (-5.8056 + 3.2240 \ \text{Log}_{10}d)$$

—a log-normal dose response function[12] where ϕ indicates the standard normal distribution function.

Low dose sublinear

$$(17) \qquad P_3(d) = 1 - \exp(-9.7 \times 10^{-5}d^2 - 1.7 \times 10^{-6}d^3),$$

—a multistage model;[10]

Low dose linear

$$(18) \quad P_4(d) = 1 - \exp(-9.5 \times 10^{-4}d - 2.5 \times 10^{-5}d^2 - 2.8 \times 10^{-6}d^3)$$

—another multistage model; and

Low dose supralinear

$$(19) \quad P_5(d) = 1 - \exp(-0.002d^{0.1} - 9.6 \times 10^{-5}d^2 - 1.7 \times 10^{-6}d^3)$$

—a modified multistage model.

These five dose-response models agree closely at the experimental doses in Table 1. The graph in Figure 3 further indicates that these are nearly indistinguishable in dose range from 0 to about 60 μg/week. (Crump[13] furnishes methods for constructing optional designs for rejecting a class of dose-response functions in favor of a particular member not in that class. These methods could be used to systematically study the problem of discriminating among the dose-response models [Equations No. 12-14]).

Table 1: Comparison of Observed and Expected Responses from Skin-Painting Experiment of Lee and O'Neill*

Dose Rate (μg/Week)	Animals Tested	Animals Responding	. . Expected Responses Using Equation . .				
			15	16	17	18	19
6	300	0	0	0.15	1.2	2.2	1.0
12	300	4	2.5	3.0	5.0	5.9	5.7
24	300	27	22.2	26.4	22.8	21.9	23.5
48	300	99	105.5	100.8	101.8	101.4	101.3

*Source: Lee and O'Neill[11]

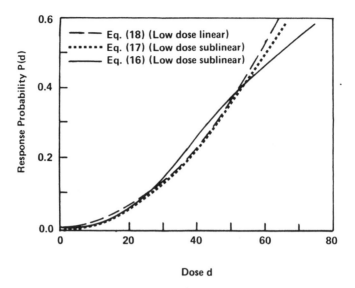

Figure 3: Dose-response functions. Source: Ricci *et al.*[7]

However, the dose-response functions predict very different results at low doses, which is illustrated by Figure 4. These curves consist of log-log graphs of extra risk *versus* dose for these functions. The dose-response curves diverge rapidly for doses below 10 μg/week, since the threshold model predicts no extra risk at all below a dose of 6 μg/week, while the probit model from the low dose sublinear class predicts an extra risk of about 10^{-10} per lifetime at a dose of about 0.8 μg/week.

The foregoing example illustrates the major difficulty with low dose extrapolation. Each of the models is similar between the 10% and the 90% response range; however, the distributions have different responses in their tails and consequently may differ by as much as several orders of magnitude in the results of low dose extrapolation. The dependence of low dose behavior on the particular model means that the choice of model is a difficult critical decision that is based on many uncertainties. For example, there usually does not exist sufficient biological support for the use of any of the distributions. A large number of observations is usually needed to detect the difference between models. A good fit of the model to the data may not mean that it is optimal for extrapolation, since there may not be responses at low doses to determine the shape of P(d) at low doses.

The choice of a model is often based on general statistical theoretical considerations. P(d) should be concave in d for small d>0. A linear low dose behavior P(d) − P(0) = αd for small d>0 can be supported by using the Taylor series expansion of p(d) near d = 0:

$$(20) \qquad P(d) - P(0) = P^{(1)}(0)d + \frac{P^{(2)}(0)}{2!}d^2 + \ldots$$

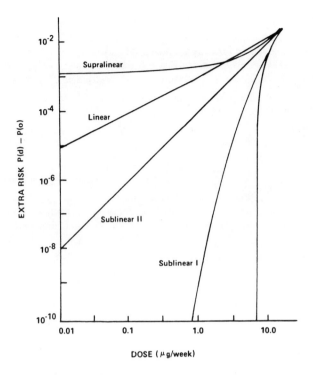

Figure 4: Low dose properties of five dose-response functions. Results of alternative extrapolation models for the same experimental data. NOTE: Dose-response functions were developed for data from a benzo-[a]pyrene carcinogenesis experiment in mice conducted by Lee and O'Neill.[11]

with the argument that $p^{(1)}(0) > 0$ (see References 7 and 14 for examples of such arguments). If the low dose behavior is not linear, it should be described by

$$(21) \qquad p(d) - p(0) = \frac{p^{(\ell)}(0) \; d^{\ell}}{\ell !},$$
$$\text{for small } d > 0, \text{ for some } m = 1, 2, \dots .$$

For example, the k-hit model gives,

$$(22) \qquad P(d) - P(0) \doteq \theta d^{k}, \qquad \text{for small } d > 0,$$

The function $P(d) - P(0)$ is linear at $k = 1$ (1-hit model) and changes to an almost threshold-like function at low doses as k increases.

The Guess and Crump[9,10] model acts like a hit model because the model mathematical formulation has an exponential of a non-negative coefficient polynomial of arbitrary degree. The flexibility and generality of the model enables different high dose behavior as the higher order terms become more dominant at higher doses.

The Guess and Crump[10] model has been applied to both real and hypothetical data sets.[15] Analyses of the hypothetical data sets reveal that it is difficult to reject the linear model in large samples even if P(d) is highly nonlinear. Further, P(d) with a small linear term and some higher order terms may result in extrapolations that may greatly underestimate the true risk.

These results indicate the difficulties in the estimation and testing of tail behaviors.

SPONTANEOUS RATES

The dichotomous dose-response models just described were based on the assumption that at zero dose, $P(0) = 0$. If $P(0) \neq 0$, the response is a spontaneous occurrence. Abbott,[16] and Albert and Altshuler[17] have suggested methods to include spontaneous responses. Abbott's correction,[16] assumes independence between the stimulus and the spontaneous response. Let C denote the proportion of individuals responding spontaneously without treatment, then P(d), assuming independent actions, would be

$$(23) \qquad P(d) = C + (1 - C) P_1(d)$$

where $P_1(d)$ is the proportion responding to the administered dose.

Albert and Altshuler[17] proposed that if the uncontaminated environment contains an additive background level d_0, then the response rate P(d) for a dose of d will be given by

$$(24) \qquad P(d) = P_1(d + d_0).$$

For the single hit model the independent and the additive background assumptions lead to the same mathematical form.

The combination of independent and additive background gives

$$(25) \qquad P(d) = C + (1-C)P(d+d_0).$$

The background is already included in the multistage model through a parameter q_0. With an independent background assumption only, the multi-stage model, for example, may be expressed in the form

$$(26) \qquad P(d) = 1-\exp \left\{- \sum_{i=0}^{k} q_i d^i\right\} \quad (q_i > 0),$$

where $q_0 = -\log(1-C)$. With an additive background assumption only, the multistage model may be expressed as

$$P(d) = 1 -\exp \left\{- \sum_{i=0}^{k} B_i d^i\right\} \quad (q_i > 0),$$

$$(27) \qquad \text{where } B_0 = \sum_{i=1}^{k} q_i d_0^i \text{ and } B_r = \sum_{s=r}^{k} q_s \binom{s}{r} d_0^{s-r} (r=1,\ldots,k).$$

Generally, it is not possible to discriminate between the independent and additivity assumptions from experimental data. The assumptions of independence and/or additional background can give significantly different results in low-dose extrapolation. Hoel[18] examines excess risk differences, assuming an independent or additive background for a log-normal dose-response model. His results, given in Table 2, clearly show substantial difference in excess risk for the same dose. The low dose linearity of the additivity assumption[19] is obvious. Hoel also found low dose linearity in models containing a mixture of independent and additive background response. An exception was when the background mechanism is totally independent of the dose-induced mechanism.

Table 2: Excess Risk, P(d) - P(0), for Log-Normal Dose-Response Model Assuming Independent or Additive Background*

	. . . . Excess Risk	
Dose (d)	Independent	Additive -
10^0	4.0×10^{-1}	4.0×10^{-1}
10^{-1}	1.5×10^{-2}	5.2×10^{-2}
10^{-2}	1.6×10^{-5}	5.2×10^{-3}
10^{-3}	3.8×10^{-10}	5.1×10^{-4}
10^{-4}	1.8×10^{-16}	5.1×10^{-5}

*$P(0) = 0.1$; log-normal model slope = 2 (from Hoel[10]).

CONFIDENCE INTERVALS

The outcome of a low dose extrapolation is usually expressed as estimates of the risk from a given environmental dose d_e or as "virtually safe doses" (VSDs). Both the "additional risk"

$$(28) \qquad A(d_e) = P(d_e;\underline{\theta}) - P(0;\underline{\theta})$$

and the "extra risk"

$$(29) \qquad R(d_e) = [P(d_e;\underline{\theta}) - P(0;\underline{\theta}]/[1 - P(0;\underline{\theta})]$$

have been suggested as appropriate measures of risk. The extra risk may be interpreted as the probability of a response at dose d_e conditional on the fact that no response would have resulted from zero dose. In the absence of background risk [$P(0) = 0$], additional and extra risk are identical. A VSD represents the dose corresponding to a specific small level of risk and may be defined in terms of either extra or additional risk. Krewski and Van Ryzin[20] showed that for the Weibull, gamma multihit, and multistage models the difference between VSDs defined in terms of additional or extra risk is typically small, provided the background level of tumor response is no greater than 25%.

If animals respond independently and the probability that an animal in the ith group is a responder is $P(d_i; \theta)$, then the likelihood of the quantal data from a bioassay is

$$(30) \qquad \ell(\underline{\theta}) = \prod_{i=1}^{g} \binom{n_i}{x_i} P(d_i;\underline{\theta})^{x_i} [1-P(d_i;\underline{\theta})]^{n_i-x_i}.$$

The maximum likelihood estimate (MLE) $\hat{\theta}$ of the parameter vector θ is defined as the value for θ which maximizes the likelihood. These maximizations generally are obtained using sophisticated computer programs. Maximal likelihood estimates of functions of the parameter vector θ are determined as the same function of the MLE $\hat{\theta}$. For example, the MLE of the extra risk is

$$(31) \qquad [P(d;\hat{\underline{\theta}}) - P(0;\hat{\underline{\theta}}]/[1 - P(0;\hat{\underline{\theta}})]$$

and the MLE $\hat{d}$ of the VSD corresponding to an extra risk of π is given by the solution to the equation $R(\hat{d}) = \pi$.

Standard asymptotic maximum likelihood theory can be used to obtain asymptotic distributions for parameters of interest in the low dose extrapolation problem which, in turn, can be used to determine approximate confidence limits for these parameters.[20] Since others have already recorded the details of these calculations and our purpose is to examine the practical applications of these approaches, we will not present the explicit formulas here. Krewski and Van Ryzin[20] consider the asymptotic distribution of $\hat{A}(d_e)$, (the MLE of additional risk at a dose d_e) and of $\hat{d}$, $\log(\hat{d})$, and $1/\hat{d}$ where $\hat{d}$ is the MLE of the VSD corresponding to a given additional risk. They also derive sufficient conditions under which the asymptotic results hold and relate these conditions to the probit, logit, Weibull, gamma multi-hit, and multistage models. Guess and Crump[21] and Crump *et al.*[8] present similar results explicitly for the multistage model.

Both theoretical and practical difficulties arise when these methods are applied to the low dose extrapolation problem. If the true value of one of the parameters in the multistage model is zero, the MLEs are no longer asymptotically normal.[8] Also, the choice made for k in this model strongly affects the confidence limits.

Crump and Masterman[22] observed that lower confidence limits on the VSD under the gamma multihit model, computed using asymptotic MLE theory, sometimes appear far too large. For example, for a carcinogenicity data set involving exposure to sodium saccharin a particular set of parameter values which was consistent with the data (the chi-square goodness-of-fit p-value being greater than 0.1) predicted a VSD which was a factor of 18,000 less than the lower 97.5 confidence limit for the VSD computed using asymptotic normal theory developed by Rai and Van Ryzin.[23] Similar observations have been made by Haseman and Hoel.[24] Another disquieting feature of this approach is that the limits are not invariant under parameter transformations.

LIMITS BASED UPON THE ASYMPTOTIC DISTRIBUTION OF THE LIKELIHOOD RATIO

Denote by $L(\theta)$ the logarithm of the likelihood $\ell(\theta)$. Let $\hat{L} = \log\ell(\hat{\theta})$ denote the logarithm of the likelihood evaluated at the MLE, and let $\hat{L}(\theta_1)$ denote the constrained maximum of the log-likelihood subject to a fixed value for a particular scalar parameter θ_1. Then, under appropriate conditions, $2[\hat{L} - \hat{L}(\theta_1)]$ has an asymptotic chi-square distribution with one degree of freedom whenever θ_1 is the true parameter value. This distribution can be used to construct approximate confidence limits for θ_1. The value θ_u greater than the MLE $\hat{\theta}_1$ which satisfies the equation

$$(32) \qquad 2[\hat{L} - \hat{L}(\theta_u)] = x^2_{1-2\alpha}$$

is a $100(1-\alpha)\%$ upper confidence limit for θ_1, where x^2_p denotes the 100p percentage point of the chi-square distribution with one degree of freedom. Lower confidence limits are similarly constructed.

This approach can also be used to construct confidence for a function of a single parameter. For monotone functions, the method is simple; if f is an increasing function and θ_u is an upper limit for a parameter θ_1, then $f(\theta_u)$ is an upper limit for $f(\theta_1)$. Mantel et al.[12] used this method to obtain lower confidence limits for the VSD for extra risk under the probit model. Since they fixed b = 1, the extra risk is given by $\phi(a + \log_{10}d)$, which is an increasing function of the parameter a and does not involve the background parameter c. (ϕ is the normal distribution function.) Mantel et al. therefore used

$$(33) \qquad \text{antilog}_{10}[\phi^{-1}(\pi) - a_u]$$

as a $100(1-\alpha)\%$ lower confidence limit for the VSD corresponding to an extra risk of π, where a_u is the corresponding upper confidence limit for the parameter as computed using the above approach.

Crump[9] developed a similar approach for the multistage model. For this model the extra risk is given by

$$(34) \qquad 1 - \exp(-q_1 d - \ldots - q_k d^k),$$

which is a function of the parameters $q_1 \ldots, q_k$. However, at low doses the extra risk can be approximated by $q_1 d$ whenever $q_1 > 0$. An approximate upper confidence limit for the extra risk at a small dose d_e is therefore estimated by $q_u d_e$, where q_u is upper limit for q_1 computed using the above approach. Similarly, π/q_u represents an approximate lower limit for the VSD corresponding to an extra risk of π.

This method will not be accurate for risk levels high enough so that the linearization is not a good approximation to the multistage dose-response. For doses in the nonlinear region of the dose-response curve, an upper limit on extra risk computed in this fashion can even lie below the MLE estimate. Further, it cannot be used without modification to compute two-sided confidence intervals because frequently Equation No. 32 will not be satisfied even if q_1 is decreased to zero.

There is a more general version of this approach which does not have either of these drawbacks. It can be shown that under appropriate regularity conditions

$$(35) \qquad \max_{\underline{\theta}} [R(d_e;\underline{\theta}): 2[l(\hat{\underline{\theta}}) - l(\underline{\theta})] \leq x^2_{1-2\alpha}]$$

is an asymptotic $100(1-\alpha)\%$ upper limit for the extra risk at an environmental dose d_e and

$$(36) \qquad \min_{\underline{\theta}} [d: R(d;\underline{\theta}) = \pi, 2[l(\hat{\underline{\theta}}) - l(\underline{\theta})] \leq x^2_{1-2\alpha}]$$

is an approximate $100(1 - \alpha)\%$ lower limit for the VSD corresponding to an extra risk of π. Similar confidence limits can, of course, be developed using the concept of additional risk.

BOOTSTRAP METHODS FOR CONFIDENCE INTERVALS

Let $P^*(d)$ be some estimate of the dose response function derived from the experimental data $X_1, \ldots, X_q$, and let $X_1^*, \ldots, X_g^*$ be independent random variables with X_i^* having a binomial distribution with parameters N_i and $P^*(d_i)$. Note that $X_1^*, \ldots, X_g^*$ may be thought of as the numbers of affected animals in the various dose groups of a hypothetical experiment with exactly the same design as the true experiment (*i.e.*, same dose levels and numbers of animals on test); the only difference between the hypothetical experiment and the real experiment is $P^*(d)$ rather than $P(d)$. Given $P^*(d)$, the complete distribution of $X_1^*, \ldots, X_g^*$ is determined, as well as the distribution of "bootstrap estimators" such as the estimate of the VSD obtained by the method of maximum likelihood applied to $X_1^*, \ldots, X_g^*$ rather than $X_1, \ldots, X_g$. These distributions may be used to estimate the accuracy of parameter estimates (*i.e.*, their standard deviation) and to construct approximate confidence intervals for parameters. These methods, known as bootstrap procedures, have been discussed in general in a series of papers by Efron.[25-27] The distribution function of a bootstrap estimator given $P^*(d)$ is known as the bootstrap distribution function CDF$_*$.

Although these bootstrap distributions are completely known, at least in principle, they generally must be approximated by Monte Carlo methods. The hypothetical experiment producing the outcomes $X_1^*, \ldots, X_g^*$ is repeated M times by computer simulation and the resulting empirical distribution of the bootstrap estimator is used to approximate CDF$_*$; By the Law of Large Numbers, CDF$_*$ is approximated arbitrarily closely as M increases.

Crump *et al.*[18] proposed the use of "envelope curves" in connection with the multistage model as a substitute for confidence limits based upon the asymptotic theory of MLEs. These curves are generated by computer simulation of 100 independent replications of the same experiment. Each of the 100 data sets involve the same set of test doses and the same numbers of animals tested at each dose as the actual experiment. The response probability at each test dose is the maximum likelihood estimate obtained from the experimental data. From each of the 100 simulated data sets a maximum likelihood dose-response curve is calculated. The value of the upper 97.5% envelope curve for additional risk at a dose d, to use a specific example, is defined as the third largest of the 100 values of additional risk at dose d. Crump *et al.*[8] showed that these envelope curves sometimes agreed quite closely with confidence limits based upon asymptotic maximum likelihood theory. Although the limits depend upon the particular values simulated, they can be made as accurate as desired by simulating more than 100 sets of data.

These envelope curves represent approximations to the empirical distribution function CDF$_*$ of the bootstrap estimator of additional risk obtained by letting $P^*(d_i)$ be the maximum likelihood estimate of risk at dose d_i. The upper 97.5% envelope curve is what Efron[27] calls an upper 97.5% confidence bound computed by the percentile method. Efron[26,27] gives three general arguments supporting the use of the percentile method for constructing confidence limits. None of these arguments, to use Efron's terminology, is "overwhelming" and Efron recommends further investigation of the percentile method.

GOODNESS-OF-FIT

Statistical goodness-of-fit tests are applied to determine if a given model gives a "reasonable" fit to the experimental data.

The chi-square statistic

$$(37) \qquad \chi^2 = \Sigma (x_i - n_i \hat{P}_i)^2 / (n_i \hat{P}_i \hat{Q}_i)$$

can be used in the assessment of the goodness-of-fit of the probit, logit, extreme value, and gamma multi-hit models but may not hold for the multistage model. Recall that the one-hit model is a special case of the extreme value and gamma multi-hit models.[13,28]

For the multistage model, an alternative Monte Carlo goodness-of-fit test based on bootstrapping the likelihood function[25] has been proposed by Crump et al.[8]

The level of significance in a goodness-of-fit test is defined by

$$p = Pr\{\chi^2 > \chi^2_{obs}\},$$

where χ^2_{obs} is calculated from equation 37. χ^2_{obs} refers to a value obtained from the observed data. The level of significance called the "p-value" measures the consistency of the model with the data. Small values indicate lack of fit.

EXAMPLES OF CALCULATIONS

Examples of the procedures for the Multistage model and the Probit model on the chloroform data discussed earlier are given in Tables 3 and 4. The dose levels in Table 3 are weighted averages derived from the dosing data presented earlier.

The calculations for the multistage model were made using the computer program GLOBAL 82. The probit calculations were made using the Mantel-Bryan program written by Dr. Charles Brown of the National Cancer Institute. Both of these methods calculate confidence limits using the asymptotic distribution of the likelihood ratio. The calculation presented in Table 4 can easily be used to obtain 95% lower limits for doses corresponding to various levels of extra risk. Consider, for example, the female data which both models fit adequately. The 95% upper limit for q_1 is 1.17×10^{-2}. The corresponding lower limit in the dose corresponding to an extra risk of 10^{-5} is $10^{-5}/1.17 \times 10^{-2} = 8.5 \times 10^{-4}$ mg/kg/day. The corresponding lower limit for the log-normal model is

$$\text{antilog}_{10}[\Phi^{-1}(10^{-5}) - a] = \text{antilog}_{10}[-4.265 - (-0.912)]$$

$$(38) \qquad \qquad = 4.4 \times 10^{-4} \text{mg/kg/day}.$$

Table 3: Tumors in B6C3F1 Mice from NCI Bioassay of Chloroform[a,b]

Observations	Treatment A					
	Male				Female	
	Matched Controls	98.9 mg/kg/day	197.8 mg/kg/day	Matched Controls	170.3 mg/kg/day	340.7 mg/kg/day
Total tumor-bearing animals/animals[c]	4/18 22%	26/50 52%	44/45 98%	2/20 10%	37/45 82%	39/41 95%
p value[d]	0.0000[f]	–	–	0.0000[e]	–	–
Time to tumor (weeks)[e]	72	66	54	27	66	67
Hepatocellular carcinoma/animals[c]	1/18 6%	18/50 36%	44/45 98%	0/20 0%	36/45 80%	39/41 95%
p value[d]	0.0000[f]	–	–	–	0.0000[f,g]	0.0000[f,g]
Time to tumor (weeks)[e]	72	80	54	–	66	67
Kidney epithelial tumors/animals[c]	1/18 6%	1/50 2%	2/45 4%	0/20 0%	0/45 0%	0/40 0%
p value[d]	0.4873	–	–	1.000	–	–
Time to tumor (weeks)[e]	92	92	92	–	–	–
Thyroid tumors/animals[c]	0/17 0%	0/48 0%	0/43 0%	0/20 0%	0/41 0%	0/36 0%
p value[d]	1.000	–	–	1.000	–	–
Time to tumor (weeks)[e]	–	–	–	–	–	–
Survival at terminal sacrifice (92 weeks)	50%	65%	65%	75%	75%	20%

[a]Source: NCI.[1]

[b]Oral dose of chloroform in corn oil administered by gavage five times per week.

[c]Based on animals whose tissues were examined from a specific organ.

[d]One-tailed p value from Armitage test for linear trend in proportions, unless otherwise stated.

[e]Time to detection of first tumor (at death).

[f]Statistically significant ($p < 0.05$).

[g]Data departure from linear trend (for departure statistic; $p < 0.05$). Fisher Exact Test is used comparing controls to a dose level. Bonferroni correction for simultaneous comparison of controls is included.

Table 4: Results from Fitting the Multistage and Log-Normal Models to
the Data from Table 3 on the Incidence of Hepatocellular Carcinoma
in Male and Female B6C3F1 Mice

. . . . Multistage. . . . .

Male Data
    MLE estimates: $q_0 = 3.75(-2)$[a], $q_1 = 0.0$, $q_2 = 6.23(-5)$
    95% upper limit on $q_1 = 2.03(-3)$
    Chi-square goodness of fit[b] p-value = 0.03
Female Data
    MLE estimates: $q_0 = 0.0$, $q_1 = 9.21(-3)$, $q_2 = 0.0$
    95% upper limit on $q_1 = 1.17(-2)$
    Chi-square goodness of fit p-value = 0.99

. . . . .Log-Normal . . . .

Male Data
    MLE estimates: $c = 0.048$, $a = -1.77$
    95% upper limit on $a = -1.54$
    Chi-square goodness of fit p-value = 0.19
Female Data
    MLE estimates: $c = 0.0$, $a = -1.22$
    95% upper limit on $a = -0.921$
    Chi-square goodness of fit p-value = 0.19

[a]$3.75(-2)$ means 3.75×10^{-2}.
[b]This goodness-of-fit test is described in Crump.[9]

Although for a risk of 10^{-5} the dose lower limits calculated from these two models only differ by about a factor of two, for smaller values of extra risk, the limits on dose derived from the log-normal model will be considerably greater than those derived from the multistage model. This is because the multistage model is linear at low doses whereas the log-normal model is sublinear.

TOXICOKINETICS AND RISK ASSESSMENT

The models described in this chapter, do not explicitly relate the exposure dose (the amount of chemical to which an individual is exposed) to the tissue dose (the amount of the ultimate carcinogen which reaches the target tissue). It may be more appropriate to utilize the tissue dose rather than the exposure dose since the tissue dose may be the "effective" dose. To estimate the tissue dose may require knowledge of the kinetics of the storage and excretion of the chemical, detoxification of the chemical, and the metabolic activation of the chemical to the ultimate carcinogen.

A problem in the application of pharmacokinetic principles to low dose risk assessment is that chemical pathways may change as the administered chemical dose decreases. Saturation kinetics may occur at high doses and may be described by a nonlinear equation.[29-31] Dose dependent nonlinearities in general, are often expressed as $v = V_{max}d/(K_M + d)$, where v is the rate of product formation of the kinetic process, and K_M is the value of the concentration, d, at which the process rate is half maximal. This equation is usually called a Michaelis-Menten equation.

Gehring *et al.*[32] conducted an experiment with rats to determine the relationship between exposure to vinyl chloride and the amount of vinyl chloride metabolized. Rats were exposed for six hours to atmospheres containing various concentrations of radioactive-labeled vinyl chloride. Immediately after exposure the rats were killed and the total amount of radioactivity of each carcass was used to estimate the total amount of metabolized vinyl chloride. The results of this experiment are shown in Figure 5. Gehring *et al.* found that the relationship between the exposure dose S, in units of μg of vinyl chloride per liter of air (1 ppm of vinyl chloride = 2.56 μg of vinyl chloride per liter of air), and the metabolized dose v, in units of μg of vinyl chloride metabolized per six hour exposure, was not linear, but could be described by a transformation of the Michaelis-Menten equation to a linear version.

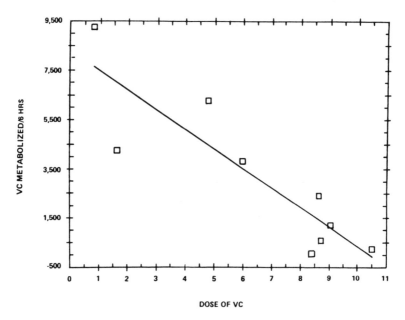

Figure 5: Relationship in rats between exposure dose of vinyl chloride (VC) and amount metabolized. Determined from radioactivity in the carcass. Source: Table 1 of Gehring *et al.*[32]

The experimental findings of Maltoni[33] on the relationship between exposure to vinyl chloride and induction of angiosarcomas in rats, shown in Table 5, relate tumor incidence to dose. Maltoni exposed rats for four hours daily, five days weekly for 52 weeks to various concentrations of vinyl chloride. Gehring *et al.*[32] calculated expected metabolized doses from Maltoni's exposure doses with the curve of Figure 5 by multiplying the result by $\frac{2}{3}$ (the $\frac{2}{3}$ figure accounts for the fact that Maltoni exposed his rats for four hours per day whereas Gehring *et al.* exposed their rats for six hours).

Table 5: Data from Vinyl Chloride Bioassay for Carcinogenicity of Maltoni[a]

Exposure Concentration S (ppm of vinyl chloride)	Metabolized Dose v (μg of vinyl chloride metabolized/4 hrs)[b]	Number of Animals Surviving for 26 Weeks	Number of Animals with Liver Angiosarcoma
0	0	58	0
50	730	59	1
250	2,435	59	4
500	3,413	59	7
2,500	5,030	59	13
6,000	5,403	60	13
10,000	5,521	61	9

[a]Source: Maltoni[33]
[b]From Gehring *et al.*[32]

In Figure 6 are displayed the plots of tumor incidence *versus* both the exposure dose (triangles) and the metabolized dose (squares). At exposure dose (triangles), tumor incidence increases rapidly with increasing dose for doses ≤500 ppm, reaches a plateau of 22% and then falls off to 15% at a dose 10,000 ppm. On the other hand, the plot of tumor incidence *versus* metabolized dose (squares) appears linear. A simple linear model shown in the figure or a maximum likelihood estimated one-hit model $P(d) = 1 - \exp(-.038 \times 10^{-4} d)$ (not shown) describes the data quite adequately. The usual chi-square goodness-of-fit statistic is 2.5, $p \geqslant 0.5$ at 5 degrees of freedom. With exposure dose, the corresponding statistic is 19.4, $p < .002$. These results demonstrate that effective dose may be the dose for risk assessment and that uncertainties for extrapolation may be reduced.

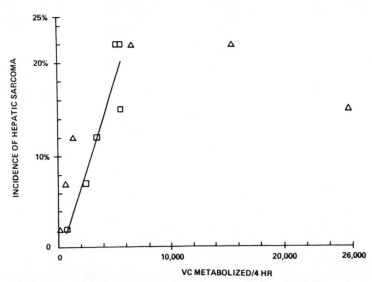

Figure 6: Incidence of liver angiosarcoma plotted against two dose variables. Data taken from Table 5. □ = metabolized dose of vinyl chloride (VC); Δ = exposure dose of VC.

However, a major limitation to the use of such toxicokinetic models is the lack of data for estimating the parameters of the models. The experiments necessary to generate such data, such as the experiment of Gehring et al.,[32] may be becoming more prevalent.

Other surrogates of effective dose are being suggested. Evidence suggests that a measure of DNA alkylation is an appropriate measure of dose at the site of action and that mutation frequency is quantitatively related to the number of alkylations of certain centers of DNA.[34] A model of Gehring and Blau[29] estimates the electrophilic alkylation of DNA from exposure dose. It denotes excretion of the chemical, activation to a reactive metabolite, detoxification of the reactive metabolite, covalent binding of the reactive metabolite to both genetic and nongenetic material, and the repair and replication of covalently bound genetic material. A schematic representation of this model is given in Figure 7.

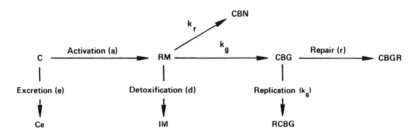

Figure 7: Schematic representation of a model proposed by Gehring and Blau.[29] In this model, excretion (e), activation (a), detoxification (d) and repair occur in accordance with dose-dependent (Michaelis-Menten) kinetics while the remaining reactions are represented by apparent first-order kinetics. C = Chemical; RM = Reactive Metabolite; Ce = Excreted Chemical; IM = Inactive Metabolite; CBN = Covalent Binding; Nongenetic; CBG = Covalent Binding, Genetic; CBGR = Repaired Covalently Bound Genetic Material; RCBG = Retained Genetic Program, Critical and Noncritical.

From the solutions of a set of differential equations describing Figure 7, Figure 8 displays graphs obtained by Gehring and Blau of the ultimate relative amounts of covalently bound noncritical material (CBN^{∞}/C_0), critical material but repaired $CBGR^{\infty}/C_0$), and replicated critical material ($RCBG^{\infty}/C_0$) *versus* the input dose C_0. Conclusions from these curves include:

(a) At low doses the graphs of CBN^{∞}, $CBGR^{\infty}$ and $RCBG^{\infty}$ *versus* C_0 are low dose linear because the graphs in Figure 8 are all flat for values of C_0 below 10^{-5}.

(b) A "hockey stick" phenomenon, where the striking part of the stick formed by the nearly flat curve below the saturation concentration and the handle formed by the steep increase once the protective mechanisms are saturated,[35] holds for the amount of replicated critical material RCBG. RCBG increases slowly with initial concentration up to 10^{-4} mols/kg and more rapidly for initial concentrations above this value.

(c) The "hockey stick" dose-response curve has some important implications for low dose extrapolation since the low dose risk may be overestimated or underestimated. If the risk at doses far below 10^{-4} mols/kg is estimated by drawing a straight line from the point on the graph corresponding to an initial concentration of 10^{-1} mols/kg, then the low dose risk might be vastly *overestimated*. If it might be surmised that a threshold exists for initial concentrations of 10^{-3} mols/kg, or that the low dose curve shape is low dose sublinear, then the low dose risk is *underestimated* if in fact the curve is linear with a very shallow slope for doses below 10^{-4} mols/kg.

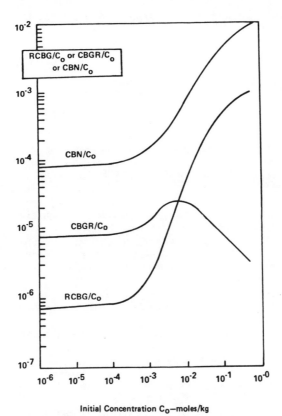

Figure 8: Hypothetical relative amounts of a chemical bound covalently to critical and non-critical material. Source: Gehring and Blau.[29] CBN/C_o = covalently bound to noncritical material; $CBGR/C_o$ = covalently bound to critical, but repaired material; $RCBG/C_o$ = covalently bound to replicated, critical material.

A better understanding of pharmacokinetic mechanisms should contribute greatly to our ability to estimate the magnitude of effects from low doses. There is a need for pharmacokinetic data which would permit estimation of the parameters in pharmacokinetic models. For estimating risks to humans from animal experiments, such data should be available on both the experimental animal species and humans or a species metabolically similar to humans.

REFERENCES

1. National Cancer Institute, Bioassay of chloroform for possible carcinogenicity. U.S. Department of Health, Education and Welfare, Publication No. (NIH), PB-264018 (1978)
2. Chand, N., and Hoel, D.G., in: *Reliability and Biometry* (F. Proschlan and R. Serfling, eds.), pp 681–700, Society for Industrial and Applied Mathematics, Philadelphia (1974)
3. Finney, D.J., *Probit Analysis* (3rd edition), London: Cambridge University Press (1971)
4. Ashton, W.D., *The Log Transformation*, London: Griffin (1972)
5. Gumbel, E.J., *Statistics of Extremes*, New York: Columbia University Press (1958)
6. Rai, K., and Van Ryzin, J., A generalized multi-hit dose response model for low-dose extrapolation. *Biometrics* (in press)
7. Ricci, P.F., Crouch, E.A.C., and Crump, K.S., *Sourcebook on Technological Risk Assessment*, Prentice Hall (in preparation)
8. Crump, K.S., Guess, H.A., and Deal, K., Confidence intervals and tests of hypotheses concerning dose-response relations inferred from animal carcinogenicity data. *Biometrics* 33: 437–451 (1977)
9. Crump, K.S., in: *Health Risk Analysis* (C.R. Richmond, P.J. Walsh, and D. Copenhaver, eds.), pp 381–392. Proceedings of the Third Life Sciences Symposium, Health Risk Analysis, Gatlinburg, Tennessee (1981)
10. Guess, H.A., and Crump, K.S., Low-dose-rate extrapolation of data from animal carcinogenicity experiments—analysis of a new statistical technique. *Math Biosciences* 32: 15–36 (1976)
11. Lee, P.N., and O'Neill, J.A., The effect both of time and dose applied on tumour incidence rate in benzopyrene skin painting experiments. *Br. J. Cancer* 25: 759–770 (1971)
12. Mantel, N., Bohidar, N.R., Brown, C.C., Cominera, J.L., and Tukey, J.W., An improved Mantel-Bryan procedure for "safety" testing of carcinogens. *Cancer Res.* 35: 865–872 (1975)
13. Crump, K.S., Designs for discriminating between binary dose response models with applications to animal carcinogenicity experiments. *Commun. in Statistics* 11: 375–393 (1982)
14. Peto, R., Carcinogenic effects of chronic exposure to very low levels of toxic substances. *Environ. Health Perspect.* 22: 155–159 (1978)
15. Guess, H.A., and Crump, K.S., Can we use animal data to estimate "safe" doses for chemical carcinogens? *Env. Hlth. Quantitative Methods*, SIAM, Philadelphia (1977)
16. Abbott, W.S., A method of computing the effectiveness of an insecticide. *J. Econ. Ent.* 18: 265–267 (1925)

17. Albert, R.E., Altshuler, B., Considerations relating to the formulation of limits for unavoidable population exposures to environmental carcinogens. *Radionuclide Carcinogenesis*, AEC Symposium series. Conf. 72050, National Technical Information Service, Springfield, VA (1973)

18. Hoel, D.G., Incorporation of background response in dose-response models. *Fed. Proc.* 39: 67–69 (1980)

19. Crump, K.S., Hoel, D.G., Langley, C.H., and Peto, R., Fundamental carcinogenic processes and their implications for low-dose risk assessment. *Cancer Res.* 36: 2973–2979 (1976)

20. Krewski, D., and Van Ryzin, J., in: *Statistics and Related Topics* (M. Csorgo *et al.*, eds.), pp 201–231, Elsevier/North Holland Publishing Co., Amsterdam (1981)

21. Guess, H.A., and Crump, K.S., Maximum likelihood estimation of dose-response functions subject to absolutely monotonic constraints. *Ann. Statistics* 6: 101–111 (1978)

22. Crump, K.S., and Masterman, M.D., in: *Environmental Contaminants in Food*. Office of Technology Assessment, Congress of the United States, Washington, DC, pp 154–165 (1979)

23. Rai, K., and Van Ryzin, J., in: *Energy and Health* (N. Breslow, and A. Whittemore, eds.), pp 99–117, SIAM, Philadelphia (1979)

24. Haseman, J.K., and Hoel, D.G., Some practical problems arising from use of the gamma multihit model for risk estimation. *J. Toxicol. Environ. Health* 8: 379–386 (1980)

25. Efron, B., Bootstrap methods: Another look at the jackknife. *Ann. Statistics* 7: 1–26 (1979a)

26. Efron, B., Computers and the theory of statistics: thinking the unthinkable. *SIAM REVIEW* 21: 460–480 (1979b)

27. Efron, B., Censored data and the bootstrap. *J. Am. Statistical Assoc.* 76: 312–319 (1981)

28. Chambers, E.A., and Cox, D.R., Discrimination between alternative binary response models. *Biometrika* 53: 573–578 (1967)

29. Gehring, P.J., and Blau, G.E., Mechanisms of carcinogenesis: dose-response. *J. Environ. Pathol. Toxicol.* 1: 163–179 (1977)

30. Gillette, J.R., Application of pharmacokinetic principles in the extrapolation of animal data to humans. *Clin. Toxicol.* 9: 709–722 (1976)

31. Reitz, R.H., Gehring, P.J., and Park, C.N., Carcinogenic risk estimation of chloroform. An alternative to EPA's procedures. *Fd. Cosmet Toxicol.* 16: 511–514 (1978)

32. Gehring, P.J., Watanabe, P.G., and Park, C.N., Resolution of dose-response toxicity data for chemicals requiring metabolic activation: Example–vinyl chloride. *Toxicol. Appl. Pharmacol.* 44: 581–591 (1978)

33. Maltoni, C., in: *Origins of Human Cancer* (H. Hiatt, ed.), pp 119–146 (1977)

34. Ehrenberg, L.S., in: *The Banbury Report* (V.K. McElheny, and S. Abrahamson, eds.), pp 157–190, Cold Spring Harbor Laboratory, Lloyd Harbor, New York (1979)

35. Cornfield, J., Carcinogenic risk assessment. *Science* 198: 693–699 (1977)

25

Risk Assessment: Biological Considerations

Joseph V. Rodricks
Duncan Turnbull

ENVIRON
Washington, D.C.

INTRODUCTION

In the past decade, it has become apparent that substances found to display carcinogenic properties occur with unexpectedly high frequency in food, air, water, the workplace, consumer products, and in medicinal agents. It would seem essential that a systematic means be found to take into account the biological properties of these substances when deciding whether and to what extent human exposure to them should be restricted. Risk assessment is the most highly systematized means available to incorporate information on the biological properties of carcinogens into this process.

The goal of risk assessment is to estimate the probability that cancer will occur in human populations under their conditions of exposure to a carcinogen. Equipped with such knowledge, decision-makers could examine the question of whether an estimated risk were a sufficiently large threat to the public health to deserve control and, if it were, to determine the most appropriate means for its control. Such decisions would be difficult even if the estimated risks upon which they were based were known to be accurate. They are, of course, made exceedingly difficult because risks estimated by the best methodology currently available are uncertain, and their relation to the true risk is generally unknown.

Under circumstances of high scientific uncertainty, the natural tendency of decision-makers is to focus on those aspects of science that appear to be most readily quantifiable. In the context of carcinogenesis risk assessment, this usually takes the form of excessive concern with numerical estimates of risk derived from the application of a mathematical model to dose-response data, and lack of attention to the underlying biological data and assumptions upon which the numerical estimates are based. This tendency is reinforced by the propensity of risk assessors to present only quantitative estimates, without carefully delineating those factors, many of which are non-quantifiable, that may reveal the likely range of uncertainty in the estimated risk.

One of the objectives of this chapter is to encourage the fuller use of biological information in risk assessment, and to suggest some ways in which this might be accomplished. A second objective is to describe the types of decisions concerning the biological data that need to be made in order to complete a risk assessment. The very important problem of selecting models for high-to-low dose extrapolation is treated separately, in Chapter 24.

Neither this chapter nor the chapter on models treats the very important problem of human exposure assessment. Nothing can be said about risk without knowledge of the magnitude, duration, and frequency of human exposure to the carcinogenic agent under evaluation. Moreover, exposure assessment frequently contributes substantially to the uncertainty in risk estimates. A critical evaluation of human exposure is thus an essential component of risk assessment, and the importance of this subject should not be underestimated.

ELEMENTS OF CARCINOGENESIS RISK ASSESSMENT

Risk assessment is a multi-step process; the major steps (excluding those related to human exposure assessment) are the following[1]:

(1) Collection, organization, and critical evaluation of all experimental and epidemiological studies that pertain to the likelihood that an agent is a carcinogen in humans.

(2) Critical evaluation of the total data base to characterize the strength of the scientific evidence of human carcinogenicity.

(3) Selection of data sets for high-to-low dose extrapolation and estimation of risks per unit of low dose exposure.

(4) Extrapolation of estimated low dose (unit) risks from animals to humans (or from one population group to another, if the risk estimate is based on epidemiological data).

(5) Statement of biological and statistical uncertainties in the estimated risks.

Many of the previous chapters in this book have been devoted to the first step listed above. The remaining sections of this chapter will thus be devoted to steps 2 to 5; that is, it will be assumed that all data pertinent to the question of the carcinogenicity of a substance have been collected and that each study has been critically evaluated. This chapter thus first deals with step 2, which concerns evaluation of the total data base.

EVALUATION OF TOTAL DATA BASE

Introduction

The quality and quantity of data available for making judgments about the likely carcinogenicity of an agent in humans vary widely among different agents. Because of this, it would seem appropriate to provide an evaluation of the *strength of the scientific evidence* upon which the characterization of likely carcinogenicity in humans is made. This characterization is an essential element of risk assessment, because it conveys to the users of risk assessments the degree of uncertainty associated with the data base. Moreover, if this approach is taken, the risk assessor is relieved of the responsibility of deciding how much evidence is needed before a substance is labeled a "carcinogen" for policy purposes. This approach does, of course, place upon the risk assessor the difficult burden of accurately and usefully characterizing the total evidence. In this section a general approach to this task is outlined; it is intended only to suggest a mode of thinking about the subject of weighing evidence of carcinogenicity, and not as a formal scheme. Some approaches proposed by others are also described. It is important to keep in mind that the goal of this stage of risk assessment is not to make any statement about risk to humans; it is only to characterize the strength of the evidence implicating a substance as a carcinogen in humans.

Factors in Evaluation

It would appear that several features of the total data base require examination before the evidence it provides can be accurately characterized. After critical evaluation of each pertinent study, it should be possible to describe the degree of data *replication, reproducibility*, and *concordance*.[2]

- A finding is said to be *replicated* if it is seen in experiments of identical design.

- A finding is said to be *reproducible* if it is seen in the same species under different conditions (*e.g.*, in different strains, sexes or dose groups).

- Experimental and epidemiological findings are said to be *concordant* if they are consistent across species.

As a general scientific principle, it would seem that as the degree of data replication, reproducibility, and concordance increases, it becomes more certain that a substance has the capacity to display carcinogenic properties in humans. It is important to add, however, that this conclusion also rests upon general biological knowledge regarding the known or expected degree of correspondence between observations of carcinogenicity in experimental animals and expected responses in humans.[3]

A critical element in judging the degree of data replicability, reproducibility, and concordance is the attention given an apparent lack of these factors for a given data set. In some cases, for example, several data sets may, upon superficial examination, appear to lack reproducibility, but more careful examination may reveal that the apparent lack of reproducibility is not a true deficiency. Thus, it is always important to attempt to learn whether the apparent lack of reproducibility is in fact due to differences in study design and conduct, rather than to true differences in response. It is generally inappropriate, for example, to characterize toxicity tests as "positive" or "negative", and then to conclude that the degree of reproducibility of a given effect is low or absent simply because some tests yielded "positive" results and others yielded "negative" results. This oversimplification of test results can be avoided if each of the studies has been subjected to critical evaluation so that the differences in various tests (*e.g.*, in extent of examination of test animals, sample size, duration and magnitude of exposure, etc.) are fully known. This type of careful examination should also be applied when assessing the degree of replication; and it becomes especially important when assessing the degree of concordance. Judging the degree of concordance of responses across various species is probably the most difficult aspect of data evaluation, so that it becomes especially important to avoid the type of oversimplification described above when evaluating this factor.

A final factor that should be kept in mind when judging total data sets concerns the difference between absence of data and absence of replication, reproducibility, and concordance. Thus, a distinction should be made between cases in which there is positive evidence to show that an effect is not reproducible, and those in which an effect has not been reproduced because no attempt has been made to do so. Clearly, the failure to reproduce an effect (assuming that it is a true failure) may raise serious doubts about the carcinogenic properties of a substance, whereas the simple absence of data concerning the reproducibility of an effect should not similarly raise such suspicions.

The Evaluative Process

Ordinarily, the individual sets of data—epidemiological and experimental bioassay data—are each fully evaluated, and then an attempt can be made to characterize the entire body of data. Thus, for example, expert evaluation of epidemiological data may, for a given agent, result in various types of characterizations of the total data set. In some cases, exposure to the agent may be said to be causally related to some form(s) of human cancer. It may be that the data establish strong or suggestive evidence of an association between exposure and human cancer, but do not establish causal links. It may be that the data are inadequate for any conclusive statement. And, for some data sets, there may be no evidence of an association within the limits of detection of the combined studies.[2,3]

A similar set of conclusions may be reached after evaluation of the entire set of data from animal bioassays. Evidence of animal carcinogenicity might be very strong (*e.g.*, data exhibiting a high degree of concordance and reproducibility, with perhaps additional evidence of tumor production at several sites, and with a high degree of malignancy produced in a relatively short period of time); moderately strong (*e.g.*, data exhibiting a moderate degree of reproducibility and concordance); limited (*e.g.*, low degree or absence of reproducibility and concordance, with an increase only in benign tumors); or inconclusive (*e.g.*, absence of replication). Data may also be inadequate for evaluation and, in some cases, they may be clearly negative, with a high degree of reproducibility and concordance.

Data from short-term studies or on metabolism might be used to modify conclusions reached on the basis of epidemiological and long-term bioassay data. Consistent findings of genotoxicity might, for example, raise the degree of suspicion about an agent for which data from studies in animals are inconclusive or inadequate. Substantial evidence of differences in metabolic patterns between test animals and humans might serve to weaken inferences about carcinogenicity in humans based on data from studies in animals. Data from short-term studies might be used in many different ways to modify conclusions reached on the basis of data from long-term animal and epidemiological studies. Expert analysis is needed to determine how such data may affect the total evidence of carcinogenicity.

Following expert evaluation of each of the individual sets of data, it becomes necessary to render a judgment about the entire body of carcinogenesis information. Each agent must be considered separately, because the nature, quality, and quantity of available data will be unique for each agent.

The goal of the evaluation might be envisioned as development of conclusions of the following type:

(1) The available evidence is as certain as current science can achieve that the agent has the capacity to display carcinogenic properties in humans.

(2) There is substantial scientific evidence to support the hypothesis that the agent has the capacity to display carcinogenic properties in humans.

(3) There is a moderate degree of scientific evidence to support the hypothesis that the agent has the capacity to display carcinogenic properties in humans.

(4) There is limited scientific evidence to support the hypothesis that the agent has the capacity to display carcinogenic properties in humans.

(5) The available scientific evidence is inadequate to determine whether the agent has the capacity to display carcinogenic properties in humans.

(6) There is limited scientific evidence to support the hypothesis that the agent has no capacity to display carcinogenic properties in humans.

(7) There is substantial scientific evidence to support the hypothesis that the agent has no capacity to display carcinogenic properties in humans.

These conclusions might be reached under various data combinations. Conclusion 1 would probably be reached only if the epidemiological evidence revealed a causal link and if the evidence from studies in animals was of considerable strength. Conclusion 2 might be reached if the epidemiological data revealed a strong association and the evidence from animals was at least moderately strong. Some analysts would no doubt reach conclusion 2 if the animal data were very strong, even if the epidemiological evidence was weak or inadequate.

The purpose here is not to prescribe a specific formal scheme for categorization of evidence of carcinogenicity. Various analysts might easily weight and combine evidence in different ways. The major point of this discussion is to encourage analysts to give considerable attention to the total body of data and to think about the language that most appropriately reflects the state of scientific knowledge about a substance. It is suggested, however, that the types of conclusions presented above are highly useful ways of describing evidence, and have the attractive feature of avoiding simplistic "yes-no" categorizations of evidence of carcinogenicity. Whatever scheme is adopted, the analyst should attempt to be as explicit as possible about how any conclusions were reached.[1,2]

Formal Schemes for Ranking Evidence of Carcinogenicity

Squire has proposed a method for ranking animal carcinogens "according to the strength of the experimental evidence and according to biological factors considered in assessing carcinogenic potency or potential human risk".[4] His aim was to achieve a regulatory classification for a carcinogen using the information provided by a standard two-species animal bioassay of the National Cancer Institute/National Toxicology Program (NCI/NTP) type plus short-term tests. In the proposed scheme, numerical scores are assigned to the various types of evidence. Most of the factors upon which the scores are based are similar to those described in the foregoing discussion. The regulatory classification depends on the total score.

It is important to note that the Squire scheme includes consideration of carcinogenic potency. It would appear that such an inclusion might inappropriately confuse the "strength of the evidence of carcinogenicity" with the "strength of the carcinogen". The Squire scheme is not designed to include epidemiological information, although the latter could probably be easily added.

Griesemer and Cueto[5] developed a scheme for classifying the degree of evidence for the carcinogenicity of chemicals in animals, using National Cancer Institute bioassays as their data source. Nine categories of evidence were proposed, ranging from "very strong evidence for carcinogenicity in two species" through "sufficient" or "equivocal evidence" in one or more species to "no evidence for carcinogenicity in two animal species". The scheme includes consideration of factors such as the adequacy of the design and conduct of the test and the type of carcinogenic response observed. The following factors are considered in determining the strength of the evidence, but numerical weightings are not assigned:

- The number of species or strains with an increased incidence of neoplasms;

- The number and types of positive results in different experiments, considering differences in routes of administration, doses, and/or sexes; and

- The degree of response, considering incidence, histological type, multiplicity of sites, and/or early onset of neoplasms.

This scheme presents a useful description of a procedure for considering evidence of carcinogenicity provided by the animal bioassay, but it was not designed as a procedure for determining the degree to which the evidence predicts that a substance is likely to be a carcinogen in humans.

The International Agency for Research on Cancer (IARC)[3] has published a description of its approach to evaluating the potential carcinogenic hazards of chemicals to man. The assessment is based primarily on evidence from studies in humans and animals, although mutagenicity and chemical structure can also be considered. The combined evidence is used to arrive at a statement regarding the carcinogenicity of a compound in animals and in humans. IARC describes a procedure for weighting the evidence. There are four categories for evidence from studies in animals:

Sufficient evidence is indicated by an increased incidence of malignant tumors: (a) in multiple species or strains, or (b) in multiple experiments (preferably with different routes of administration or using different dose levels), or (c) to an unusual degree with regard to incidence, site or type of tumor, or age at onset.

Limited evidence indicates that the data suggest a carcinogenic effect but are limited because: (a) the studies involve a single species, strain, or experiment; or (b) the experiments are restricted by inadequate dosage levels, inadequate duration of exposure to the agent, inadequate period of follow-up, poor survival, too few animals, or inadequate reporting; or (c) the neoplasms produced often occur spontaneously or are difficult to classify as malignant by histological criteria alone (*e.g.*, lung and liver tumors in mice).

Inadequate evidence means that because of major qualitative or quantitative limitations, the studies cannot be interpreted as showing either the presence or absence of a carcinogenic effect.

Negative evidence indicates that within the limits of the tests used, the chemical is not carcinogenic.

Three categories of evidence from studies in humans are described:

Sufficient evidence of carcinogenicity is indicated by a causal association between exposure and human cancer.

Limited evidence means that a possible carcinogenic effect in humans is indicated, although the data are not sufficient to demonstrate a causal association.

Inadequate evidence indicates that the data are qualitatively or quantitatively insufficient to allow any conclusion regarding carcinogenicity for humans.

On the basis of the available evidence, the suspected carcinogen is placed in one of four groups:

Group 1   Sufficient evidence is available from human studies.

Group 2A   Almost sufficient or suggestive evidence is available in humans or animals.

Group 2B   As in Group 2A, but the evidence is less strong.

Group 3   Classification is not possible.

It is evident that the IARC approach depends heavily on scientific judgment and that the way in which individual factors are considered is not formalized. For example, the critical determination of how much and what kind of evidence is used to distinguish between Groups 2A and 2B is not discussed. Also, the IARC scheme does not weigh negative evidence against positive evidence.

The approaches for identifying and classifying carcinogens described above have a number of factors in common, but differ in the degree of detail utilized in the weighting of these factors. Generally recognized are the use of animal models to predict potential effects in humans, the correlation between a stronger response in animals (more tumors, more species, more sexes) and the likelihood of human carcinogenicity, and the utility of short-term testing to provide supporting but not sufficient evidence. All the approaches identify the need for case-by-case review of the studies by qualified scientists.

SELECTION OF DATA FOR RISK ASSESSMENT

Introduction

For some substances there will be available only a single set of animal bioassay data, and there is no choice but to use that data set for risk assessment. For other substances there will be many sets of data, some from studies in animals and others from epidemiological investigations. The available data sets for most substances fall between these extremes. Given these circumstances, the risk assessor is frequently faced with the problem of deciding which of the available data sets is best suited for the next step in risk assessment—high-to-low dose extrapolation. In this section are described some of the issues that need to be considered in data selection.

Options for Data Selection

The choice of data sets for use in extrapolation may involve both scientific and policy considerations. For example, a policy decision may be made that only human data be used for risk extrapolation, or that the data set predicting the highest risk to humans be used.[2] While there may be some justification for such decisions it must be recognized that they are not necessarily consistent with the best scientific reasons for data selection. The major options for data selection are listed below. A brief discussion of the merits and limitations of each follows.

(1) Human data, where available, may be selected. Various criteria may then be needed for selecting among human data sets if more than one is available. Criteria may include factors such as the selection of the data set giving the highest estimate of relative risk, the set with the "best" study design, the largest study population, the highest degree of statistical significance, or the most reliable estimates of exposure to the carcinogen and cancer incidence.

(2) Selection may be limited to animal data. Once again, it will often be necessary to select among data sets. Selection may be on the

basis of the most sensitive species, the species most "relevant" to humans, or the "best" study.

(3) Selected sets of human and animal data may be used to provide a range of risk estimates and to determine the quantitative degree of data concordance.

(4) All adequate data may be used, incorporating a statistical procedure to weight different studies according to their quality or relevance to obtain a "best" estimate of human risk.

Merits and Limitations of Data Selection Options

The use of human data alone has the advantage of providing the most relevant dose-response relationships since it avoids the problems inherent in interspecies extrapolation. However, for most chemicals that display carcinogenic properties, adequate epidemiological data are seldom available. Even when some epidemiological data exist, use of these data for risk extrapolation is often difficult. By their nature, epidemiological studies are not controlled so that comparability between exposed and control groups cannot be assured. Quantitative estimates of exposure are often difficult to make, particularly in retrospective studies where documentation of levels of exposure is often scanty. When the type of cancer induced by the carcinogen occurs commonly, a low incidence of exposure-related cancers may not be detectable. Also, because of the long latency involved in the development of cancers, epidemiological methods cannot be applied to newly introduced chemicals.[2,6,7,8]

The use of studies in animals for risk assessment has the advantage that such studies can be better controlled and provide a better defined dose-response relationship than epidemiological studies and do not require such a long latent period before results are known. However, the use of animal data introduces the complex problems of interspecies extrapolation. Selection of the most sensitive species is generally a policy decision to provide the most conservative estimate of risk, *i.e.*, the estimate predicting the highest risk. Deciding which animal data set is most "relevant" to human risk may not be possible when a different route of exposure is involved in humans and animals, or if comparative data on metabolism, pharmacokinetics, etc. are not available. It seems clear, however, that if appropriate biological data are available to permit selection of the animal model most likely to predict human responses, then data from this model should be used and given more weight than data from other models.

Although the "best" animal study may provide the most accurate estimate of the dose-response curve for that species, the relationship between risks estimated from these data and true human risks is generally no better known than for other animal data.[2,8,9]

To make use of the different strengths of animal and epidemiological data, it might be reasonable to use data from a well-conducted study in animals to quantify the risk and epidemiological data to confirm the relevance of the animal data; perhaps using negative epidemiological data (*i.e.*, data giving no indication of carcinogenicity) to predict an upper limit on human risk. Use of this procedure will give a range of risks and further interpretation may be needed to assess its relevance to the human population of interest.

Incorporation of data from all adequate studies has the advantage of considering all data in estimating a range of risks. As with the previous case, interpretation of the range of risks estimated will generally be required. Procedures that give weight to different data sets to produce a single maximum likelihood estimate of unit risk based on all data have been proposed by Crouch and Wilson[10] and DuMouchel and Harris.[11] However, these procedures involve much greater technical complications than are inherent in other procedures, and it is unclear if these increased complications are justified by an improvement in reliability.

A somewhat less complicated procedure which does not incorporate all available data, but rather evaluates all data sets for "quality" and then uses the set with the highest "quality" for risk assessment has been proposed by Crump *et al.*[12] This procedure does not automatically select either human data or data on the most sensitive species. Rather, studies are ranked according to how well they fit a set of criteria concerning the thoroughness of the experimental design and conduct and its consistency with the expected route of human exposure.

Commonly Used Procedures for Data Selection

Until recently, the most widely used procedure for data selection was the choice of either epidemiological data, or if adequate epidemiological data were not available, data on the most sensitive species, *i.e.*, that predicting the highest risk.[2,8,13] The justification often given for the choice of the most sensitive species is that the human population is likely to encompass a wider range of susceptibilities to cancer than any small group of more or less inbred experimental animals and may, thus, include individuals or subgroups as sensitive as the most sensitive group of animals tested.[2,9] The Interagency Regulatory Liaison Group (IRLG) noted that "Use of data from less sensitive species is justifiable only if there are strong reasons to believe that the most sensitive animal model is completely irrelevant to any segment of the exposed human populations". The U.S. Environmental Protection Agency (EPA)[13] selected "the data set which gives the highest estimate of lifetime risk," but noted that "efforts are made to exclude data sets which produce spuriously high risk estimates because of a small number of animals."

In its Cancer Policy, the Occupational Safety and Health Administration (OSHA)[8] discussed the use of risk assessment but concluded that "the uncertainties involved in extrapolation from high-dose animal experiments to predict low-dose risks to humans are far too large at present to justify using the estimates as the basis for quantitative risk/benefit analysis." OSHA did, however, consider that "in the few cases where epidemiological studies provide good dose-response data in exposed humans, it is reasonable to make quantitative estimates of risks at low exposure levels."

More recently, the use of all adequate available data has been advocated to give an indication of the range of possible risks.[11,12,14] It is not always clear how this is to be accomplished.

Use of Negative Data

Most of the foregoing discussion on data selection has been concerned with selection among sets of positive data, *i.e.*, data demonstrating a significant association between exposure and an increase in tumor incidence. Often, however, the situation arises that there exists for a chemical both positive evidence of carcinogenicity and negative evidence, where no significant increase in tumor incidence was related to exposure. For example, there may be positive evidence in studies in animals and non-positive evidence in epidemiological studies. Although such results may appear to be in conflict, the apparent qualitative difference in response may, in some cases, reflect simply a quantitative difference in sensitivity of the studies because of differences in dose levels, lengths of exposure, background tumor incidences, sizes of study populations, etc. It may be useful in such situations to consider the statistical power of the non-positive data, *i.e.*, the smallest increase in tumor incidence that could be detected by the study as statistically significant, and to compare this with the increase predicted by the positive data at the dose level of the non-positive study. If the increase predicted by the positive study is less than the non-positive study was capable of detecting as significant, then the two sets of data may not be inconsistent. If, however, such an analysis reveals that the predicted increase should have been detectable by the non-positive study, then some reason other than differences in study sensitivity is needed to explain the inconsistency. This type of analysis may considerably assist analysis of apparently nonconcordant data.[8,10]

Uncertainty Introduced into Risk Assessment by Data Selection

Risk assessment is, by its nature, an uncertain science and any procedure that limits the data used for risk assessment contributes to that uncertainty, unless there is good reason to believe that data eliminated from consideration are not relevant to human risk. Rarely can we be so confident.

In some cases, elimination of data from consideration (for example, selection of data from the most sensitive species only) can be supported on the basis of conservative public health policy criteria. But it must be realized that such a decision is a policy decision and does not necessarily provide a good estimate of human risk.[1] It may rather give a false impression of the accuracy of the estimate. Conversely, the use of all available data appropriate for risk assessment to generate a range of risk estimates helps to make explicit the uncertainty in the assessment.

Utilization of Selected Data

Once one or more sets of data which define the relationship between dose and carcinogenic response at some (usually, high) dose level(s) are chosen, high-to-low dose extrapolation performed using one or more of the procedures discussed by Silvers and Crump in this volume will produce an estimate of risk per unit dose (unit risk) or a range of such unit risks at low dose levels. Such unit risks apply strictly to the species from which the data on carcinogenicity were developed. Modification of the unit risks may be needed for extrapolation across species boundaries, which is the subject of the next section.

CONSIDERATIONS IN EXTRAPOLATION OF RISKS FROM ANIMALS TO HUMANS

Introduction: Issues Involved in Dose Adjustment and Interspecies Scaling

A number of difficult issues are associated with interspecies extrapolation.

First, doses can be expressed using several different units (*e.g.*, quantity administered per unit body-weight, quantity administered per unit body-surface area, or concentration in the diet). Although the relationship between these measures of dose are known for a given species, they depend on body size, food consumption, metabolic rate, and other scaling factors. Hence, the relationship between the different measures of dose vary considerably from species to species. It is not clear which measure of dose, if any, should be assumed to produce the same risk in different species.[10,12,15]

Second, humans live much longer than experimental animals, and it is not clear how this should be taken into account in interspecies extrapolation. At one extreme, it could be assumed that dose rates in mg/kg/day would produce equivalent cancer risks in different species; at another extreme, it could be assumed that dose rates in mg/kg/lifetime would be equivalent.

Third, the relationship between the dose administered to an animal and the quantity reaching target organs and tissues depends on metabolic and pharmacokinetic factors that control the absorption, retention, distribution and metabolism of the chemical in the body.[16,17] These factors may vary considerably between species, and may also depend on other factors such as the route of administration and the vehicle in which the chemical is administered.

In this section, each of these three major issues will be discussed.

Measure of Dose

The expression of a dose requires specification of three measures: the amount of the substance administered, the size of the organism receiving the substance, and a temporal descriptor. There are several possibilities for each of these measures. The most widely used measures for the quantity of the chemical administered are weight (mg), volume (ml), concentration (ppm or mg/m^3), and moles.

The measures of the size of the organism include weight (kg), surface area (m^2), amount of DNA per cell, and blood volume (ml). Weight and surface area are the only two measures that are frequently used, with weight being the more common. The timing of dosage may be incorporated in terms of average lifetime daily dose, average daily dose during the period of exposure, maximum daily dose, or cumulative lifetime dose. Risk assessors have not demonstrated a clear preference for one of these measures of timing of exposure, although toxicologists usually report their studies in terms of the amount of substance actually administered on a given day. The list of examples given here is not exhaustive, but can be combined to yield 64 (4 x 4 x 4) possible definitions of dose.[18]

The problem is illustrated in Table 1, which tabulates conversion factors for 5 species under different measures of dose rate. Inspection of the table reveals that the two extreme dose scale assumptions are mg/kg/day and mg/kg/lifetime. Thus, if the risk assessor assumed that humans and mice were at equal risk on the basis of a dose expressed in mg/kg/day, but the two species were actually at equal risk on the basis of mg/kg/lifetime dose, then the use of mg/kg/day would lead to an underestimate of risk of about 40-fold (25,500 ÷ 639, *see* Table 1). Conversely, adoption of mg/kg/lifetime would overestimate risk by the same factor if mg/kg/day were, in fact, the most accurate measure.

Table 1: Conversion Factors Between Various Measures of Dose Rate of
a Chemical Administered in the Diet

Species	mg/kg Body Weight/Day	ppm in Diet	mg/m^2 Body Surface/Day	mg/kg Body Weight/Lifetime
Mouse	1	5.0	3.0	639
Hamster	1	12.5	4.1	480
Rat	1	16.7	5.2	730
Dog	1	40.0	19.4	3,650
Man	1	46.7	37.0	25,500

Note: The figures tabulated for each species are those equivalent to ingestion
of 1 mg/kg body weight/day. Data were derived from References 18–20.

There are very little empirical data available to assist selection of appropriate interspecies measures of dose for carcinogens. Freireich *et al.*[19] used toxicity data on 18 anticancer drugs to analyze the quantitative relationship in response between humans and other mammals. The maximum tolerated dose (MTD) was the measure of risk used for humans, dogs, and monkeys, while the LD_{10} was the measure for mice and rats. The route of administration in almost all cases was intraperitoneal or intravenous. Potency was expressed as cumulative doses adjusted to daily doses for 5 days of administration in units of mg/m^2 body surface area. When the average MTDs for humans were plotted on a logarithmic scale against the average MTDs or LD_{10}s for each species, their magnitudes were found to be closely correlated, and the points for each species fell roughly about a line indicating equivalence with the human dose. When the average LD_{10}s for mice were plotted against the human MTDs in units of mg/kg body weight, the regression line was offset from equivalence by a factor of 12, which corresponds almost exactly to the ratio of the correction factors (kg/m^2) used to convert doses for humans and mice from mg/kg to mg/m^2. This study thus suggests that expression of dose in terms of body surface area is appropriate for interspecies extrapolation. It should be noted, however, that this study does not concern carcinogenic risk, and its results may therefore not be pertinent to the issue under examination here.

The National Academy of Sciences[20] compared the carcinogenic potency in humans and animals of six known human carcinogens for which there were sufficient data for at least rough estimation of human exposure and corresponding increase in cancer incidence [benzidine, chlornaphazine, diethylstilbestrol (DES), aflatoxin B$_1$, vinyl chloride, and cigarette smoke]. This selection criterion could theoretically have imposed a bias toward chemicals to which humans are relatively sensitive, thus exaggerating the sensitivity of humans in comparison to laboratory animals.[18] The doses were expressed in units of mg/kg body weight/lifetime. Studies in animals involving a variety of different protocols were examined, and the study showing the greatest sensitivity to each substance was selected. For three of the six substances (benzidine, chlornaphazine, and cigarette smoke) the human response to a given lifetime average dose was found to be similar to the response predicted by the slope of the dose-response curve of the most sensitive animal species exposed to the same lifetime average dose. For the remaining three substances, the animal responses predicted human responses 10 to 500 times higher than had been observed. The report concluded:

> Thus, as a working hypothesis, in the absence of countervailing
> evidence for the specific agent in question, it appears reason-
> able to assume that the lifetime cancer incidence induced by
> chronic exposure in man can be approximated by the lifetime
> incidence induced by similar exposure in laboratory animals at
> the same total dose per unit body weight.[20]

The tendency of the animal responses to over-estimate human risk, and the possible bias introduced by the selection of chemicals to which humans may be particularly sensitive, suggest that average daily dose may be a more appropriate comparative measure than average lifetime dose.

Crouch and Wilson[15] compared carcinogenic potency estimates between mice and rats using mg/kg/day as the unit of dosage. The maximum likelihood estimate of the dose-response slope parameter β in the one-hit model for the tumor site giving the largest value was used as the measure of carcinogenic potency for each species. The National Cancer Institute's bioassays in rats and mice for 90 substances provided the sets of data for the comparison of potencies in B6C3F1 mice, Osborne-Mendel rats, Fischer 344 rats, and Sprague-Dawley rats, and of males and females of the individual strains. In each case, the potencies expressed in units of response per unit dose in mg/kg body weight were strongly correlated across species and sexes.

These authors also assembled estimates of carcinogenic potency in mg/kg in humans and in rats or mice for 13 chemicals. The studies yielding the potency estimates were much less uniform in design than those used in the previous portion of the study. Nevertheless, the human and rodent potencies were found to be correlated, although not as strongly as those of mice and rats. Humans were found to be approximately five times more "sensitive" to these substances than rodents, when sensitivity was defined as response per unit increment of dose in mg/kg. However, this result could be due to the heterogeneity and imprecision of the data sets, rather than to true interspecies differences.

Following the suggestion of Mantel and Schneiderman[21] EPA has adopted lifetime average mg/m² surface area/day as the dosage unit it would consider equivalent across species in quantifying human risks for its water quality criteria documents.[13] Mantel and Schneiderman proposed the idea of using doses in units of surface area, not on the grounds of any empirical evidence, but solely on the basis of the assumption that the locus of action of any drug is on some surface.[21]

Because of the numerous factors influencing the comparability of potency estimates (experimental error, route of administration, model in which potency was estimated, dosing schedule, chemical-specific interactions with animals, etc.), the compilation of a data set to determine the best measure of dose for interspecies extrapolation would be exceedingly difficult.[18] It is also possible that there is, in fact, no universally equivalent unit of dose. Further, the most extreme difference resulting from the use of mg/kg rather than mg/m², for instance, would be a factor of 12 for estimation of human risk from mouse data; in view of the overall uncertainty surrounding risk estimates, a factor of this magnitude may not be of prime importance.[18] Since for so many other reasons estimates of carcinogenic risk to humans cannot be regarded as accurate predictors of human risk, it would seem wise to use a particular unit uniformly so that estimated risk for various substances would be comparable for ranking purposes. The unit of mg/kg/day is most commonly used by experimentalists and for general toxicity evaluations, and, since this unit has some empirical support, it may be the most appropriate.[12,18]

Routes of Absorption

It is sometimes necessary to use data from a study in one species exposed by one route to estimate risk to the same or a different species exposed by a different route. If data on absorption rates are available for the various routes of concern, then it becomes possible to estimate the equivalent doses arising from these routes. In the absence of relevant absorption data, it is common practice to adopt conservative assumptions about the extent of absorption or to use data from closely related substances.[9] If such inter-route dose estimates are made, it is important to specify the assumptions adopted, and perhaps to test the effect upon the risk estimate of adopting alternative assumptions.

Metabolism and Pharmacokinetics Data

The dose of a compound available internally to cause an effect may be substantially different from the administered dose. A large number of factors can affect the actual amount of compound that is present at a site of action within the body.[16,17] The differences between species as well as between strains within a species in the pharmacokinetics of a compound may cause large differences in the response to a carcinogen. The quantitative relationship between administered dose and target site dose may also change as a function of dose. Ideally, risk assessment should be based on target site dose (or concentration) rather than on administered dose, both for cross-species comparisons and for high-to-low dose extrapolation within a species.

Most compounds are metabolized by a process which usually detoxifies the compound and allows it to be excreted more rapidly. Many chemical carcinogens, however, are metabolically activated to their ultimate carcinogenic forms. Williams[22] has discussed variations in metabolic pathways found between species. Although all species tend to show the same general pattern of metabolism of foreign compounds, he states:

> If any foreign compound (or xenobiotic) is administered to more than one species, although one can now predict the pathways of xenobiotic metabolism, it is almost certain that species differences in the amounts of predicted metabolites formed and excreted will be found and in some cases gross differences in the actual routes of metabolism will be found.

Numerous reports have shown that interspecies differences in response to carcinogens are related to the nature and concentration of reactive metabolites which interact with macromolecules of the target cell. Schumann et al.[23] showed that perchloroethylene was metabolized and its metabolite bound more readily in the mouse liver than in the rat liver; this suggested that the higher degree of binding might explain the observation that perchloroethylene was carcinogenic in the mouse and not in the rat. In a paper that has become a classic, Miller *et al.*[24] found that the mouse, but not the guinea pig could metabolize 2-acetyl-aminofluorene (AAF) to N-hydroxy-AAF. N-hydroxy-AAF caused tumors in both mice and guinea pigs while AAF produced tumors in mice only. Thus, the guinea pig is insensitive to the potential carcinogenic effect of AAF because it is unable to metabolize AAF to the proximate carcinogen, N-hydroxy-AAF.

Any such knowledge should be incorporated into a risk assessment when deciding which animal model might be most suited for interspecies extrapolation. Even if metabolic data are only suggestive, they can still be used to decide which animal model(s) should be given greater weight in the overall assessment of risk. This type of analysis, which might only be qualitative in nature, is an essential component of a risk assessment. It is one of the factors that can be used to give greater perspective to the meaning of numerical estimates of risk.[25]

The pharmacokinetics of a compound within an animal can be described by a number of different mathematical models in which the body of the animal may be modeled as consisting of several compartments. More complex models may be required to describe the pharmacokinetics of carcinogenic chemicals that require metabolic activation to exert their carcinogenic effect. For example, Gehring and Blau[26] have presented a model that involves 8 differential equations. Their scheme was developed for a hypothetical chemical carcinogen which undergoes activation to a reactive electrophilic metabolite and subsequent irreversible, covalent binding to genetic material.

Models such as these are useful for obtaining a more precise estimation of the actual exposure of the target tissue to a carcinogen. The simplest model can give an estimation of the body burden or tissue concentration of the chemical compound over time. A more complex model can give an estimation of the amount of interaction between the ultimate carcinogen and the proposed receptor, in this case, the DNA of the cell. To use these models, appropriate data must be obtained from the species of animal under investigation. The complexity of the studies needed to obtain these data depends on the complexity of the model to be used.

Even if such data can be obtained only for experimental animals, they might be extremely useful in estimating low dose risks for the animal population.

Gehring and Blau[26] have discussed the possible effect on the pharmacokinetics of a chemical of conducting studies at high dose levels. They state:

> As long as pharmacokinetics of a chemical remain linear, any increase in dose will result in an equivalent increase in the concentration of the chemical in tissue at any point in time. However, many metabolic and excretory processes are saturable, and as doses of chemicals begin to saturate or overwhelm these processes, it may be expected that there will be a disproportionate increase in the concentration in tissues and consequently, toxicity (*see* Gehring *et al.* 1976). For these processes, non-linear pharmacokinetics apply which can be described by the Michaelis-Menten equation.

$$-dC/dt = VmC/(Km + C)$$

In this equation dC/dt is the rate of change in the concentration of the chemical at time t, C is the concentration of chemical at time t, Vm is the maximum rate of the process and Km,
the Michaelis constant, is equal to the concentration of the
chemical at which the rate of the process is equal to one-half
Vm.

When the concentration of the chemical is much smaller than Km, the change in
concentration of the chemical over time is proportional to the chemical concentration. When the concentration of the chemical is much larger than Km the
change in its concentration is dependent solely on the parameter Vm. This implies that the results of carcinogenicity studies performed at high dose levels,
where non-linear pharmacokinetics may exist, may not be accurately extrapolated to lower dose levels using the administered dose as the measure of dose
in the high-to-low dose extrapolation.

To demonstrate the importance of these considerations, Gehring *et al.*[27]
used tumor incidence data from a vinyl chloride inhalation carcinogenicity study
in rats together with pharmacokinetic data to examine the dose-response relationship. They found that the metabolism of vinyl chloride was not linearly proportional to the dose administered and could be fitted to the model described
above. A good linear fit for all the data was found for probit response *versus* the
logarithm of the amount of vinyl chloride metabolized. There was not a good
linear fit when the probit response was plotted against administered dose. They
suggested that the amount of metabolized vinyl chloride was a better measure of
dose than administered dose.

Use of pharmacokinetic data in interspecies risk extrapolation requires that
the pharmacokinetic parameters be known for all the relevant species. It is unlikely that the pharmacokinetics of most industrially used compounds can be
determined for humans, although they probably can be acquired for certain
classes such as drugs and food additives. Although it is desirable to utilize pharmacokinetic data wherever they are available, their major utility is likely to be
limited to the type of high-to-low dose extrapolation within an animal species
that has been described above for vinyl chloride.

Approaches to Defining the Uncertainty of Interspecies Extrapolation

Recently, two approaches were proposed to express mathematically the uncertainty associated with risk estimates involving interspecies extrapolation.

Crouch and Wilson[10] have proposed an approach to risk assessment that
yields a probability distribution for risk. Rather than simply multiplying an estimate of potency (or its upper limit) by an estimate of exposure to derive an expected (or "worst-case") risk, their method incorporates a probability distribution of a species-to-species (animal-to-human) conversion factor, K_{ha}, a probability distribution of possible exposures, d, and a probability distribution of animal potency β_a, to derive a probability distribution of human risk, β_h:

$$\beta_h = K_{ha}\beta_a d$$

Theoretically, this scheme is applicable to any functional expression of a dose-
response relationship.

The dose-response model chosen and the set of experimental data selected determine the animal potency and its probability distribution. Concerning the species sensitivity factor, Crouch and Wilson assert "by comparing tests performed with many chemicals in two species (1 and 2) we may define a 'best value' for K_{12} (the species-to-species conversion factor) for those particular species, together with the probability distribution for variations in K_{12}." Derivation of such a quantitative definition of differences in potency from species to species from existing data, however, is not likely to be easy, particularly when one of the species of interest is the human where the data will be very limited.

To use their scheme, Crouch and Wilson have specified several assumptions. In particular, for ease of computation, they suggested that all the probability distributions in their model may be assumed to be lognormal. They proposed that the measure of dose should be average lifetime dose in units of mg/kg/day and that the data should be fitted to the one-hit model. They also proposed selecting the set of data yielding the highest estimate of potency and suggested that reporting the upper 98th percentile on the derived risk distribution will encourage further experimentation to reduce the uncertainty.

DuMouchel and Harris[11] have proposed a Bayesian statistical method that simultaneously incorporates potency estimates on a number of substances derived in parallel sets of testing systems to obtain an estimate of carcinogenic potency in humans for a substance for which epidemiology results are not available. This procedure might also be used to quantify the uncertainty associated with potency estimates due to experimental sampling error, unknown conversion factors among species, and the uncertain relevance of each type of experiment to the others.

Although both of these approaches appear promising and merit further development, they have not yet been developed to the point where they could be used for routine risk estimation. Both require that several assumptions be made about dose-response relationships and about the form of the probability distributions and involve a degree of statistical detail in the information to be used in the model that is lacking for most carcinogens.

BIOLOGICAL THRESHOLDS

None of the commonly used extrapolation models discussed by Silvers and Crump in this volume incorporate a threshold dose. By a threshold dose we mean a finite dose level of a carcinogen below which the risk of cancer is zero. In some cases, however, these models are used to define a dose level that is the practical equivalent of a threshold, a "virtually safe dose" to use the expression of Mantel and Bryan,[28] at which the risk is very low.

Arguments have, however, been advanced that true thresholds may exist for some carcinogens for biological reasons. Some of these are listed below:

(1) A small dose of a carcinogen might be totally metabolized to a noncarcinogen,[29,30] or the body's immune system or DNA repair system might be capable of defending against small insults. How-

ever, this would require a totally perfect detoxification or defense system for a true (absolute) threshold.

(2) Some carcinogens may act indirectly by causing some gross physiological change, such as repeated necrosis and reactive hyperplasia, or hormonal imbalance that is necessary for development of neoplasia but which would not occur at very low doses.

(3) Because the mean cancer latency period has been shown to be inversely related to dose of some chemicals, Jones and Grendon[31] have suggested that there must be a practical threshold because at very low doses the latency period would exceed the life span of the organism. However, although the *mean* latency period may exceed the life span at low doses, this does not necessarily mean that no tumor would develop within the life span of an organism, only that the probability is low.[32,33]

If any such thresholds were shown to exist, identification of safe exposure levels could be achieved by the traditional methods of identification of a no-effect-level and application of a safety or uncertainty margin as used with noncarcinogens.[7,9]

PRESENTATION OF RISK ASSESSMENT

When all of the factors discussed above have been taken into consideration, and low dose extrapolation and, if necessary, interspecies extrapolation have been conducted, it is important that the results be presented not simply in the form of a quantitative estimate of risk, but be accompanied by a summary of the qualitative information underlying the estimate. This should include:[25]

(1) A statement about the degree of confidence in the finding that the substance is carcinogenic, and a synopsis of the nature and strength of supporting evidence.

(2) A statement about any information concerning the mechanism of action of the carcinogen, and the confidence with which the mechanism is known. A statement about the influence of this knowledge on low dose risk estimation and interspecies extrapolation should also be included, with a view of the uncertainties.

(3) A statement about the dose-response relationships and the reasons for selection of data and mathematical models for high-to-low dose extrapolations, accompanied by a statement regarding the uncertainties.

(4) A statement about the human dose estimates and the uncertainties associated with them.

(5) A description of the population at risk, including its size and other characteristics that may influence risk.

REFERENCES

1. National Research Council Committee on the Institutional Means for Assessment of Risks to Public Health, *Risk Assessment in the Federal Government: Managing the Process*, Washington: National Academy Press (1983)
2. Interagency Regulatory Liaison Group (IRLG), Scientific bases for identification of potential carcinogens and estimation of risks. *J. Natl. Cancer Inst.* 63: 244-268 (1979)
3. International Agency for Research on Cancer (IARC), Chemicals and industrial processes associated with cancer in humans. *IARC Monograph Supplement 1* (1979)
4. Squire, R., Ranking animal carcinogens: A proposed regulatory approach. *Science* 214: 877-880 (1981)
5. Griesemer, R.A., and Cueto, C., Toward a classification scheme for degrees of experimental evidence for the carcinogenicity of chemicals for animals. *IARC Scientific Publications No.* 27: 259-281 (1980)
6. Carcinogen Assessment Group (CAG), Preliminary Report on *Population Risk to Ambient Benzene Exposures*, Washington: U.S. Environmental Protection Agency (1978)
7. Food Safety Council, Proposed system for food safety assessment. *Fd. Cosmet. Toxicol.* 16, Supplement 2:1-136 (1978). Revised report published June 1980 by the Food Safety Council, Washington, D.C.
8. Occupational Safety and Health Administration (OSHA), Identification, Classification and Regulation of Potential Occupational Carcinogens. Final Rule. *Fed. Register* 45: 5001-5296 (1980)
9. National Academy of Sciences (NAS), *Drinking Water and Health. Vol. III*. Washington: National Academy Press (1980)
10. Crouch, E., and Wilson, R., Regulation of carcinogens. *Risk Analysis* 1: 47-66 (1981)
11. DuMouchel, W.H., and Harris, J.E., *Bayes Methods for Combining Cancer Experiments in Humans and Other Species*, Technical Report No. 124, Massachusetts: Department of Mathematics, Massachusetts Institute of Technology (1981)
12. Crump, K.S., Howe, R.B., and Fiering, M.B., *Approaches to Carcinogenic, Mutagenic, and Teratogenic Risk Assessment.* Prepared by Science Research Systems, Ruston, Louisiana for Meta Systems, Inc., Cambridge, Massachusetts. Prepared for U.S. Environmental Protection Agency, Contract No. 68-01-5975, Washington (1980)
13. U.S. Environmental Protection Agency (USEPA), Water Quality Criteria Documents; Availability. Appendix C—Guidelines and Methodology Used in the Preparation of Health Effect Assessment Chapters of the Consent Decree Water Criteria Documents. *Fed. Register* 45: 79347-79357 (1980)
14. European Chemical Industry, Ecology and Toxicology Centre, *A Contribution to the Strategy for the Identification and Control of Occupational Carcinogens*, Monograph No. 2. Brussels, Belgium: European Chemical Industry (1980)
15. Crouch, E., and Wilson, R., Interspecies comparison of carcinogenic potency. *J. Toxicol. Environ. Health* 5: 1095-1118 (1979)
16. Gehring, P.J., Watanabe, P.G., and Blau, G.E., Risk assessment of environmental carcinogens utilizing pharmacokinetic parameters. *Ann. N.Y. Acad. Sci.* 329: 137-152 (1979)

17. Gehring, P.J., Watanabe, P.G., and Young, J.D., in: *Origins of Human Cancer (Book A: Incidence of Cancer in Humans)*. (Hiatt, H.H., Watson, J.D., and Winston, J.A., eds.), pp 187-203, Cold Spring Harbor: Cold Spring Harbor Laboratory (1977)

18. Dixon, R.L., Problems in extrapolating toxicity data from laboratory animals to man. *Environ. Health Perspect.* 13: 43-56 (1976)

19. Freireich, E.J., Gehan, E.A., Rall, D.P., Schmidt, L.H., and Skipper, H.E., Quantitative comparison of toxicity of anticancer agents in mouse, rat, hamster, dog, monkey, and man. *Cancer Chemotherapy Reports* 50: 219-244 (1966)

20. National Academy of Sciences (NAS), *Pest Control: An Assessment of Present and Alternative Technologies. Vol. I. Contemporary Pest Control Practices and Prospects: The Report of the Executive Committee*. Washington: National Academy of Sciences (1975)

21. Mantel, N., and Schneiderman, M.A., Estimating "safe" levels—A hazardous undertaking. *Cancer Res.* 35: 1379-1386 (1975)

22. Williams, R.T., Species variations in the pathways of drug metabolism. *Environ. Health Perspect.* 22: 133-138 (1978)

23. Schumann, A.M., Quast, J.E., and Watanabe, P.G., The pharmacokinetics and macromolecular interactions of perchloroethylene in mice and rats as related to oncogenicity. *Toxicol. Appl. Pharmacol.* 55: 207-219 (1980)

24. Miller, E.C., Miller, J.A., and Enomoto, M., The comparative carcinogenicities of 2-acetylaminofluorene and its N-hydroxy metabolite in mice, hamsters, and guinea pigs. *Cancer Res.* 24: 2018-2031 (1964)

25. Rodricks, J., and Taylor, R., Application of risk assessment to food safety decision making. *Regulatory Toxicol. Pharmacol.* 3: 275-307 (1983)

26. Gehring, P.J., and Blau, G.E., Mechanisms of carcinogenesis: Dose response. *J. Environ. Pathol. Toxicol.* 1: 163-179 (1977)

27. Gehring, P.J., Watanabe, P.G., and Park, C.N., Resolution of dose-response toxicity data for chemicals requiring metabolic activation: Example—vinyl chloride. *Toxicol. Appl. Pharmacol.* 44: 581-591 (1978)

28. Mantel, N., and Bryan, W., "Safety" testing of carcinogenic agents. *J. Natl. Cancer Inst.* 27: 455-470 (1961)

29. Cornfield, J., Carcinogenic risk assessment. *Science* 193: 693-699 (1977)

30. Falk, H.L., Biologic evidence for the existence of thresholds in chemical carcinogenesis. *Environ. Health Perspect.* 22: 167-170 (1978)

31. Jones, H.G., and Grendon, A., Environmental factors in the origin of cancer and estimations of the possible hazard to man. *Fd. Cosmet. Toxicol.* 13: 251-268 (1975)

32. Guess, H.A., and Hoel, D.G., The effect of dose on cancer latency period. *J. Environ. Pathol. Toxicol.* 1: 279-286 (1977)

33. Peto, R., Carcinogenic effects of chronic exposure to very low levels of toxic substances. *Environ. Health Perspect.* 22: 155-159 (1978)

Part IX

Regulatory Implications

26

Regulatory Implications: Perspective of the U.S. Environmental Protection Agency

Richard N. Hill

U.S. Environmental Protection Agency
Washington, D.C.

INTRODUCTION

The U.S. Environmental Protection Agency (EPA) was created in 1970 as an outgrowth of the "ecology consciousness" of the 1960's. The nucleus of the Agency was formed from an array of existing organizations covering a broad range of concerns including water quality, animal protection, exposure to radiation, and the use of pesticides. At that time, the general perception of EPA was that of an agency charged with the protection of the environment. However, with time, greater emphasis has been placed upon public health concerns resulting from chemical exposure.

In contrast to some of the other regulatory agencies that were formed to examine the effects of specific types of chemical exposures (*i.e.*, drugs, food additives and occupational exposures), EPA's scope is broader and includes a host of potential environmental exposures to chemical substances. Various programs empowered by Congressional acts have developed within EPA around potential routes of exposure (*i.e.*, air, water and drinking water), the problems of solid waste and waste disposal sites, the use of pesticides and toxic industrial substances, and potential contamination of and exposure to radioactive substances.

Each program within EPA is involved in assessing the potential adverse health effects of exposure to toxic chemicals and managing the risks posed by these substances. Assessment of the potential carcinogenic effects of chemicals is an integral part of each program's activities.

This chapter will trace the evolution of the Agency's involvement with the management of potential carcinogenic risks from chemical exposures and will outline future directions of assessments at the Agency.

EARLY ENCOUNTERS WITH CARCINOGENICITY

From the beginning of the EPA in 1970 to the middle of the decade, a principal undertaking at the EPA was the evaluation of the potential hazards of pesticides, namely DDT, aldrin/dieldrin, and heptachlor/chlordane. These evaluations led to a series of administrative hearings (largely adversarial in nature) to cancel the uses of these substances in the United States. Comments made by various scientists on the carcinogenicity of chemicals were extracted from some of the hearing records and compiled into a List of Principles for future Agency use. Because these statements had been taken out of context and were easily misinterpreted or were stated too simplistically, they became the brunt of much scientific criticism. For instance, the British journal, *Lancet*, published an editorial entitled, "Seventeen Principles About Cancer or Something".[1]

These Principles—the Agency's first attempt to articulate a cancer policy—inadequately stated the procedure used in the Agency's determination of potential carcinogenicity. For example, they failed to establish the nature and strength of the data supporting a determination of carcinogenicity. They failed to acknowledge the difference in potency among carcinogens. They did not incorporate the vital links which describe the ways in which exposure to agents alters potential carcinogenic risks. In addition, some people interpreted the Principles as espousing a "zero-risk" stance, similar to that embodied in the Food and Drug Administration's famed Delaney clause for carcinogenic food additives, even though EPA had attempted to balance risks and benefits in each of the pesticide decisions as is required by the governing legislation.

To establish a firmer technical position for the regulation of carcinogens the Agency initiated an effort to develop guidance to be used in reviewing chemicals for carcinogenicity. This effort culminated in the publication in 1976 of the *Interim Procedures and Guidelines*[2] for the identification of chemical carcinogens which have been in effect ever since.

ASSESSMENT GUIDELINES

EPA's method for evaluating carcinogenic risks employs a two-step process. The first involves an estimation of the likelihood that a chemical may pose a potential carcinogenic risk in humans. For those agents that may be carcinogenic, the second stage is carried out, namely an estimate of the public health impact of exposures to the agent.

The first phase of the assessment involves a qualitative review of all data bearing on the potential carcinogenicity of the chemical. It involves the evaluation of human epidemiological studies and long-term experimental studies in animals, supplemented with investigations of short-term test results, comparative metabolism studies and structure-activity relationships. The review culminates in a weight-of-evidence judgment of the likelihood that a chemical may be carcinogenic in humans.

Assuming a chemical is carcinogenic in humans, then one proceeds to the second part of the risk assessment, the quantitative estimation of the consequences of exposure to the agent. Due to the paucity of relevant human data, quantitative measures are most often based upon data from long-term studies in experimental animals. In these cases two types of extrapolations are usually performed. The first is an extrapolation of the cancer incidence from the relatively high doses employed in animal studies to the low doses anticipated from human contact with the chemical. Various mathematical models are used to estimate the tumor incidence at specific levels of exposure. A second extrapolation attempts to relate the effects seen in animals with those anticipated in humans since they differ in such things as weight, metabolic rate, and life span.

ASSESSMENT IN PRACTICE

At the time of publication of the interim guidelines in 1976, the Agency established the Carcinogen Assessment Group (CAG) to prepare technical risk assessments for the program offices. Operational procedures were developed for the implementation of the guidelines, and certain modifications have been introduced over time. The most important of these are discussed.

Weight-of-the-Evidence

In the Guidelines it was recognized that the weight-of-evidence varies considerably among different compounds. It ranges from definitive human studies supported by animal experiments on the same compounds (this is the best evidence possible) to short-term tests and special carcinogen screening tests, which are considered to provide only suggestive evidence for carcinogenicity.

Early on CAG used the summary adjective "substantial" to describe situations where some human or animal evidence of carcinogenicity existed and "suggestive" or "inadequate" to describe chemicals where the evidence was not as strong. In recent times, CAG has explored using the criteria established by the International Agency for Research on Cancer[3] which categorizes information on the strength of evidence separately for humans and animals.

Dose Extrapolation Models

Although the preamble to the *Interim Procedures and Guidelines* pointed out that "evidence has accumulated that the no-threshold concept can. . .be applicable to chemical carcinogens," the body of the document stated that the assessments would employ a "variety of risk extrapolation models, *e.g.*, the linear non-threshold model and the log probit model." In practice, however, CAG moved to a position of expressing risks from a single model, initially the one-hit model and more recently the 95% upper confidence limit of the multistage model.[4] Both of these models are considered as placing an upper bound on risk at a given exposure; at low doses, both show linear non-threshold characteristics. In actuality the "real" risk may lie anywhere between the upper bound and zero. Unfortunately, not enough information is available to determine where in this range the "real" risk lies.

Genotoxic *versus* Non-Genotoxic

As described earlier, EPA has been quantitatively evaluating carcinogens in a rather uniform fashion. Dose-response information is being entered into an extrapolation model to estimate risks at a given low level of exposure. Usually, a linear model is used because we recognize that carcinogenic mechanisms are unknown and such models put a ceiling on what the risks might be. Others might claim, however, that implicit in a scheme that evaluates chemicals in a similar way is the assumption that all carcinogens operate through the same mechanism or at least by paths that result in the same dose-response relationships; however, one could argue that carcinogens do not all act in the same way.

Evidence has accumulated that some carcinogenic chemicals produce mutagenic and other "genotoxic" effects in short-term tests. Other substances which are carcinogenic in long-term studies in animals fail to show this genotoxic potential. Such a finding suggests that carcinogens may act through at least two different mechanisms that may be differentiated on the basis of current short-term tests. If this were true, then risks imposed by these two classes of carcinogens may be evaluated differently. One might conceive that genotoxic carcinogens may induce effects following a single "hit" of a cellular receptor and thus, any dose of the compound may be associated with some finite risk. Non-genotoxic agents on the other hand, may induce effects by more "traditional" means of toxicity (*e.g.*, cellular toxicity, hormonal action) and could be evaluated by applying predetermined safety factors to doses that in studies in animals were not associated with an adverse effect.

Two years ago CAG developed a proposal to categorize chemicals based on their behavior in short-term tests and to evaluate the risks from these agents in two different ways. A group of scientists from outside the Agency and representing a range of perspectives were asked to comment on the proposal. A wide diversity of opinion was apparent reflecting a lack of consensus in the scientific community. Therefore, the Agency was led to conclude that it would be premature to proceed at that time with such a scheme. This difficulty in differentiating among carcinogenic substances by the use of short-term tests is also illustrated in the conclusions of two international groups.[5,6]

Other Assessments

In 1976, the EPA's program offices lacked the expertise to perform carcinogenic risk assessments, and this activity was conducted by CAG. Over the years, however, changes have occurred. Offices have become active in various aspects of assessments. Several are now involved with the evaluations of human exposure to carcinogenic substances, and the Pesticides and Toxic Substances offices are now performing their own qualitative as well as quantitative risk assessments. Although the entry of different groups into the assessment arena has stimulated thinking about new approaches, it has also increased the challenge of maintaining a consistent Agency approach to the assessment of risk from chemical carcinogens.

THE ASSESSMENT FUTURE

It can be safely stated that risk assessment will be an enduring concept for some time to come. Assessments are currently being conducted by each of the

Federal chemical regulatory agencies, and the National Academy of Sciences has just published a report which supports the role of risk assessment in the decision-making process.[7] The National Academy study goes on to recommend the development of guidelines to focus Federal reviews of chemicals for carcinogenicity along consistent lines.

To this end, projects have been initiated to lay out guidance for the performance of risk assessments for chemical carcinogens. For instance, there is an activity currently underway coordinated by the President's Office of Science and Technology to update the Federal regulatory agencies' position on carcinogenesis which had originally been published in 1979.[8] A final report expected in 1985 will provide a current summary of the scientific aspects of carcinogenicity (*e.g.*, mechanisms of action, short-term testing) and evaluation procedures along with a series of broad-based principles to guide agencies in their reviews of potential cancer-causing substances.

In addition, there is an effort to update EPA's 1976 interim guidelines of carcinogenic risk assessments. All EPA program offices have provided input to this activity prior to its publication for broad public comment in 1984.

Still other groups have provided statements bearing on aspects of carcinogenic risk assessment. For example, the National Cancer Advisory Board has just issued a report[9] on the use of quantitative assessment of carcinogenic risks to supplement their 1977 publication on the qualitative criteria for determining carcinogenic activity of chemicals.[10] Other examples include the multi-year project of the Food Safety Council to prepare guidance for the testing and evaluation of substances coming under the purview of the Food and Drug Administration[11] and the report of the Administrative Conference of the United States.[12] These efforts point out the extent of activity centered on the regulations of carcinogens at the Federal level.

More recently, State governments have become quite active in the area of risk assessment. The State of California has issued a policy statement[13] covering the procedures they will employ in evaluating carcinogens. In late 1983, EPA sponsored a well attended conference for States that dealt with risk assessments for toxic substances. One can imagine that the trend of involvement of States in the assessment of local problems will continue for some time.

All of the above activities help to illustrate the keen interest given to cancer on behalf of government bodies. It also reflects the continued public concern over this dreaded set of diseases and its implications for human health.

UNCERTAINTIES

Whatever approach is taken toward qualitative and quantitative assessment of carcinogenic risk, they all seem to share an abundance of ignorance and a dearth of information in certain key areas. In the area of hazard assessment, seldom do we have the type and depth of animal data we would prefer, let alone precise epidemiological information. At best we almost always are faced with the non-trivial task of making judgments about humans based on animal data. In exposure assessment, we in the environmental area are faced with estimating not only the direct exposures one might receive from the source of concern, (*e.g.*, exposures to pesticide applicators), but we must also consider indirect exposures which might result from transformation and transport of the chemical through the environment back to the individual (*e.g.*, accumulation through drinking water or the food chain). Finally, in quantitative assessment, we are hampered by the lack of detailed information on carcinogenic mechanisms which would give insight into the ultimate shape of the dose-response curve in the low-dose range; without this information one must pick, somewhat arbitrarily, among risk extrapolating models or attempt to place a conservative or upper bound on what the real risks might be. Perhaps in the case of a prescription drug we have come closest to the goal of adequate information on a chemical—combined human and experimental animal testing of the agent, knowledge to some degree of the dose-response characteristics, information on the handling of the compound by the human body, and some knowledge of the amount of chemical used in treatment.

Shortcomings in the data on a specific chemical, in our knowledge about carcinogenic mechanisms, and in our understanding of the shape of the dose-response curve in the low-dose range erect a number of barriers to our ability to proceed readily with evaluations of chemicals. To help with these reviews, agencies make assumptions and develop science policies. For instance, we assume that people weigh 70 kg; although that may be true for the "physiological man," most persons are at some other weight. People realize, however, that as a starting point 70 kg is not unreasonable. Many other questions are scientific in nature, but their answers cannot be ascertained presently. In the absence of knowledge about the true state of nature, certain interim decisions or science policies are made. An example includes the following: For the purpose of estimating the carcinogenic potential of an agent at a given anatomical site, the frequency of animals with benign tumors of a given histogenic type will be combined with the frequency of animals with malignant tumors of the same type. On the one hand it could be argued that this science policy is invalid, since a benign tumor is not a malignancy, and it usually does not lead to death. On the other hand, some benign neoplasms are very difficult to differentiate from their malignant counterparts (*e.g.*, thyroid tumors) and in other cases benign tumors seem to represent a transitional state leading to malignancy. Thus, although science policies should have some technical support for their existence, they are by their very nature judgmental items; hence, much controversy surrounds many of these policies, since there is a lack of consensus on how to proceed. Oftentimes regulatory agencies have adopted policy positions that are conservative; that is, they err on the side of protection of public health.

Hope for more informed assessments is to be found in the progress that is being made in basic studies on the mechanisms of carcinogenesis, comparative metabolic analyses, pharmacokinetic studies, and the nature and form of dose-response relationships. A long neglected area which calls for increased attention, since it represents literally half the contribution to risk assessment, is exposure assessment. More extensive, more precise monitoring data, coupled with validated exposure models hold the promise of more realistic estimation of human exposure. Tissue residue levels of certain chemicals in humans can be readily measured. Means of coupling this information with that in experimental animals need to be investigated.

In addition to fundamental research and a better understanding of human exposure information, research should be directed toward a number of applied topics which may influence significantly the way we conduct risk assessments. Each would involve the "filling in" of data gaps so that we have a better understanding of the power and shortcomings of currently available tools to assess carcinogenic substances. For instance, about a score of human carcinogens are known. Let's study them in greater detail: Make certain there are good long-term studies in experimental animals to complement the information in humans; assess the degree to which there is anatomical site agreement among animals and humans; compare tumor sites following different routes of exposure; determine to the extent possible the exposures in humans that were associated with carcinogenic responses; test the compounds in batteries of short-term tests; look at comparative metabolic differences between humans and animals; and estimate, where possible, the quantitative differences in the responsiveness of humans compared with animals.

In summary, the Environmental Protection Agency in the course of a little over a decade has made real strides forward in its evaluation of chemicals for carcinogenicity and estimation of the health consequences of such exposures. Public interest continues in the area of control of carcinogenic risks, but we are still faced with a myriad of scientific questions which cloud our ability to produce truly credible statements. Until carcinogenic processes and human exposures become better characterized and chemicals are studied more in-depth, carcinogenic risk assessment will remain to a large extent judgmental in nature and be surrounded by controversy.

Acknowledgments

Ideas for this paper were adapted from a speech given by the author at the American Chemical Society annual meeting in Washington, DC, August 31, 1983, at a Symposium on Federal Regulation of Carcinogens. The material in this paper reflects the impression of the author and are not meant to be a statement on behalf of the U.S. Environmental Protection Agency.

Many helpful suggestions were received from Donald Barnes and Robert McGaughy.

REFERENCES

1. Editorial, Seventeen Principles About Cancer, or Something. *Lancet* i: 571-573 (1976)
2. Environmental Protection Agency, Interim procedures and guidelines for health risks and economic impact assessments of suspected carcinogens. *Fed. Register* 42: 21402-21405 (1976)
3. International Agency for Research on Cancer, *IARC Monographs on the Evaluation of the Carcinogenic Risk of Chemicals to Humans*, Supplement 4, Lyon: IARC (1982)
4. Environmental Protection Agency, Water quality criteria (final). *Fed. Register* 45: 79316-79379 (1980)
5. Upton, A.C., Clayson, D.B., Jansen, J.D., Rosenkranz, H., and Williams, G., Report of ICPEMC task group on the differentiation between genotoxic and non-genotoxic carcinogens. *Mutation Res.* 133: 1-49 (1984)

6. International Agency for Research on Cancer, *Approaches to Classifying Chemical Carcinogens According to Mechanisms of Action,* Report No. 83/001 Lyon: IARC (1983)
7. Committee on the Institutional Means for Assessment of Risks to Public Health, *Risk Assessment in the Federal Government: Managing the Process,* National Research Council, Washington, DC: National Academy Press (1983)
8. Interagency Regulatory Liaison Group, Scientific bases for identification of potential carcinogens and estimation of risks. *J. Natl. Cancer Inst.* 63: 243–68 (1979)
9. National Cancer Advisory Board, *Policy of Risk of the Health Effects of Hazardous Exposures to Populations,* A Report of the Subcommittee on Environmental Carcinogenesis, Bethesda, MD: National Cancer Advisory Board, National Cancer Institute (1983)
10. National Cancer Advisory Board, General Criteria for assessing the evidence for carcinogenicity of chemical substances: report of the Subcommittee on Environmental Carcinogenesis, National Cancer Advisory Board. *J. Natl. Cancer Inst.* 58: 461–465 (1977)
11. Food Safety Council, *Proposed System for Food Safety Assessment,* Washington, DC: Food Safety Council (1980)
12. Administrative Conference of the United States, *Federal Regulation of Cancer-Causing Chemicals,* Washington, DC: Administrative Conference of the United States (1982)
13. State of California, *Carcinogen Identification Policy: A Statement of Science as a Basis of Policy,* (Section I & II and *Carcinogen Policy* (Section 3), Sacramento, CA: State of California, Health and Welfare Agency, Department of Health Services (1982)

27

New Approaches to the Regulation of Carcinogens in Foods: The Food and Drug Administration

Robert J. Scheuplein
Herbert Blumenthal
W. Gary Flamm

Food and Drug Administration
Washington, D.C.

INTRODUCTION

A principal task of the Bureau of Foods of the Food and Drug Administration (FDA) is to evaluate the toxicity and establish safe use levels for food additives and contaminants. Food additives are now almost essential to the supply, storage, distribution and palatability of our food and contaminants are the unavoidable residues of new technologies and economizing in methods of food production.

The wider distribution of additives and contaminants coupled with the increased sensitivity of methods of chemical analysis occurring during the last two decades have generated new problems in the evaluation of the safety of food. One of these concerns is the potential risk of cancer from exposure to very low levels of substances found to be carcinogenic or mutagenic in laboratory studies. The problem is not new, but it is beginning to be realized that previous solutions, namely those that envisage the total elimination of carcinogens at all levels from our food supply, as exemplified by the Delaney Clause, are no longer practicable.

This chapter traces the history and impact of the Food, Drug, and Cosmetic Act (FD&C Act) on the regulation of food safety in the United States. It describes, in particular, the development of regulations of food-borne carcinogens through the enactment of the Delaney Clause up to the present debate over quantitative risk assessment. We have tried to identify the role that changes in technology have played along with refinements in methods of toxicological assessment in the evolution of regulatory policy.

HISTORICAL OVERVIEW OF FOOD SAFETY REGULATION IN THE UNITED STATES

1906-1957

The historic mission of the Bureau of Foods has been to prevent the adulteration of food. The first attempt at Federal control of food, was a bill introduced on January 20, 1879, "for preventing the adulteration of articles of food and drink". During this period Americans were becoming concerned over the safety of their food supply for several reasons, all relating to the fact that much of the food was no longer produced in the home or in the neighborhood, and incidents of adulteration were increasing. Unwholesome imports were being "dumped" into the United States and domestic food was being debased by the intentional substitution of inferior substances. Damage was concealed and some food was simply filthy. These concerns culminated in the 1906 Act which aimed at the elimination of these acts of adulteration of otherwise natural wholesome food. Proponents of the 1906 Act were also alarmed by the accumulating number of unfamiliar chemicals that were "added" to preserve food and improve its appearance and texture, a problem created by the necessity to store food longer and transport it farther. The notion of adulteration, originally intended to apply more to intentional debasement of food for profit, came to embrace the presence of "unsafe chemical additives" that seemed to be added more for the producer's convenience than the consumer's. The 1906 statute's central idea seems to have been the prevention of acts by food producers, motivated either by greed, carelessness or ignorance, that caused ordinarily wholesome food to become unsafe or that resulted in its deceptive representation. There was no expressed intent of improving the safety of natural food as selected and prepared by individuals. If greater health could be had through better nutrition or a better section of foodstuffs, this was not perceived in 1906 as a matter for Federal intervention.

The 1938 Act and its interpretation by FDA substantially broadened FDA's mission in the direction of protecting the consumer from unsafe food *per se* rather than acting solely in response to an act of food adulteration by a food manufacturer or distributor. Section 402 (a)(1) for the first time contained a provision that prohibited the marketing of even a traditional food that was "ordinarily injurious." No intervening human act of adulteration was required. A distinction was made, however, in the safety standard that was to apply to naturally occurring "poisonous or deleterious substances" as compared to intentionally added substances. Natural constituents in food, such as oxalic acid in rhubarb or solanine in potatoes, could be deemed adulterants only if the food contained them in sufficient quantity to be considered "ordinarily injurious". FDA has used this provision to regulate very few substances, most notably poisonous mushrooms and Burma beans. FDA has never attempted to restrict the marketing of a traditional food because it contained a "non-added" carcinogen. If FDA wished, for example, to bring the nitrosamines in some natural substances, the hydrazines in mushrooms or the safroles in spices under the ambit of this provision, the Agency would have to demonstrate a real probability (not a mere possibility) of harm to a significant percentage of ordinary consumers.

"Added" constituents, on the other hand, were made subject to the far stiffer "may render injurious" standard under the same Section 402 (a)(1). Under this provision, FDA need show only the existence of some significant possibility that the food could be injurious to the health of a consumer. The courts[1] have stated, "if . . . , it cannot by any possibility, when the facts are reasonably considered, injure the health of any consumer, such food, though having a small addition of poisonous or deleterious ingredients, may not be condemned under the Act." Until recently FDA took the position that the presence of an added carcinogen at any level inherently violated this provision.[2] In the 1950's two artificial sweetners, dulcin (4-ethoxyphenylurea) and P-4000 (5-nitro-2-propoxy-aniline) were prohibited under Section 402 (a)(1) after studies indicated that they produced tumors in animals.

FDA has historically interpreted the term "added" quite broadly. Thus, environmental contaminants, such as mercury or PCB's, that are not "inherent" constituents of food, but may be present in amounts that exceed those naturally present because of additional contamination from the environment, are regulated as "added" substances. Similarly, the mold toxin, aflatoxin, on corn or peanuts is regulated as an "added" substance because, although contamination with aflatoxin may occur as the result of a natural process, aflatoxin is not an inherent constituent of the food. The 1938 Act authorized FDA, for the first time, to permit the presence of "safe" levels of poisonous and deleterious added substances in certain justifiable instances. If such substances were necessary in the production of food or if they were unavoidable even under the best food manufacturing practices, the Act authorized the FDA to set regulations limiting the quantity of such substances to the extent found necessary to protect the public health. FDA has taken the position that it may, under this section of the Act, establish tolerances for environmental contaminants that find their way into food. The tolerance is established by considering the contaminant's toxicity, the extent to which its occurrence can be controlled, and the capability of analytical methods to measure the contaminant and enable enforcement of the tolerance. This provision, Section 406, as interpreted by FDA, comes closest to an explicit risk-benefit provision that exists in the FD&C Act. Unfortunately, the inherent reasonableness of this provision proved of little immediate benefit. Under both the 1906 and 1938 Acts, the burden of providing needed information remained with FDA. It was up to FDA to become aware of possible toxicological problems, to conduct the appropriate safety studies, to establish the appropriate tolerance and to provide assurance that this amount would not be exceeded, taking into account the diverse dietary habits of the American public. Limitations in FDA personnel and resources mitigated against the frequent use of this provision. Another major limitation was the lack of sophistication in the art of toxicological and carcinogenicity testing. This can be illustrated by the outcome of a Congressional mandate in the 1938 Act to ". . . promulgate regulations providing for the listing of coal-tar colors which are harmless and suitable for use in food . . ." Based mainly on acute toxicity studies, over one hundred colors in common use had been certified as "harmless" immediately after 1938.

However, prompted by growing public concern over the toxicity and possible carcinogenicity of coal-tar colors, FDA began a more extensive testing program. The 90-day studies that were typically used at the time were readily capable of demonstrating positive toxic effects, but dosage schedules were often not adequate for the establishment of safe levels. In addition, information on current and anticipated exposure of humans from unknown uses was lacking. As a consequence, many colors were prohibited because FDA, finding them to be toxic in 90-day studies, could not, with sufficient certainty, predict the likely long-term, cumulative effects of color consumption.[3]

The statutory provisions described (see Table 1), extensively supplemented by others, still exist and embody the Agency's basic food safety requirements. They permit greater risk or less assurance of safety for substances of greater perceived value (*i.e.*, traditional food); they permit less risk for inherently unnecessary substances (*i.e.*, additives), while tolerating intermediate risk for necessary or unavoidable substances (*i.e.*, contaminants).

Table 1: Basic (Pre-1958) Statutory Food Safety Standards

Food Categories	Statutory Safety Standards*
Traditional Foods	**Sec. 402 (a)(1)**
Possibly containing naturally occurring poisonous or deleterious substances (could include carcinogens).	The food is adulterated if the substance renders the food *ordinarily injurious to health.*
Added Substances	**Sec. 402 (a)(1)**
Possibly poisonous and deleterious substances (could include carcinogens).	The food is adulterated if the substance *may render the food injurious to health.*
Unavoidable Added Substances	**Sec. 406**
Substances either required in the production of food or unavoidable by good manufacturing practice (could include carcinogens).	The food is adulterated if the amount of substance *exceeds the tolerance* which attempts to balance the need to protect the public health with the unavoidability or essentiality of the substance.

The reader is referred to the quoted sections of the FD&C Act for the precise phraseology of the various provisions.

1958-Present

The original triad of provisions discussed above has been amended several times since 1938, usually to separate out a particular class of added substances for special regulatory attention. For example, Congress required the registration and licensing of pesticides under The Pesticide and Chemical Act of 1954. In 1958, the Food Additives Amendment established a similar preclearance scheme for substances directly added to formulated foods or for substances used in processing or in packaging that could migrate into food or otherwise affect its characteristics. However, the Food Additives Amendment did not apply to all intentionally added ingredients or to all potential migrants. An exception was made for GRAS ("generally recognized as safe") substances and for substances that were approved either by FDA or the U.S. Department of Agriculture (U.S.D.A.) prior to 1958. GRAS substances included a large class of traditional additives (*e.g.*, sugar, salt . . . etc.), in common use and others later to be established as GRAS by panels of scientific experts. "Prior sanctioned" substances were in effect "grandfathered" on the basis of previous approvals or advisory statements by U.S.D.A. and/or F.D.A. Despite such exceptions, the Food Additives Amendment reversed the legal burden of proof demanded under the law and fundamentally changed the regulation of food additives in the United States. FDA was no longer required to show that a marketed food additive might be injurious to consumers; instead, the sponsor had to provide experimental evidence to FDA demonstrating that the additive is safe for its intended use prior to receiving approval for marketing.

The safety standard for food additives, Sec. 402 (a)(1) and Sec. 409, was a demonstration of a "reasonable certainty of no harm" under anticipated and reasonably foreseeable levels of exposure. Carcinogenic food additives were, in addition, banned under the Delaney Clause. The Color Additive Amendments of 1960 established very similar rules for color additives, including a Delaney Clause.

From this brief discussion it is evident that current United States food safety requirements are an amalgam of several provisions of the FD&C Act that have been enacted at different times since 1938. The amendments in 1958 and subsequently have tended to produce specialized regulatory requirements for different functional categories of additives at the cost of some internal consistency in the treatment of comparable risks. Each set of category-specific provisions operates essentially without regard to the treatment accorded other classes of food constituents.[4]

THE REGULATION OF CARCINOGENS

Regulatory History

Before 1958, carcinogens were not legally distinguished from other toxic or poisonous and deleterious substances. When the Delaney Clause was enacted in 1958, career scientists at FDA regarded it as neither particularly helpful nor harmful, but merely redundant. No one then believed that a food additive would be declared safe under the general safety provisions if it was an animal carcinogen. Furthermore, the Delaney Clause was a weaker provision in one important respect. While a suspicion of carcinogenicity could be sufficient to undermine a showing of safety, the Delaney Clause required a frank finding of carcinogenicity. As a result, from 1958 to 1975, many more substances were prohibited as food or color additives under the authorization of the general safety provisions than under the Delaney Clause. The Delaney Clause was first formally invoked in

April, 1967 for Flectol H (1,2-dihydro-2,2,4-trimethylquinoline) and next in December, 1969 for 4,4'-methylene bis(2-chloroaniline); both substances had previously been approved for use in food packaging adhesives.

The FDA's removal of safrole (in December, 1960), oil of calamus (in May, 1968), cyclamate (in October, 1969), diethylstilbestrol (DES) in cattle and sheep (in 1972-1973), diethylpyrocarbonate (in August, 1972), mercaptoimidazoline (in November, 1973), FD&C Violet No. 1 (in April, 1973) and FD&C Red No. 2 (in February, 1976) were taken under the Agency's general (or transitional) safety provisions. Only after 1976 did the Delaney Clause come to be relied on or referred to more frequently, notably for DES (in January, 1976), nitrofurans (in May, 1976), acrylonitrile copolymers used to make beverage containers (in March, 1977) and, of course, saccharin (in April, 1977).

Changing Perceptions of the Carcinogenic Hazard

During the 1970's the number of regulatory actions on carcinogens in foods and cosmetics increased. Perhaps two scientific trends were primarily responsible: First, the sensitivity of analytical methods improved and the instrumentation to carry out these analyses became widely available; second, many more long-term animal bioassays were being conducted—notably, by the National Cancer Institute's (NCI) Carcinogen Testing Program. To the average person the result of this "progress" was increased confusion and dismay. Hearing about the carcinogenic hazards from corn, peanuts, milk, grain, canned food, hamburger, poultry, beef, fish, hot dogs and even scotch and beer, large segments of the public began to wonder whether anything was safe anymore. Others began to question the soundness of a regulatory policy that threatened to remove useful and popular articles from commerce on the basis of what appeared to them to be very low and even trivial levels of risk.

The initial concern in 1958 over carcinogens developed against the background of scientific knowledge of cancer, or more accurately, the uncertainty in that knowledge that existed at the time. Listed below is a summary[3] of what that knowledge was then considered to be:

1. Although cancer can be caused by extraneous agents, not all members of the exposed population will develop cancer. Those that are most susceptible can be identified only by experience.

2. Even a powerful carcinogen requires weeks or months to elicit cancer in mice or rats and probably requires years in man.

3. No change need be recognizable in the organ or tissue destined to become cancerous before the cancer itself.

4. Experience in the laboratory does not predict unequivocally the reaction of humans to the same agent. On the other hand, those few chemical and physical agents known to produce cancer in man, with the possible exception of inorganic arsenical compounds, have elicited cancers in animals.

5. No one at this time can tell how much or how little of a carcinogen would be required to produce cancer in any

human being, or how long it would take for the cancer to develop.

6. The effect of certain chemical carcinogens can be markedly increased by other compounds with little or no carcinogenic power.

7. The accumulated evidence suggests the irreversibility of the cancerous response once it has been initiated and further suggests a cumulative effect.

8. The most potent carcinogens, by their very strength, are almost sure to be discovered clinically. It is assuredly the less potent carcinogens that are most important in human cancer and provide the real problem for evaluation. A major objective of experimental carcinogenesis is, therefore, the bioassay for the presence of weak carcinogens.

9. Chemical configuration alone cannot be used to predict the ability of a new compound to produce cancer.

10. Possession (by a substance) of a biological effect, known to be associated with a particular type of cancer, may be of importance in assessing potential carcinogenicity. Examples are: estrogenic activity, goitrogenic activity, and production of liver cirrhosis.

These comprised the central principles concerning the prediction of carcinogenic response, as understood at the time. Most oncologists would agree that, with some modifications and additions, perhaps to items numbers 5 and 8, it is still a fair statement of what we believe to be true today. The effect of dose was also considered, but perhaps less tolerantly than it might have been if the consequences of today's analytical technology had been more clearly foreseen.

During the Color Additive Hearing of 1960, the Secretary's testimony in support of the Delaney Clause stated in part:

We have no basis for asking Congress to give us discretion to establish a safe tolerance for a substance which definitely has been shown to produce cancer when added to the diet of test animals. We simply have no basis in which such discretion could be exercised because no one can tell us with any assurance at all how to establish a safe dose of any cancer-producing substance.[5]

The House Report accompanying the reported bill summarized the Committee's position:

In view of the uncertainty surrounding the determination of safe tolerances for carcinogens, the Committee decided that the Delaney anti-cancer provision in the reported bill should be retained without change.[6]

The awareness of growing regulatory problems gradually increased, but as late as May of 1974, FDA continued to support officially the Delaney Clause, but with some reservations:

... we are not prepared to state that the Delaney Clause has had a deleterious effect, to date, upon the food supply, nor could we suggest any particular change in the anti-cancer clauses.

We believe that the growth of knowledge in carcinogenesis may eventually permit safe levels of carcinogenic additives to be determined, but that day is not yet here. We also believe that the elected representatives of the people may some day be called upon to permit exceptions to the clause for additives which may be important to the food supply and yet for which there is evidence of carcinogenicity. [Dr. Alexander Schmidt, Commissioner of Food and Drugs.] [7]

The statement proved prophetic. In November of 1977, Congress enacted the Saccharin Study and Labeling Act (PL-95-203) which, in effect, created an indefinite exception for saccharin. [8] Other problems occurred with lead (in tin cans), lead acetate (in hair dyes), carcinogenic impurities (in color additives and packaging materials), and DES and nitrites (in meat). Recognizing that such problems were consuming a disproportionate and increasing share of the Agency's resources, that the public health benefits resulting from banning very low levels of carcinogens were doubtful at best, that the Agency's credibility was being harmed, and that it appeared to be possible to establish crude but nonetheless "safe" tolerances for carcinogens, the FDA, at the 1983 Food Safety Hearings, asked Congress for authorization to use a risk assessment approach for trace amounts of added carcinogens in food.

The motivation for this change in regulatory approach was not primarily scientific. No scientific breakthrough had suddenly provided the knowledge that now permitted "safe" tolerances for carcinogens to be determined with certainty. Much had indeed been learned in the 20 or more intervening years about the mechanism of cancer. The existence of at least a two-stage carcinogenic process was substantially verified, the importance of modifications in DNA in the initiation step was discovered, as was the need for metabolic activation to electrophiles. The existance of DNA repair processes was established, new methods of "screening" for carcinogens, such as the "Ames test", were being developed and tested, and much more. But this knowledge, however valuable and crucial to an eventual understanding and possible control of cancer, was not of great regulatory significance. Much more information was needed to be able to establish safe tolerances for exposure of humans to carcinogens from first principles. The crucial event that occurred during the intervening two decades was not a scientific breakthrough, but rather a continuous advance in technology. The improved "sensitivity" of analytical instrumentation and techniques eventually allowed the detection of carcinogens at the parts per billion and even the parts per trillion level and virtually assured finding carcinogens both in new and in familiar food and color additives. However, the ability to *detect* a substance does not always mean it can be reliably identified and confirmed. The reliability of identifying and quantitating substances decreases exponentially as the concentration decreases. [9] Moreover, the vastly improved ability to *detect* substances, often in artificially ideal conditions, does not automatically mean that comparably precise or reliable chemical measurements are available in practice. Electronic noise in measuring instruments, the leaching of impurities from containers, background contamination, and the difficulties in separating and isolating substances in complex food matrices generally mean that the improvements in analytical science are more effective in finding problems than in enabling regulators to deal with them.[9]

In 1958, Congress did not foresee the widespread presence of trace amounts of carcinogens in food, the possibility that common food substances might themselves be shown to contain carcinogens or the occurrence in humans of carcinogens as essential nutrients or as an outcome of normal metabolism. Congress did not anticipate the extent to which substances then regarded either as absent from foods, or as non-carcinogenic on the basis of weaker technology, would later prove to be present and to be animal carcinogens (*i.e.*, saccharin, nitrites, lead, etc.). In short, the acknowledged scientific uncertainty surrounding carcinogenesis was larger and less amenable to the apparently prudent solution Congress proposed, than it could have foreseen.

Risk Assessment of Carcinogens

In the early 1940's some investigators had proposed quantitative analysis of dose-response data[10] from carcinogens and even systems of grading carcinogenic potency.[11,12] By 1970 there were hundreds of studies in animals that supported quantitative dose-response behavior, at least to the extent that lower doses in the same strain of rodent consistently produced lower tumor incidence. Methods of using the dose-response behavior for assessing human risk from carcinogens at very low exposures were proposed in 1961 by Mantel and Bryan[13] and were soon extended by others.[14-18] However, the two crucial quantitative extrapolation steps, *i.e.*, (a) high dose to low dose, and (b) animals to humans have not been equally well developed. The use of conservative assumptions was and still is generally regarded as a necessary prudence to bridge over gaps in our understanding of the effects of differing species sensitivities, metabolic responses, diets, patterns of consumption, etc., between man and animals as well as the occurrence of additive or synergistic effects. All of these provide opportunities for error aside from the question of the accuracy of the dose-response extrapolation model. Despite these difficulties, support gradually developed for the notion that while scientific advances still could not provide a basis for establishing an absolutely safe threshold, they might provide a basis on which discretion could be exercised in establishing tolerances for carcinogens at the cost of acceptably low and, within bounds, ascertainable risks.

The National Academy of Sciences Panel on Risk Assessment and Management has recently affirmed the value of risk assessment despite the uncertainties involved. Their report[26] recognizes that the regulator must often build inferential bridges to temporarily fill information gaps in the more uncertain steps in risk assessment. The Panel recommended greater use of uniform guidelines by the Federal regulatory agencies to improve public understanding and foster consistency in risk assessment and prevent oversights and judgments that are inconsistent with current science. The recent OSTP (Office of Science and Technology Policy) chemical carcinogen document[27] implements that suggestion in the form of broad interagency guidelines for assessing cancer risks from chemicals.

Another factor supporting the use of risk assessment was the much larger risk from unregulated exposures to added carcinogens. The estimated dietary intake of nitrosamines in the United States is from 1 μg/day to 10 μg/day and it is approximately the same in Western Europe and at least as great in China and Japan.[19] Our exposure to polynuclear aromatic hydrocarbons (PNA's) from a variety of sources is at least this great.[20] We have learned that traditional methods of preparing and preserving food contaminate it with both classes of carcinogens (*e.g.*, charboiling and smoking with PNA's, and pickling with nitrosamines). When the upper bound of human risk from these exposures is estimated from data obtained from studies in animals by the same techniques proposed for food additives (*e.g.*, linear extrapolation) the risk exceeds 10^{-4} (*i.e.*, one in ten thousand in a lifetime). This is just the tip of the iceberg; the spectrum of natural carcinogenic contaminants at low levels in food is far larger than these two examples can suggest. These "added" carcinogens are officially ignored because the exposures are ubiquitous and they would be extraordinarily difficult if not impossible to control and regulate. Finally, there is the risk from the diet itself; a risk not necessarily quantitatively attributable to the level of carcinogenic contamination, but possibly more the promotional character of some major nutrients. A recent report[21] of the National Academy of Sciences on Diet, Nutrition, and Cancer states:

> . . . Judging from the observed differences in cancer rates among populations with different diets, it is highly likely that the United States will eventually have the option of adopting a diet that reduces its incidence of cancer by approximately one-third.

The impact of all this information gradually created a distinction between the regulatory consequences forced by the Delaney prohibition against carcinogenic additives at any level and "safe" tolerances which now seemed feasible under the "reasonable certainty of no harm" standard of the general safety provisions. The focus of the distinction was primarily the low level cancer risk from small amounts of carcinogenic drug residues in animals, migrants from food packaging materials, and contaminants in direct food and color additives. The wisdom of banning these useful additives, which could be expected to produce only miniscule levels of carcinogens in food, seemed open to question. Control of these substances appeared manageable through risk-assessment procedures. Under current law FDA has very limited administrative discretion to deal with low level cancer risks from additives. Quantitative risk assessment of carcinogens has played a significant role in the development and use of FDA's administrative authority. However, because of the uncertainty in the accuracy of risk-assessment procedures and the level constraint still imposed by the Delaney Clause, FDA's approach to risk-assessment has been cautious and limited.

FDA first suggested the use of risk-assessment in 1973 for a proposed rule dealing with drug residues in animals.[22] This was later issued as a regulation in February of 1977.[23] Because of a special exemption proviso added to the law as part of the Drug Amendments of 1962, the use of risk-assessment in this instance was not considered to be in violation of the Delaney Clause. That provision, the DES proviso, permitted the use of carcinogenic drugs for use in animals raised for food production if "no residue" was found in the edible tissue

[Sec. 512(d)(1)(H)]. This proviso makes the detection of residues of the drug in edible animal tissue rather than its *administration* to animals or *addition* to animal feed the critical inquiry.[4] It also means permitting some carcinogenic residue, namely, the amount present below the limit of the official method of detection. For some years FDA insisted that the protection of human health from carcinogenic drugs in animals required that the most sensitive methods be used as soon as they were available—thus, continually reducing the apparent "zero residue" level. This was called the "sensitivity of method" regulation or SOM. Finally in 1979, concluding that the continually moving regulatory target made little sense when cancer risks of that order were coming to be regarded as insignificant, FDA adopted a fixed "insignificant risk" level of 10^{-6} / lifetime (by linear extrapolation) regardless of the capability of analytical techniques to detect residues at this level or below.[24]

With the increasing ability of analytical methods to operate at lower levels and the Delaney prohibition against additives at any level, the anticancer provisions were operating like the early models of the SOM regulation. Legally permissible carcinogen levels were being driven down to current analytical limits. This was a special problem for color additives and food packaging materials, many of which can contain potentially carcinogenic contaminants. Time seemed to be running out rapidly for many of these products. If Section 409 or 706 of the Food, Drug, and Cosmetic Act were to be literally and fully enforced, it was difficult to imagine how many of them would continue to remain on the market.

In response to the growing problem with low-level carcinogenic impurities, FDA proposed its "Constituents Policy" under which these impurities would be regulated under the general safety provisions of the Act by risk-assessment procedures.[25] The language of the Delaney provision being silent on the impurity question lent itself to interpretation on this issue. FDA proposed that the word "additive" in the Delaney phrase (" . . . no such additive shall be deemed to be safe if it is found to induce cancer . . .") should be interpreted to mean the "additive as a whole" including the trace constituents that may accompany it. Therefore, if the additive as a whole, when tested in feeding studies in animals, is not found to be carcinogenic, it does not come under the ambit of the Delaney Clause, despite the fact that a trace constituent(s), when tested by itself at higher doses, is known to be carcinogenic. The constituent is not ignored however; it is regulated by "risk-assessment" under the general safety provisions of the Act. FDA has, for the present, used 10^{-6} /lifetime (by linear extrapolation) as the cutoff for a significant risk level. The "Constituents Policy" is currently under review and no one knows its future. In the absence of a change in the statute, however, some administrative flexibility along these lines appears essential. FDA believes that some use of "dose-response" in the regulation of carcinogens comes closer to preserving the original intent of the Delaney Clause, that is, of distinguishing carcinogenic from non-carcinogenic additives, than an interpretation that would, given current analytical capabilities, result in the indiscriminate banning of virtually all additives regardless of dose.

Risk Assessment—Its Value

Many foods contain carcinogens. Our regulatory task is hopeless without some method of distinguishing between large and small risks. Risk assessment, at least as currently practiced, embodies two implicit axioms. The first is the certainty of some risk from chemicals (everyone now seems to recognize that absolute safety is unattainable), and the second is the uncertainty in its measurement. If carcinogenic risk were avoidable, risk assessment would be unnecessary; if carcinogenic risk could be measured easily, risk assessment would be trivial. The scientific basis of quantitative risk assessment at present is weak, particularly the extrapolation from animals to humans. However, when combined with other evidence and used in a conservative manner chosen in a way that is not likely to understate the risk, it can be a valuable regulatory tool. It provides a measure of orderliness, openness and equity in the regulation of carcinogens. FDA has accepted it for a part but not for the whole of the regulatory process and applies it cautiously and on a limited basis because of its scientific disabilities as well as current legal proscriptions.

The law and the need to act promptly require FDA to make decisions, usually in a climate of scientific uncertainty.[2] Quantitative risk assessment is not, at present, a fully adequate procedure, but this cannot be expected when scientific information is lacking. It is, however, the only alternative to inaction available presently.

REFERENCES

1. U.S. *versus* Lexington Mill & Elevator Co. 232 U.S. 399 (1914)
2. Hutt, P.B., Food and regulation, *Fd. Drug Cosmet. Law J.* 33: 501-558 (1978)
3. Certified Color Industry Committee, *et al. versus* Folsom, USCA 236 F 2d866 (1956)
4. Merrill, R.A., Regulation of Carcinogens in Food: A legislator's guide to the food safety provisions of the Federal Food, Drug, and Cosmetic Act, *Mich. Law Rev.* 77: 171-250 (1978)
5. Color Additives: Hearings on H R 7624 and S2197. Before the House Committee on Interstate and Foreign Commerce, 86th Congress, 2nd Session 61 (1960)
6. H. R. Rep. No. 1761 86th 2nd. Sess., (1960)
7. Food and Drug Administration "Study of the Delaney Clause and other Anti-Cancer Clauses:" Hearings on Environmental and Consumer Protection Appropriations for 1975, Before the House Subcommittee, of the Committee on Appropriations, 93rd Congress 2nd Session, May (1974)
8. National Academy of Sciences, Food Safety Policy: Scientific and Societal Consideration, Part 2 (March 1979)
9. Horwitz, W., Today's chemical realities. *J. Assoc. Off. Anal. Chem.* 66: 1295-1301 (1983)
10. Bryan, W.R., and Shimkin, M.D., Quantitative analysis of dose-response data obtained with three carcinogenic hydrocarbons in strain C3H male mice. *J. Natl. Cancer Inst.* 3: 503-531 (1943)
11. Berenblum, I., Systems of grading carcinogenic potency. *Cancer Res.* 5: 561-564 (1945)
12. Druckrey, H., Quantitative Grundlagen der Krebsergeugung. *Klin. Wschr.* 22: 532-540 (1943)
13. Mantel, N., and Bryan, W.R., "Safety" testing of carcinogenic agents. *J. Natl. Cancer Inst.* 27: 455-470 (1961)

14. Albert, R.E., and Altshuler, B., in: *Radionuclide Carcinogenesis* (J.E. Ballou, D.D. Mahlum, and C.L. Sanders, eds.), pp 233-253, AEC Symposium Series, Conference-72050, NTIS, Springfield, VA (1973)

15. Friedman, L., in: *Assessment of the Carcinogenicity and Mutagenicity of Chemicals,* World Health Organization Technical Report No. 546, pp 14-19 (1974)

16. Hoel, P.G., Gaylor, D.W., Kirschstein, R.L., Saffiotti, U., and Schneiderman, M.A., Estimation of risks of irreversible delayed toxicity. *J. Toxicol. Environ. Health.* 1: 133-151 (1975)

17. Guess, H., Crump, K., and Peto, R., Uncertainty estimates for low-dose-rate extrapolation of animal carcinogenicity data. *Cancer Res.* 37: 3475-3483 (1977)

18. Hartley, H.O., and Sielken, R.L., Estimation of "safe doses" in carcinogenic experiments. *Biometrics* 33: 1-30 (1977)

19. IARC, Monographs on the Evaluation of the Carcinogenic Risk of Chemicals to Humans: Some N-Nitroso Compounds, Vol. 17, World Health Organization (1978)

20. Howard, J.W., and Fazio, T., Review of polycyclic aromatic hydrocarbons in foods. *J. Assoc. Off. Anal. Chem.* 63: 1077–1104 (1980)

21. National Research Council, Report of the Committee on Diet, Nutrition, and Cancer, Assembly of Life Sciences, Diet, Nutrition and Cancer, pp 1-13 (1982)

22. Chemical Compounds in Food-Producing Animals, *Fed. Register* 38: 19226-19227 (July 19, 1973)

23. Chemical Compounds in Food Producing Animals, *Fed. Register* 42: 10412-10437 (Feb. 1977)

24. *Chemical Compounds in Food Producing Animals, Fed. Register* 44: 17070-17114 (March 1979)

25. D&C Green No. 6, *Fed. Register* 47: 14141-14142 (April 2, 1982)

26. National Research Council, Report of the Committee on the Institutional Means for Assessment of Risks to Public Health, Commission of Life Sciences. Risk Assessment in the Federal Government; Managing the Process (March 1983)

27. Office of Science and Technology Policy, Chemical Carcinogens; Notice of Review of the Science and its Associated Principles, *Fed. Register* 49: 21594-21661 (May 1984)

28

Workplace Carcinogens: Regulatory Implications of Investigations*

Robert P. Beliles

Occupational Safety and Health Administration
Washington, D.C.

INTRODUCTION

In 1775 Percivall Pott reported the induction of scrotal cancer in chimney sweeps due to topical occupational exposure to a carcinogen. A little over 100 years later, in 1895, Rehn described bladder cancer in dyestuff workers. This was the first description of systemic cancer in humans developing from occupational exposure to chemical carcinogens. In 1915, Yamagiwa and Ichikawa demonstrated the induction of cancer in animals. These three events comprise the foundation on which the field of occupational carcinogenesis is based.

The Occupational Safety and Health Act (OSH Act) of 1970 established the Occupational Safety and Health Administration (OSHA) in the Department of Labor to set standards which most adequately assure, to the extent feasible and on the best available evidence, that no employee will suffer material impairment of health or functional capacity even if such employee has regular exposure for the period of his working life. Until the passage of the OSH Act, occupational safety and health had been in the hands of the States, except in a few special areas, such as railroading and mining. The result had been ragged and uneven enforcement. The National Institute for Occupational Safety and Health (NIOSH) was created in the same Act to provide research support to OSHA in setting such standards. To OSHA was left the tasks of not only setting standards but also enforcing them.

Unlike the OSH Act, the Federal Insecticide, Fungicide and Rodenticide

---

*This article was written by Robert P. Beliles in his private capacity. No official support or endorsement by the Occupational Safety and Health Administration or any other agency of the Federal Government is intended or should be inferred.

Act (FIFRA) administered by the U.S. Environmental Protection Agency (EPA) is responsible for the regulation of pesticides, except with regard to their manufacture. FIFRA requires registration of a pesticide and labeling to establish the conditions of use. The Toxic Substances Control Act (TSCA), on the other hand, has a much wider scope. While excluding compounds used for certain purposes, it gives EPA the responsibility to act, in the face of unreasonable risks of injury to health or the environment, on the manufacture, processing, distribution in commerce, use, or disposal of chemicals.

The National Environmental Policy Act (NEPA) of 1969 required regulations to be analyzed for environmental impact. A series of executive orders culminating in 1981 with Executive Order 12291 reiterated this obligation, required inflationary impact analysis, cost-benefit analysis, alternative approaches, and gave the Office of Management and Budget (OMB) review and veto powers over regulations.

In this chapter, I will review the development of Federal standards that deal with carcinogenic chemicals in the workplace, the major court decisions that were rendered when such standards were promulgated, and the laws under which workplace carcinogens are regulated. In addition, the possible future mode of regulatory activity on chemical carcinogens that are found in the workplace will be discussed.

HISTORY OF FEDERAL REGULATIONS OF WORKPLACE CARCINOGENS

OSHA, in accordance with the provisions of the 1970 Act, adopted the Federal and consensus standards that were available in 1971. Most of the standards had been developed by the American National Standards Institute (ANSI) or were Threshold Limit Values (TLV) of the American Conference of Governmental Industrial Hygienists (ACGIH). The latter were not complete standards, but merely a series of recommended exposure limits. The adoption of consensus standards was only allowed for a limited period of time by the OSH Act.

Asbestos

Asbestos was the first material for which a complete health standard was issued by OSHA.[1] The original action on asbestos was the adoption of a permissible exposure limit (PEL) of 12 fibers/cc. This was adopted as a consensus standard from a 1969 Federal standard issued under the Walsh-Healey Public Contracts Act. Asbestos was widely used because of its fire-resistant properties. It is also useful in friction devices such as brake linings. In response to a petition from the AFL-CIO, OSHA published on December 7, 1971, an Emergency Temporary Standard (ETS) reducing the PEL to 5 fibers/cc, measured as an 8-hour time weighted average (TWA). In addition, a short-term exposure limit of 10 fibers/cc for periods not to exceed a total of 15 minutes per hour for up to five hours in an 8-hour day was included. On June 7th of the following year the Agency published the final Standard, with an effective date of July 7, 1973. The Standard retained the 5 fibers/cc 8-hour TWA and had a ceiling level of 10 fibers/cc. The PEL was to be reduced by July 1, 1976 to 2 fibers/cc under additional provisions of the Standard. More important, however, is the detail of other requirements of this Standard. The Standard defined asbestos; specified compliance requirements covering engineering controls, work practices, the conditions of use for respirators, special clothing, change rooms and lockers, laundering of clothing, air monitoring, caution signs and labels, housekeeping, waste disposal; and required medical surveillance and recordkeeping. In addition to being the first complete standard adopted by OSHA, the asbestos standard may have reduced the exposure of more workers to a carcinogenic agent than any other regulation promulgated by that agency. It has been estimated that as many as 2.5 million workers may have been exposed to this material.

In 1975, a new asbestos standard was proposed.[2] Provisions of this proposal included lowering the PEL to 0.5 fibers/cc and developing a separate standard for the construction industry. The National Institute for Occupational Safety and Health (NIOSH) and a NIOSH/OSHA joint committee both recommended lowering the PEL to 0.1 fibers/cc in 1976 and again in 1979. These recommendations which have gone unheeded, were based on the fact that the standard of 1972 was based largely on the assumption that it would prevent asbestosis and hopefully thereby the asbestos-associated cancer. This has not been the case. While very high exposure to asbestos causes asbestosis, lower levels, particularly in smokers, markedly increase the incidence of lung cancer. At even lower levels, mesothelioma is induced. The use of asbestos has dropped from a high of 800,000 tons to less than 300,000 tons over the last few years. The general recognition that exposure to asbestos is hazardous, the fear of third party suits, and the general slowdown in the economy may have been at least as important in this decline as the adoption of the standard or the proposal of an even more stringent one.

"Fourteen Carcinogens"

One group of carcinogens, the so-called "14 carcinogens", was regulated by a single rulemaking.[3] These are listed in Table 1. The activity on these standards began on May 22, 1972. At that time OSHA requested NIOSH to provide information on nine compounds alleged to be carcinogens. On January 4, 1974, a petition for an ETS was received from the Oil, Chemical and Atomic Workers and the Health Research Group requesting the Agency to regulate 10 compounds. An ETS was promulgated on 14 carcinogenic substances on May 3, 1973. A proposal was issued in August of that year and a hearing was held in September. The final standards were issued on January 29, 1974. These standards were for work practices and did not contain permissible exposure limits. They outlined a series of requirements designed to limit worker exposure to the carcinogens and to monitor closely those workers that might be exposed. All the compounds that were regulated as a result of this rulemaking were listed in the appendix of the 1968 ACGIH TLVs, except for 1-naphthylamine. When OSHA adopted the 1968 ACGIH TLVs by incorporating the Walsh-Healey Act, it was claimed that the ACGIH appendix containing the carcinogens and a recommended zero exposure limit had not been adopted and could not therefore be adopted by OSHA without specific rulemaking. Actually, 15 compounds were under consideration, but dimethyl sulfate was not included because documentation of its carcinogenicity was judged by OSHA to be inadequate. These 14-carcinogen standards were similar in many respects. In the Scope and Application section, an exclusion was

Table 1: The "Fourteen Carcinogens" Regulated
in a Single Rulemaking in 1974

2-Acetylaminofluorene*
4-Aminobiphenyl*
Benzidine*
Bis(chloromethyl) ether*
Chloromethyl methyl ether
3,3'-Dichlorobenzidine*
4-Dimethylaminoazobenzene*
Ethyleneimine
4,4'-Methylenebis(2-chlorobenzenamine)
1-Naphthylamine
2-Naphthylamine*
4-Nitrobiphenyl*
N-Nitrosodimethylamine*
β-Propiolactone*

*Those included in the petition from the Oil, Chemical and
Atomic Workers and the Health Research Group.

provided for compounds shipped in sealed containers and, generally, for mixtures containing less than 0.1% of the carcinogen. The Definitions section explained the wording of the Standard, and was, for the most part, very general and would be useful in understanding the language of almost any standard. The Standards established and defined a regulated area in which the compounds could be used. They specified washing of the hands, face and arms before exiting and showering after the last exit of the day from the regulated area; they required the wearing of protective clothing. In this section of the Standards special attention was given to rules for research and quality control activities. Additional rules were provided for those activities that could be considered of an animal support nature. The general requirements of the section on regulated areas required that certain signs be placed at the entrance to the regulated areas (*i.e.*, CANCER-SUSPECT AGENT, AUTHORIZED PERSONNEL ONLY). This section also required that a daily roster of persons entering the regulated area be maintained. It mandated that air-supplied hood respirators be used at all times, and prohibited smoking or eating in the regulated area. Another section was devoted to specific requirements for signs, information, and training. The Reports sections of the Standard required reports of incidents in which employees were exposed to or treated for exposure to the regulated carcinogens. In the final section of these Standards, medical surveillance and the keeping of records was made mandatory.

2-Acetylaminofluorene

The basis for the regulation of 2-acetylaminofluorene (2-AAF) was the finding of a positive carcinogenic effect in rats, mice, dogs, rabbits, hamsters and fowl. The metabolism of this compound to its more potent metabolite was discussed. 2-AAF was developed originally for use as a pesticide but was never marketed because of the experimental findings related to its carcinogenic potential. It is widely used now as a positive control in experimental studies on carcinogenicity. About 1,000 workers conducting laboratory research may be exposed to this material. The exclusion provision for mixtures containing 2-AAF is 1.0%.

4-Aminobiphenyl

The induction of bladder cancer in man by 4-aminobiphenyl (4-ABP, also known as 4-aminodiphenyl) and its high potency for tumor induction in dogs, mice and rabbits were cited as the basis for regulating this compound. Exposure to 4-ABP may occur in the course of its use in the synthesis of other materials. However, the use of substitutes for 4-ABP as antioxidants in the rubber industry has greatly reduced exposure of workers to the carcinogen.

4-Nitrobiphenyl

The positive evidence regarding the carcinogenic potential of 4-nitrobiphenyl was limited to the induction of bladder cancer in dogs. In addition, its *in vivo* conversion to 4-ABP was used as a basis for establishing the carcinogenicity of this material. It is no longer produced in or imported into the United States. The British have banned the use or manufacture of the compound. Apparently, it was used exclusively in the manufacture of 4-ABP.

Benzidine

Regulation of benzidine as a carcinogen was based on the high incidence of bladder cancer in workers exposed to the chemical, supported by the induction of cancer by this chemical in rats, dogs, hamsters, and mice. Of the experimental animals, only dogs developed bladder cancer following exposure to benzidine. Benzidine is used in the manufacture of many dyes. The number of workers exposed to benzidine is probably between 500 and 2,000. The carcinogenicity of several derivatives of benzidine is currently under investigation.

3,3'-Dichlorobenzidine

3,3'-Dichlorobenzidine (DCB) was used as a curing agent for urethane plastics and in the production of certain pigments. In 1974 NIOSH estimated that 1,100 people were exposed to this chemical. The potential carcinogenicity of DCB in humans was based on extrapolation from animal studies. Epidemiological studies suggested that this chemical may be a carcinogen in humans. However, workers exposed to 3,3'-dichlorobenzidine had also been exposed to other carcinogenic materials. Positive carcinogenicity findings in hamsters, mice and rats were nevertheless convincing enough for the Agency to regulate this material as a potential carcinogen in humans.

β-Propiolactone

The production of β-propiolactone (BPL) in the United States is very limited.[4] This chemical was used mainly in the manufacture of acrylic acid and its esters, but the majority of the workers who may have been exposed to BPL were in the health care industry and hospitals, where it was used as a sterilant. While there were no data indicating that BPL was carcinogenic in humans, the evidence was clear that this highly reactive material was carcinogenic in experimental animals provided it did not react with other materials before altering the living cells. Injections of mice and rats with BPL produced significant increases in the number of tumors. Skin application of BPL to hamsters also increased markedly the incidence of skin tumors in treated animals. It is interesting to note that in regulating this pesticide, OSHA did not defer to EPA for control under FIFRA, nor were any legal objections raised on this point.

4-Dimethylaminoazobenzene

The carcinogenic potential of 4-dimethylaminoazobenzene (DAB) had been shown in rats, dogs, trout and neonatal mice. The similarity in metabolism of related compounds in dogs and man was also taken into consideration in the regulation of this compound. OSHA set an exclusion limit of 1.0% for mixtures containing DAB. It was estimated that 2,500 workers were exposed in its use as a coloring agent and as a chemical indicator.

2-Naphthylamine

For over 50 years 2-naphthylamine (2-NA) was used primarily as an intermediate in dyes, and as an antioxidant in the rubber industry. Epidemiological studies have shown that the chemical is clearly a bladder carcinogen in humans. Urinary bladder cancer has also been induced experimentally with 2-NA in dogs, monkeys and hamsters. Tumors at other sites were also induced by administration of the chemical to rats and mice. The Standard for 2-NA excludes 2-NA when it occurs as the result of destructive distillation, such as from coke ovens.

1-Naphthylamine

The major use of 1-naphthylamine (1-NA) was as an antioxidant. Other uses included as a color developer, and as an intermediate in the manufacture of other compounds including some herbicides. The structural and metabolic similarities of 1-NA to 2-NA were the major bases for the regulation of this compound. It was noted that in most studies where an effort had been made to study 1-NA alone, it was highly likely that some contamination with 2-NA was present.

Bis(chloromethyl) Ether

Bis(chloromethyl) ether (BCME) is used in the synthesis of other chemicals and in the manufacture of plastics and resins. In addition to epidemiological studies showing that BCME causes lung cancer in workers, animal studies had also indicated that the compound was carcinogenic. At the time the Standard was promulgated, it had been shown that airborne concentrations of BCME as low as 0.1 ppm produced lung cancer in mice and rats. The chemical was also known to produce cancer by dermal application or by subcutaneous injection.

Chloromethyl Methyl Ether

While epidemiological studies had suggested that chloromethyl methyl ether (CMME) was a carcinogen in humans, the possibility that there was some concomitant exposure to BCME could not be overlooked. Technical grades of CMME are contaminated with 1% to 8% of BCME.[4] Thus, experiments in animals using purified CMME were cited as the primary bases for regulation of this compound.

N-Nitrosodimethylamine

The carcinogenicity of N-nitrosodimethylamine (DMNA) had been established by experimental investigations in several species of animals. Rats developed liver and renal tumors and respiratory tract tumors when exposed to airborne DMNA. In addition, a positive carcinogenic response had been documented in mice, hamsters, guinea pigs, rabbits, and several species of fish following exposure to DMNA. DMNA is not now produced in the United States. While DMNA was used as a solvent in fibers and plastics, as an antioxidant and as a lubricant additive, its greatest use was as an intermediate in the production of liquid rocket fuel.

Ethyleneimine

Two separate positive carcinogenicity studies, one in mice and another in rats, were cited as the primary basis for the regulation of ethyleneimine. Tumors in the rat study were injection site sarcomas. Because of its high reactivity, this compound was useful in a large number of organic syntheses. The end products were widely used in the paper and textile industries.

4,4'-Methylenebis(2-chlorobenzenamine)

A curing agent used in the polyurethane plastics industry, 4,4'-methylenebis(2-chlorobenzenamine) (MBOCA), was among the original "14 carcinogens". The basis for regulation of this compound was the experimental induction of urinary bladder tumors in dogs, the induction of lung, liver, mammary gland and zymbal gland tumors in rats, and the induction of liver tumors in mice. The Standard contained special provisions, including the elimination of the requirement for regulated areas when premixing solutions of MBOCA and prepolymer, if the chemical interaction already had been started. Of the 14 Standards, only the MBOCA Standard was successfully opposed by industry in legal action. This action resulted in the Standard being remanded to the Agency, which withdrew it in 1976 on procedural grounds. However, several States still regulate MBOCA in the workplace.

Vinyl Chloride

In January of 1974, OSHA was informed by NIOSH that the B.F. Goodrich Chemical Co. reported that several of its employees had died from angiosarcoma, perhaps as the result of occupational exposure to vinyl chloride (VC).[5] A joint inspection of the B.F. Goodrich Plant in Louisville, KY, by OSHA, NIOSH and the Kentucky Department of Labor resulted in a fact-finding hearing held on February 15, 1974. Preliminary information on the induction of angiosarcoma in rats exposed to 250 ppm of VC in a laboratory in Italy was presented. An ETS reducing the PEL from a ceiling of 500 ppm to 50 ppm and providing other requirements including monitoring and respiratory protection, was promulgated on April 5, 1974. Before the proposed standard was issued, data were presented to the Agency by the Industrial Bio-Test Laboratories (IBT) showing that in an ongoing study, two of 200 mice exposed to 50 ppm of VC for seven months had developed angiosarcomas of the liver. The proposed standard issued on May 10, 1974 called for the limitation of employee exposure to VC to "no detectable level" based on an analytical method sensitive to 1 ppm. A lengthy hearing was subsequently held at which time additional information regarding the carcinogenicity of VC was presented. This included findings of carcinogenicity in hamsters, establishment of a dose-response relationship in the Italian study, and a significant increase in cancer at sites other than the liver in experimental animals in the IBT study. For example, although in the first 11 months of the IBT study 100 mice died (64 of these were not examined), liver tumors were present in 36%, lung tumors in 58% and skin tumors in 25% of the remaining 36 mice. Opposition to the adoption of the VC Standard focused on the fact that no tumors had been found in experimental animals at airborne concentrations of VC below 50 ppm (levels lower than 50 ppm had not been tested at that time), that worker exposure to higher levels had not resulted in a significant increase in cancer and that the metabolism of VC might have a significant influence on the development of the carcinogenic response. On October 4, 1974, the final standard on occupational exposure to VC was published. The comprehensive Standard contained a PEL of 1 ppm as an 8-hour TWA, a 15 minute limit on exposure above 5 ppm, and an action level of 0.5 ppm which triggered compliance with other requirements. The effective date of the Standard was to be January 1, 1975, but this was held in abeyance until April 1, 1975, because of a suit brought by the plastics manufacturers, the primary users of this chemical. It was estimated that over 350,000 workers could have been exposed to VC at the time the Standard was issued.

Coke Oven Emissions

The final standard for coke oven emissions[6] was issued on October 22, 1976. This was the first, and to date the only, OSHA health standard on a carcinogen to deal with an industrial process in contrast to a single chemical. The Standard that had been previously applied to the area covered by the coke oven emissions standard was the coal tar pitch volatiles (CTPV) standard, which had been taken from the ACGIH 1968 TLV list. Under this Standard the airborne concentration of CTPV (as the benzene soluble fraction) was limited to 2 mg/m^3. On June 8, 1975, the American Iron and Steel Institute (AISI) petitioned OSHA to develop a distinct standard applicable to coke oven emissions. In July of that year, the United Steelworkers of America requested the Agency to issue a more stringent standard to cover coke oven emissions. OSHA denied both requests and asked NIOSH to undertake further investigation of the area. In addition, the Agency published guidelines for protective measures that could be undertaken in the interim. A Standards Advisory Committee on Coke Oven Emissions was established by OSHA. This group recommended the adoption of a full standard because of the special problems inherent in industries in which coke oven emissions were present. A proposed standard for coke oven emissions was published in the Federal Register on July 31, 1975. The process regulated by this standard begins when bituminous coal is made into coke producing a clean uniform fuel that is widely used in the manufacture of steel. The coking process heats coal to high temperatures; an oxygen deficit prevents complete combustion. In modern coke ovens, the gases (carbon monoxide, sulfur oxides, coal tars, and others) escape through the cracks in the coke oven doors or piping. This chemical brew is highly toxic. The coal tars, in particular, have been identified as potent carcinogens for more than 100 years. The composition of the coal, temperature of the oven, and other factors change the composition of the gases. Analytically, these gases are characterized in terms of the portion which is soluble in benzene. (The coke oven emissions standard is especially important with regard to the risk assessment requirements developing out of the 1980 Supreme Court decision on benzene; the Supreme Court said in that decision that the Agency had done a rudimentary, but an acceptable risk assessment in the course of establishing the final coke oven emissions standard.) This Standard established a PEL of 0.15 mg/cubic meter of CTPV in the coke oven facilities. The PEL was based on epidemiological studies which showed an increase in lung cancer among workers exposed in this particular industrial segment, but technological feasibility limited lowering the permissible concentration further. However, other provisions of the Standard such as the requirements for protective clothing, respirators, and medical surveillance provided additional protection over and above the previously invoked CTPV PEL. In the preamble to the coke oven emissions standard, OSHA had estimated that the more stringent standard would prevent 240 excess cases of lung cancer each year. The Third Circuit Court of Appeals upheld the relevant parts of the Standard. Industry then appealed to the Supreme Court, which agreed to hear the case. When the Court mentioned, in the decision on benzene, that the risk estimate in the coke oven emissions standard was acceptable, industry withdrew its appeal before the case could be argued.

1,2-Dibromo-3-Chloropropane

On March 17, 1978, OSHA issued a final standard for occupational exposure to 1,2-dibromo-3-chloropropane (DBCP) based on evidence that exposure to this chemical, an agricultural nematocide, presented a hazard of sterility and of cancer.[7] The Standard excluded from the scope the use of the material as a pesticide or the storage, transportation, or sale of DBCP in sealed containers because other Federal agencies had jurisdiction in those areas. The PEL under this standard was 1 ppb as an 8-hour TWA. In addition, eye and skin contact were prohibited. In the Medical Surveillance section, radioimmunoassay for FSH, LH, and total estrogen was required in females. The reproductive data which served as the basis of this standard were derived from animal experiments performed as early as 1961 showing testicular effects and additional more recent evidence in man. However, what led to the consideration of this chemical as a candidate for regulatory activity was a 1977 finding of markedly decreased sperm counts in workers exposed to the chemical. The evidence of carcinogenicity was based on positive findings in rats and mice in bioassays conducted by the National Cancer Institute. Positive findings of *in vitro* mutagenic responses were cited as further evidence of potential carcinogenicity. The Agency stated ". . . that a substance which causes cancer in animals must be considered, as a policy matter, as posing a carcinogenic risk to workers." The preamble noted this view, and it was not challenged during the course of the proceedings. It was estimated by OSHA that 1,600 to 2,900 workers were to be affected by this standard. Formal rulemaking activity on this standard began with the issuance of an ETS on September 9, 1977. However, OSHA alerted manufacturers of the potential hazard to workers on August 12, 1977. The Agency was petitioned by a union on August 23, 1977, to lower the PEL to 1 ppb. EPA on October 27, 1977 issued a suspension order which revoked the registration of DBCP for use on all food crops and a conditional suspension limiting its use for other purposes to certified applicators and requiring them to wear respirators and protective clothing. There had been no national consensus standard for DBCP. The adoption of this standard did not result in an immediate legal challenge as has been the case with many of OSHA's standards.

Arsenic

In 1971, OSHA adopted the consensus standards for airborne concentrations of arsenic and its compounds of 0.5 mg/cubic meter and 1.0 mg/cubic meter for lead arsenate and calcium arsenate.[8] These were based on the 1968 ACGIH TLV's. In a 1973 NIOSH criteria document, a PEL of 50 micrograms/cubic meter was recommended. In September of 1974, OSHA conducted informal hearings on the potential health hazard of arsenic in the workplace. In November of the same year NIOSH recommended a PEL of 2 micrograms/cubic meter based on new data indicating the carcinogenicity of arsenic in the workplace. On January 21, 1975, OSHA issued a proposed standard for inorganic arsenic in which the PEL was 4 micrograms/cubic meter. The record was reopened in June of the following year to receive new information on feasibility and new scientific data. On May 5, 1978 the Agency published a final arsenic standard. This comprehensive Standard established a PEL of 10 micrograms/cubic meter. In addition, the Standard provided for an action level of 5 micrograms/cubic meter, and excluded from the scope arsenic and its compounds when used as pesticides, including their use as wood preservatives. Reports that arsenic induced lung cancer in workers in several occupational settings were the basis of the Standard. The PEL was set at 10 micrograms/cubic meter because the Agency determined that lower levels could not be met.

After the Supreme Court's decision on benzene, OSHA asked the Ninth Circuit Court to remand the Standard to the Agency for the purpose of determining the significance of risk.[9] The Standard had been challenged by industry shortly after its issuance and was before the Court at that time. The Agency proposed a risk assessment based on epidemiological studies in copper smelters and the pesticide manufacturing industry. Hearings were held on that effort and other assessments were reviewed. The Chemical Manufacturers Association (CMA) represented industry and challenged the risk assessment performed by the Agency. They initially tried to maintain that it had not been demonstrated that arsenic was a carcinogen. OSHA affirmed the risk at the previous PEL and showed that the new PEL (10 micrograms/cubic meter) reduced the risk of cancer in exposed workers. These findings were published in the Federal Register on January 14, 1983.

Acrylonitrile

Before the rulemaking began on acrylonitrile (Vinyl cyanide), the PEL was 20 ppm as an 8-hour TWA.[10] This value had been adopted from the 1968 ACGIH

TLV. Acrylonitrile (AN) is used in the manufacture of plastics, resins, rubber and a wide variety of synthetic fibers, as well as an intermediate for a number of other types of chemicals. In March 1977, the Chemical Manufacturers Association forwarded to OSHA information on the interim results of a rat study in which AN had been given in the drinking water. Shortly thereafter the Agency also received information that indicated that AN produced similar carcinogenic responses when given to rats via inhalation. In May of that year the Agency received information suggesting that positive carcinogenic effects were seen in an ongoing epidemiological study. OSHA published a request for information. In December of the same year NIOSH concluded that workers might indeed be at risk from exposure to AN. OSHA issued an ETS on January 17, 1978, establishing a PEL of 2 ppm with a 15 minute short-term exposure limit of 10 ppm. On October 3, 1978, the final standard was issued. The provision with regard to exposure level was similar to that in the ETS, but in addition, an action level of 1 ppm was established. OSHA set the PEL based on the judgment that it provided significant protection of workers and was the lowest feasible level that employers could achieve. At the time the Standard was issued OSHA estimated that 5,130 workers were affected by the Standard, but as many as 270,000 workers are potentially exposed. This Standard was not challenged in court.

Ethylene Oxide

A recent action (April 21, 1983) of OSHA was a proposal of an occupational exposure standard[11] for ethylene oxide (ETO). The PEL was lowered in the final standard (June 22, 1984) from 50 ppm to 1 ppm. The risk assessment, the second undertaken by the Agency since the Supreme Court's decision on benzene, was based on a chronic inhalation exposure of rats which showed a dose-related carcinogenic effect. The known action (alkylation), positive mutagenic responses, positive adverse reproductive effects both in animals and man, and strongly suggestive epidemiological studies all attested to the threat of this chemical's adverse effects in humans. While the primary (99%) use of ETO is as an intermediate in the manufacture of other compounds, mainly ethylene glycol, ETO is also used as a sterilant and fumigant primarily for certain types of medical supplies and in hospitals where the greatest numbers of workers are exposed. The Agency was directed by the U.S. Court of Appeals to issue an ETO proposed standard within 30 days as a result of a suit involving the failure of the Agency to respond to a petition for an ETS. More important was the opinion of the Court that OSHA could not yield jurisdiction to EPA under FIFRA with regard to the sterilant use of ETO at least in some industrial segments. The Court stated that OSHA coverage was not preempted in "areas—such as the health care industry—where EPA has apparently exercised minimal, if any regulatory authority . . .". This ruling by the Court could have great significance in the future. It is the second time OSHA has regulated a pesticidal use of a material. The first time, of course, was in the case of BPL. Interestingly, both these actions involve the use of a sterilant in the health care industry. In the past the Agency has deferred to EPA when the chemical was used as an agricultural pesticide (*i.e.*, arsenic and DBCP). However, the Court's decision, if it stands, opens the door for OSHA regulation of pesticides used in non-agricultural industrial segments.

Ethylene Dibromide

On October 7, 1983, OSHA issued a proposed standard which would reduce the PEL of ethylene dibromide (EDB) from 20 ppm to 0.1 ppm.[12] EDB is used in the manufacture of leaded gasoline, as an intermediate in the manufacture of other compounds, as a solvent for gums, waxes and resins, and as a fumigating agent for some types of agricultural products and equipment. Under this proposal the agricultural use would not be covered, but the offgassing exposure in the workplace would. The use as a pesticide was to be handled by EPA. That agency had issued a notice on EDB a few days earlier. OSHA and EPA were trying to coordinate their activities on EDB, but the action by OSHA was delayed by OMB. The exposure to EDB in storage, distribution, handling or retail sales of leaded gasoline will apparently not be covered by either agency. The estimate of risk to EDB was based on inhalation studies in experimental animals which showed an increase in cancer. In addition, the proposed short-term exposure limit (STEL) of 0.5 ppm was based on the reproductive effects of the compound. It is interesting to note that California had previously adopted an occupational exposure limit of 0.13 ppm.

Beryllium and Trichloroethylene

OSHA has proposed two standards on carcinogenic materials which have neither been nor are likely to become final regulations, namely for beryllium and trichloroethylene. A review of this OSHA activity may be of interest. On October 17, 1975, OSHA published a proposal for a standard on beryllium.[13] At that time the PEL was 2.0 micrograms/cubic meter. A ceiling of 5.0 micrograms/cubic meter and a 30 minute short-term exposure limit of 25 micrograms/cubic meter were proposed. These were adopted from the 1970 ANSI standards. The proposed standard included an 8-hour TWA of 1.0 micrograms/cubic meter and a ceiling of 5 micrograms/cubic meter. The industrial uses of beryllium include alloys of other metals such as copper, with which it produces a harder alloy, and in nuclear reactors, the electronics industry, and in the aerospace industry. OSHA cited what it said was "overwhelming animal data" regarding the carcinogenicity of beryllium and characterized the epidemiological data as consistent with the animal data, but "not determinative in itself". While the difference between the proposed PEL and the current one was small, it was felt that the worker would be provided additional protection through the other requirements of the proposed standard such as medical surveillance and hygiene facilities. In the hearing that followed the publication of the proposal, a number of unusual things occurred. One industry witness cast doubt on the validity of work conducted by his department chairman. In addition, he also denied the validity of some publications which he himself had authored. NIOSH was said to have prevented the appearance of certain industry witnesses who were concurrently working under contract to NIOSH. In addition, certain government witnesses were charged by their own co-authors with gerrymandering data. While there has been no formal statement from OSHA, it would seem that the peculiar nature of the record, along with the minimum change in the proposed PEL, were likely reasons for the standard never having been adopted.

On October 20, 1975, OSHA issued a proposal for an occupational exposure standard on trichloroethylene (TCE).[14] This chemical is widely used as an industrial degreasing agent and as a dry cleaning fluid. The proposal was in part prompted by a preliminary report from the National Cancer Institute (NCI) that TCE was carcinogenic in mice. While the proposed standard was to maintain the 100 ppm PEL adopted from the 1967 ANSI standard, it did eliminate the five minute 300 ppm peak and reduced the 200 ppm ceiling to 150 ppm. Before the rulemaking progressed further, it became apparent that the test material in the NCI study contained epichlorohydrin, a known carcinogen; the rulemaking was subsequently dropped.

Benzene

The current standard for benzene was adopted in 1971 from the ANSI standards.[15] It is an 8-hour TWA of 10 ppm, with a ceiling of 25 ppm and a maximum peak concentration not to exceed 50 ppm for longer than 10 minutes in any 8-hour work period. This standard was based on the induction of blood dyscrasias. No association of leukemia with exposure to benzene was known at that time. Benzene is produced as a by-product in petroleum refining and in the coke oven industry. It was widely used as a solvent and is a starting or intermediate material in the synthesis of numerous chemicals. Excluding the retail gasoline trade where exposure may occur from the inclusion of benzene in domestic gasoline at a concentration of about two percent, as many as 3 million workers may be exposed to this chemical. In April of 1976, OSHA was requested to issue an ETS. This request was originally denied. Following a revised NIOSH recommendation and preliminary conclusions of an epidemiological study showing a relationship between leukemia and exposure to benzene, the Agency issued an ETS on May 3, 1977. Although the ETS was challenged in court, the Agency promulgated a new standard on February 10, 1978. The PEL for benzene was 1 ppm as an 8-hour TWA, with a 15 minute short-term exposure limit of 5 ppm. The other provisions of the Standard included a prohibition against skin contact. In July of 1980, the Supreme Court vacated the new benzene standard largely, but not solely, on the grounds that OSHA had failed to demonstrate that significant health risks existed under the old standard. It is probably of great political significance that the Agency went out of its way in the benzene standard to stress that it felt that a risk assessment was neither possible nor necessary.

THE FUTURE AND IMPLICATIONS OF CARCINOGENICITY TESTING

The Supreme Court's decision on the benzene standard had profound effects on the OSHA Cancer Policy[16] which had been published on January 22, 1980. The purpose of this Policy, which was preceded by extensive hearings and a massive record of testimony from various experts and interested parties, was to: (a) Establish a method of setting priorities for the chemicals or processes on which the Agency would work; (b) identify and resolve questions which seemed to have come up in all previous hearings on standards, thereby enabling the Agency to promulgate standards more rapidly; and (c) set out certain standard provisions for the regulation of carcinogens. The Policy did not regulate any specific substance. The Cancer Policy established criteria by which the Agency would judge whether or not a material is a carcinogen. This was very important since OSHA was not empowered by the 1970 Act to require any investigation by industry. Furthermore, the Agency was not supposed to do any research, but was to rely on NIOSH for this function. This arrangement is very awkward, since OSHA is part of the Department of Labor and NIOSH is a part of the National Institutes of Health, specifically, under the Center for Disease Control.

Since the Supreme Court's decision on benzene seemed to direct the Agency to do a risk assessment and the Cancer Policy indicates that the Agency does not deem this necessary, a reassessment of the Cancer Policy is clearly necessary. In particular, it would seem that the Agency must decide on how to define a significant risk. The decision on benzene specifically mentioned the Cancer Policy in holding that the Agency must assume the "threshold responsibility of establishing the need for more stringent standards" rather than relying on a special policy for carcinogens. It is not at all clear what exact procedures the Court had in mind in the ruling on the benzene standard. The decision was a five to four vote, and one of the Justices cast his vote on grounds other than that the Agency must show significant risk. However, it would seem that the Supreme Court was generally referring to setting of the PEL, and not to all parts of the Standard, in its discussion of significant risk.

This becomes most clear in the Supreme Court's decision on the cotton dust standard. In this decision the Supreme Court rejected the use of cost-benefit analysis in setting exposure levels (PEL's). In the Cotton Dust Decision, the Supreme Court also indicated that feasibility is that which is capable of being done—technologically and not economically. The Court contended that in passing the OSH Act the Congress was fully aware that OSHA standards would impose real and substantial costs of compliance on industry and the Congress believed that such expenses were part of the costs of doing business.

Some confusion on what constitutes a risk assessment may have been at least partially resolved by a recent publication by the National Research Council.[17] In this report risk assessment was defined as having four components: Hazard identification; dose-response assessments (quantitative risk analysis or determination of the rate of cancer in exposed persons); exposure assessment (the concentration and duration to which people are exposed and the number of persons involved); and risk characterization (the application of the first three along with the attendant uncertainty).

Congress enacted TSCA in recognition of the loopholes existing in the statutes.[18] Congress was concerned that new chemicals could be manufactured and used without any governmental review. Only DBCP and 1-naphthylamine have been regulated by OSHA in the absence of any pre-existing consensus regulations. TSCA has sweeping authority to collect scientific and economic data concerning chemicals. The type of information gathered by EPA includes chemical production and use, and health and environmental testing data. TSCA also requires that manufacturers inform the EPA when studies in animals or humans indicate that a product may present a risk of injury to health or the environment. This type of information could be of great assistance to OSHA since the OSH Act only requires the submission of the most serious human based data.

The introduction of quantitative risk assessments into the regulatory scheme will require that additional information be obtained, perhaps not on every compound, to answer a few basic questions on the proper use and design of mathematical models and to better understand the results they generate. For example, the regulatory agencies need information on the effect of cessation of exposure on risk and how to estimate that effect.

There appear to be three different types of responses that may occur when exposure to a carcinogen stops. In some cases the risk may decline, as with cessation of cigarette smoking. On the other hand, it is apparent that with some agents and tumor types, the risk continues to increase following the end of treatment. This is the apparent case with 2-AAF and liver tumors in experimental animals, but not with all tumor types induced by this compound. Additionally, epidemiological studies with asbestos indicate that low cumulative doses cause a shift to occur in the most frequent tumor type from lung cancer to mesothelioma. Another important problem is the effect of intermittent exposures *versus* continuous low level exposures. Finally, a long-standing but as yet unresolved problem is whether a previous exposure to a carcinogen increases the risk from cancer when a worker is further exposed to other potential carcinogens in the course of employment. It is highly likely, for example, that some sterilizer operators exposed to BPL were subsequently exposed to ETO when BPL was phased out as a sterilant. Likewise, in some manufacturing facilities, it is likely that workers exposed to DBCP were then exposed to EDB when the production of DBCP was ended.

Part of the problem in the past has been that OSHA lacked an appropriate plan for the development of health standards on carcinogens. The Agency acted in the face of petitions or crisis situations such as in the situation with VC. The Cancer Policy was a beginning in the direction of comprehensive planning, in that it was intended to identify and establish a priority list of compounds which the Agency would consider for rulemaking activity. There are now several such lists which the Agency could consider as a basis for action. For example, the National Toxicology Program (NTP) publishes a list of compounds in its Annual Report on Carcinogens. The ACGIH indication of carcinogens in the workplace might also be useful. It has the additional advantage in that the materials listed are occupational rather than environmental hazards. Another list is that prepared by the International Agency for Research on Cancer (IARC). Based on these lists OSHA now could determine those agents that are present in workplaces in the United States and eliminate the need for the Agency to determine further that the material is a carcinogen.

One might think that the number of workers exposed to a particular compound would be an important consideration when undertaking regulatory activity by OSHA. However, this historical review reveals that this has little influence in the activity of the Agency. While it is unlikely that in the near future the Agency will regulate compounds with only 1,000 exposed workers, as was the case with 2-AAF, it is also unlikely that the chemical hazards that expose two to three million workers will be regulated without considerable effort on the part of scientific, political, legislative, and judicial factions. A combination of factors account for this lethargy, chief among them being the economy and the political inclination of the country, along with the extreme influence of trade organizations.

Although OSHA does not have the authority to conduct research, the Agency may nominate compounds for testing by the National Toxicology Program. The nominations of such compounds should focus on those chemicals which appear to be workplace carcinogens, but for which the evidence thus far is not suitable for use in quantitative risk analysis. OSHA also has input into the Interagency Testing Committee which provides the Agency another avenue for obtaining the type of data that it feels is needed for regulatory activity.

Only in the last year has EPA used TSCA to effect an improvement in the health of the industrial worker. EPA has recently issued an advance notice of proposed rulemaking on MBOCA. This is the only one of the "14 carcinogens" regulated by OSHA for which the Standard was not upheld by the courts.

EPA also has begun to take similar action on 4,4'-methylenedianiline (MDA). MDA is used primarily as a chemical intermediate in the production of isocyanates and polyisocyanates which are used in the manufacture of polyurethane. MDA is also used as a curing agent for epoxy resins, as a dye intermediate and as a corrosion inhibitor. The ultimate outcome of these EPA actions will be very interesting since TSCA is a balancing act; that is, a number of factors including economic impact must be balanced against the benefits of a particular action. This is in contrast to the Supreme Court's interpretation of the OSH Act, which holds that OSHA-promulgated standards, at least health regulations, should be based solely on consideration of feasibility and on the demonstration of significant risk and its reduction. Historically, this type of intra-agency cooperative effort is evident only in the simultaneous actions taken with regard to DBCP and EDB. However, TSCA requires that the Administrator of EPA formally notify OSHA, by publication in the Federal Register, when a finding of unreasonable risk is made on a chemical that is present in the workplace. Upon such notification the Assistant Secretary must respond formally.

This review, if nothing else, should clearly indicate that OSHA has moved slowly and haltingly in the regulation of carcinogens in the workplace. For example, the standard for arsenic was four years in the making (1974–1978) and is still being defended by the Agency. Those regulations it has promulgated have, for the most part, been based on data from bioassays conducted in animals. Only the regulations on asbestos and arsenic had limited consideration of animal data. While the standard for coke oven emissions was based on epidemiological data, the fact that bioassays had shown that various components were consistently positive was also taken into consideration.

Regulations in the future will probably continue to be based on bioassays conducted in animals because of the nature of epidemiological studies, and their confounding factors, such as uncertain exposure concentrations and the interaction of other environmental factors (*i.e.*, smoking). This will be the case even more frequently in the future because of the requirement for risk assessment. However, the indication that the worker is affected will certainly be a driving force for regulation, as it was in the case of vinyl chloride. Unlike the situation which existed with vinyl chloride, an imperfect study, such as the IBT study, is unlikely to be considered an acceptable basis for establishing a dose-response curve and for the calculation of risks. Fortunately, the quality of current long-term bioassays is much improved. Inhalation studies will likely be of the greatest use, since this is the route most frequently encountered in the occupational setting. The use of other types of data, such as short-term mutagenicity studies, will not be the primary basis of regulations by OSHA. However, these data may be very useful in establishing the carcinogenic potential of a compound, especially if only one positive long-term bioassay result is available. In addition, mutagenicity studies will be useful in determining whether the carcinogenic material is genotoxic or epigenetic or, as is probable in many cases, has both capabilities.

The implication of scientific information on the health of the industrial workers is now represented during rulemaking to the regulatory agencies largely by trade organizations. Regulatory agencies must make a greater effort to ensure that the entire scientific community is fully aware of the regulatory activity and the need for expert information and input. Without this activity and interchange, the worker will continue to be exposed to an ever-increasing number of carcinogenic materials, the interactions among which are not understood and the scientific community will find itself farther and farther removed from the decision-making process.

REFERENCES

1. Occupational Safety and Health Administration, Standard for Exposure to Asbestos Dust. *Fed. Register* 37:11318–11322 (1972)
2. Occupational Safety and Health Administration, Occupational Exposure to Asbestos: Notice of Proposed Rulemaking. *Fed. Register* 40: 47652–47665 (1975)
3. Occupational Safety and Health Administration, Occupational Safety and Health Standards: Carcinogens. *Fed. Register* 39: 3756–3797 (1974)
4. National Toxicology Program, Third Annual Report on Carcinogens: December 1982 (1983)
5. Occupational Safety and Health Administration, Standard for Exposure to Vinyl Chloride. *Fed. Register* 39: 35890–35898 (1974)
6. Occupational Safety and Health Administration, Exposure to Coke Oven Emissions. *Fed. Register* 41: 46742–46790 (1976)
7. Occupational Safety and Health Administration, Occupational Exposure to 1,2-Dibromo-3-Chloropropane (DBCP): Final Rule. *Fed. Register* 43: 11514–11533 (1978)
8. Occupational Safety and Health Administration, Occupational Exposure to Inorganic Arsenic: Final Standard. *Fed. Register* 43: 19584–19631 (1978)
9. Occupational Safety and Health Administration, Occupational Exposure to Inorganic Arsenic: Supplemental Statement of Reasons for Final Rule. *Fed. Register* 48: 1864–1903 (1983)
10. Occupational Safety and Health Administration, Occupational Exposure to Acrylonitrile (Vinyl Cyanide): Final Standard. *Fed. Register* 43: 45762–45814 (1978)
11. Occupational Safety and Health Administration, Occupational Exposure to Ethylene Oxide: Proposed Rule. *Fed. Register* 48: 17284–17319 (1983)
12. Occupational Safety and Health Administration, Occupational Exposure to Ethylene Dibromide: Notice of Proposed Rulemaking. *Fed. Register* 48: 45956–46003 (1983)
13. Occupational Safety and Health Administration, Occupational Exposure to Beryllium: Notices of Proposed Rulemaking. *Fed. Register* 40: 48814–48827 (1975)

14. Occupational Safety and Health Administration, Occupational Exposure to Trichloroethylene: Notice of Proposed Rulemaking. *Fed. Register* 40: 49032–49045 (1975)
15. Occupational Safety and Health Administration, Occupational Exposure to Benzene: Permanent Standard for the Regulation of Benzene. *Fed. Register* 43: 5918–5970 (1977)
16. Occupational Safety and Health Administration, Identification, Classification and Regulation of Potential Occupational Carcinogens: Final Rule. *Fed. Register* 45: 5002–5296 (1980)
17. National Research Council, Risk Assessment in the Federal Government: Managing the Process. National Academy Press, Washington, DC (1983)
18. Druley, R.M., and Ordway, G.L., The Toxic Substances Control Act. The Bureau of National Affairs, Inc. Washington, DC (1977)

29

Evaluation of Carcinogens: Perspective of the Consumer Product Safety Commission*

Andrew G. Ulsamer
Paul D. White
Peter W. Preuss

Consumer Product Safety Commission
Bethesda, Maryland

INTRODUCTION

The Consumer Product Safety Commission (CPSC) has jurisdiction over a wide variety of chemical-containing products to which consumers may be exposed. These include paints and other coating products, aerosols, cleaners, dyes, textile finishes, pressed wood products, insulation, and plastics. The jurisdiction of the Commission excludes foods, drugs and cosmetics, pesticides, fungicides, and rodenticides.

To protect consumers from exposure to chemical products which are likely to cause injury, illness or death, the Commission has available to it two primary statutes: The Federal Hazardous Substances Act (FHSA) and the Consumer Product Safety Act (CPSA). These statutes allow the Commission to exercise a number of regulatory options in carrying out its mandate including disseminating product information, labeling consumer products, establishing performance or other standards (either mandatory or voluntary) and banning hazardous products. For a recent legal review of the Commission's regulatory authority and its application to chemical hazards, *see* Merrill.[1]

Over the years the Commission has considered regulatory alternatives for a number of chemical consumer products including those containing vinyl chloride, TRIS [tris(2,3-dibromopropyl)phosphate], benzene, benzidine congener dyes, formaldehyde, asbestos, nitrosamines, and diethylhexyl phthalate. This

---

*The opinions expressed in this article are those of the authors and do not necessarily reflect the official positions and policies of the Consumer Product Safety Commission.

chapter reviews the Commission's authority to regulate carcinogens, cites regulatory history, discusses the process CPSC follows in evaluating hazards posed by chemical carcinogens, and presents examples of how the Commission has dealt with several chemical carcinogens in recent years, showing the evolution of the process from a reactive process to an active one.

REGULATORY AUTHORITY

The Commission's ability to regulate carcinogens and other hazardous substances is derived from sections 7, 8, 9, 15, and 27 (e) of the CPSA and sections 2 (q) and 3 (a) of the FHSA. Section 7 of the CPSA authorizes the Commission to "promulgate consumer product safety standards" when it finds such a standard to "be reasonably necessary to prevent or reduce an unreasonable risk of injury" associated with exposure to a consumer product. If, however, the Commission finds that "no feasible consumer product safety standard . . . . . would adequately protect the public from the unreasonable risk of injury," it may then declare the product a banned hazardous substance under section 8 of the Act. The language of section 2 (q) of the FHSA is similar to that of section 8 of the CPSA.

Both Acts require that the Commission consider and weigh the risk, potential costs and benefits, and alternative actions before promulgating a rule; the rule must additionally be necessary and in the public interest. The Commission also has available to it section 27 (e) of the CPSA under which it can require manufacturers to provide technical and performance data about products presenting a hazard to consumers using them.

Prior to beginning a rulemaking process under sections 7, 8, or 9 of the CPSA or under section 2 (q) of the FHSA that relates to "a risk of cancer, birth defects or gene mutations from a consumer product," the Commission is required under amendments (sections 28 and 31) added to the CPSA in 1981 to convene a Chronic Hazard Advisory Panel (CHAP). The Panel consists of seven members appointed by the Commission from nominees submitted by the President of the National Academy of Sciences. The members of the Panel must have expertise in the area under consideration and may not be employees of the Federal government or receive compensation from or have a substantial financial interest in any manufacturer, distributor or retailer of a consumer product. The Panel reviews "the scientific data and other relevant information . . . . to determine if any substance in a product is a carcinogen, mutagen or a teratogen (and if it is, to estimate, if feasible, the probable harm it poses to human health) and to report its determination to the Commission". The Commission must then consider the Panel's report and incorporate it into both the advanced notice of the rule and the final rule.

Finally, the Commission has available to it, under section 15 of the CPSA, a wide variety of remedies ranging from a public notice of defect by the manufacturer to ordering the manufacturer to correct the defect for products posing a "substantial product hazard". A "substantial product hazard" can result either from the failure of a manufacturer to comply with an applicable rule dealing with the safe use of consumer products or from a defect in the consumer product itself.

CARCINOGEN POLICY—PAST AND PRESENT

Historical Aspects

The Commission does not presently have a formal written policy for classifying and dealing with carcinogens. Such a policy was established on an interim basis in 1978 (with concomitant solicitation of comments).[1,2] This interim policy classified carcinogens and suspect carcinogens into four categories (A through D): A) Those substances for which there was "strong evidence of carcinogenicity" from human epidemiological studies, long-term animal studies or a combination of long-term animal studies and *in vitro* tests; B) those substances for which there was suggestive evidence of carcinogenicity from human or animal studies or from short-term tests; C) those substances which are "members of a class or family of chemicals, many members of which are known to be carcinogens" or substances with "very limited evidence of carcinogenicity"; D) those substances previously classified as either A, B or C but for which subsequent evidence did not indicate a "carcinogenic potential". Substances in Category A would have been subject to regulation depending on the degree of exposure, human uptake, availability, cost and toxicity of substitutes, potential economic and social effects, environmental assessment and risk factors. Substances in Categories B and C would have been recommended for additional testing and could, in the interim, have been subject to warning statements or labeling, if appropriate. The Commission considered applying its interim cancer policy almost immediately to perchloroethylene but was successfully sued by Dow Chemical U.S.A. for failure to provide adequate notice of, and opportunity to comment on, the cancer policy. The interim cancer policy was subsequently withdrawn.[1,3]

Interagency Carcinogen Evaluation Efforts

At about the time that the CPSC withdrew its interim policy on carcinogens, the Interagency Regulatory Liaison Group (IRLG) was formed to coordinate scientific and policy activities among five Federal regulatory agencies (the Consumer Product Safety Commission, the Environmental Protection Agency, the Food and Drug Administration, the Occupational Safety and Health Administration, and the U.S. Department of Agriculture) responsible for the health and safety regulation of chemicals. The IRLG established the development of guidelines for the evaluation of carcinogenic risks as one of its initial priorities. The CPSC decided to participate in this effort and made no further attempt to develop a new cancer policy of its own. The effort of the IRLG differed from the CPSC interim cancer policy in that it was directed towards developing scientific guidelines for evaluating potential carcinogens rather than establishing a fixed set of criteria to categorize carcinogens. A working group of member agency scientists supplemented with scientists from the National Cancer Institute developed a series of guidelines which were published in the *Journal of the National Cancer Institute* in 1979.[4] Prior to adopting these guidelines as a formal component of regulatory evaluation, they were published in the *Federal Register* and public comments were solicited on their appropriateness and applicability. Public comments were received, but before analysis of the comments could be completed, the IRLG was disbanded in 1981.

Shortly thereafter (1982) a new coordinating group was established under the direction of the Office of Science and Technology Policy in the White House. This new group, composed of scientists from the various Federal regulatory and research agencies, established the development of state-of-the-art guidelines for carcinogen evaluation as a goal. Through this effort the group sought to identify and discuss, the major issues, in greater detail than in the IRLG document, and strove to emphasize the examination of recent scientific progress and its implications for identification and assessment of carcinogens. This effort was completed during 1984 and is presently undergoing Agency review.

The CPSC has profited from the coordinated Federal efforts for evaluation of carcinogens. The documents and discussions that have resulted have been valuable to the CPSC and other agency scientists by providing a consensus on a substantial body of knowledge.

Chemical Screening Process

The Commission's approach for dealing with chemical carcinogens has two broad levels of evaluation. Initially, a chemical screening group reviews health and use information on chemicals for which data on chronic health effects have become available. Chemicals possessing both demonstrated adverse health effects and the potential for consumer exposure are selected for further in-depth evaluation. Based on the results of this evaluation some of the chemicals may undergo a second level of evaluation and become individual projects. At the project level, detailed hazard, exposure, risk and economic analyses are performed as warranted. Chemicals which are carcinogenic may also enter the process via petitions submitted to the Commission by outside parties.[5]

Chemicals which enter the screening process have been tested or evaluated for chronic health effects including carcinogenicity, mutagenicity, teratogenicity, other reproductive effects, and neurotoxicity. In practice, the majority of evaluations to date have been devoted to examining chemicals which are potential carcinogens. Several sources of information are consulted to identify chemicals for the screening process including the National Toxicology Program's (NTP) Carcinogen Bioassay Program and the monographs of the International Agency for Research on Cancer. The screening process also examines reports of chemicals tested by industry and other private groups, or forwarded to CPSC either directly or through cooperation with the Environmental Protection Agency (EPA). Lists of chemicals of potential health concern developed by the EPA, the National Institute for Occupational Safety and Health (NIOSH), and the Occupational Safety and Health Administration (OSHA) are examined and compared to lists developed by the Program. While no comprehensive review of the scientific literature is attempted, reports and published articles discussing chemical hazard testing are also entered into the screening process.

Chemicals selected for evaluation from the various sources listed above are entered into a data base, the System for Tracking the Inventory of Chemicals (STIC), which serves as the core of the CPSC screening process. Approximately 1,000 chemicals have been entered into the STIC. Chemicals in the STIC are prioritized by an interdisciplinary working group which selects those that further merit toxicity or economic review. To date, about 40 chemicals have progressed to the point of having both health and economics reviews. For these chemicals, key primary and secondary references are used to define chemical and physical properties, metabolic and pharmacokinetic data, as well as data on human and animal toxicity. The economic reviews provide data on the production volumes of chemicals, the fraction of production used in consumer products, products using the chemical in question and the amount of the chemical present in product formulations. These data provide the basis for a screening recommendation on whether the potential chronic health risks of a chemical warrant in-depth review as individual projects.

In-Depth Chemical Evaluation

An in-depth evaluation of the biological hazard posed by a chemical entails a critical analysis of the relevant primary literature to determine if, on balance, the data indicate that a chronic hazard is likely to exist for exposed humans. The degree to which different studies support or conflict with each other is assessed. The health review does not attempt to determine whether studies fit specific criteria, but rather addresses the level of confidence that the staff has in the biological data on a case-by-case basis and the applicability of the data to humans. The process of preparing health evaluation documents at the CPSC thus has much in common with that utilized by other Federal agencies or academic institutions.

It is in the chemical exposure assessment that differences between Federal agencies become apparent and it is this area which probably most distinguishes the CPSC's efforts from the activities of other agencies. Accordingly, exposure assessments will be discussed in some detail here.

Performing an exposure assessment is frequently one of the most resource demanding phases of CPSC's evaluation of a chemical hazard. It is noteworthy that most of the contract funds for Health Sciences are used for this purpose. The range of uses of single chemical compounds in consumer products is great and the ways in which consumers utilize any given product may vary considerably. For example, the techniques required for assessing exposure to a gas that may be emitted from building materials into home air on a continuous basis are quite different from those used to assess intermittant exposure from a point source. Exposure may also involve the dermal or oral routes depending on the use scenarios. As a result, CPSC approaches exposure assessments on a case-by-case basis with most reviews requiring original experimental or theoretical work. Overall, the general activity of exposure assessment can be described as a four step process:

1. Determine the release of a compound from products and estimate the quantity of release. The degree of difficulty of this step can vary greatly. For example, a preliminary assessment may be straightforward if, for example, the compound of interest is volatile and contained in an aerosol product. It may require extensive experimental study if the compound is contained in a plastic matrix that is subjected to a variety of uses and environments. More often than not, in CPSC's experience, extensive experimental studies are required to determine exposure levels. Even if the substance is readily available from a consumer product, additional studies may be required to determine if the substances can enter the body and in what form.

2. Relate the quantity of the chemical released to the level of human ex-

posure from use of the products. A series of analyses are required for this step. First, use patterns for the products must be determined; the most typical use patterns and those that could lead to lower or higher degrees of exposure must be considered. Staff experience, information from industry, and consumer surveys can provide this information. Then, for a specific use, the data on chemical release must be used to estimate the actual amount of contact that the user may have with the chemical. Thus, for a chemical emitted into the home air, data on release rate, use patterns, home or room volume, air exchange rate, suppression factors and "sinks" must be combined, to the extent feasible, in a mathematical model to estimate the average and extremes of levels in the air. Modeling results are confirmed wherever possible by field validation studies.

3. Determine the degree and rate of entry of the material into the body and its metabolic fate. This step can be relatively straightforward if the chemical in question is volatile and the toxicity information was obtained by inhalation exposure. On the other hand, in the case of dermal exposure, data on absorption of a compound are frequently lacking. In that case experimental studies, such as painting the skin of an experimental animal with a radiolabeled form of the compound of interest, may be conducted. Finally, if the product in question releases non-violatile particulates, the problem becomes even more complex. The form in which the chemical enters the body and its metabolic fate thereafter are other factors that also need to be considered.

4. Combine the data from steps one through three to assess the degree of human exposure to a compound.

While these four steps are presented as one sequence, exposure estimation is often an interactive procedure. For example, available limited information may be used to make preliminary estimates of risk which may (if sufficiently low) eliminate concern about exposure or may be successively refined by gathering data where they are most needed.

Assessing exposure from chemicals in consumer products is a developing science which makes innovative use of standard physical and chemical data, demands development of new experimental procedures, and combines relatively "hard" experimental data with "soft" data on widely varying human behavior patterns. While each exposure assessment is a new undertaking, certain basic techniques (such as air level modeling) are finding repeated application. Perhaps in the next several years the knowledge now being gained will lead to more readily standardized and more easily performed exposure assessments.

Data from the biological hazard evaluation and the exposure assessment can form the basis for a quantitative assessment of the human health risk. The Commission staff performs risk estimates from exposure to carcinogens when the underlying hazard and exposure data are of sufficient quality and quantity to support a meaningful assessment. The CPSC does not have a formal set of procedures that are utilized for risk assessment. The models selected and the assumptions adopted for a particular risk assessment are chosen after consideration of all relevant data. In performing risk assessments, the CPSC staff has generally presented a range of estimates that are obtained by using different assumptions or models. One or more of the models that predict linearity of risk *versus* dose at low doses have been used in risk assessments, where appropriate, by the CPSC primarily because of the cogent arguments for low dose linearity when compounds may interact with background carcinogenic processes.[6] Other types of models have been included in risk assessments involving chemicals where such interaction may not occur, as in the case of diethylhexyl phthalate.[7] In preparing risk assessment documents, the CPSC staff has placed emphasis on clearly stating the assumptions used in deriving the numerical estimates and in indicating the substantial uncertainties associated with them.

In concert with a health hazard evaluation the Commission will often conduct other work. For example, an economic evaluation is needed to address product alternatives that can reduce chemical exposures; or specific product engineering questions may arise. Most significantly, CPSC is now required to obtain the advice of a Chronic Hazard Advisory Panel (CHAP) before beginning regulatory action on a chemical. The timing of a Commission decision to convene a CHAP typically occurs after the staff review of a chemical hazard. The analysis conducted by a CHAP then can supplement and buttress internal CPSC evaluation efforts.

CHEMICAL CARCINOGENS EVALUATED BY CPSC

Thus far we have discussed the legal framework under which CPSC can regulate carcinogens as well as the Commission's policies for dealing with carcinogens, the uniqueness of the products regulated and, in general, the types of data required. In order to provide the reader with some sense as to how these factors come together in CPSC's regulation of carcinogens, it may be useful to discuss the specific actions taken by the Commission with regard to various carcinogens. This will, of necessity, be a relatively short list of examples as the Commission has dealt on an in-depth basis only with six individual carcinogens and two classes of carcinogens, each of which has presented different types of data.

Vinyl Chloride

The initial foray of the CPSC into the regulation of carcinogens involved vinyl chloride, a chemical used as a propellant in self-pressurized (aerosol) products. The Commission voted in 1974 to declare self-pressurized household products containing vinyl chloride as banned hazardous substances under the FHSA.[8] In this instance the Commission relied upon health hazard data gathered by OSHA to support its ban. The two lines of evidence cited by the Commission in support of its action were: 1) Human data showing an increased incidence of liver angiosarcomas in workers in plants manufacturing polyvinyl chloride and/or vinyl chloride monomers; and 2) animal data showing that the inhalation of vinyl chloride caused rats to develop various tumors including liver angiosarcomas. Manufacturers of self-pressurized household products containing vinyl chloride were required to identify themselves to the Commission and provide information on sales, use patterns and health-related data. The Commission also required that manufacturers repurchase any products containing vinyl chloride from consumers.

The rule was subsequently overturned on procedural grounds, but by then the manufacture of self-pressurized household products containing vinyl chloride had ceased. The Commission subsequently published a revised rule to assure that such products did not re-enter the marketplace.[9] This first regulation of a carcinogen by the Commission was noteworthy in that the Commission did not perform its own health assessment, did not perform an exposure assessment, and made no attempt to estimate risk.

Tris(2,3-Dibromopropyl) Phosphate

The Commission's second attempt to ban the use of a carcinogen in consumer products involved tris(2,3-dibromopropyl) phosphate (TRIS). TRIS was used to treat children's sleepwear and other wearing apparel made with polyester, acetate or triacetate in order to meet flammability requirements for children's sleepwear. In 1977, a bioassay conducted by the National Cancer Institute (NCI) demonstrated that TRIS administered in the diet caused liver, kidney, stomach and lung tumors in mice and kidney tumors in rats.[10] TRIS was also shown to be mutagenic in several short-term tests including the Ames test.[11] No human carcinogenicity data were available.

As part of its investigation of the hazards posed by exposure to TRIS, the Commission performed a series of studies demonstrating that ^{14}C-TRIS could penetrate the skin of rats and rabbits either by itself or following release from impregnated cloth.[12,13] These latter studies were particularly relevant to polyester fabric where TRIS was padded on as a fabric after-treatment. The Commission utilized available data to estimate the potential exposure from the mouthing of TRIS-treated apparel by young children.[14] Data from this exposure assessment and the NCI's bioassay were utilized along with methodology developed by Brown *et al.*[14] (single hit and log probit models) to estimate the increased risk of kidney cancer from TRIS in exposed children. Thus, in this instance, the Commission performed its own analysis of the hazard presented by a carcinogen and established a pattern of analysis which has been followed in all subsequent evaluations of carcinogens. The hazard and risk analyses for TRIS were somewhat abbreviated and lacked the sophistication of later assessments, but the exposure analysis was fairly complete even by present standards. A regulatory decision was made declaring unwashed (washing removes readily available TRIS) or unsold TRIS-treated children's wearing apparel a banned hazardous substance under the FHSA, but not to require a recall as in the case of vinyl chloride.[14] The Commission's ruling was subsequently set aside on procedural grounds by a U.S. District Court. The Commission later adopted a statement of policy that TRIS-treated children's garments were banned hazardous substances for enforcement purposes.[15]

Benzene

In 1978, the Commission proposed to ban benzene as an intentional ingredient or as a contaminant (at 0.1% or above) in consumer products with the exception of gasoline and laboratory solvents.[16] As a basis for this ban under the CPSA, the Commission cited an increased risk of blood disorders, chromosomal abnormalities and leukemia. The Commission was particularly concerned about consumer exposure to benzene in paint removers and rubber cements. Gasoline was exempted because it was considered more appropriately to be under the jurisdiction of OSHA, EPA or the National Highway Traffic Safety Administration. There was, additionally, concern about the major economic impact of regulating benzene in gasoline. The choice of less than 0.1% benzene as a contaminant was based on existing economic information as well as on analytical data derived from a product survey. The Commission performed both an exposure assessment and a risk assessment to support the proposed regulation. The hazard evaluation relied upon both human (primarily) and animal data and was based upon a report prepared by a consultant for the Commission (a more extensive review was subsequently prepared by the Health Sciences staff as the Commission's evaluation proceeded).[16] As in the case with TRIS, the exposure assessment attempted to be as realistic as possible and ultimately involved chamber studies to measure actual concentrations of benzene in air from the use of benzene-containing paint strippers.[17,18] Based on a projection of ten uses of 5 hours each in a lifetime, an increase in the risk of leukemia was predicted from the use of paint strippers.[16] The effects of the proposed ban on the cost, utility and availability of benzene-containing products were also considered. The Commission did not finalize its proposed rule on benzene because, by 1980, in response to the Commission's action and other factors, the use of benzene in consumer products was virtually nonexistent. The proposed ban was withdrawn in 1981.[19]

Benzidine Congener Dyes

A similar course of action to that of benzene was followed in the case of benzidine congener dyes. These dyes became a Commission project as a result of a petition from various arts and crafts groups in 1978.[20] They were used extensively in consumer (home use) dyes as well as in commercial dyeing. The Commission conducted an extensive hazard evaluation of these dyes, some of which were known carcinogens.[20] Included in their evaluation were the findings of studies performed by the NTP at the Commission's request.[21] These studies demonstrated that benzidine congener dyes (*i.e.*, those diazo dyes with either benzidine, o-anisidine or o-tolidine as the core molecule) were capable of being metabolized by Fischer 344 rats to their respective bases, all of which are carcinogenic in animals and one of which, benzidine, is a human carcinogen.

The Commission was originally concerned about exposure to these dyes via ingestion, inhalation and dermal absorption. Subsequent studies indicated that inhalation of consumer dyes presented a rather small risk to consumers because of the small amounts of dye actually becoming airborne during pouring. There were a number of instances of dye ingestion by children, but the major potential route of exposure was projected to occur via dermal absorption from consumer-dyed clothing. The Commission determined that selected benzidine congener dyes were released from consumer-dyed apparel items under simulated conditions of use.[21] Additionally, the Commission determined that there was essentially no breakdown of these dyes by bacteria typically found on human skin.[21] Finally, the Commission initiated studies to determine whether radiolabeled benzidine congener dyes could penetrate rabbit skin. Within the limits of the test, the representative dyes tested were found not to be able to penetrate rabbit skin in measurable amounts even under occluded conditions.[21] Since use of these dyes had virtually ceased in the consumer and commercial dye markets by 1982 (with cessation of the former essentially eliminating the risk of ingestion), no regulatory action was deemed necessary.

Asbestos

The Commission took its first action on asbestos in 1977 when it banned the use of asbestos-containing patching compounds (mostly for dry wall use) and artificial fireplace embers containing free form asbestos.[22] In developing this regulation, the Commission reviewed the occupational data on the risks of cancer from exposure to asbestos and reports of mesothelioma resulting from non-occupational exposure to asbestos. For patching compounds, controlled studies of exposure of workmen during installation of dry wall demonstrated that exposures to asbestos above the occupational limits occurred. No exposure data for emberizing compounds were available, so the Commission estimated the potential degree of exposure using the nature of the product and its intended use. A risk assessment using human data was performed to quantitate consumer risk from the use of patching compounds.[22]

In 1979, the Commission undertook a second major project on asbestos involving hairdryers containing asbestos heat shields.[23] CPSC contracted with the National Institute for Occupational Safety and Health to measure the quantities of asbestos released from these hair dryers;[24] measurable asbestos release was demonstrated. Instead of undertaking a formal rulemaking under Section 15 of CPSA, the CPSC negotiated with hairdryer manufacturers, and developed voluntary agreements under which manufacturers stopped the use of asbestos shields and provided refunds or product replacements to past purchasers of these products.

CPSC continued its investigation of asbestos by publishing an Advanced Notice of Proposed Rulemaking indicating CPSC's plans to initiate regulation of products which could expose consumers to asbestos. Many relevant comments and a great deal of information were received from manufacturers and others.[25] The Commission followed this notice with a General Order requiring manufacturers of a selected list of products, mostly appliances, to inform the CPSC of the use of asbestos in their products.[26] Upon review of the data obtained, the CPSC staff determined that the uses reported were not likely to lead to consumer exposures to asbestos. The CPSC subsequently initiated a study (still in progress) to measure asbestos released from a number of products containing bulk asbestos which are still in the marketplace in small quantities.

In conjunction with this work the CPSC convened a Chronic Hazard Advisory Panel to review data on the hazards of exposure to asbestos. This expert panel met over a six month period and prepared a final report to CPSC in July, 1983.[27] This report, together with product testing data, will enable the Commission to decide on the appropriateness of regulatory action on the remaining uses of asbestos in consumer products. The Commission is also studying the problem of asbestos installed in older homes.[28]

Formaldehyde

The investigation of formaldehyde represents perhaps the single largest expenditure of Commission resources for evaluation of chemical hazard and risk. The Commission was particularly concerned by the large number of complaints received from residents of homes insulated with urea-formaldehyde foam insulation (UFFI).[29] A variety of health effects, primarily acute, was described. These ranged from irritation of eyes, nose and throat to nausea, dizziness, and head-aches, to lower respiratory disorders and allergic reactions. In early 1980 the Commission considered the possibility of a labeling rule warning consumers of the adverse health effects that could result from the installation of this product into the walls of their homes and then, in fact, proposed such a rule.[29]

The Commission requested the National Academy of Sciences (NAS) to re-view the available data on formaldehyde[30] and also began its own extensive re-view of the literature.[31] The Commission's concern was heightened by the an-nouncement of the initial findings of the Chemical Industry Institute of Toxi-cology (CIIT) showing that rats exposed to formaldehyde gas developed a rare form of nasal cancer.[31] The assistance of the NTP was requested in forming a panel of Federal government scientific experts to evaluate the chronic effects of formaldehyde (an area not addressed by the NAS report which was completed prior to the availability of the CIIT data). The Federal panel determined that formaldehyde was a carcinogen in rats, that it was mutagenic, and that it should be presumed to pose a carcinogenic risk to man (direct evidence of carcinogen-icity in man was inconclusive).[32] The panel also suggested that the Commission use the multistage model in any risk assessments it might wish to perform. Based on its analysis of all available data, including the Federal Panel and the NAS re-ports, as well as the infeasibility of developing a standard, and its own extensive exposure studies, the Commission proposed in early 1981 to ban UFFI.[31] The specific concerns cited were that UFFI presented an unreasonable risk of injury to exposed consumers from irritation, sensitization and cancer, and that there was no feasible standard which would adequately protect the public. The ban applied both to residences and to schools. For a recent review of the health ef-forts of formaldehyde, *see* Ulsamer *et al.*[33]

In addition to its extensive hazard assessment, the Commission determined the release of formaldehyde from UFFI foamed into simulated wall cavities by major manufacturers under ideal conditions.[6] All products tested were found to emit formaldehyde and to continue to do so over an 18-month period. The Com-mission also determined that formaldehyde emissions increased dramatically as the temperature increased.[6] Levels in homes were projected by modeling and agreed well with a large body of data on formaldehyde levels in existing UFFI homes.[6] These latter data clearly demonstrated that installation of UFFI signifi-cantly increased formaldehyde levels over those found in homes without UFFI. The risk assessment performed by the Commission staff projected an upper estimate of risk of 51 additional cancers/million people exposed from installa-tion of UFFI using the upper confidence limit of the multistage model. The Commission also determined that substitute forms of insulation were available for almost all UFFI-use situations and that the cost of these alternates was prob-ably less than UFFI with comparable or superior effectiveness. The cost of ban-ning UFFI to the industry, some of whom installed other types of insulation, was found not to outweigh the benefits of a ban. The Commission voted to ban UFFI under Section 8 of the CPSA in early 1982 following a review of submitted comments. This ban was subsequently overturned by the 5th Circuit Court of Appeals following an industry suit in April, 1983.[34] The Court's decision was based on both scientific and procedural grounds (*i.e.*, use of CPSA rather than FHSA). The Court agreed that there was a problem but stated that the Commission failed to quantify precisely either the acute or chronic risk. With regard to the Commission's chronic risk assessment, the Court stated that virtually all of the available data (including the CIIT study and the exposure data) were inadequate to allow a *precise* quantitation of risk. A thorough discussion of this decision may be found in a recent review article by Ashford *et al.*[35] Although the Court's decision contained numerous major scientific errors, which caused the Department of Justice to petition for a rehearing, the Court refused to be persuaded by the arguments offered and made only a minor correction in its ruling. The Justice Department subsequently decided not to appeal the case to the Supreme Court.

More recently, the Formaldehyde Consensus Workshop (October 2-6, 1983) preliminarily concluded that: The CIIT study is adequate for risk assessment; use of the upper limit of the multistage model is one method of choice for estimating the increased risk of cancer from formaldehyde exposure; existing data clearly show that UFFI homes have higher levels of ambient formaldehyde than non-UFFI homes; and that, although people (depending on the level of exposure) experience irritation reactions from exposure to formaldehyde, the data are inadequate for quantitatively assessing the risk of experiencing such acute effects. The Commission is presently monitoring the UFFI industry for signs of resurgence and is convening a CHAP to examine the chronic effects of exposure to formaldehyde prior to any possible regulatory decision either on UFFI, or on other formaldehyde-containing products.[36]

The Commission is also examining the release of formaldehyde from pressed wood products and the potential health effects that may result from such exposure.

Diethylhexyl Phthalate and Nitrosamines

Two final examples of the Commission's experience with carcinogens involve diethylhexyl phthalate (DEHP) and nitrosamines. DEHP is used as a plasticizer in polyvinyl chloride products. The Commission was most concerned about exposure of infants via dermal absorption (*i.e.*, from crib bumpers and mattresses as well as from playpen liners) and ingestion (*e.g.*, pacifiers, teething rings and toys). DEHP has been shown to be carcinogenic in rats and mice but has not been shown to be genotoxic based upon the data evaluated in the Commission's extensive hazard assessment. The exposure assessment involved determination of phthalate transfer from products where dermal exposure is likely to occur, using simulated dermal exposure (*i.e.*, fabric treated with lanolin that is rubbed over the vinyl products) as well as simulated mouthing (*i.e.*, using artificial and real saliva as well as a gas-driven piston to simulate gumming).[7] The Commission additionally determined that radiolabel from ^{14}C-DEHP can penetrate rabbit skin. These data, as well as those obtained from the simulated dermal exposure study, were then modeled to estimate exposure. The subsequent risk assessment projected an increase, under some scenarios, in cancer for infants exposed to DEHP-containing products. Since DEHP has not been demonstrated to be genotoxic, several risk models were chosen to cover both possibilities (*i.e.*, genotoxic *versus* non-genotoxic). For the genotoxicity case, the multistage model upper confidence limit was chosen; for the non-genotoxicity case, the probit model was chosen. The latter model was used in two modes: The first assumed additivity with background and the second assumed independence of background. Background as used here refers to ongoing carcinogenic processes in the body as well as exposure to other carcinogenic substances. Based on the hazard assessment and the range of risk estimates provided, the Commission voted to convene a CHAP.

In the case of nitrosamines in pacifiers, the Commission has also performed extensive exposure testing demonstrating the release of nitrosamines from pacifiers into artificial saliva.[37] The Commission analyzed the available hazard data which clearly demonstrated that nitrosamines are animal carcinogens and mutagens. The amount of nitrosamines released from individual pacifiers varies since these chemicals are not added directly to the rubber but rather are formed from amine precursors used as accelerators and stabilizers. The available cancer data, unfortunately, are less than ideal for purposes of estimating risk for a number of reasons. These include less than lifetime exposure, use of single doses, and the fact that all animals developed cancer. In addition, although newborn animals appear to be more sensitive to the carcinogenic effects of nitrosamines than older animals, there is no way at present to factor this into the risk assessment. Nor is there any way at present to factor in the increased risk from nitrosatable amines released from the pacifiers concomitantly with the nitrosamines. The Commission accordingly decided to proceed without a risk assessment and issued an enforcement policy under the FHSA which took effect on January 1, 1984.[38] This policy, which the Commission announced jointly with FDA on December 27, 1983, (the FDA policy dealt with rubber baby nipples), establishes an action level, based on present technology, of 60 ppb nitrosamine (as measured following extraction by methylene chloride).

SUMMARY AND CONCLUSIONS

From what has been presented above, it is apparent that the Commission's involvement with carcinogens is a relatively recent one. It is also clear that it is an evolving process that has moved from a fairly simple level, relying heavily on the work of other Federal agencies, to a much more complex level that may entail several years of work to gather and evaluate the data necessary to project the degree of hazard posed by a particular chemical. In lieu of a formal cancer policy, the Commission has evaluated each carcinogen on a case-by-case basis using accepted scientific principles. The Commission has also worked closely with other Federal agencies toward the development of uniform methodologies for the evaluation of carcinogens and the assessment of risk from exposure to carcinogens. It is in this latter area, exposure, that the CPSC frequently finds itself in a unique situation. The products regulated by the Commission are distinct from those considered by other agencies and the development of the methodologies required to assess exposures from such products is a major part of the Commission's efforts to deal with carcinogens.

Agency efforts to deal with human exposure to carcinogens are becoming ever more complicated and time consuming. This is the result of both the amount and complexity of the data being evaluated and of the degree of scientific evidence required by changing legal and policy requirements. Beyond the scientific issues, one must also consider the costs of regulation to both the consumer and the industry against the projected benefits, the necessity of having a product on the market, and the availability of substitutes (and the hazards posed thereby). There is the distinct danger that the process may become so costly and involved, that very few carcinogens may ultimately be regulated. It is clear that a balancing of varied interests will have to be accomplished in order to adequately protect the public good and at the same time to avoid excessive regulation. In this regard the reestablishment of formal interagency cooperation in dealing with carcinogenic substances is a step in the right direction.

REFERENCES

1. Merrill, R.A., CPSC Regulation of cancer risks in consumer products: 1972–1981. *Virginia Law Review* 67: 1261-1375 (1981)
2. Consumer Product Safety Commission Interim Policy and Procedure for Classifying, Evaluating and Regulating Carcinogens in Consumer Products. *Fed. Register* 43: 25,658-25,665 (1978)
3. Consumer Product Safety Commission Interim Policy and Procedure for Carcinogens: Withdrawal of Statement of Policy and Procedure. *Fed. Register* 44: 23,821-23,822 (1979)
4. Interagency Regulatory Liaison Group, Work Group on Risk Assessment, Scientific Bases for Identification of Potential Carcinogens and Estimation of Risks. *J. Natl. Cancer Inst.* 63: 241-268 (1979)
5. Preuss, P.W., The elimination of carcinogenic risks in consumer products. *Ann. N.Y. Acad. Sci.* 363: 63-78 (1981)
6. Cohn, M.S., Revised carcinogenic risk assessment of urea-formaldehyde foam insulation: Estimates of cancer risk due to inhalation of formaldehyde released by UFFI. *Fed. Register* 47: 14,366-14,421 (1982)
7. Cohn, M.S., Risk Assessment on Di(2-ethylhexyl)phthalate in Children's Products. Briefing Package Prepared by the Chronic Hazards Program Staff (Aug., 1983)
8. Consumer Product Safety Commission, Self-pressurized household substances containing vinyl chloride monomer. Classification as banned hazardous substance. *Fed. Register* 39: 30,112-30,114 (1974)
9. Consumer Product Safety Commission, Self-pressurized household substances containing vinyl chloride monomer. Withdrawal of classification as banned hazardous substance. *Fed. Register* 43: 12,308-12,310 (1978)
10. Department of Health, Education and Welfare, Bioassay of TRIS (2,3-Dibromopropyl)phosphate for Possible Carcinogenicity. *DHEW Publication No. (NIH) 78-1326, Technical Report Series* No. 76 (1978).
11. Blum, A., and Ames, B.N., Flame-retardant additives as possible cancer hazards. *Science* 195: 17-23 (1977)
12. Ulsamer, A.G., Osterberg, R.E., and McLaughlin, J., Flame retardant chemicals in textiles. *Clin. Toxicol.* 17: 101-131 (1981)
13. Ulsamer, A.G., Porter, W.K., and Osterberg, R.E., Percutaneous absorption of radiolabeled TRIS from flame-retarded fabric. *J. Environ. Pathol. Toxicol.* 1: 543-549 (1978)
14. Consumer Product Safety Commission, Children's wearing apparel containing TRIS: Interpretation as a banned hazardous substance. *Fed. Register* 42: 18,849-18,854 (1977)

15. Consumer Product Safety Commission, TRIS, TRIS-treated wearing apparel and other products containing TRIS. *Fed. Register* 42: 61,621-61,622 (1977)
16. Consumer Product Safety Commission, Proposed rule to regulate consumer products containing benzene as an intentional ingredient or as a contaminant under the CPSA. *Fed. Register* 43: 21,837-21,854 (1978)
17. Callahan, J.F., Dorsey, R.W., Crouse, C.L., and Feeney, J.J., Final report on chamber descriptions, operating parameters, and test results obtained in studies designed to measure the volatilization rate of benzene spiked paint removers under both static and dynamic air flow conditions. Prepared for the Consumer Product Safety Commission under CPSC-IAG-80-1376, Task Order #2 by the Toxicology Research Branch, Research Division, Chemical Systems Laboratory, Aberdeen Proving Ground (June 22, 1981)
18. Johnson, W.C., Final report on chemical analysis used in tests designed to measure the volatilization rate of benzene spiked paint removers under both static and dynamic air flow conditions. Prepared for the Consumer Product Safety Commission under CPSC-IAG-80-1376, Task Order #2 by the Analytical Branch, Research Division, Chemical Systems Laboratory, Aberdeen Proving Ground (Mar. 9, 1981)
19. Consumer Product Safety Commission, Benzene-containing consumer products; proposed withdrawal of proposed rule. *Fed. Register* 46: 3034-3036 (1981)
20. Fausett, R.S., Briefing package on benzidine congener dyes prepared by the Chronic Chemical Hazards Program Staff (Sept. 24, 1980)
21. Gerber, A.I., Benzidine congener dyes—final recommendations. Prepared by the Chemical Hazards Program Staff (April 26, 1983)
22. Consumer Product Safety Commission, Consumer patching compounds and artificial emberizing materials (embers and ash) containing respirable free-form asbestos; Final rule. *Fed. Register* 42: 63,354-63,365 (1977)
23. Consumer Product Safety Commission, Hair driers containing asbestos; Proposed rule to regulate under the Consumer Product Safety Act. *Fed. Register* 44: 28,828-28,830 (1979)
24. Geraci, C.E., Baron, P.A., Carter, J.W., and Smith, O.L., Testing of hair driers for asbestos emissions, Report for the Consumer Product Safety Commission (Sept., 1979)
25. Consumer Product Safety Commission, Consumer products containing asbestos; Advanced Notice of Proposed Rulemaking. *Fed. Register* 44: 60057-60068 (1979)
26. Consumer Product Safety Commission, Consumer products containing asbestos; General order for submission of information. *Fed. Register* 45: 84384-84388 (1980)
27. Asbestos CHAP Report, Chronic Hazard Advisory Panel on Asbestos, Report to the U.S. Consumer Product Safety Commission (July, 1983)
28. Consumer Product Safety Commission and Environmental Protection Agency, Asbestos in the home (August, 1982)
29. Consumer Product Safety Commission, Urea-formaldehyde foam insulation: Proposed notice to purchasers. Fed. Register 45: 39,434-39,444 (1980)
30. National Research Council, Formaldehyde—an assessment of its health effects. Washington, D.C.: National Academy of Sciences, 38 pp. (1980)
31. Consumer Product Safety Commission, Urea-formaldehyde foam insulation; proposed ban; denial of petition. *Fed. Register* 46: 11,188-11,211 (1981)
32. Griesemer, R.A., Ulsamer, A.G., Arcos, J.C., Beall, J.R., Blair, A.E., Collins,

T.F.X., *et al.*, Report of the Federal panel on formaldehyde. *Environ. Health Perspect.* 43: 139–168 (1982)

33. Ulsamer, A.G., Beall, J.R., Kang, H.K., and Frazier, J.A., in: *Hazard Assessment of Chemicals* 3: 337–400 (1984)

34. Fifth Circuit Court, Gulf South Insulation *vs.* Consumer Product Safety Commission. 701 Fed. Rep. 2nd Ser. 1137 (1983)

35. Ashford, N.A., Ryan, C.W., and Caldart, C.C., Law and science policy in federal regulation of formaldehyde. *Science* 222: 894–900 (1983)

36. Consumer Product Safety Commission, CPSC still concerned about formaldehyde health risks. Press Release (Oct. 21, 1983)

37. Schmeltzer, D., Nitrosamines in pacifiers, ongoing investigation and proposed voluntary standard. Briefing Package prepared by the Directorate for Compliance and Administrative Litigation (Oct. 13, 1983)

38. Consumer Product Safety Commission, Children's products containing nitrosamines; enforcement policy. *Fed. Register* 48: 56988–56990 (1983)

30

International Aspects of Testing for Carcinogenicity and Regulation: A Selected Bibliography

William H. Farland

U.S. Environmental Protection Agency
Washington, D.C.

INTRODUCTION

The last decade has seen a change in a large number of national legislations relating to the control of chemical risks throughout the world. In addition, international organizations such as the World Health Organization (WHO) and the Organization for Economic Cooperation and Development (OECD) have begun the task of assembling data and providing guidance on the testing of such chemicals for potential health and environmental effects, including cancer. In general, such activities have been stimulated by the facts that 1) the scope of the laws tends to emphasize manufactured or imported chemical substances; 2) the laws take a broad approach to the protection of human health and the environment rather than focusing on individual effects; and 3) the laws often seek to anticipate risks posed by exposure to chemicals and focus on the means to assess "new" chemicals and "new" risks posed by existing chemicals. The OECD, in a number of publications, lists the following laws as belonging to this new generation of legislation on environmental chemicals:

Canada: Environmental Contaminants Act, 23-24 Elizabeth II, 2nd December, 1975, Canada Gazette Pt. III Vol 1, No. 12.

Denmark: Act No. 212 of 23rd May, 1979, on Chemical Substances and Products (Lov om kemiske stoffer og produkter), Lovtidende A, 538.

France: Act No. 77-771 of 12th July, 1977, on the control of chemicals (Loi sur le controle des produits chimiques), J.O. of 13th July, 1977, as amended by Act No. 82-905 of 21st October, 1982.

Germany: Act on Protection against Dangerous Substances (Chemicals Act–Chemikaliengesetz) of 16th September, 1980, Bundesgesetzblatt I, 1718.

Japan: Law concerning the examination and regulation of manufacture, etc. of chemical substances (1973, Law No. 117).

Netherlands: Draft Chemical Substances Act (Ontwerp wet millieugevaarlijke stoffen) of December 1981 (not yet enacted).

New Zealand: Toxic Substances Act 1979 (No. 27, of 19th October, 1979).

Norway: Act on Products Control (Lov om produktkontroll) No. 79 of 11th June, 1976 (Lovtidend p. 441).

Sweden: Act on Products Hazardous to Health and to the Environment (Lag om halso- och miljofarliga varor) of 27th April, 1973 (SFS 1973: 329).

Switzerland: Federal Law on Trade in Toxic Substances (Toxicity Law–Giftgesetz) of 21st March, 1969, SR 814.80.

United Kingdom: Health and Safety at Work etc. Act 1974 (ch. 37, of 31st July, 1974), and Control of Pollution Act 1974 (ch. 40, of 31st July, 1974).

United States: Toxic Substances Control Act, 1976, 90 Stat, 2003, of October 11, 1976.

European Communities: Council Directive of 18 September 1979, amending for the sixth time Directive 67/548/EED on the approximation of the laws, regulations and administrative provisions relating to the classification, packaging and labelling of dangerous substances (79/831/EEC).

Of particular interest in the context of testing for carcinogens is the fact that these laws have tended away from a rigid approach to the categorization of risk and reflect a need for more flexible and scientifically sound approaches to risk assessment.

Such flexibility of approach has led to a proliferation of methodologies for prioritizing, evaluating and characterizing hazards from chemicals such as carcinogenicity and has raised the question of international harmonization of assessment methods. Such harmonization, while viewed as a noble goal, faces obstacles based on the legal findings required to take any of a number of control actions under these various laws. The strongest hope for eventual harmony of assessments (first, of chemical hazards, and second and with more difficulty, of chemical risks) comes from the development of a unified understanding of the scientific basis for such assessments. At issue is guidance on performance and relative utility of short-term, predictive tests for specific effects, chronic studies in animals and epidemiology in both scientific and regulatory decision-making. In this regard, the completed activities of the Chemicals Testing Program and the ongoing activities of the Updating Program, both under the OECD, provide excellent examples of international efforts to obtain a coordinated view of the scientific problems associated with chemical evaluation, and to reach consensus conclusions on their potential solutions.

The following selected list may provide the interested reader with a perspective on the nature of some of the problems relevant to carcinogen testing faced by the international community. These references are meant to complement the more specific work which is cited in previous chapters.

SELECTED BIBLIOGRAPHY

1. Anon, International programme for the evaluation of short-term tests for carcinogenicity. *Mutation Res.* 54: 203–206 (1978)
2. Berenblum, I. (ed.), *Carcinogenicity Testing (IUCC Technical Report Series, No. 2)*, International Union Against Cancer, Geneva, Switzerland (1969)
3. Commission of European Communities Publication, *Decision-Making Process in the Evaluation of New Chemicals in the EC and the USA*. Published for the CEC by the Instituto Superiore della Sanita, Rome, Italy (1982)
4. Commission of European Communities Publication, *Quality Assurance of Toxicological Data*, CEC, Luxembourg (1982)
5. Committee of the Health Council Publication, *The Evaluation of the Carcinogenicity of Chemical Substances*, Ministry of Public Health and Environment, Leidschendam, Netherlands (1979)
6. Dayan, A.D., and Brinblecomb, L.W. (eds.), *Carcinogenicity Testing: Principles and Problems*, MTP Press Ltd, Lancaster, UK (1978)
7. Health and Welfare Canada Publication, *The Testing of Chemicals for Carcinogenicity, Mutagenicity and Teratogenicity*, Department of Health and Welfare, Ottawa, Canada (1973)
8. Henschler, D., *Kriterien zur Bewertung cancerogener Stoffe (Evaluation Criteria for Carcinogenic Substances)*. *Sichere Arbeit* 31 (3): 6–12 (1978)
9. Holmberg, B., Rantanen, J.J., and Arrhenius, E., *Provning och utvardering av carcinogen aktivitet–riktlinjer och synpunkter (Testing and Evaluating Carcinogenic Activity–Rules and Considerations*, Arbetarskyddsstyrelsen, Selna, Sweden (1979)
10. IARC Monographs on the Evaluation of the Carcinogenic Risk of Chemicals to Humans, Supplement 2, *Long-term and short-term screening assays for carcinogens: A critical appraisal*, International Agency for Research on Cancer, Lyon, France (1980)
11. INSERM Publication, *Carcinogenic Risk and Strategies for Intervention*, INSERM Symposia Series, Vol. 74, Paris, France (1979)
12. Institute of Occupational Health Symposium, *Prevention of Occupational Cancer–International Symposium*, International Labor Office, Geneva, Switzerland (1982)
13. Montesano, R., Bartsch, H., and Tomatis, L. (eds.), *Molecular and Cellular Aspects of Carcinogen Screening Tests (IARC Scientific Publication No. 27)* (1980)
14. OECD Publication, *OECD Guidelines for Testing of Chemicals*, Organization for Economic Cooperation and Development, Paris, France (1981)

15. Schlegel, H., Berufskrebs (Occupational Cancer). *Schweizerische Rundschau fur Medizin (Praxis)* 70 (20): 892–897 (1981)

16. Smagghe, G. and Millischer, R., Les experiences toxicologiques (Toxicological Experimentation). *Cahiers de Medicine Interprofessionnelle* 21 (82): 33–49 (1981)

17. WHO Publication, *Principles and Methods for Evaluating the Toxicity of Chemicals (Environmental Health Criteria 6)*, Part 1, Geneva, Switzerland (1978)

Part X

Industry Perspective

31

An Industrial Perspective on Testing for Carcinogenicity

Donald E. Stevenson

Shell Development Company
Houston, Texas

Paul F. Deisler, Jr.

Shell Oil Company
Houston, Texas

INTRODUCTION

Industry is as diverse as society itself. Indeed, industry is an integral part of society, it permeates and affects in one way or another every segment of society, and it is a chief economic supporter of society.

Industry's diversity makes it difficult, perhaps impossible, to present a "unified industry" view on cancer or carcinogenicity testing. Some industries and individual companies, for example, have been aware for many years of the potential for their operations to produce adverse health effects in employees or consumers and have taken various precautions. Others, not having encountered specific problems, have become aware of such problems only more recently.

Industry is comprised of enterprises which employ people and other resources to create products and services of value. It is often equated with manufacturing activity, although in reality a broader range of functions is included. Since the Industrial Revolution there has been a continuing movement of the work force from agriculture into manufacturing and then into service industries. Most recently, information-based industries have been increasing rapidly. These trends are similar for all developed countries, although the rates vary. This evolution is accompanied by economic and social changes which affect the way people work and may also be expected to change patterns of health and disease.

Many people work in small establishments where the level of sophistication and understanding of health issues may be lower than in larger establishments which can support a range of health professionals. Clearly, the perspective on health matters will vary according to the industry, the activities of an organization within an industry, the segment of the industry under consideration, and the location and size of the operating units. Some industries are capital intensive with few employees per unit of output, whereas others are people intensive. The biggest employers in manufacturing are food and kindred products, apparel and textiles, metal products and machinery, electrical equipment and transportation equipment. Petroleum and coal products, together, constitute one of the smallest employment groups, reflecting the capital intensity of much of their operations whereas chemicals and allied products are of intermediate size. The known health issues vary greatly between the various industrial classifications.

Commercial organizations may face issues which relate solely to their own products, particularly if these are proprietary and patented as is the case for drugs and pesticides. In other cases, several organizations may have similar products or may be involved with a specific segment of an industry — a producer of raw materials, a fabricator or processor, an applicator or a distributor. Where there is a commonality of interest there is usually an organization such as a trade association which functions on behalf of its members. In the United States alone there are many such organizations, some of which are heavily involved in both regulatory activities and in the sponsoring of health research or in the provision of health related information to their members. Since these organizations cover specific industrial sectors, their views will not always be in agreement.

Industry is subject to the same political, social and legal processes as other members of society. Because of the nature, size and continuity of its segments, industry is often regarded as a prime instigator of societal problems and is frequently under attack from other sectors of society. Certainly, industry is easier to regulate than some other sectors of society and this often appears to be the reason why regulatory actions aimed at the reduction of cancer are directed at industry rather than at society as a whole. Furthermore, the public perceives that any additional cost should be borne by industry rather than by themselves, although such cost beating only applies in the short term. A broader effort to reduce cancer would require major changes in individual habits such as eating or smoking which far overshadow industry in their contribution to total cancer.[1,2]

Ease of regulation and progress in the reduction of cancer are not synonymous.

THE GROWTH OF INDUSTRY'S INVOLVEMENT IN
CARCINOGENICITY TESTING

The eighteenth and nineteenth centuries, when the Industrial Revolution occurred, were characterized by urbanization of the population. The major health concerns were infectious diseases and, in industry, the direct toxic effects of such commonly used materials as products containing lead, mercury, arsenic, and phosphorus. Life expectancy in the mid-eighteenth century was about 50 years and cancer was not regarded then as a major cause of death. Hunter[3] provides an account of industrial activities in previous centuries and outlines the types of exposure conditions which occurred before the regulation of industrial activities. During the twentieth century, infectious diseases have been controlled to the extent that today they cause fewer deaths in the United States than accidents and violence. Life expectancy has risen and now, cardiovascular diseases and cancer together cause over two-thirds of all deaths in the United States with camcer causing nearly one-fifth of all mortalities.

Cancer research and carcinogenicity testing reflect the growing awareness of cancer as a major cause of death. Many of the earliest reported cancers related to specific causes were associated with industrial activity, although among the first definitive accounts were instances found in consumers and in workers in a service industry. In 1761, John Gill correlated the use of snuff with the onset of nasal polyps and cancer and in 1775, Sir Percivall Pott described scrotal cancer in chimney sweeps. A hundred years later, other occupations were found to be associated with an increased incidence of scrotal and skin cancer, particularly those which involved extensive contact with pitch, coal, tar, or shale oils.

During the first half of this century an increased cancer risk was shown in occupations involved in uranium mining, the use of radium, nickel refining, chromate manufacture, formulation of arsenicals, working with asbestos, and manufacturing of aromatic dyes. More recently, woodworkers using hardwoods, boot and shoe operators, and other industrially-exposed groups have been shown to have excess nasal cancer. The International Agency for Research on Cancer (IARC)[4] recognized seven industrial processes and 23 chemicals and groups of chemicals as probably linked to carcinogenicity in humans. Materials such as vinyl chloride, bis(chloromethyl)ether and benzene, among others, have been linked to various forms of cancer. A study of these lists is of great interest because any strategy of carcinogenicity testing and regulation should be measured against its ability to detect those carcinogens which have already been identified.

Legislation aimed at controlling health hazards has grown during this century, culminating in the *Occupational Safety and Health Act (1970)*, the *Toxic Substances Control Act (1976)*, as well as legislation covering clean air and water, the disposal of toxic wastes and other environmental toxicity areas. The 1970s were peak years for enacting legislation. Subsequently, activity has centered around regulations and other activities associated with the new legislation. Revisions of existing legislation and new areas of legislation dealing with liability and exposures to toxic substances are now being explored.

Industrial organizations have also developed individual approaches to health and safety as a result of specific issues. Thus today, almost all major industrial concerns have an internal focus for such activities. General toxicity testing did not necessarily follow regulatory initiatives in chronological order in industry, nor did carcinogenicity testing. Efforts to organize the Chemical Industry Institute of Toxicology (CIIT) began in 1974, before the Toxic Substances Control Act (TSCA) was passed. Although the organizational efforts occurred at a time when the congressional debates leading to the ultimate passage of the Act were in progress, the Institute's founders did not then, any more than the Institute does now, have regulatory response in mind as part of its charter. The Institute was founded to provide a scientific presence of outstanding excellence in the field of the toxicology of common or commodity chemicals, funded by the chemical industry and others. Its motivation was to be proactive and not merely reactive in determining the factors bearing on the hazard or safety of such chemicals. Its aim was to inform the public of these findings and to permit the chemical industry to, in the words of the Institute's founding chairman Dr. M.E. Pruitt, "find its own next vinyl chloride" and take the necessary precautionary actions. Indeed, as a well-known example, the Institute has carried out its first chairman's dictum in its studies of formaldehyde[5] and of many other common chemicals.

A second example of jointly sponsored industry efforts which predates the passage of TSCA by many years is the lengthy program of toxicologic studies of crude oils and their fractions and of typical refinery streams and products — highly complex mixtures — funded by the American Petroleum Institute (API). In many of these studies, the focus has been on carcinogenicity. The Institute had traditionally gathered statistics and developed useful literature in the field of accident prevention, fire prevention, and general safety. The early toxicity studies, given the existing knowledge of the carcinogenicity of tars and other materials, were a natural extension of these activities into the field of health safety. Today, the API continues its work to provide general health safety information to its members and to provide the soundest type of information for responding to regulatory requirements under TSCA.

In building their internal forces to carry out and manage their toxicologic testing and research programs, companies in the process industries and the toxicologists themselves have had to go through significant adjustments. For example, agricultural chemical manufacturers, because of the nature of their products and their early regulation, have had a long association with toxicology and toxicologists; indeed, the two fields — the manufacture of the chemicals and toxicology itself — have together grown rapidly over the last two or three decades and have had an opportunity to learn how to communicate with each other. To most other chemical manufacturers, with a few exceptions, and also to oil refiners, the acquisition of their own, internal staffs of toxicologists and related scientists, with or without their own laboratories is a much newer phenomenon. It has taken place largely within the last decade as a result of the fast developing science, the implementation of TSCA's regulatory requirements, the growing legislative load in the toxics area, and the highly litigious atmosphere prevailing in the country.

It has been our experience that there now prevails a general acceptance of the continuing need for toxicologic studies of the highest quality, that the maintenance of the scientific integrity of the scientists is highly important, that the results of testing cannot be predicted, and that a company's organization should be such that the scientist's findings can readily reach the decision making levels where they must be heard so that correct decisions can be reached. Industry scientists who identify adverse health effects of chemicals have a legal obligation to report their findings to their corporation for a decision as to whether the Environmental Protection Agency (EPA) should be notified under TSCA Section 8(e); moreover, if they disagree with that decision they have the legal right to report directly to the EPA. It must be recognized that these same scientists and other health professionals are the very people who are central to answering questions regarding the meaning of their results for human health and the conditions under which products can be manufactured, distributed and used safely. The roles of toxicologists and related health professionals working in industry in today's legal and regulatory atmosphere is a very important one to understand.[6,7]

TESTING: NEEDS, STRATEGIES AND APPROACHES

The approach to carcinogenicity testing which emerged from the 1960's and 1970's was epitomized by a statement in the National Cancer Institute's *Guidelines for Carcinogen Bioassay in Small Rodents:*[8] "Most human cancers are believed to be caused by exposure to extrinsic factors, among which chemical agents are thought to be a major contribution. These factors must be identified, evaluated and controlled if the incidence of human cancer is to be reduced."

This viewpoint may now be regarded as simplistic and obsolete. It is now clear that it cannot ever lead to an appreciable reduction of the total incidence of cancer.[1,2] It has also proved to be very expensive and less informative than was hoped. There is increasing recognition that many of the carcinogens and mutagens to which humans are exposed may be produced incidentally to daily living[9] and have no connection with industry.

If the products of industry affect human health, then an in depth analysis of which populations are exposed to what products, and the degree of likely exposure, is important. Unfortunately, such information is generally unavailable, incomplete, or may be misleading. It is common to find statements in articles on this topic that about 60,000 chemicals are commonly used in industry, that this list is growing by some thousands each year, and that the total number of known chemicals is about three or more million. Furthermore, in order to test all these products at the rate of "x" hundred per year, it would take "y" years to complete — which would take us well into the twenty-first century, if not beyond.

Hoerger[10] pointed out that less than 2% of the commercial chemicals listed in the TSCA inventory represent more than 80% of the production tonnage and that 70% are produced in annual amounts of less than 100,000 pounds. Mobility of employment, the use of replacement substances and many other factors also limit potential exposures to only a proportion of the working life.

The number of about 60,000 chemicals is based on the TSCA inventory list which was drawn up to identify products and chemicals known in 1977. There were practical reasons related to potential future testing requirements for having products listed. The inventory included trade names and a variety of common names so that there is appreciable duplication in the list, *e.g.*, where very similar products are sold by corporations using their own identifying names. In other cases a single product may have several hundred constituents, *e.g.*, gasoline with hundreds of identified constituents, where the composition will vary between suppliers, but, in many cases, without any likely major change in potential hazard.

The use of tonnage as a surrogate for potential exposure can be misleading. The selection of ethyltoluene and trimethylbenzene for proposed testing under TSCA Section 4 was partly based on tonnage. However the vast amounts of these chemicals that are sold are in gasoline where they are very dilute and thus, actual individual exposures are minute. Moreover, the ultimate fate of these substances is to be burned, which further decreases significant exposure. It does not seem sensible to test individual constituents of complex mixtures as a first priority, particularly since such results cannot be used to predict the toxicity of mixtures under conditions of normal exposure. Rather, thorough testing of a limited number of mixtures is called for.

A further problem with using tonnage is that over the years manufacturing practices have changed and even though the tonnage manufactured may have increased, the frequencies and levels of exposure will have decreased. Benzene is a good example. When questions were raised concerning benzene and leukemia and myelotoxicity in the 1960's and 1970's, many chemists were very skeptical; anecdotal information on high personal exposures was universal. Benzene was used for removing stains on clothing, filling cigarette lighters, cleaning glassware and removing grease from hands as well as for more orthodox uses in solvents, in glues, and in pyrolysis gasoline, with up to 25% in some brands in foreign countries. Recognition of the potential health effects and the setting of standards has greatly reduced exposure to the chemical. Exposures to benzene and to many other products has also been reduced as a result of evolving improvements in manufacturing plant design and industrial hygiene practices.

Another consideration in devising testing strategies is the national statistics on cancer. These show that over the last fifty years the age-adjusted incidence of cancer has been very stable, excepting some obvious trends such as the increase in lung tumors and the decrease in tumors of the stomach which are generally explained by changes in smoking and eating habits. During the same period of time, changes in industry have been very large, not only changes in practices and increases in tonnages, but switches of employment from one sector to another and types of goods manufactured and marketed. If industrial activities were responsible for a high proportion of cancer, then large changes in the national statistics would be expected, contrary to actual observations. Historically, industrially related cancer has been detected in small, highly exposed populations, often by clinical observations in single workplaces rather than by large scale epidemiology studies. The follow-up of individual cases, particularly of cancer at unusual sites or of occurrences of neoplasms at an early age, may still prove to be a very valuable source of information.

Thus, graphs which simply plot chemical tonnage *versus* time to suggest that cancer will also increase due to higher exposures are misleading and there is no "cancer epidemic" caused by exposure to industrially derived chemical substances: Such a situation would require drastic and urgent action. There are, however, such things as potential human carcinogens requiring identification, evaluation and control.

Now having some idea of the size and urgency of the problem, we need a strategy for identifying those areas where action will lead to the greatest reduction most quickly and feasibly. Deisler[11] and Deisler *et al*[12] have outlined a step-wise approach to accomplish this in the context of industry. Despite the fact that most of industry is a minor contributor to the total cancer burden, to the extent that it does contribute, the contribution must be reduced.

For some years, the relationship between carcinogenesis in man and animal was a question of belief rather than scientific understanding, although it is now evident that the problems of extrapolation are being perceived more broadly than was true ten years ago. It was then argued that all human carcinogens (with the possible exception of arsenic) were also carcinogenic to animals and that the many other compounds which were known to produce tumors in rats or mice would also produce tumors in man. It was also argued that only about 10% of all chemicals would be found to be carcinogenic and replacement was unlikely to be a problem. It is now realized that of the chemicals tested, a much higher percentage have produced positive results in one system or another — perhaps as high as 30% to 40%. It is now also realized that where the same compound has been tested on different strains of the same species, qualitatively or quantitatively different results were obtained. We are not arguing against the use of animal studies, but rather that the results obtained must be used with great caution and understanding.[13]

During the last ten years there has been a growing awareness that short-term tests may also have a place in indicating potential carcinogens, although indirectly and inferentially.[14,15] As described elsewhere in this book, these tests range from simple biochemical or bacterial assays, to *in vivo* studies of genetic or other endpoints in animals. Just as in animal testing, the results obtained provide valuable information, but similarly there are exceptions and uncertainties to create many dilemmas. These short-term tests do have two desirable features — the quantity of test material required and the time to conduct a test. The potential for being misled may still be high.

The importance of a knowledge of metabolism was emphasized when it was realized that many carcinogens were in fact inactive until converted metabolically to more active forms. The ultimate carcinogens were found to be electrophilic reactants which could bind covalently with macromolecules.[16] There may be important comparative differences in the metabolism of substances by different species and organs which will affect the activity of the chemical. Wright[17] pointed out that there may also be important differences between metabolism *in vivo* and *in vitro*, particularly when enzyme inducers are used to pretreat animals for the preparation of microsomal or S9 fractions for use as activation systems.

THE USE OF TEST RESULTS IN CHARACTERIZING AND ABATING CARCINOGENIC RISKS

The way data are analyzed in the course of risk assessment is as important and deserves as much care and consideration as how the data are obtained. In particular, when considering what to do to abate risk, the 'risk manager' deserves and needs the best analysis of the data unbiased by non-scientific value judgments or policy constraints. For example, a risk assessment based on the use of the most sensitive species may prove to be without value in assessing potential human risk and control measures may be accordingly unrealistic.

For extrapolation, the probit, logit, Weibull, one-hit, multi-hit and multi-stage models are commonly used [*see* References 18 and 19]. The last three have been derived on the basis of overly simple mechanistic considerations which are far more likely not to fail to apply in the case of any specific substance.[20] Thus, all extrapolation models so far in use must be considered simply as flexible, useful, but empirical fitting models, one or more of which will usually give a good fit to data in the experimental dose region. Such results are useful in interpolation but, for the extrapolations of several orders of magnitude needed to go from dose levels typical of animal tests to lower dose levels more like the exposures to which people might be subjected, the different models diverge widely.[18,21] Whether such extrapolations actually provide useful knowledge of risks at low doses is questionable,[11,13,22] and the answer to the question of how well *the test animal's own risks* can be estimated by extrapolation is this: very, very poorly.

It is clear, in fact, that information is needed of a biochemical, metabolic and pharmacokinetic nature to decrease the uncertainty of extrapolation by indicating how animals might respond, compared to the various extrapolations, to place limits on the zone in which the correct values of response rate might lie, or, if sufficient knowledge is obtained, to permit the derivation of an extrapolation model reflecting what is known about the mechanism of action of the test substance. Recently, the derivation of such a function has been published to illustrate, among other things, the dependence of the shape of the dose-response curve on the rate constants of the reactions involved.[23] This model, while hypothetical in nature, is based, in part, on observation of the actions of actual carcinogens.

Developing such a model for animals, while difficult, is facilitated by the fact that direct, controlled, experimentation is possible. That this is not possible for humans for the great bulk of chemical substances leaves a final gap that we have so far been unable to fill by known, ethical means. This is not entirely the case for medicinal drugs, where the risks and benefits are borne by the same individual and where certain experimentation is possible under ethical and legal conditions of informed consent.

In comparing the ranges of estimates of human risk derived by considering both quantitative and qualitative information, extrapolated across species and to low doses characteristic of human exposures, with epidemiologic data when they are available, and considering the large uncertainties inherent in both kinds of results being compared, it is clear that it is not possible to say, *a priori* and in general, which kind of information should carry more weight. Case-by-case analysis is needed with no preconceptions. Although thresholds for carcinogenesis have not been accepted in regulatory practice, Schaeffer[24] concluded that they are consistent with other areas of science and are likely to occur with carcinogens. As he says aptly, "a no-threshold hypothesis is a statement of pessimism". A true generalization is not possible at this time and a search for thresholds in specific cases may be a valuable step forward in protecting human health. This is not a hypothetical argument since research has produced instances of true thresholds and strongly indicates the existence of others. Terephthalic acid is an example of the former[25] while formaldehyde is an example of the latter.[5] In recent years, and especially since the Occupational Safety and Health Administration (OSHA) first proposed a cancer policy[26] for the generic regulation of carcinogens in the work place, certain industry associations have proposed cancer policies of their own. One example of such a policy is that developed by the Food Safety Council (FSC),[18] and another is that developed by the American Industrial Health Council (AIHC).[27]

The AIHC came into being in 1977 as an ad hoc committee of the Synthetic Organic Chemicals Manufacturers Association. Its purpose was to study and respond to the just-proposed OSHA cancer policy and to offer workable alternatives to OSHA where these appeared necessary. It soon became evident that cancer was an issue transcending the interests of a single regulatory agency and by July of 1978, the AIHC became a free-standing trade association of about a hundred companies from many different segments of industry.

Since that time, the AIHC has pursued its mission of developing and proposing the means whereby sound science may be used to provide the best basis for regulatory decisions. This is an extremely important area to industry since many earlier initiatives by regulatory agencies [for example, OSHA,[26] the Interagency Regulatory Liaison Group (IRLG),[28] EPA,[29] the Consumer Products Safety Commission (CPSC)[30]] set policy constraints on the full use of scientific analysis and judgement. The precedence of positive animal data over negative human data was advocated, as was the confounding of science and policy by the inclusion of requirements that thresholds of action should be assumed not to exist for carcinogenesis; that extrapolations should include linearity of response at low doses; that such extrapolations should be made to determine the so-called "upper bound" of risk; and that, only data from the most sensitive animals should be used — despite the fact that such extrapolations can be up to several orders of magnitude in error on the high side in estimating animal response at low doses. Moreover, the estimated responses most likely would have little to do with human responses. The largest experiment ever made, the ED_{01} experiment[31] does not support low dose linearity down to the low doses it employed.[32] These regulatory policy proposals amount to including entirely arbitrary, large, multiple safety factors inside and inextricably intertwined with a so-called "scientific" estimation of risk, instead of first estimating the most likely risk scientifically and then, as a matter of regulatory policy, applying appropriate safety factors. The inherent arbitrariness of these proposals, their *de facto* failure to distinguish degrees of risk, their incommensurability with other important factors in selecting risk abatement options such as cost-effectiveness, and their failure to utilize fully what scientific knowledge is available are among the qualities that industry associations set out to rectify. The confusion of roles of the scientists and the regulators also needed rectification.

The AIHC's basic policy is set forth in one of its documents[27] and summarized elsewhere.[12] Six key principles are proposed by the AIHC to ensure a successful regulatory outcome: (a) the need to regulate should be established on a sound scientific basis before initiating the regulatory process; (b) it is important to distinguish the role of independent scientific evaluation from that of regulatory decision-making; (c) in any regulatory process, it is necessary to maintain the flexibility to accommodate the development of knowledge; (d) mechanisms for validating the data used and how they are used scientifically need to be part of the regulatory process; (e) it is necessary to have a logical decision process to follow in proceeding from initial hazard identification to final regulatory response; and (f) the regulatory function must manage the overall regulatory process.

To ensure that valid science is used as a basis for regulation and used soundly, the AIHC proposed a number of mechanisms. These included strengthening of individual agency scientific capabilities, pre-regulatory symposia or workshops to capture the latest state of knowledge before beginning the regulatory process, and public and peer review through scientific panels.

The Food Safety Council also advocated the principles of the independent and sound utilization of good science as well as peer review. The utilization of a scientific panel is likewise advocated; where the Food Safety Council differs from the AIHC is in its advocacy of an additional special panel to assist the regulator in reaching a sound regulatory decision. The AIHC leaves that portion of the regulatory process to the usual, established processes involving notification, public hearings, and the like.

The AIHC's fifth principle calls for a logical decision process. AIHC has consequently proposed a stage-wise process as has the National Research Council (NRC) in their study.[34] Figure 1 shows both processes schematically on a comparable basis, omitting the data input features, although these should not be forgotten. In both proposals the process begins with the question, is there a need to regulate in the first place? (see the arrows with question marks in the Figure). In the Hazard Identification stage, all the available data — not just animal data — are gathered and examined, and validated as to their quality and relevance for determining whether hazard exists. Here, "Hazard" is used to mean the potential to do harm, not whether harm may in fact occur. This is a different definition from that used by toxicologists where "toxicity" is the innate potential to cause harm and "hazard" reflects the likelihood of harm actually occurring. Hazard, in the sense in which it is used here, could apply broadly to dangers not resulting from toxicity such as fires, explosions or accidents; the likelihood of harm is expressed by "risk" — and expresses the probability of a specific type of adverse effect with a particular degree of seriousness. In the present instance, the hazard is cancer.

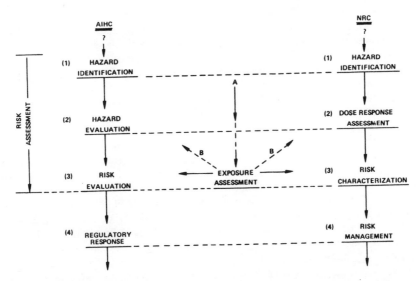

Figure 1: A comparison of the risk assessment and response processes proposed by AIHC and NRC.

The first stage is a significant decision step. If a hazard is not identified there is no reason to proceed with the rest of the risk assessment (the first three steps, taken together) unless new data later require a review of that decision. In this stage, too, it may become clear whether an identified hazard applies to humans. In the second stage, the qualitative evaluation of the hazard may indicate its inapplicability to humans and the decision can then be made not to follow the process further. In the third stage, if the risk is insignificant or non-existent, it is unnecessary to proceed to the fourth stage. Careful attention to these decisions can conserve scarce resources for use in identifying true hazards and abating their risks.

The Hazard Evaluation stage is the one on which both quantitative and qualitative factors are used to predict the ranges of types and sizes of responses that one would expect from a "laboratory human" under controlled conditions of low levels of exposure. What these levels might be are obtained by an initial assessment of real exposures (see the dashed arrows, labelled B in Fig. 1), the Exposure Assessment activity having usually already begun, as indicated by the arrow marked A in the Figure. Exposure Assessment is a stage identified explicitly in the NRC study which is not in the decision chain but which is an important adjunct to it. The need for exposure information and the analysis of its meaning was called for in the AIHC proposals, but it was not identified as a named activity, under one heading. AIHC has now adopted this step, as is done by the NRC.

In the second stage, the qualitative evaluation of the animal data which has passed the screen of the first stage is examined to determine its applicablity to humans. Gray areas abound here, and there is much room for exercising careful scientific judgment.

Although the second stage proposed by the NRC is entitled "Dose-Response Assessment" and so might be taken by some to mean that it is solely a quantitative assessment stage, such is not the case. The report, itself, makes it clear that qualitative responses are fully included in the assessment.

With the information from the second stage and from the Exposure Evaluation stage, the third stage, Risk Evaluation (AIHC) or Risk Characterization (NRC) may now be carried out.

In the third stage, the ideal outcome is to determine or describe whether and to what extent the potential hazard may be realized under real world exposure conditions. The risk may be characterized descriptively, its characterization may include statements of the best estimate of the probability of the hazard occurring, or it may be characterized as significant or insignificant, for example, in its recent notice on the inorganic arsenic standard[35] characterized the risk of lung cancer as "significant" for anyone exposed to the prior standard (500 $\mu g/m^3$) for a forty-five year working life. Acceptability of the risk may or may not be an explicit criterion in characterizing the risk; thus in the case of OSHA it is not, but in the case of the Food and Drug Administration (FDA) a risk of cancer above one in a million in a lifetime for indirect additives in food is unacceptable.[36] Indeed, in the inorganic arsenic example OSHA discusses the significance of the level of risk estimated at the level of the new standard (10 $\mu g/m^3$), eight per thousand employees, in relation to other risks and to the Supreme Court's view[37] that a reasonable person might consider the risk significant at one per thousand and take steps to decrease or eliminate it. OSHA finds the new standard to pose a significant risk but, on the basis of feasibility studies, leaves the standard at 10 $\mu g/m^3$. OSHA does not discuss acceptability directly.

Thus, at the end of the third stage risk may be characterized as insignificant, significant or acceptable depending on the regulatory agency and the mandates under which it operates. Clearly, the setting of a standard at a significant risk level may occur, where the reasons for what amount to acceptance of a significant risk lie not within the third stage but within the fourth stage. In any event, what the AIHC and the NRC both advocate is that the risk be characterized as being the most likely risk, that the assumptions and premises used in arriving at the conclusion be fully displayed, and that the ranges and uncertainties, quantitative and/or qualitative be given. As the regulator enters the fourth stage, Regulatory Response (AIHC) or Risk Management (NRC) in which technical, societal, economic and other factors must be considered in developing options for abating risk, this complete way of characterizing risk assures that the regulator is as fully informed as possible on the risks involved.

Having discussed the AIHC's proposals in some depth we must hasten to add that other industry associations have developed positions and views on science and regulation. The API, for example, supported major studies at the Brookings Institute.[38] A recent paper from this group describes some of the experiences the API underwent in the benzene regulatory actions starting in the late 1970's and presents a process for risk assessment and management.[39] There are many differences in detail as one examines the various views. However, the need to improve the utilization of science, unconstrained by prior policy decisions, is clearly visible throughout.

Individual companies have developed their own processes for assessing risks and responding to them by setting internal standards, warning employees and instructing them in safety practices, and notifying customers by letter, by labeling, and by their product safety literature. The DuPont Company, for example has set numerous internal workplace standards,[40] below those specified by OSHA where necessary. Numerous companies set workplace standards for ethylene oxide several years ago, well below OSHA's standard.[41] To set such standards, companies must have internal procedures not unlike a form of regulatory process, capable of justifying actions which can be costly to the managements involved. Some companies have, in fact, published papers giving the principles and even some of the procedures they follow. Examples of these are an extensive paper by authors from the Proctor and Gamble Company,[42] as well as papers from the Monsanto Company[43,44] and our own company.[33]

In our own case we follow a four stage process much like that of the AIHC, with several differences: (a) At the end of the third stage, after having displayed the ranges of the most likely quantitative estimates of the probabilities of an individual suffering at least one adverse effect in a lifetime as a function of dose (or equivalent exposure), together with all assumptions made in the dose and inter-species extrapolations, and having considered the relevant qualitative factors, the risk is characterized as high, low or insignificant; (b) in our case, the fourth stage is entitled "Risk Response" since it is the stage in which we decide on our options for risk abatement depending on the existing level of risk; (c) where we are able to quantify the range (which may be more than an order of magnitude wide) within which we believe the risk lies at a given exposure level, we determine its level by comparison with a quantitative yardstick, described elsewhere,[11] which defines the probability-boundaries between the risk regions; and (d) we do not, because it is a societal decision we are not equipped to make, decide whether a risk is acceptable or not. Pragmatically, if a risk is judged to lie in the high zone, a strategy is developed to lower that risk, so that it ultimately lies no higher than the low risk zone; if the risk is found to lie in the low zone, reasonable steps are taken to lower the risk further; and if the risk is judged insignificant, no action is needed. Even with quantitative data of high quality, judging whether a risk is in the low or in the insignificant zone is often not possible, so blunt are our risk assessment tools.

Where we are unable to quantify the risk at all, but have identified a hazard and done a qualitative evaluation, we would treat the risk as though it was in the low risk zone, taking reasonable steps to lower it further while launching the work needed to improve our assessment of the risk. Thus, progress toward safety need not await quantification.

In any event, we comply with existing standards and set our own more stringent standards where we judge existing standards to be inadequate. We may also set our own standard where none already exists. From our knowledge of the views of other companies, this view is a common one. Practically speaking, then, we cannot know that the risks we achieve are "acceptable" in a societal sense. We can, however, say that our process, our risk categorization, and our response to risk do increase the safety of our workplaces and, through notification of our own findings and actions, they should have a beneficial effect on our customers' workplaces as well. It was through the use of this technique some years ago that we decided to set our own ethylene oxide standard; we now use the technique on a regular basis to review the safety of other materials. Clearly, from the above discussion it can be seen that there is no uniformity of view from one industry association to another when it comes to specific recommendations on exactly how science is best brought into the regulatory arena, on the best process to use, or even on a common nomenclature for similar activities. There is, however, a general agreement that the sound and full use of science together with careful, balanced, logical assessment is the right way to achieve sound regulation. Between companies, too, each espouses its own methods in making health safety decisions, but the need to make such decisions when sound data so indicate, even in advance of regulatory actions, is clearly understood and acted upon.

It is our belief that industry is making substantial progress in the matter of health safety and the reduction of cancer risk, that it has learned to appreciate and understand this area, that it expends substantial resources both on learning more and on applying its knowledge, and that it has contributed significantly to the national understanding of these problems and will continue to make important contributions as its knowledge-base grows.

AREAS FOR FUTURE CONSIDERATION

We agree with the statement by Weisburger and Williams[45] that the classical procedures for testing potential carcinogens in animals have not changed substantially in the last fifty years. In the past it has been the practice to take the data at face value and to regulate those substances which yielded a statistically significant excess of cancer. While this approach is justified with agents that are obviously carcinogenic, such as yielding a high incidence of cancer at a given site in several species in a short time, there are many cases where the results remain equivocal even after lengthy reviews and re-reviews.

Much of the debate on carcinogenicity testing has bogged down in situations where many of the features of the protocol are unsatisfactory or where there is a dispute as to the significance of the pathology. The most notorious example of this is the mouse hepatoma, which accounts for a very significant proportion of all positive assays.

It has been our personal experience that working within the framework of Risk Assessment, as outlined in this chapter, has had an important impact on the type of information which is utilized to evaluate hazard to man and then to determine the risks, if any, which should be abated.

Information on the chemical composition and purity of substances under investigation is very important. Exposure to certain chemicals may be substantially less when they comprise a small part of complex mixtures. Even though this type of information may not be available on new products, exposure may be predicted by simulating anticipated uses. Such information should be obtained and evaluated for use in planning experimental programs.

Clearly, the central issues of carcinogenicity testing are the relevance of animal data and the methods of extrapolation to man. We advocate strongly the importance of gathering and using information which relates directly to man[46] where such information can be obtained ethically. Direct observations are only possible in a few instances such as with chemotherapeutic drugs for the treatment of cancer. However, there is increasing emphasis on the use of human tissues to measure specific endpoints, such as metabolites, DNA adducts and chromosomal or gene mutations. There are many sources of human material which are considered ethically and legally acceptable, including biopsy material incidental to clinical treatment, autopsy samples, blood and other tissues. There are many human cell lines, although cultures of human epithelial cells — the targets of most human cancer — remain a challenge.

Parallel studies using animal and human tissues will become increasingly important to investigate the mechanism of action of carcinogens *e.g.*, whether a substance is an initiator, promoter, immunosupressant, and what might be the pathways of activation and detoxification, and possible differences in the kinetics of absorption, metabolism, and excretion. There almost always are differences between species in the metabolism of foreign compounds which can be important in evaluating possible hazards to man. We must be prepared to utilize the advances which have been made in the knowledge of the etiology of cancer during the last decade.

It is important that all the available information is utilized to assess carcinogenic hazard and that appropriate weight be given to each type of information. Where there is information on several species, simply to pick the most sensitive species means that information is not being utilized and results are being seriously distorted. It also means that a conservatism is being built inextricably into the evaluation which may not be understood by the risk manager. There may be several layers of conservatism which may lead to a completely illogical result.

The public has become increasingly skeptical of much of the scientific endeavor in the area of carcinogenicity testing – the ever increasing numbers of animals used, media stories of poor quality or inadequate testing, the difficulty in dealing with information on products which are part of everyday life. Like the public, industry finds it difficult to operate in an environment where the rules are perceived to be arbitrary and the outcome of experimentation highly dependent on chance and where interpretation may be a matter of social belief rather than scientific analysis.

The best service that could be afforded to industry by those engaged in carcinogenicity testing, is to be aware of, and to understand the context in which their results will be utilized and to endeavor to produce the information which is most relevant for the qualitative and quantitative evaluation of hazards of carcinogens to man. This applies both to the unraveling of the causes of existing cancers and to the study of the properties of specific substances whose properties are as yet unknown. In this way, science can best help the risk manager to . . . "look into the night and distinguish the real forms from the shadows".[47]

REFERENCES

1. Doll, R., and Peto, R., The causes of cancer: Quantitative estimates of avoidable risks of cancer in the United States today. *J. Natl. Cancer Inst.* 66: 1192-1308 (1981)
2. Higginson, J., and Muir, C.S., Environmental carcinogenesis: Misconceptions and limitations to cancer control. *J. Natl. Cancer Inst.* 63: 1291-1298 (1979)
3. Hunter, D., *The Diseases of Occupation*, London: Hodder and Stoughton (1978)
4. International Agency for Research on Cancer, *IARC Monographs on the Evaluation of the Carcinogenic Risk of Chemicals to Humans, Supplement 4.* Lyon (1982)
5. Gibson, J.E., *Formaldehyde Toxicity*, New York: Hemisphere Publishing Corp., (1983)
6. Deisler, P.F. Jr., Toxicology in business decision making. *Reg. Toxicol. Pharmacol.* 2: 335-344 (1982)
7. Scala, R.A., The duty to report hazards: A toxicologist's view. *Bull. N.Y. Acad. Med.* 54: 774-781 (1978)
8. National Cancer Institute, *Guidelines for Carcinogen Bioassay in Small Rodents.* Carcinogenesis Technical Report Series No. 1, U.S. Dept. of Health, Education and Welfare (1976)
9. Ames, B.N., Dietary carcinogens and anticarcinogens. *Science* 221: 1256-1264 (1983)
10. Hoerger, F.D., in: *Banbury Report No 9: Quantification of Occupational Cancer.* Cold Spring Harbor Laboratory (1981)
11. Deisler, P.F. Jr., A goal-oriented approach to reducing industrially related carcinogenesis risks. *Drug Metabol. Rev.* 13: 875-911 (1982)
12. Deisler, P.F. Jr., Science, regulations and the safe handling of chemicals. *Reg. Toxicol. Pharmacol.* 3: 60-70 (1983)
13. Stevenson, D.E., Thorpe, E., and Hunt, P.F., in: *Carcinogenicity testing, principles and problems* (A.D. Dyan and R.W. Brimblecombe, eds.), MTP Press, Lancaster, England (1978)

14. Ames, B.N., Durston, W.E., Yamasaki, E. and Lee, F.D., Carcinogens are mutagens. Simple test system combining liver homogenates for activation and bacteria for detection. *Proc. Natl. Acad. Sci. USA* 70: 2281-2285 (1973)

15. Ames, B.N., McCann, J., and Yamasaki, E., Methods for detecting carcinogens and mutagens with the Salmonella/Mammalian microsome mutagenicity test. *Mutat. Res.* 31: 347-363 (1975)

16. Miller, E.C., and Miller, J.A., in: *Chemical Carcinogens* (C.S. Searle, ed.), ACS Monograph 173, Amer. Chem. Soc. Washington, DC (1976)

17. Wright, A.S., Metabolism in chemical mutagenesis and chemical carcinogenesis. *Mutat. Res.* 75: 215-241 (1980)

18. Food Safety Council, *Proposed System For Food Safety Assessment, Report of the Scientific Committee of the Food Safety Council*, pp 137-160, Washington, DC (1980)

19. Park, C.N., and Snee, R.D., Quantitative risk assessment: State-of-the-art for carcinogenesis. *Fund. Appl. Toxicol.* 3: 320–333 (1983)

20. Squire, R.A., Ranking carcinogens: A proposed regulatory approach. *Science* 214: 877-880 (1981)

21. Bruce, R.D., Low dose extrapolation and risk assessment. *Chemical Times & Trends*, pp 19-23 (October, 1980)

22. Wong, S., Low dose extrapolation: Inference and design under the multistage model. Communication to the American Statistical Society (in press)

23. Hoel, D.G., Kaplan, N., and Anderson, M.W., Implication of non-linear kinetics on risk estimation in carcinogenesis. *Science* 214: 1032-1037 (1983)

24. Schaeffer, D., Thresholds for carcinogenesis and their significance to medical practice. *Medical Hypothesis* 10: 175-184 (1983)

25. Chin, T.Y., Tyl, R.W., Popp, J.A., and Heck, H. d'A, Chemical urolithiasis 1. Characteristics of bladder stone induction by terephthalic acid and dimethyl terephthalate in weaning Fischer-344 rats. *Toxicol. Appl. Pharmacol.* 58: 307–321 (1981)

26. Occupational Safety and Health Administration (OSHA), Administration, identification, classification and regulation of toxic substances posing a potential occupational carcinogenic risk, proposed rule and notice of hearing. *Fed. Register* 42: 54149–54239 (1977)

27. American Industrial Health Council (AIHC), *Chronic Health Hazards: Carcinogenesis, Mutagenesis, Teratogenesis; A Framework for Sound Science in Federal Decisionmaking.* A statement by AIHC (1981)

28. Interagency Regulatory Liaison Group (ILRG), Scientific basis for identification of potential carcinogens and estimation of risk. *Fed. Register* 44: 39858-39979 (1979)

29. Environmental Protection Agency (EPA), National emission standards for hazardous air pollutants. Proposed policy and procedures for identifying, assessing and regulating air-borne substances posing a risk of cancer. *Fed. Register* 44: 58642-58670 (1979)

30. Consumer Product Safety Commission (CPSC), Classifying, evaluating and regulating carcinogens in consumer products. *Fed. Register* 43: 25658 (1978)

31. Staffa, J.A., and Mehlman, M.A., (eds.), *J. Environ. Pathol. Toxicol.* 3 (3) — Special Issue (1980)

32. Carlborg, F.W., 2-Acetylaminofluorene and the Weibull Model. *Fd. Cosmet. Toxicol.* 19: 367-371 (1981)

33. Deisler, P.F. Jr., Berger, J.E., and Brunner, R.L., A systematic approach to reducing the risk of industrially related cancer. *Reg. Toxicol. Pharmacol.* 3: 26-37 (1983)
34. National Research Council, *Risk Assessment in the Federal Government: Managing the Process,* National Academy Press, Washington, DC (1983)
35. Occupational Safety and Health Administration (OSHA), Occupational exposure to inorganic arsenic. *Fed. Register* 48: 1864-1903 (1983)
36. Food and Drug Administration (FDA), Chemical compounds in food-producing animals. *Fed. Register* 44: 17070-17121 (1979)
37. United States Supreme Court, Industrial Union Department; AFL-CIO *vs* American Petroleum Institute *et al.* No 78-911, decided July 2, 1980
38. Lave, L.B., (ed.), *Quantitative Risk Assessment in Regulation,* Washington, DC: The Brookings Institute (1982)
39. Swanson, S., An evaluation of quantitative risk assessment in health hazards. *Proc. 11th World Petroleum Congress* (1983)
40. Reinhardt, C.F., Industry's approach: A common-sense approach to toxicological research. *J. Amer. College Toxicol.* 2: 51-55 (1983)
41. Occupational Safety and Health Administration (OSHA), Occupational exposure to ethylene oxide. *Fed. Register* 48: 17284-17319 (1983)
42. Beck, L.W., Maki, A.W., Artman, N.R., and Wilson, E.R., Outline and criteria for evaluating the safety of new chemicals. *Reg. Toxicol. and Pharmacol.* 1: 19-58 (1981)
43. Hanley, J.W., Monsanto's early warning system. *Harvard Business Review,* pp 107-116 (Nov-Dec, 1981)
44. McCarville, W.J., Approaches used by industry for assessing exposure to commercial chemicals — the Monsanto example. *Toxic Substances J.* 4: 199-209 (1982)
45. Weisburger, J.H., and Williams, G.M., Carcinogen testing: Current problems and new approaches. *Science* 214: 401-407 (1981)
46. Hayes, W.J. Jr., in: *Pesticide Chemistry, Human Welfare and Environment* (J. Miyamoto, and P.C. Kearney, eds.), Vol. 3, Pergamon Press, Oxford (1980)
47. Todhunter, J.A., Risk management strategy under the Toxic Substances Control Act and the Federal Insecticide, Fungicide and Rodenticide Act. *Reg. Toxicol. Pharmacol.* 3: 163-171 (1983)

Index

Absorption, 540
and molecular weight, 7
Accidents, 44–45
Acetamide, 18, 23
4-Acetylaminodiphenylsulfide, 10
2-Acetylaminofluorene (2-AAF),
10, 21, 153, 155, 156, 160,
169, 201, 240, 286, 316,
443, 469, 541, 572
Acetylators
rapid, 124
slow, 124
N-Acetyltransferase, 124
Acid leaching, 388
Acridine orange, 10
Acrylamide, 182, 202
Acrylonitrile, 578
Actinomycin D, 22, 467
Acylating agents, 14-16, 18
Adrenal gland
subcapsular cell hyperplasia
of, 298
AF2, 330
Aflatoxin, 21, 36, 122, 123, 182,
201, 330, 558
AIN-76a, 258
Alcohol, 29, 37
Aldehyde dehydrogenase, 6
Aldrin, 17, 549
Aliphatic azo-compounds, 16
Alkylating agents, 14–16, 20, 106
Alkylation, 522

Alkylbenzene sulfonates, 23
Alphafetoprotein (AFP), 438
application, 442
function, 439
purification, 440
radiolabeling, 441
Altered-foci, 158
and hepatocellular carcinoma,
168
Alveolar buds, 217
American Industrial Health Council
(AIHC), 615, 616, 617, 618
American Institute of Nutrition
(AIN), 257
American National Standards
Institute (ANSI), 570
American Petroleum Institute
(API), 611
Ames test, 61, 84, 152, 167, 391, 594
1-Aminoanthracene, 243
2-Aminoanthracene, 144, 243
Aminoazo dyes, 120
o-Aminoazotoluene, 161, 201
3-Aminobenzamide, 155
4-Aminobiphenyl, 240, 573
2-Aminofluorene (2-AF), 124, 182
Aminotriazole, 10
Amosite, 385, 387, 390, 392, 395,
396, 401, 402
Amphiboles, 386
Amyloidosis, 328, 336
Angiosarcoma, 36, 361, 520

Aniline mustard, 182
Animal selection, 255
Anthralin, 235, 243, 469
Antibody dilution curve, 441
Anticarcinogenic factors, 48
Anticarcinogens, 246, 471
Antimetabolites, 22, 106
Antineoplastic agents, 21
Aplysiatoxin, 235
2-Aralkyl-5-nitrofurans, 10
Arochlor 1254, 73, 87
Aromatic amides, 106, 225
Aromatic amines, 8-10, 106, 318
    N-acetylation, 8
    O-acetylation, 8-9
    aryl moieties, 8
    N-hydroxylation, 8
Aromatic dyes, 610
Aromatics, polyhalogenated, 7
Arsenic, 578
Arsenicals, 610
Arylamidonium ion, 9
Arylamines, 317
Aryldialkyltriazenes, 16
Aryl hydrocarbon hydroxylase
    (AHH), 217, 393
Aryl moieties, 8
Asbestos, 18, 46, 332, 333, 384,
    385, 386, 387, 389, 406,
    407, 570, 587, 596, 610
    and chromosomal aberrations,
        390
    as co-carcinogen, 392-394
    and lung cancer, 36, 43
    substitutes, 408
Asbestosis, 395
Assays,
    Ames, 61, 84
    cellular transformation, 63,
        130-150
    chromosomal damage, 61-63
    cytogenetics, 61-63, 100-115
    DNA damage and repair, 63,
        116-129
    gene mutation, 61
    for genotoxicity, 59
    intercellular communication,
        422, 437
    micronucleus, 62
    peroxisome proliferation, 482
    rat liver foci, 152-178
    sister chromatid exchange, 58,
        61, 102-105

    spot, 91
    suspension, 92
    with potential utility, 421-500
Na$^+$/K$^+$ ATPase, 61, 158
Attapulgite, 384, 408
Audit, 372, 373
Auramine, 10
Aza-aromatics, 120
Azaserine, 20, 155, 201, 316, 458
Aziridines, 16, 182, 198
Azobenzene, 202
Azo reductase, 7
Azoxy compounds, 16

Barbiturates, 46
"Bay region," 11, 12, 14
Benefits, 549
Benzene, 36, 163, 578, 581, 587,
    594, 610, 613
Benzenediamines (SBD), 313, 317
Benzethonium chloride, 23
Benzidine, 91, 95, 106, 120, 124,
    538, 573, 587, 595
Benzo[a]phenanthrene, 11
Benzo(a)pyrene, 11, 21, 89, 106,
    121, 154, 155, 161, 163,
    198, 218, 333, 392, 405
Benzo(e)pyrene, 235, 243
Benzo[f]fluoranthene, 11
Benzoyl chloride, 18, 199
Benzoyl peroxide, 235, 239, 243
Beryllium, 580
Bile acids, 23, 47, 429
Bioassays,
    for asbestos, 384-419
        in vitro, 388-394
        in vivo, 395-403
    for insoluble materials, 389-419
    limited, 151-250
    long-term animal, 251-382, 529
Bio-availability, 7
Biphenyls, polyhalogenated, 17
Bis-chloroethylnitrosourea, 22
Bis-chloromethyl ether, 7, 8, 15,
    38, 574, 610
Bleomycin, 332
Bonferroni, 365
Bootstrap methods, 516
Bracken fern, 315
Bromodeoxyuridine, 202
Bromoform, 199
1,3-Butadiene,
    and hemangioma, 300

1,3-Butadiene (con't)
  and hemangiosarcoma, 300
Butylated hydroxyanisole, 206,
  243
Butylated hydroxytoluene, 206,
  243, 429
Butylated hydroxytoluene-hydroperoxide, 243
N-Butyl-N-(4-hydroxybutyl)-
  nitrosamine, 330

Cages, 259
  labeling, 275
  and rack configuration, 275
Canadian Ministry of Health and
  Welfare, 286
Cancer
  bladder, 30
  breast, 30, 48, 49, 222
    and pregnancy, 48
  causes, 29-31
  and chemicals, 32
  childhood, 45-46
  colon, 40
  endometrial, 49
  esophagus, 39
  laryngeal, 331
  lung, 29, 36, 39, 40, 43
    and smoking, 39
  mammary, 222
  multifactorial origin, 29
  registry, 39
  skin, 38, 40
  stomach, 38, 40
Carbamates, 16, 23, 182, 198,
  235
Carbonium ion, 12, 14, 15
Carbon tetrachloride, 17, 21, 154
  and hepatocarcinogenicity, 23
Carcinogen Assessment Group
  (CAG), 550, 551
Carcinogenesis
  endogenous, 46-49
  general principles, 3-6
  occupational, 37-40
  respiratory, 331-332
  solid state, 385
  two-stage theory of, 60
"Carcinogenic factors," 29
Carcinogenic index, 185
Carcinogenicity
  evidence of, 379-380
    limited, 33
    ranking, 531-532
    sufficient, 33
  foreign body
    and physical shape, 18
    and size, 18
  industry perspective, 608, 624
  international aspects, 603-606
  modification, 7-8
  promoters of, 21, 23, 29, 144
Carcinogenic response
  comparison
    between species, 312-318
    between strains, 312-318
"Carcinogenic risk factors," 29
"Carcinogenic stimulus," 29
Carcinogens
  acid-catalyzed hydrolysis, 6
  alkali-catalyzed hydrolysis, 6
  direct acting, 6
  epigenetic, 4, 18, 482
    and cell membrane, 21
    intercellular communication, 4
    peroxisome proliferation, 4
  foreign body, 4, 18
  genotoxic, 4
    covalent binding, 4
    metabolic activation, 6
Carnitine acetyltransferase, 491, 494
Carrageenan, 330
Case-control, 37, 41-42
Catalase, 484, 489, 491, 493, 494
Cedar wood shavings, 183
Cell cycle, 105
  G_0 phase, 106
  G_1 phase, 62, 106, 464, 466, 473
  G_2 phase, 62, 104
  S phase, 62, 104, 464, 466
Cell lines, 465, 466
  Chinese hamster lung (V79), 105
  Chinese hamster ovary (CHO),
    105
  human fibroblasts (WI-38), 105
  human lymphocytes, 105
  mouse lymphoid (L5178Y), 105
  BHK-21 Syrian baby hamster
    kidney, 137
  Syrian hamster embryo, 130
Cell proliferation, 154
Cell transformation, 20, 63, 130
  assays for, 130-150
    comparison of, 141, 142
    modifications, 143, 144
Chelating agents, 23

Chemical Industry Institute of Toxicology (CIIT), 253, 254, 256, 597, 610
Chemical Manufacturers Association (CMA), 579
Chemical reactivity, 7
Chemicals
    exogenous, 31
    halogenated aliphatics, 91
    volatile, 91
"Chemical trauma," 23
Chemotherapeutic agents, 31, 182, 200
Chlordane, 17, 549
Chlorinated ethanes, 121
Chlorinated ethylenes, 121
Chlorinated hydrocarbons, 106
Chlornaphazine, 538
4-Chlorobiphenyl, 17
2-Chloroethyl ether, 199
Chloroform, 17, 163, 167, 199, 243, 504, 518
    and hepatocarcinogenicity, 23
Chloromethyl ethers, 235, 574
Chloroquine, 243
Chlorpromazine, 243
Chromate manufacture, 610
Chromosomal aberrations, 391
    and asbestos, 390
    and radiation, 101
    tests for, 101–104
        advantages, 107–108
        disadvantages, 108
Chromosomal alterations, 58, 60
Chromosome banding techniques, 103
Chronic Hazard Advisory Panel (CHAP), 588, 593
Chrysarobin, 235, 243
Crysotile, 385, 388, 390, 392, 395, 396, 398, 400, 401, 402
Cigarette smoking, 31, 42, 46, 120, 331, 538, 583
    and lung cancer, 29
Cinnamyl alcohol, 200
Clara cells, 180, 296
Clastogenic compounds, 20
Clinical observations, 261
Clofibrate, 18, 494
Coal-tar colors, 558
Co-carcinogenic factors, 332
Cochran-Armitage trend test, 363

Cohort, 36, 37, 42–44
    prospective, 37
    retrospective, 37
Coke oven emissions, 235, 576
Colchicine, 469
Confidence intervals, 513
    bootstrap methods, 516
Consumer Product Safety Act (CPSA), 587, 588
Consumer Product Safety Commission (CPSC), 587–602
    carcinogen policy, 589, 616
Controls
    concurrent, 377
    historic, 377
    program historic, 378
    specific laboratory historic, 377
Cordycepin, 467
Correlations
    with carcinogenicity, 94–95
    mutagenicity and carcinogenicity, 60
Coumarin, 330
Covalent binding, 4
Criteria
    functional, 3, 19–23
    guilt by association, 3
    structural, 3, 18–19
Crocidolite, 385, 390, 392, 395, 396, 401, 402, 404
Culture
    metabolizing mammalian cells in, 86–87
Cumene hydroperoxide, 243
Cumene peroxide, 243
Cycasin, 21
Cyclamate, 561
Cyclophosphamide, 21–22, 144
Cyprotein acetate, 171
Cytogenetic tests, 100–115
Cytotoxicity, 425

Data
    evaluation, 185
    limitations, 76
    metabolism, 540
    negative, 535
    pathology, 354–355
    pharmacokinetics, 540
    reporting, 93
    and risk assessment, 536
    selection, 534

Data (con't)
  utilization, 536
Daunomycin, 22
DDT, 17, 21, 22, 330, 429, 431
  549
Decanoyl peroxide, 243
Dehydroepiandrosterone, 49
Delaney clause, 549, 556, 560,
  561, 562, 565, 566
Dialkyldithiocarbamate, 23
Diaminodiphenylmethane
  (DDPM), 456
Dibenz[a,h]anthracene, 11, 198
Dibenzo[a,h]pyrene, 11
Dibenzo[a,i]pyrene, 11
Dibenzodioxins, 17
1,2-Dibromo-3-chloropropane,
  17, 23, 577
1,2-Dibromoethane, 17, 23, 199
3,3'-Dichlorobenzidine, 573
1,2-Dichloroethanes, 143
3,5-Dichloro(N-1, 1-dimethyl-2-
  propynyl)benzamide (DCB),
  161
Dieldrin, 21, 161, 549
Diepoxybutane, 202
Diet, 29, 47–48
  choline-deficient, 155, 156,
    445, 458
  closed formula, 258
  fat, 29, 222, 223
  fiber, 29, 47
  food additives, 47
  and lifestyle, 46–49
  methionine-low, 155, 156
  non-purified, 258
  open formula, 258
  and risk of cancer, 47
  unrefined, 258
Di-(2-ethylhexyl)phthalate (DEHP),
  18, 485, 494, 587, 593, 598
Diethylnitrosamine (DEN), 154,
  155, 156, 161, 167, 168,
  170, 332, 454, 466, 467,
  469
Diethylpyrocarbonate, 561
Diethylstilbestrol (DES), 46, 106,
  107, 221, 315, 333, 334,
  538, 561, 563
  and pregnancy, 334
Differences
  qualitative, 77
  quantitative, 77

α-Difluoromethylornithine (DFMO),
  466, 470, 473
Dihydrosafrole, 313
4-Dimethylaminoazobenzene, 10,
  89, 106, 574
3,2'-Dimethyl-4-aminobiphenyl,
  121
7,12-Dimethylbenz(a)anthracene,
  121, 154, 163, 198, 216, 219,
  220, 223, 225, 231, 244, 313,
  335, 406, 469
Dimethylcarbamoyl chloride, 106,
  332
Dimethylformamide, 106
Dimethylhydrazine, 123, 154, 155,
  163, 240, 402
Dimethylnitrosamine (DMN), 19,
  21, 89, 90, 240
  and hepatocarcinogenicity, 23
Dimethyl sulfate, 571
Dimethylsulfoxide (DMSO), 184,
  431
Dinitrotoluene, 121
p-Dioxane, 18, 23, 163, 167, 170,
  202
Dioxin, 329, 336
Dipalmitoylphosphatidylcholine,
  405
DNA adducts, 102, 135, 154, 164,
  621
DNA repair, 20, 58, 60, 63, 116–129
  tests for, 116–129
Dose, 254
  measure of, 537
Dose-response functions, 506
  low dose linear, 507
  low dose sublinear, 508
  low dose supralinear, 508
  threshold, 507
Dumps, 45
Dyes
  benzidine, 91, 95

Ear marks, 275
π-Electron shift, 10
Electrophiles, "soft" and "hard," 4
  concept, 4
Emission
  coke oven, 235, 576
  diesel, 120
  roof tar pot, 120
Envelope curves, 516

Environmental Protection Agency
(EPA), 77, 78, 141, 535, 539,
548, 570, 582, 584, 590, 611
Enzymes, 6, 7
N-acetyl transferase, 124
aryl hydrocarbon hydroxylase,
217, 393
ATPase, 61, 158
epoxide hydrase, 11
glucose-6-phosphatase, 158
hypoxanthine-guanine-phosphoribosyl transferase
(HGPRT), 61, 424
lactate dehydrogenase, 389
and metabolic activation, 6
ornithine decarboxylase (ODC),
393
thymidine kinase (TK), 61
Epichlorohydrin, 17, 106, 199,
240, 243, 581
Epidemiology, 28-55, 527, 529
background, 28
techniques, 33-35
Epithelial cell transformation
assay, 134
Epoxide hydrase, 11
Epoxides, 15-16
Erionite, 385, 386, 391, 404, 408
Escherichia coli (WP2), 61
Estimated maximum tolerated
dose (EMTD), 380
Estrogens, 29, 49
Ethane methanesulfonate, 226
Ethanol, 158, 332, 431
Ethionine, 20, 106, 155, 451
Ethyl bromoacetate, 199
Ethylene dibromide, 580
Ethyleneimine, 575
Ethylene oxide, 579
Ethylenethiourea, 22, 106
Ethyl methanesulfonate, 23
2-Ethyl-N-nitrosourea (ENU), 313,
316
Ethyltoluene, 611
Evaluation
hazard, 618
statistical, 92-93
Evidence, carcinogenicity
limited, 33
sufficient, 33
Exposure
duration of, 256
low levels of, 49-50

Extrapolation, 49-50, 503, 527,
533, 542, 543, 544, 615
animals to humans, 74-75, 283
considerations, 536
interspecies, 534, 536, 537, 539,
541, 542
low dose, 510

False negatives, 202, 361, 378, 425
False positives, 202, 359, 360, 361,
362, 378, 425, 431
FANFT, 202
Fat, 47
FD & C Red No. 2, 561
FD & C Violet No. 1, 561
Federal Hazardous Substances Act
(FHSA), 587, 588
Feed, 257
Ferroactinolite, 387, 398
Fiber, 47
mineral, 43
size, 387
Fibrogenesis, 389
"Fisher rat leukemia," 305
Fisher's Exact Probability test, 361,
362, 363, 365, 366
Flectol H, 561
Fluorodeoxyuridine, 202
1-Fluoro-2,4-dinitrobenzene, 243
Foci
altered, 158
ATPase-deficient, 160, 161, 163,
167, 171
GGT-positive, 160, 163
G-6-Pase-deficient, 160, 161
incidence, 160
iron-deficient, 158-161
BALB/c-3T3 Focus assay, 134-135
C3H-10T½ Focus assay, 135-136
Food additives, 182, 200, 330, 548,
556
Food and Drug Administration (FDA),
286, 345, 549, 556, 618
history, 556
Food Safety Council (FSC), 254,
615, 617
Formaldehyde, 7, 91, 329, 587, 596,
597, 611
"Fourteen carcinogens," 571
Frequency, 370

Gamma-glutamyltranspeptidase (GGT),
155, 156, 158, 160, 169, 335, 443

Gap junctions, 422, 424, 431
Gender, 163
"Generally recognized as safe"
    (GRAS), 560
Genetic monitoring, 257
Gene-Tox Program, 76-78, 141
Genotoxic agents, 58-82
Genotoxicity, 550
    and carcinogenicity, 58-150
    intraspecies differences, 124
Glucocorticoid receptors, 180
Glucose-6-phosphatase, 158
Glutathione transferase, 6
Good Laboratory Practices
    (GLPs), 345, 353, 373
Goodness-of-fit, 517
Growth factor, 465
Guidelines, 549

Haloalkanes, 16-17
Haloalkenes, 17
Haloethers, 15
Halogenated hydrocarbons, 16
Hamster, 286, 327, 390, 572
    cheek pouch, 335
    gall bladder, 334
    kidney, 333
    and long-term animal bio-
        assay, 326-344
    pancreas, 334
    skin, 334
    trachea, 333
Hazard, 617, 618
    evaluation, 618
Health quality, 257
Hepatocarcinogenicity, 23, 48,
    153
    initiation, 153
    promotion, 156
Hepatocarcinogens, 120, 160,
    167, 171, 440, 442, 485,
    and alphafetoprotein, 438
    and peroxisome proliferation,
        482
Hepatocellular proliferation, 443
Hepatocyte primary culture/DNA
    repair test, 116-129
    exposure
        in vivo, 121
        vapor, 121
    and hepatocarcinogens, 120
    modifications, 120-124

reliability, 120
species differences, 123
xenobiotics in, 120, 122-124
Hepatocytes, 121, 122, 123, 124,
    144, 443
    guinea pig, 121
    hamster, 121, 122, 123
    man, 121
    mouse, 121
    rabbit, 121, 124
    rat, 121
Heptachlor, 17, 549
Heteroatomic moieties, 10
Hexachlorobenzene, 158
Hexachlorocyclohexane, 199
Hexamethylphosphoramide, 106
Histopathology, 219, 261, 279, 353
Hormones, 464
    dependence, 221
    imbalance, 22
Host-mediated systems, 86
"Hot spots," 36
Human cell focus assay, 133-134
Husbandry, 257, 329
Hydralazine, 124
Hydrazine, 106, 123, 330, 558
Hydrazo-compounds, 16
Hydrocarbons
    halogenated, 16
    polyhalogenated, 16
Hydrogen bond reactors, 23
Hydrogen peroxide, 243
Hydrophilic groups
    and solubility, 7
Hydroquinone, 243
N-Hydroxy-2-acetylaminofluorene,
    201, 225, 541
Hyperplasia
    of adrenal gland, 298
    of bile duct, 309
    of uterus, 299
Hyperplastic ileitis, 328
Hypolipidemic compounds, 485
Hypoxanthine-guanine-phospho-
    ribosyl transferase (HGPRT),
    61, 424
    and intercellular communication,
    424

Immunoglobulin, 102
Immunosuppressive agents, 22, 46
"Incumbrance area," 12

Indole alkaloids, 235
Induction period, 30
Industry perspective, 607, 624
Initiation, 60, 153
Initiators, 60, 160, 239, 240, 424
    and mouse skin, 233, 234
Interaction
    antagonistic, 46
    synergistic, 46
Interagency Regulatory Liaison
    Group (IRLG), 327, 589,
    616
Intercalation, 10, 15, 20
Intercellular communication, 4,
    21, 422–437
    and gap junctions, 424
    interpretation, 428
    limitations, 428
International Agency for Research
    on Cancer (IARC), 532
International Collaborative Pro-
    gram, 78–79
International Commission for
    Protection Against Environ-
    mental Mutagens and Carcin-
    ogens (ICPEMC), 79
Interpolation, 615
In vitro assays, 388–394
    intercellular communication,
    422, 437
Iodoacetic acid, 469
Iododeoxyuridine, 202
Isoniazid, 46

Kepone, 17, 21, 23
"K-region," 11, 14

Lactate dehydrogenase, 389
Lactones, 16
Latent period, 38, 219, 370
Lauryl peroxide, 243
Lead, 163, 563
Leukemia, 294, 300, 305, 307
    and benzene, 36
Lifestyle, 38, 48, 49
Life table methods, 370
Lighting, 259
Limited bioassays, 151, 250
"Limited negatives," 76
Lindane, 17, 21
Lipid peroxidation, 222
Lipoxygenase, 469
List of Principles, 549

Log P, 7
Long-term animal bioassay, 251, 382
    conduct, 268–281
    design, 253–263
    hamsters in, 326–344
    interpretation of, 372–382
    B6C3F1 mice in, 282–325
    F344 rats in, 282–325
    species in, 283
    statistical evaluation of, 358–371
    strains in, 283
Love Canal, 45
Lung tumors, 385
    bioassay for, 179–214
        chemicals tested, 182, 187–197
        false negatives, 202
        false positives, 202
        relative carcinogenicity, 203–
        204
    in strain A mice, 179–214
Luteoskyrin, 21
Lymphocytic chorio-meningitis
    virus, 328
Lymphoma
    follicular cell, 294
    mixed, 294
    pleomorphic, 294
Lyngbyatoxin, 235

Malonaldehyde, 243
Mammary carcinogenesis
    and fat, 222
Mammary gland, rat, 215–229
    carcinogens of, 216–220
Mammary tumor virus (MTV), 289
Mapping
    correlation, 36
    and lung cancer, 36
Marker, 438, 464, 467
Maximum likelihood estimate (MLE),
    514, 515, 516
Maximum tolerated dose (MTD), 77,
    254, 380, 489, 496, 538
Medication, 46
Melphalan, 199
Mercaptoimidazoline, 561
Mesothelioma, 43, 385, 387, 388,
    397, 407, 409
    and asbestos, 43
Mestranol, 158
Metabolic activation, 6, 10, 13, 17,
    73, 74, 86–89, 141, 143–145
    azo dyes, 10

Metabolic cooperation, 21, 424
  false negatives, 425
  false positives, 425
  and gap junctions, 424
  and promoters, 425
  protocol, 425
Metabolism
  reductive, 91
Metals, 106, 141, 182, 199
Methionine, 106
Methotrexate, 22
Methyl(acetoxymethyl)nitros-
    amine, 315
3-Methylcholanthrene, 11, 21, 87,
    144, 182, 198, 218, 244,
    334, 393, 406
3'-Methyl-4-dimethylaminoazo-
    benzene (3'MDAB), 451
4,4'-Methylenebis(2-chlorobenz-
    amine), 575
4,4'-Methylenedianiline (MDA),
    584
Methylglyoxal-bis(guanylhydra-
    zone) (MGBG), 466
N-7-Methylguanine, 167
O^6-Methylguanine, 167
Methylmethanesulfonate, 202
N-Methyl-N'-nitro-N-nitroso-
    guanidine (MNNG), 144,
    154, 163, 240
3-Methyl-4-nitroquinoline-N-
    oxide, 106
4-(Methylnitrosamino)-1-(3-
    pyridyl)-1-butanone (NNK),
    198
N-δ-(N-Methyl-N-nitrosocarbamoyl)-
    L-ornithine, 330
N-Methyl-N-nitrosourea (MNU),
    154, 163, 219, 220, 225
Mezerein, 243, 245, 470
Mica, 384, 386
B6C3F1 Mice
  characteristics, 289
  comparison
    with other species, 317
    with other strains, 313
  lesions
    age-associated, 298
    in long-term bioassays, 282–325
  neoplasms
    induced, 299–300
    spontaneous, 290–298
  origin of, 288

Mice
  B6C3F1, 282–325
  nude, 134
Mirex, 17
Mitochondrial respiration
  inhibitors of, 21
Mitogen, 156
Mitomycin C, 22
Mitotic inhibitors, 22
Mixed-function oxidases, 6
  inducers of, 21
Models, 541, 550
  Guess and Crump, 506, 511
  log-normal, 513
  modified multistage, 509
  multi-hit, 614
  multistage, 509, 512, 515, 517,
    614
  one-hit, 512, 521, 614
  probit, 517, 614
  stochastic, 506
  tolerance distribution, 505
  Weibull, 506, 614
Moieties
  aryl, 8
  heteroatomic, 10
Molecular weight, 7
Monoacetylputrescine, 465
Monoacetylspermidine, 465
Monocyclic aromatic
  amides, 120
  amines, 120
Morphometry, 491
Mortality
  adjustments, 367–369
  differential. . .tests, 370
  occupational, 36
Murine pneumonia, 331
Mustard
  aniline, 182
  nitrogen, 182
  uracil, 199
Mutagens
  conjugated, 91
Mutational theory, 100
Mycotoxins, 106, 120

β-Naphthoflavone, 87
1-Naphthylamine, 106, 182, 201,
    571, 574
2-Naphthylamine, 10, 21, 106,
    182, 201, 240, 547

National Cancer Institute (NCI),
255, 256, 257, 258, 283,
299, 318, 326, 345, 504,
539, 581
National Institute for Occupational Safety and Health
(NIOSH), 569, 590
National Toxicology Program
(NTP), 145, 152, 256,
257, 258, 275, 286, 288,
299, 318, 326, 345, 353,
590
Necropsy, 219, 261, 278, 347
"Negative" study, 50
Neoplasms
alveolar/bronchiolar, 296
hepatocellular, 290, 310, 311,
313, 318
interstitial cell of testis, 301
lymphoreticular, 294
of mammary gland, 305
of pituitary, 304
of urinary bladder, 311
Neoplastic nodule, 310, 311
Nickel
refining, 610
subsulfide, 316, 317
Nicotine, 326, 331
NIH-shift, 11
Nitrilotriacetic acid, 314
4-Nitrobiphenyl, 121, 573
Nitrofurans, 561
Nitrogen mustards, 15, 182, 199
1-Nitropyrene, 202
4-Nitroquinoline-N-oxide, 106,
240
Nitrosamides, 220, 225
Nitrosamines, 20, 106, 120, 144,
182, 331, 565, 587, 598
N-Nitroso compounds, 16
N-Nitrosodimethylamine, 575
N-Nitrosoethylurea (ENU), 199,
240
N-Nitrosomethylurea (NMU), 199,
240
N-Nitrosomorpholine, 170
N-Nitrosonornicotine (NNN), 198
Nitrosoureas, 182
Nitrotoluenes, 182, 201
Nucleotide base analogs, 182
Nude mice, 134

Occupational Safety and Health
Act, 610

Occupational Safety and Health
Administration (OSHA),
535, 569, 590, 615, 618
Ochratoxin A, 21
Office of Science and Technology
Policy, 590
Oil of calamus, 561
Oncogenes, 102
Oral contraceptives, 49
Organ homogenates, 87–88
Organization for Economic Cooper-
ation and Development
(OECD), 603
Organohalides, 182, 199
Organ weights, 261, 347
Ornithine decarboxylase (ODC), 393,
406, 464, 466, 467
and carcinogenesis, 465
and ultraviolet light, 470
and vitamin A, 471
Oval cells, 445, 448, 456, 458
Ovarian cysts, 299
Oxidative phosphorylation
uncouplers of, 21

Pairwise tests, 361
Partial hepatectomy, 154, 155, 158,
164, 168, 170, 443, 451
Partition coefficient, 7
Peer review, 373
Perchloroethylene, 317, 540, 541
Perfluoro-n-decanoic acid, 330
Peroxisome proliferation, 21, 160,
485
chemicals tested in, 488, 489
and hepatocarcinogens, 482
Peroxisomes, 484
Pesticides, polyhalogenated, 17
Peto's trend, 363, 366
Pharmacokinetics, 541, 542
Phenacetin, 46
Phenanthrene, 243
Phenanthrenequinone, 243
Phenobarbital, 21, 73, 87, 153, 156,
158, 159, 160, 161, 170, 171,
430, 431, 469
Phenytoin, 46
Phorbol esters, 23, 235, 425
Phosgene, 17
Phospholipase, 469
Physical state, 7
Pollution, ambient, 44–45
Polyamines, 464, 465, 466
inhibitors of, 466, 467, 470

Polybrominated biphenyls (PBB),
    17, 21, 429
Polychlorinated biphenyl (PCBs),
    17, 21, 22, 558
Polycyclic aromatic hydrocarbons
    (PAH), 47, 77, 120, 141, 154,
    182, 198, 220, 224, 233, 235,
    467, 565
  amides, 120
  amines, 120
  and metabolic activation, 13
Polynuclear compounds, 11-14
  aromatic hydrocarbons, 106
  and methyl substitution, 11
Potency, 538, 539
Praziquantel, 330
Predictive formalism, 2
Pregnancy, 29, 46, 48, 334
  and smoking, 46
Procarbazine, 123
Procarcinogens, 143
Progesterone, 49, 171
Progressive renal disease, 314
Prolactin, 49, 222, 223
Promoters, 60, 77, 144, 160, 163,
    167, 235, 240, 424, 425,
    429, 430, 467
  and ornithine decarboxylase, 468
  and SENCAR mice, 240, 243
  and skin carcinogenicity, 235,
    236
Promotion, 156
1,3-Propanesultone, 240
β-Propiolactone, 8, 163, 202, 573
Propylene oxide, 300
Prostaglandins, 222
  synthetase, 6
Pulmonary tumors
  in chemically-treated mice, 196
  in control mice, 186
Putrescine, 464, 465, 466, 473
Pyrene, 106, 122
Pyrolizidine alkaloids, 91, 120

Quaboin, 243
Quality assessment, 346, 353, 356
Quality assurance, 263, 345-357
Quarantine, 274
Quartz, 385
Quazepam, 330
Quercetin, 48, 182, 330
  and hepatocarcinogenesis, 48
Quinolines, 235

Radiation, 28, 29, 62, 101, 215,
    226, 470, 548
Radioimmunoassay, 441
Radium, 610
Randomization, 260, 274
F344 Rats
  characteristics, 300
  comparison
    with other strains, 314
    with other species, 317
  lesions
    age-associated, 308-310
    in long-term bioassays, 282-325
  neoplasms
    induced, 310-312
    spontaneous, 300-308
  origin of, 288
  and progressive renal disease,
    314
Rat liver foci, 152
  assay
    chemicals tested, 164-166
    protocol, 156
    uses, 167
Rat mammary carcinoma model
  attributes, 220
  chemicals active in, 224
  limitations, 220
  modifications, 222
Rauscher leukemia virus-Fischer
    rat embryo (RLV/RE), 138-
    139
Reactive intermediate, electro-
    philic, 6
  and carcinogenicity, 6
Records
  industrial, 43
  linkage, 43
Redundant variable, 359
Regulatory implications
  Consumer Product Safety Com-
    mission, 587-602
  Environmental Protection
    Agency, 548-555
  Food and Drug Administration,
    556-568
  international aspects, 603-606
  Occupational Safety and Health
    Administration, 569-586
Retinoic acid, 243
Retinoids, 464, 471
  and ornithine decarboxylase,
    472

Risk, 549, 604, 617
    characterization, 618
    evaluation, 618
    industrial, 36
    occupational, 36
Risk assessment, 406–410, 501–
        546, 553, 564, 604, 614
    biological considerations, 526–
        546
    data for, 533, 536
    future, 551
    guidelines, 549
    in practice, 550
    and toxicokinetics, 519
    value, 566
Rotenone, 330
Rough endoplasmic reticulum
        (RER), 21
Route, 255, 375

Saccharin, 18, 21, 158, 206, 316,
        317, 429, 431, 561, 563,
        564
Safety, 263
Safrole, 106, 123, 161, 163, 558
Salmonella mutagenicity assay, 83–
        99
    variations of, 90–92
Sanitation, 260
Schedules
    cage and rack rotation, 276
    chemical reanalysis, 276
    dosage analysis, 276
    weighing, 276
SENCAR mice
    initiators used, 239
    promoters in, 240–243
    and skin tumorigenesis, 230–
        250
Sensitivity, 76, 236
Serpentines, 386
Sex steroids, 167
Short-term exposure limit (STEL),
        580
Short-term tests, 551
    advantages, 64–73
    limitations, 64–77
Significance
    biological, 377
    physiological, 376–377
    statistical, 376
    toxicological, 376

Silica, 384, 385, 386
Silylating agents, 182, 200
Simian adenovirus SA7-Syrian
        hamster embryo cells
        (SA7/SHE), 139–140
Sister-chromatid exchange
    tests for, 102–105
        advantages, 108
        disadvantages, 108
Skin tumors, 230
Social class, 38
Solid state carcinogenesis, 385
Solubility, 7
Specificity, 76
Spermatogenesis
    inhibitors of, 23
Spermidine, 464, 465, 466
Spermine, 465
Spontaneous rates, 512
Spot test, 91
Standardized Incidence Ratio (SIR),
        40
Standardized Mortality Ratio (SMR),
        38
Standard Operating Procedures
        (SOPs), 274, 276, 353
Statistical evaluation, 358
Sterigmatocystin, 240
Strain A mice, 179–214
Strains
    comparison of
        mouse, 313–314
        rat, 314–317
        Salmonella, 84–86
Structure
    -activity, 3–25
    and carcinogenicity, 1
Student's t-test, 361
Sultones, 16
Sunlight, 29, 38
Surface-active agents, 23
Surface property, 388–390
Suspension assay, 92
Syrian hamster embryo (SHE), 405
    clonal assay, 131, 133
        advantages, 132
    focus assay, 133

Talc, 408
TCDD, 17, 21, 22, 243, 431
    and hepatocarcinogenicity, 23
Teleocidin, 23, 235, 243

Temperature and humidity, 259
Teratogenic compounds, 20
"Terminal buds," 217
Tertiary butyl-hydroperoxide,
    243
Tetrachloroethylene, 199, 314
3,3',5,5'-Tetramethylbenzidine,
    106
Thioacetamide
    and hepatocarcinogenicity, 23
Thiouracil, 22
Thiourea, 18
Threshold, 544, 615
    biological, 543
Threshold Limit Values (TLV),
    570
Thymidine kinase (TK), 61
"Time to tumor" analyses, 370
Tobacco, 29, 37, 46, 326
Toe clipping, 275
Toxicokinetics, 519
Toxic Substances Control Act
    (TSCA), 570, 582, 610,
    611, 612
TPA, 231, 235, 245, 313, 429,
    467, 469, 470, 473
Transformed clones, 133
Tremolite, 402
Trend tests, 363, 365, 366
1,2,4,5,8,9-Tribenzopyrene, 11
Tricaprylin, 184, 186
Trichloroethylene, 143, 314,
    580, 581
2,4,6-Trichlorophenol, 170
Triethanolamine, 18, 23
Trifluoperazine, 469
Trimethylbenzene, 612
TRIS, 587, 594
Tryptophan synthesis operon, 61
Tumorigenicity

and fiber size, 387
    foreign body, 394–395
    and magnesium, 388
Tumor progression, 245
Tweens, 23, 469
Two-stage carcinogenesis, 239
    and mouse skin, 231, 232
    in SENCAR mice, 245

Ultraviolet B light
    and ornithine decarboxylase,
        470
Uracil mustard, 199
Uranium, 610
Urethane, 22, 163, 184, 186, 240

Valium, 431
Vinblastine, 22
Vincristine, 22
Vinyl bromide, 167
Vinyl chloride, 17, 29, 37, 49, 167,
    182, 206, 520, 538, 542, 575,
    587, 593, 610
    and angiosarcomas, 520
    and hemangiosarcomas, 313, 317
Vinyl fluoride, 167
Vinylidene fluoride, 167
Virtually safe doses (VSD), 513,
    515
Vitamin A, 46
    and ornithine decarboxylase,
        471

Waste disposal, 44–45
Water, 258
Weight-of-evidence, 550
World Health Organization (WHO),
    603
Wy-14,643, 454